2014
2018

Encyclopedia of
Smoking and Tobacco

Encyclopedia of Smoking and Tobacco

Arlene B. Hirschfelder

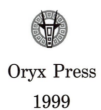

Oryx Press

1999

The rare Arabian Oryx is believed to have inspired the myth of the unicorn. This desert antelope became virtually extinct in the early 1960s. At that time, several groups of international conservationists arranged to have nine animals sent to the Phoenix Zoo to be the nucleus of a captive breeding herd. Today, the Oryx population is over 1,000, and over 500 have been returned to the Middle East.

© 1999 by Arlene B. Hirschfelder
Published by The Oryx Press
4041 North Central at Indian School Road
Phoenix, Arizona 85012-3397
http://www.oryxpress.com

Cover photo © by Doris Friedman

Published simultaneously in Canada
Printed and bound in the United States of America

∞ The paper used in this publication meets the minimum requirements of American National Standard for Information Science—Permanence of Paper for Printed Library Materials, ANSI Z39.48, 1984.

Library of Congress Cataloging-in-Publication Data

Hirschfelder, Arlene B.
    The encyclopedia of smoking and tobacco / Arlene B. Hirschfelder.
        p. cm.
    Includes bibliographical references and index.
    ISBN 1-57356-202-5 (alk. paper)
    1. Tobacco habit—United States Encyclopedias. 2. Smoking—United States Encyclopedias. 3. Tobacco industry—United States Encyclopedias. I. Title.
    HV5760.H57   1999
    362.29'6'097303—dc21
                                                    99-43450
                                                        CIP

CONTENTS

PREFACE

In the middle of the gulf between these two islands . . . . I found a man alone in a canoe who was going from . . . . Santa Maria to Fernandina. He had food and water and some dry leaves which must be a thing very much appreciated among them, because they had already brought me some of them as a present at San Salvador.

Christopher Columbus, 1492

In 1492, during his first voyage to the New World, Christopher Columbus recorded in his diary that the people he encountered smoked tobacco leaves. In the ensuing 500 years, the use of tobacco has grown enormously, but in ways unimagined by the Native American people who greeted Columbus. Tobacco has become associated worldwide with politics, religion, finance, and disease. The rapid spread of tobacco use from the Americas to Europe and the rest of the world also gave rise to the first great drug controversy of global dimensions. But beheadings by barbaric rulers, prohibitions, medical statistics, warnings by physicians and governments, and high taxes on tobacco products have all failed to end the use of cigarettes, cigars, chewing and pipe tobacco, and snuff.

Tobacco holds a special interest for Americans and pervades virtually every aspect of American life. Since John Rolfe first cultivated it in colonial Virginia in 1613, tobacco has become the sixth biggest crop in the United States. Tobacco also assumed major social, political, economic, and medical roles in American history, and has maintained those roles to the present. From the beginning of tobacco cultivation in Virginia almost 400 years ago, colonial and state governments and the United States government have enacted a variety of regulations to control the product or to influence its production and use. These efforts continue today.

During the 1990s, the subjects of tobacco and smoking have received unprecedented coverage in the print and broadcast media. Attention has focused on a broad range of issues, including catastrophic illness caused by tobacco use, secondhand smoke, and the costs of smoking to the national health care system. Proposed curbs on smoking in restaurants, sports stadiums, public transportation, and work spaces affect both smokers and the nonsmokers who breathe secondhand smoke. In 1997 and 1998, the media reported almost daily on the legal settlements that ended lawsuits brought by all 50 states against the tobacco industry for reimbursement of Medicaid costs arising from treatment of tobacco-related illness. The Food and Drug Administration's current efforts to gain regulatory control over tobacco products and the attention focused on tobacco advertising and smoking as a "pediatric disease" keep tobacco in the spotlight and continue to capture the public's interest.

Publishers in the United States and around the world have also given unprecedented coverage to the subject and weighed in with tomes on such subjects as the tobacco plant, the tobacco industry, environmental tobacco smoke, litigation, nicotine dependence, tobacco-related illnesses, tobacco collectibles, smoking cessation, and the anti-smoking policies of governments. In June 1999, amazon.com listed for sale almost 700 books under the topic "tobacco."

About This Book

The *Encyclopedia of Smoking and Tobacco* is the place to begin learning about the ancient herb that commands so much of the contemporary world's attention, and that lies at the heart of one of the great social controversies of the late twentieth century. The *Encyclopedia*'s A-to-Z format makes a vast amount of current information easily accessible. Nearly 600 entries, compiled from authoritative sources, convey information about the lively history, manufacture, and use of all forms of tobacco. As the entries reveal, tobacco and smoking held the attention of the American public, the U.S. government, and health care professionals long before issuance of Surgeon General Luther Terry's stunning report on smoking in 1964. This book will prove useful for many people, including readers of American popular culture, history buffs, teachers and students from junior high school to college, health care professionals, public policy makers, and tobacco-free and smokers' rights advocates. It is intended for people who have never smoked, chewed, or dipped, but who have become fascinated with the subject of tobacco. It is also intended for people who smoke, chew, or dip or who are considering taking up or quitting smoking. It will also be of use to those who are seeking to prevent others from getting addicted to tobacco or who are looking for information to deglamorize smoking. The *Encyclopedia* aims to provide accurate, current, and balanced information to people of all viewpoints and on both sides of the smoking debate.

Special features of this book include appendixes of contributions by key players in the contemporary American tobacco control movement, selected landmark workplace and smoking cases, an annotated list of surgeon general's reports on smoking and health issued between 1964 and 1998, and a detailed chronology of tobacco since 1492. A bibliography sends readers to some of the most authoritative books, articles, and Web sites available. Finally, the index provides readers with a full listing of topics covered by the *Encyclopedia*. Although no one volume could cover the entire range of material available about tobacco, this volume will help readers effectively navigate the oceans of information on this controversial substance.

A Note About Tobacco Company Names

A word must be added about the names of tobacco companies that appear countless times throughout the *Encyclopedia*. Since 1911, when the U.S. Supreme Court broke up the tobacco trust, several tobacco companies have dominated the industry. Owing to mergers and diversification, tobacco company names have changed many times over the years. To help straighten out the confusion, especially in entries that describe companies and their activities at a particular point in time, the series of name changes for the five largest U.S. tobacco companies are listed below:

- Philip Morris Inc., or Philip Morris USA, founded in 1919, is one of the four principal subsidiaries of Philip Morris Companies Inc.

- In 1970, R.J. Reynolds Tobacco Company, founded in 1875, became a wholly owned subsidiary of R.J. Reynolds Industries, Inc., which later changed its name to RJR Nabisco Holdings Corporation. In 1999, the company split up and shed its tobacco business.

- In 1927, Brown and Williamson Tobacco Company, founded in 1906, was purchased by the British American Tobacco Company and its name was changed to the Brown and Williamson Tobacco Corporation. Today the company is a wholly owned subsidiary of B.A.T. Industries PLC (formerly the British American Tobacco Company), a British firm. In 1994, Brown and Williamson bought the American Tobacco Company.

- The Lorillard Tobacco Company, Inc., founded in 1760, became a subsidiary of Lorillard Inc., and then became a subsidiary of Loews Corporation in 1969.
- In 1986, Liggett and Myers Tobacco Company, whose name appeared for the first time in 1873, had its name changed to Liggett Group, Inc. when the tobacco company became part of a conglomerate; in 1990, the Liggett Group, Inc. merged with Brooke Group Ltd.

A Note About Dates

The author tried to obtain birth and death dates for each person profiled in the encyclopedia. However, some dates are lost to history and others, despite the wonders of Internet, e-mail, and deft researchers, never materialized.

ACKNOWLEDGMENTS

I unearthed some of the unique historical and contemporary materials on smoking buried in archives around the nation when I visited the Arents Collection in the rare book room of the New York Public Library; the Frances E. Willard Memorial Library in Evanston, Illinois; the library at the national headquarters of the Seventh Day Adventists in Silver Spring, Maryland; the offices of Action on Smoking and Health and the Advocacy Institute in Washington, D.C., the American Lung Association in New York City, and Stop Teenage Addiction to Tobacco in Springfield, Massachusetts (now located in Boston); and, especially, the private library of Dr. John Slade.

This book also owes a debt to the federal government officials, especially Don Shopland at the National Cancer Institute, and scholars too numerous to mention who returned phone calls, snail mail, fax, and e-mails. I am especially indebted to Eva McKeon who spent the summer of 1998 helping me conduct the research a book of this nature requires. With my wish lists in hand, she ran to libraries in New York City and towns all over Bergen County, New Jersey, to retrieve books, photocopy articles, congressional documents, or whatever else I asked of her.

Finally, a special thank you to the six contributors who generously provided the essays that appear in Appendix 1.

GUIDE TO SELECTED TOPICS

Legal Aspects of Tobacco: Legislation

Media: Print and Audio-Visual

Native Americans

Organizations: Tobacco Control

Organizations: Tobacco Industry and Smokers Rights

Pipe

Action on Smoking and Health (ASH)

ASH is a national nonprofit legal-action and educational organization, headquartered in Washington, D.C., fighting for the rights of nonsmokers. It was created in February 1968 by John F. Banzhaf III, the attorney responsible for the Federal Communications Commission "fairness doctrine" ruling. Banzhaf declared ASH "both a nickname and a goal—

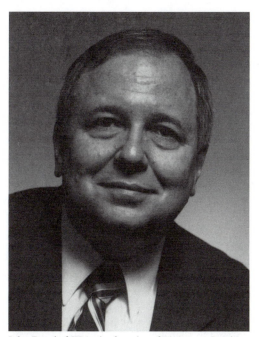

John Banzhaf III is the founder of Action on Smoking and Health. *Courtesy of Action on Smoking and Health.*

the end of cigarettes" (Soper, p. 2). ASH uses the power of law to represent nonsmokers in courts and legislative bodies and before regulatory agencies. It publishes a quarterly newsletter, *ASH Smoking and Health Report.* In the late 1990s, the newsletter gave special coverage to environmental tobacco smoke issues as well as to flaws in the $368.5 billion tobacco settlement of June 1997. The ASH Internet Web site <http://ash.org> provides up-to-the-minute news about important developments, statements by other organizations, speeches by tobacco control leaders, texts of major bills, court rulings, agency rulings, research studies, tobacco documents, tobacco contributions to politicians, and votes in Congress. *See also* FAIRNESS DOCTRINE OF THE FEDERAL COMMUNICATIONS COMMISSION (FCC); TOBACCO SETTLEMENT—JUNE 1997

References: Francis A. Soper, "John Banzhaf and the Giants," *Listen, Journal of Better Living*, vol. 21, no.7, n.d.

Adams, John Quincy (1767–1848)

The sixth president of the United States, John Quincy Adams, who broke his own smoking habit, sympathized with the anti-tobacco movement of 1830–1860. He smoked West Indian cigars during his 20s, was a connoisseur of Havana cigars, and made them "proper" and fashionable for Bostonians. *See also* CIGARS AND PRESIDENTS

Additives to Tobacco Products

Tobacco companies use additives to make tobacco products more acceptable to consumers. Some prolong life (humectants), some make the smoke milder and easier to inhale (sugars and humectants), some add flavor and aroma, some improve the delivery of nicotine (ammonia compounds), and some numb the throat (menthol and eugenol, the active ingredient in cloves). When some additives burn in cigarettes they create new chemicals by combining with other additives as well as with the tobacco.

When chewing tobacco was a national pastime in the 1800s, the number of possible sweetening recipes was infinite and manufacturers took pains to keep their formulas secret. The most important "casing" or flavoring ingredient was licorice, which was used around 1830 by some of the 119 factories in Virginia and North Carolina. But rum, sugar, tonka beans, cinnamon, nutmeg, and other spices and condiments were also added to the chew.

At the end of the 1990s, additives to tobacco products were not subject to government regulation in the United States. Since the mid-1980s, cigarette manufacturers have been required to submit a list of tobacco additives used in cigarettes to the Department of Health and Human Services, but the department is barred from publishing the list. Further, the manufacturers do not have to specify which cigarette brands use which additives. The tobacco companies are not required to disclose anything about additives to cigarette papers (such as fillers and adhesives) or to filters. In April 1994, public pressure forced the major cigarette makers to publish a version of a list containing 599 materials that might or might not be added to any brand of cigarettes. The list does not say how much of the various additives are used.

Advertising and Cigarettes and Smokeless Tobacco

The creation of mass-produced cigarettes on the BONSACK MACHINE in 1884 led to innovations in distributing and marketing them on a national scale. JAMES BUCHANAN DUKE, who had installed Bonsack machines in his factory, hired the services of advertising agencies to help him create a market for the huge number of cigarettes his company manufactured. Duke advertised in newspapers and magazines, using colorful packaging with attention-grabbing, brightly colored paper labels, catchy names, and images that attracted male smokers. He advertised on BILLBOARDS, in theater programs, and on posters tacked to storefronts. In 1889, he spent $800,000 on advertising the 834 million cigarettes he manufactured that year.

Between 1885 and 1892, Duke and dozens of other tobacco manufacturers put small lithographed picture cards in each cigarette pack to attract cigarette buyers to their brands. The small cards, arranged in series, pictured birds, dogs, flags, and flowers as well as actresses, great American Indian chiefs, presidents, and baseball players—the new national heros.

Duke used other promotions to attract smokers, including coupons in Sovereign cigarettes that could be redeemed for a ½ cent in cash. In Mecca cigarettes, postcards (without stamps) were included that were "eminently suited for the U.S. mail." Some Duke cigarette brands offered buyers coupons redeemable for miniature college pennants and Oriental rugs. Coupon programs lasted until after World War I, when most tobacco companies stopped them.

Around 1912, tobacco companies inserted "silks" in cigarette boxes. These colorful silk rectangles were aimed at women smokers (then a small minority) who bought the cigarettes, collected the silks, and stitched them onto pillows and bedspreads. Small silk rugs were also the perfect size for dollhouses. Some companies packaged miniature silk rugs in envelopes and slipped them into cigarette boxes or inserted leather patches printed with college seals.

Like Duke, RICHARD JOSHUA REYNOLDS believed in marketing and advertising his cigarettes. On October 21, 1913, his ad agency launched the first national cigarette advertising campaign in the nation for Camels, the first "modern" blended cigarette, containing "Turkish and domestic tobaccos." The multimillion-dollar ad campaign was built around the theme that Camels did not offer premiums like other cigarettes. Ads explained that the cost of the tobaccos used in the Camel blend was too great to permit anything except the product itself. People bought the message, and by 1919 Camels were the top-selling cigarette.

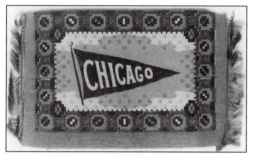

Colorful silk rectangles, like the one pictured here bearing the Chicago banner, were placed in cigarette packages as a way to promote smoking to women.

By the 1920s, women were smoking in greater numbers and advertising firms began to create ads that made smoking appear attractive to both men and women. Once people became accustomed to seeing women smoke in public, ad agencies devised ways to convince them to smoke their brands. By the second half of the 1920s, tobacco advertisers began to push their products directly at women. A 1926 CHESTERFIELD CIGARETTES ad shows a woman asking her date, who is smoking, to "Blow some my way." A storm of protest greeted the ad, but other tobacco companies soon followed suit. In 1927, Marlboro ads showed a woman's hand in silhouette holding a lit cigarette. The same year, Camel placed women in their ads, but didn't show them actually smoking until 1933. During the 1930s, even more ads were aimed at women. Major middle-class women's magazines pictured rich-looking American women, opera stars, and athletic-looking women promoting cigarette brands.

During the 1920s, cigarette manufacturers were among the most enthusiastic pioneers in using radio for coast-to-coast advertising. After magazines, radio was the second greatest national advertising medium. The AMERICAN TOBACCO COMPANY, owned by GEORGE WASHINGTON HILL, was one of the first tobacco companies to charge into radio. Two months after Lucky Strike commercials had their debut on 39 radio stations in September 1928, sales skyrocketed by 47 percent. Soon other cigarette companies shifted their ad budgets from outdoor signs to the powerful new medium.

The distribution of free cigarettes during World War I and World War II contributed to the massive growth of the smoking habit, but so did advertising campaigns. Tobacco advertisers injected ad campaigns that linked smoking, war, and patriotism directly into radio programs. Camels ran a "Thanks to Yanks" radio campaign. Contestants who correctly answered game show questions could send 2,000 Camels to the serviceman of their choice. If game contestants could not answer a question correctly, 2,000 cigarettes went into the "Thanks to Yanks" duffle bag. By January 1943, 29,250 packs of Camels had been shipped to servicemen free of charge.

Cigarette ads in magazines especially linked smoking and war. Camel ads showed men in torpedo rooms of submarines, breaking through barbed wire, and lugging antitank guns. Chesterfield had its "Workers in the War Effort" campaign. Pall Mall used military themes and Raleigh offered cheap prices on gift cigarettes sent to soldiers overseas. Tobacco companies also showed women hard at work in the national effort. Camel ran a series of ads picturing and naming women who worked in war industries. The Chesterfield campaign targeted feminine war workers. By the second half of the 1940s, tobacco companies portrayed women as wives and sweethearts waiting for returning husbands and boyfriends while they smoked.

In the late 1940s, tobacco advertisers were quick to recognize the potential of another powerful advertising medium—television. In 1947, Lucky Strike began sponsoring college football games and in 1948 the Lucky Strike "Barn Dance." In 1948, Camel sponsored the "Camel News Caravan." By the 1960s, children and teens were being exposed to hundreds of glamorous cigarette messages. In a typical week, cigarette companies spent about $3 million to air 3,000 commercials urging viewers to smoke 38 different brands.

Tobacco companies also gave financial support to professional sports teams. In 1963, R.J. REYNOLDS TOBACCO COMPANY sponsored eight different baseball teams, and the American Tobacco Company sponsored six more. Philip Morris sponsored National Football League games on CBS, Brown and Williamson Tobacco Corporation sponsored football bowl games, and Lorillard was a sponsor of the 1964 Olympics. Angry that the airwaves were saturated with an endless barrage of commercials telling children and teens that cigarette smoking was a pleasant habit with no health risks, the Federal Communications Commission (FCC) recommended and Congress acted to ban all cigarette advertising from television and radio effective January 2, 1971.

After the BROADCAST BAN ON CIGARETTE ADVERTISING, tobacco companies poured hundreds of millions of advertising dollars into billboards that associated smoking with success, athletics, social acceptance, youth, glamour, thinness, and healthy outdoor fun. Tobacco companies also poured money into the print media. In 1970, before the TV/radio ban, tobacco companies spent $50 million on magazine advertising; in 1979, the figure rose to more than $257 million.

In the 1970s, tobacco companies shifted their advertising efforts to attract more women to smoking. Virginia Slims and other cigarette advertising flooded women's magazines, newspapers, and Sunday newspaper supplements. By 1979, cigarettes were the most advertised product in some women's magazines, with as many as 20 ads in a single issue.

Cigarette makers also poured money into new promotions. In 1971, Philip Morris launched a series of tennis matches called the "Virginia Slims Invitational." Also in 1971, RJR Nabisco's "Winston Cup" auto racing began. Philip Morris sponsored the Marlboro Grand Prix, Marlboro 500, Marlboro Challenge, and Laguna Seca Marlboro Motorcycle Grand Prix.

Cameras picked up cigarette logos and ads on stock cars, stadium billboards, and clothing. Even as the Justice Department took action in the summer of 1995 against Philip Morris for its strategic placement of billboards in sports stadiums to receive air time during televised games, the company insisted it had not violated the TV ad ban.

Besides cigarettes, tobacco-sponsored sporting events put smokeless tobacco on television despite the broadcast ban. In 1991, the Federal Trade Commission (FTC) took action against the Pinkerton Tobacco Company, makers of Red Man chewing tobacco. The FTC charged the tobacco company with violating the 1986 COMPREHENSIVE SMOKELESS TOBACCO HEALTH EDUCATION ACT, which prohibited television advertising of smokeless tobacco. Pinkerton sponsored televised truck and tractor-pull events known as the "Red Man Series" and agreed to stop the display of the Red Man brand name on banners, billboards, clothing, and vehicles and to use Red Man only as part of the event's title and only if it did not resemble the Red Man logo.

In addition to billboard advertising and sports events sponsorship, cigarette makers poured millions into point-of-purchase ads and displays in drugstores, supermarkets, gas stations, and bowling alleys. Other promotions included free cigarette samples or smokeless tobacco products and gifts (T-shirts, coffee mugs, lighters, ash trays, key chains) and catalog merchandise in exchange for coupons from cigarette packs. Cigarette advertising expenditures for catalog promotions quadrupled from $184 million to $756 million between 1991 and 1993.

Besides marketing to women, tobacco companies marketed cigarettes to African Americans, Asian Americans, and Hispanic/Latino communities as well as to civil liberties, health, religious, community service, cultural nonprofit, charity, and AIDS service organizations.

A combination of factors in the 1990s affected the advertising and marketing practices of tobacco companies. These factors included the impact of advertising campaigns like R.J. Reynolds Tobacco Company's OLD JOE CAMEL on children and teens, the increase in tobacco use by children and teens, and the emergence of secret TOBACCO DOCUMENTS that showed how the tobacco companies studied the smoking habits of teens and looked for ways to attract young smokers. Further, the 1994 series of landmark nationally televised congressional hearings on tobacco industry practices examined the possibility of providing the Food and Drug Administration (FDA) with regulatory authority over tobacco products, including a proposal to classify nicotine in tobacco as a drug. The FDA proposals for regulating tobacco included regulations to restrict smoking ads that appealed to minors as did the unsuccessful tobacco settlement of June 1997.

In the tobacco settlement of November 1998 between the tobacco companies and the attorneys general of 46 states, the cigarette manufacturers agreed to marketing restrictions that included bans on billboard and transit advertisements and on the sale of clothing and merchandise with brand logos. They agreed to avoid cartoon figures in ads and to ban sponsorship of youth-oriented sporting events and concerts, but were allowed to maintain at least one sports sponsorship a year.

In the late 1990s, tobacco companies were adapting to restrictions and lining up new ways to advertise and market their products—from Internet sites to new packaging to publishing magazines like *Marlboro Unlimited*. *See also* CHILDREN AND TEENS, UNITED STATES; FOOD AND DRUG ADMINISTRATION (FDA), 1995 PROPOSAL FOR REGULATING TOBACCO; TOBACCO SETTLEMENT—JUNE 1997; TOBACCO SETTLEMENT—NOVEMBER 1998; WAXMAN HEARINGS

Advertising and Cigars

Only a small amount of conventional advertising appears for cigars, most of it in magazines. Advertisements present cigars as lavish, yet affordable, luxuries. In some ads, the history and tradition of cigar making is depicted. Many ads create a personal link with the company owners, founders, or the artisans and farmers who create the product. Sexuality permeates some of the ads.

The most important way cigars have been presented to the public has been through promotional activities. The CIGAR RESURGENCE in the United States has been closely associated with the lifestyle magazine, *CIGAR AFICIONADO*, published by Marvin R. Shanken, since the fall of 1992. The magazine's success led to *SMOKE*, another tobacco lifestyle magazine, launched in 1996 by Lockwood, a tobacco trade publisher. Another similar magazine, *Cigar Monthly*, has also appeared. These three magazines have been imitated in France (*L'Amateur de Cigare*).

Cigar dinners build word-of-mouth advertising. In 1994, *Cigar Aficionado* sponsored gala affairs and dinner parties at expensive restaurants featuring cigars, wines, and celebrity guests. Similar events have become widespread, and the magazine publicizes restaurants that offer "smoker nights."

In a 1992 issue, a list of 32 domestic and four foreign restaurant and cigar clubs offered such events. By the spring of 1997, the number of listings had grown to 591 entries in the United States and 70 listings from outside the country. Magazine subscribers receive formal invitations to events sponsored by the magazine.

Smoking clubs appeared in many communities in the mid-1990s. Among the most elaborate are cigar bars identified with the Macanudo brand of cigars. Social clubs organized around cigars have also appeared on a number of college campuses.

Cigars are featured on the World Wide Web at many sites. There are online catalogs for ordering as well as links that provide background information and ratings. The sites operated by manufacturers not only provide information and images about specific brands but also link customers with retailers who carry their products. These sites also offer discussion and news groups. *Cigar Aficionado* and *Smoke* maintain elaborate sites.

Cigars have long been available by mail order, but the resurgence in popularity of expensive cigars has prompted the introduction of new speciality catalogs for cigar users, such as one called the *Cigar Enthusiast*.

The cigar craze has also nourished a cottage industry that produces cigar accessories such as lighters, cutters, ashtrays, humidors, books, videos, cigar label lithographs, and clothing. Accessories for cigars have also been appearing in more established upscale catalogs, such as those from Herrington, Frontgate, and Hammacher Schlemmer.

Culbro (General Cigar) has a series of promotions for its White Owl and Garcia y Vega brands that involve returning proofs of purchase for branded t-shirts and other premiums. Not only has it developed a small catalog for the Garcia y Vega brand, it has launched a line of expensive sportswear geared to its premium brands. General Cigar features the Macanudo name prominently on each article of clothing, which then become advertisements for the brand. It also promotes Macanudo through furniture that features the crest design on the upholstery.

Cigars are common props on magazine covers, in fashion photography, and among movie and television stars, musicians, sports stars, and other public figures. They are also used as props in movies and advertisements for the movies. *See also* THE CIGAR AND PRESIDENTS

Advocacy Institute (AI)

The Advocacy Institute, headquartered in Washington, D.C., is a behind-the-front-line organization dedicated to strengthening the advocacy capability of the least powerful citizen groups and communities so that their voices will be heard. Founded in 1984 by MICHAEL PERTSCHUK and David Cohen, the AI brings together seasoned advocates and community-based leaders to help build their capacity to advocate for their causes. The Institute serves public interest groups engaged in a wide spectrum of issue campaigns, ranging from civil and human rights to public health, the environment, campaign financing reform, and economic justice. The mission of the AI is realized primarily through its two programs: The Capacity Building Program, which facilitates exchange—and brings groups of advocates together to work on the elements of capacity building—and the Tobacco Control Project.

Since 1987, the AI has provided strategic guidance and counseling to tobacco control advocates through the Tobacco Control Project that links advocates across the country through SCARCNet (the Smoking Control Advocacy Resource Center Network), the world's first electronic network for professional tobacco control advocates. SCARCNet, a private, nonprofit, Web-based computer communication network, brings together the tobacco control community and offers a program of strategic consultation, skills building, and connection to unfolding events and campaigns.

Through SCARCNet, advocates participate in ongoing discussions on such issues as promoting clean indoor air, restricting advertising and promotion, limiting the tobacco industry's access to youth, promoting tobacco excise taxes, and linking tobacco and politics. Supporting the policy discussions are online resources including a daily news bulletin, Action Alerts, an extensive searchable database, advocacy guides, and case studies. While the Tobacco Control Project does not engage in frontline advocacy, and does not take public positions on legislation, sign petitions, or try to set the agenda for the tobacco control movement, it provides the tools for advocates to advance that agenda.

The AI has trained thousands of advocates from around the United States and across five continents and helped launch and guide the American Stop Smoking Intervention Study (ASSIST), the first major federal program to help state advocacy efforts on tobacco.

The Institute has analyzed the role of tobacco money in politics, examined the connections between the tobacco industry and the ACLU, and analyzed strategies and tactics of the tobacco industry. It has published various media advocacy guides on tobacco and a directory of tobacco industry spokespersons, front groups, and their allies. *See also* AMERICAN CANCER SOCIETY (ACS)

Agricultural Adjustment Act of 1933

On May 12, 1933, President Franklin D. Roosevelt signed the Agricultural Adjustment Act (AAA), a law aimed at providing immediate relief to growers of crops designated as basic commodities, such as wheat, cotton, corn, and tobacco. Farmers were going broke because crop prices were dropping while costs were not.

To help farmers regain the same purchasing power they had had before World War I, the AAA offered cash payments to farmers who volunteered *not* to grow tobacco and other crops that were in oversupply. Farmers agreed to cut back their production of tobacco to help drive up prices. After the 1933 legislation was declared unconstitutional, substitute legislation authorized payments for withdrawing acreage from soil-depleting crop production, or for planting soil conserving crops. *See also* AGRICULTURAL ADJUSTMENT ACT OF 1938; AGRICULTURAL TOBACCO POLICY OF THE U.S. GOVERNMENT; SOIL CONSERVATION AND DOMESTIC ALLOTMENT ACT

Agricultural Adjustment Act of 1938

The Agricultural Adjustment Act of 1938 authorized marketing quotas, with a penalty for growers who exceeded them. The program is available for all kinds of tobacco except shade-grown wrapper and périque (an aromatic fermented Louisiana tobacco). Marketing quotas have been approved and in effect since 1938 for each crop of flue-cured, burley, and dark tobacco. Cigar binder and Ohio filler crops first came under quotas in 1951. Price supports were never applied to Pennsylvania filler and last applied to the Maryland crop in 1965 and the Connecticut-Massachusetts binder crop in 1983.

Congress found that because the tobacco, cotton, wheat, corn, and rice markets constituted the greatest basic industries of the United States and that their activities directly affected interstate and foreign commerce at every point, stable conditions were necessary for the general welfare.

Many farmers were forced to borrow money or lease land when natural causes interfered with tobacco production. And since they were widely scattered throughout the nation, farmers could not organize effectively. Federal assistance was not available to effectively control the orderly marketing of tobacco, and in 1938 farmers produced and dumped abnormally excessive tobacco supplies on the nationwide market, burdening and obstructing interstate and foreign commerce.

As a result, the U.S. Congress passed the Agricultural Adjustment Act of 1938 to amend the SOIL CONSERVATION AND DOMESTIC ALLOTMENT ACT of 1936. The new act regulated interstate and foreign commerce in tobacco (and cotton, wheat, corn, and rice) to the extent necessary to provide an orderly, adequate, and steady flow of these products by storing reserve supplies and making loans and marketing quotas. The law ensured that the agriculture secretary would assist farmers, processors, and distributors to obtain, when practical, the parity price for these commodities and parity of income, and that consumers would obtain an adequate and steady supply of these crops at fair prices.

Enacted on February 16, 1938, the law, in part, declared the following:

> Sec. 2. It is hereby declared to be the policy of Congress to continue the Soil Conservation and Domestic Allotment Act, as amended, for the purpose of conserving national resources, preventing the wasteful use of soil fertility, and of preserving, maintaining, and rebuilding the farm and ranch land resources in the national public interest; to accomplish these purposes through the encouragement of soil-building and soil-conserving crops and practices; to assist in the marketing of agricultural commodities for domestic consumption and for export; and to regulate interstate and foreign commerce in cotton, wheat, corn, tobacco, and rice to the extent necessary to provide an orderly, ad-

equate, and balanced flow of such commodities in interstate and foreign commerce through storage of reserve supplies, loans, marketing prices for such commodities and parity of income, and assisting consumers to obtain an adequate and steady supply of such commodities at fair prices.

The law provided that the secretary of agriculture announce a national marketing quota for flue-cured, burley, and other grades of tobacco for each of the next three succeeding marketing years and determine and announce the total quantity of flue-cured, burley, and other kinds of tobacco that may be marketed (and increased if necessary) to meet market demands.

The law has been amended many times since its enactment. The No Net Cost Tobacco Program Act of 1981 substantially revised the provisions of the 1938 act relating to tobacco, as did the Dairy and Tobacco Adjustment Act of 1983. *See also* Agricultural Adjustment Act of 1933; Agricultural Tobacco Policy of the U.S. Government; Consolidated Omnibus Budget Reconciliation Act (COBRA) of 1985; Omnibus Budget Reconciliation Act (OBRA) of 1993

Agricultural Tobacco Policy of the U.S. Government

During the 1930s, when Congress enacted laws aimed at rescuing farmers during the Depression years, it laid the groundwork for the U.S. tobacco program. Although the laws enacted during those years have been amended many times, the basic components remain. U.S. tobacco growers are guaranteed minimum prices through price supports in exchange for limiting production via allotments and quotas. The tobacco program is paid for by producers and purchasers through marketing assessments. Since the legislative guidelines are ongoing and precise, program adjustments usually require new legislation. A referendum is held every three years for flue-cured and burley tobacco to determine whether producers support continuing the

program; past votes have overwhelmingly supported the programs.

Under the current tobacco program, national marketing quotas are set each year. These quotas determine the maximum amount of burley and flue-cured tobacco that producers can sell that year. The national quotas are allocated among individual allotment holders. This allotment grants each holder the right to market a given amount of tobacco. Allotment holders who do not produce tobacco may lease or sell their quota to active producers within the same county.

Since the late 1980s, the U.S. tobacco program has been revised several times in response to economic, political, and international pressures. Changes were made to increase the U.S. competitive position in world markets and to significantly lower taxpayer costs for operating the program.

Expanding international markets resulted in rapidly rising marketing quotas. However, the demand for U.S. tobacco was reduced sharply in 1992 and 1993 in response to a significant surplus of less expensive tobacco in international markets and to changing manufacturing blending practices to accommodate increasing sales of generic cigarettes. U.S. cigarette manufacturers responded by importing record levels of tobacco into the United States. Faced with declining domestic sales and marketing quotas, the U.S. tobacco program was modified in 1993 to limit the volume of imported tobacco.

Demand for U.S. tobacco in the domestic market has also been adversely affected by increases in the number of smoking restrictions and bans, wholesale cigarette prices, and taxes. As a result, demand for U.S. tobacco has declined considerably from the record levels established during the early 1990s. *See also* Agricultural Adjustment Act of 1933; Agricultural Adjustment Act of 1938; Consolidated Omnibus Budget Reconciliation Act (COBRA) of 1985; Dairy and Tobacco Adjustment Act; No Net Cost Tobacco Program Act of 1981; Omnibus Budget Reconciliation Act (OBRA) of 1993; Soil Conservation and Domestic Allotment Act

Air-Cured Tobacco

Nearly all cigar tobaccos, a large portion of BURLEY TOBACCO, and other tobaccos grown in Kentucky and Tennessee are air cured. After tobacco leaves wilt, they are hung in curing barns where air circulation is good and little or no artificial heat (charcoal or gas fires) is required. Regulating ventilation controls the rate of drying. If tobacco leaves are killed by bruising, rapid drying, or too high heating, there is no way to remove natural starch in the leaf, and the tobacco becomes harsh and lifeless.

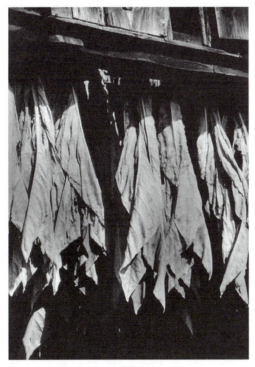

Air-cured tobacco leaves hanging in a barn. ©*Doris Friedman.*

Air-cured tobacco is divided into two groups: light and dark. The light group includes burley and Maryland, both used in manufacturing cigarettes. The dark group includes Green River and Virginia's sun-cured and one-sucker, all used mainly for producing chewing tobacco. The U.S. Department of Agriculture grades air-cured tobacco class three. *See also* TOBACCO CLASSES

Allen and Ginter

In 1872, partners John F. Allen (1814–1890) and Lewis Ginter (1824–1897) owned a Richmond, Virginia, factory under the name John F. Allen and Company that made chewing tobacco, smoking tobacco, and cigars. Around 1874, the firm went into cigarette manufacturing. The company's hand-rolled cigarettes won honors at the 1876 Centennial Celebration in Philadelphia.

By 1888, the firm, known as Allen and Ginter, produced two million cigarettes per day. The most skilled and dedicated female worker ("roller") rolled four to five cigarettes a minute, about 300 cigarettes an hour, or 3,000 in a 10-hour day. A leading supplier for the national and international markets, and anxious to keep up with the growing demand for cigarettes, Allen and Ginter sponsored a contest with a prize of $75,000 for the inventor of a machine that could roll cigarettes automatically. On March 8, 1881, James Albert Bonsack, a mechanic from Lynchburg, Virginia, patented his design for a cigarette-rolling machine and allowed Allen and Ginter to use the machine on a trial basis. At the time, it could produce over 70,000 cigarettes in a 10-hour day. After the short trial period was over, Allen and Ginter rejected the BONSACK MACHINE because they felt smokers preferred hand-made cigarettes and would dislike mass-produced ones.

Lewis Ginter of Allen and Ginter had a worldwide reputation for genius in advertising. His company put picture cards in each pack of cigarettes both as a means of advertising as well as a stiffener for the pack. The colorful cards of American Indian chiefs, military battles, baseball players, animals, and leading actresses came in numbered series to lure buyers into collecting entire sets. Allen and Ginter distributed booklets containing pictures of the cards. *See also* CIGARETTE PICTURE CARDS, UNITED STATES

American Cancer Society (ACS)

The American Cancer Society, headquartered in Atlanta, Georgia, has a prominent role in the fight against tobacco. The ACS provides smoking education, prevention, and SMOKING CESSATION programs to millions of adults and young people through some of its 3,400 local units. Each year, it distributes millions of pamphlets, posters, and other materials on smoking. It sponsors the GREAT AMERICAN SMOKEOUT, an annual event in November. The ACS also carries out smoking prevention programs in schools through teaching units and audio-visual materials it has developed.

In 1993, in partnership with the NATIONAL CANCER INSTITUTE, the ACS began a 17-state project (which grew to 30 grantees) called ASSIST (American Stop Smoking Intervention Study for Cancer Prevention), intended to attack smoking in homes, schools, health care centers, community groups, work sites, and the mass media. The statewide efforts relied on the cooperation of a variety of community groups and the society's volunteers to reach 91 million people, or a third of the population, including about 20 million smokers. In September 1999, the ASSIST program ended.

In 1998, the ACS began an aggressive anti-tobacco campaign attacking tobacco with words and images taken from the cigarette industry's own advertising (a picture of Joe Camel, a photo of tobacco industry executives being sworn in before Congress). The campaign's mission was to "expose the lies of the tobacco companies and reengage the public in the public debate" (Beatty, 1998). The $5 million budget for the ads came from the society's annual working budget, which reflects individual and some corporate donations. As many as six ads were planned; the commercials ran nationally on CNN. *See also* AMERICAN HEART ASSOCIATION (AHA); AMERICAN LUNG ASSOCIATION (ALA); HAMMOND, E. CUYLER; HORN, DANIEL; LITTLE, CLARENCE COOK

References: Sally Beatty, "Bucking Big Tobacco with Just $5 Million," *Wall Street Journal*, September 16, 1998, B.10.

American Council for Science and Health (ACSH)

The American Council for Science and Health, founded in 1978 by Elizabeth Whelan, Sc.D., and other scientists, is a con-

sumer education nonprofit organization located in New York City. It publishes *Priorities,* a quarterly journal that discusses issues related to food, drugs, chemicals, lifestyle, the environment, and health. The journal has published numerous articles regarding the health hazards of tobacco products.

In 1980, ASCH did the first of three surveys of popular magazines. It studied 10 women's magazines published from 1967 to 1979 to determine whether articles were being published about the dangers of smoking. All 10 magazines carried cigarette ads during the years under study. ACSH found a total of eight feature articles about the dangers of smoking in all 10 magazines during the survey period. ACSH also found that of the 10 magazines, 4 never carried anything about smoking during the entire 12-year period. By contrast, two magazines did carry articles—and no cigarette advertising. *Seventeen* ran 5 stories and *Good Housekeeping* ran 11 stories. "Project Censored" ranked the ACSH story one of the top 10 censored stories of 1980. (Since 1976, Project Censored is an annual national media event. Each year, 40 media watchers pick the 10 best censored stories.)

In 1982, ACSH surveyed 18 large-circulation magazines that discussed health issues. ACSH counted the health-related articles in each magazine between 1965 and 1981 and looked to see if tobacco was discussed. ACSH concluded only one-third of the magazines surveyed reported the hazards of smoking both frequently and accurately. ACSH also found that the best coverage of health hazards of smoking was in magazines that did not accept cigarette ads. Among the best magazines covering smoking and health were *Reader's Digest, Prevention,* and *Seventeen.* The worst coverage was found in *Ms., Newsweek, Parade,* and others.

In 1986, ACSH did another survey to see how well American magazines were covering the health hazards of smoking during the 1980s. It looked at the reporting of smoking as a health hazard in a select group of 20 magazines, some of which accepted cigarette ads and some of which did not. Of all the magazines surveyed, *Reader's Digest* had the best all-around coverage of the hazards of smoking, as it had for many years. ACSH awarded worst coverage to *Cosmopolitan,* which printed no articles about smoking during the survey period. ACSH concluded that magazines that accept cigarette ads were less likely to report on the health hazards of smoking.

American Health Foundation (AHF)

Founded in 1969, the American Health Foundation is a nonprofit private research organization devoted primarily to the prevention of chronic diseases, especially cancer, through an interdisciplinary research and intervention approach. The AHF, a National Cancer Institute-supported Cancer Center, is the only center engaged specifically in multidisciplinary research on cancer prevention.

The Foundation's mission is based on the concept that mortality and morbidity from cancer, heart disease, and stroke (which account for more than two-thirds of all premature deaths) can be reduced by a rational program of disease prevention. It supports the belief that chronic diseases are due to lifestyle choices that include smoking, nutritional habits, drug and alcohol abuse, lack of activity, and exposure to occupational and environmental hazards.

AHF scientists have been honored nationally and internationally for their research in the area of disease prevention. Founder ERNST L. WYNDER, M.D., who first established the link between tobacco smoking and cancer, was also editor-in-chief and founder of the international journal *Preventive Medicine,* which fosters exchange of information obtained from disease prevention research among professionals.

Some 200 researchers at AHF laboratories provided the first clear demonstration of the link between tobacco use and cancer and have identified and characterized the adverse biological effects of many of the more than 4,000 chemical compounds in cigarette smoke and smokeless tobacco. Since its inception, the AHF has been in the forefront of tobacco-related cancer research. *See also* GRAHAM, EVARTS

American Heart Association (AHA)

The American Heart Association, headquartered in Dallas, Texas, supports the elimination of smoking in all public places. It prohibits the use of all tobacco products during sessions of any meeting, conference, seminar, or assembly being held under its sponsorship and on all Association premises.

The AHA promotes smoking intervention programs at schools, workplaces, and health care sites. One of its anti-smoking programs, "Save a Sweet Heart," deals with advertising and peer pressure in the world of teenagers. *See also* SMOKING CESSATION

American Lung Association (ALA)

The American Lung Association, headquartered in New York City, has assumed a leading role in the fight against tobacco, helping smokers to quit, encouraging children not to start smoking, cleaning up the air in indoor and outdoor environments, protecting nonsmokers from secondhand smoke, and preventing lung disease caused by microorganisms. The ALA conducts public education programs, seminars, and workshops for health professionals; answers public inquiries; finances research; and works with other organizations to clean up the atmosphere.

Most ALA local units have a program specialist who provides consultant services and materials to schools for developing smoking education curricula and for implementing biofeedback and peer-teaching programs about smoking. Local units offer books, pamphlets, puzzles, posters, buttons, films, and other materials to combat smoking.

ALA has worked to ban cigarette vending machines, create stricter laws against selling cigarettes to minors, and encourage smoke-free workplaces. In the 1990s, in response to survey findings, the ALA developed a Quit Smoking Action Plan. The plan brings together state-of-the-art information including resources and products as well as personal support required for personalized smoking termination plans.

In April 1997, the ALA and the Nicotrol® franchise of nicotine replacement therapies formed an educational partnership in an effort to help more people quit smoking. The ALA provides a comprehensive behavior change program and Nicotrol provides an array of NICOTINE REPLACEMENT PRODUCTS, including an over-the-counter transdermal patch, a prescription nasal spray, and a nicotine inhaler, all designed to help smokers quit. Nicotine replacement therapy used in conjunction with a behavioral change program is considered to be the first-line therapy in SMOKING CESSATION and increases a smoker's chances of successfully quitting. *See also* AMERICAN CANCER SOCIETY (ACS); AMERICAN HEART ASSOCIATION (AHA)

American Medical Association (AMA)

The largest medical group in the U.S., with more than 300,000 physicians, the American Medical Association has made tobacco control advocacy one of its most important policy issues. In the past, however, AMA policy tolerated smoking. Many physicians had been heavy smokers in a high-stress profession. The tobacco industry distributed free cigarettes at medical meetings and conventions throughout the first half of the century and even beyond. Doctors were slow to denounce smoking to their patients. In 1957, an AMA spokesman testified at the first congressional hearings on smoking and health that a person would have to inhale 10,000 cigarettes a day to absorb a dose equivalent to what was being painted on the shaved backs of mice to test the carcinogenic potential of tobacco. This was a reference to the 1953 experiments carried out by Dr. ERNST L. WYNDER and Dr. EVARTS GRAHAM.

The AMA leadership announced soon after the release of the 1964 surgeon general's report that it had accepted a $10-million, no-strings grant from the tobacco industry for a five-year study of questions relating to smoking and health. That same year, the AMA published an educational leaflet announcing that smoking was a "threat to life" because "numerous deaths occur each year from burns and suffocation due to falling asleep while smoking." Under the heading, "Suspected Health Hazards," the AMA leaflet concluded that according to some researchers,

cigarette smoking "shortens life expectancy" and was "alleged to cause cancer of the lungs and bladder." The leaflet advised as follows: "Some equally competent physicians and research personnel are less sure of the effect of cigarette smoking on health. . . . Smoke if you feel you should, but be moderate" (Whelan, 1984).

The AMA leadership opposed the first health warning labels on cigarette packs when Congress considered the idea in 1965. The AMA stated that:

> With respect to cigarettes, cautionary labeling cannot be anticipated to serve the public interest with any particular degree of success. The health hazards of excessive smoking have been well publicized for more than 10 years and are common knowledge. Labeling will not alert even the younger cigarette smoker to any risks of which he may or may not be already aware.

In the 1970s and 1980s, the AMA changed directions, prodded by a new breed of physicians like RONALD M. DAVIS. In 1989, the AMA took a major step into the area of tobacco control advocacy when it sponsored the Tobacco Use in America Conference in Houston, Texas, which brought together tobacco control advocates and members of Congress. The 100 invited conference participants formed work groups around major policy issue areas and developed recommendations. In 1993, the AMA sponsored a second conference, in Washington, D.C., again promoting collaboration between legislators and the tobacco control community and producing a series of recommendations.

Special tobacco editions and articles in the *Journal of the American Medical Association (JAMA)*, one of the most widely read journals by U.S. physicians, are important sources of research and draw media attention to tobacco issues.

In 1994, the AMA and the Robert Wood Johnson Foundation, the nation' largest philanthropic organization dealing with health issues, announced a $10-million anti-smoking campaign called SmokeLess States to be carried out in 19 states. The Foundation provided the money and the AMA managed the distribution of that money in grants to existing anti-tobacco lobbying organizations. The AMA and the Foundation used California's successful program of using tobacco taxes to support anti-tobacco education. This program supports statewide coalitions to reduce tobacco uptake and use and increase public awareness of the role of tobacco control policy in health care reform. *See also* CALIFORNIA'S PROPOSITION 99

References: Elizabeth M. Whelan, *A Smoking Gun: How the Tobacco Industry Gets Away with Murder*, Philadelphia: George F. Stickley Co., 1984, p. 104.

American Medical Women's Association (AMWA)

Founded in 1915, the American Medical Women's Association, now headquartered in Alexandria, Virginia, is a national organization of female physicians and medical students with a membership of 10,000. A leading advocate for women's health, AMWA relocated its headquarters from New York City to Washington, D.C. in 1988 to intensify its public policy efforts. One of the women's health issues AMWA has worked to improve is smoking prevention and cessation.

In 1996, the AMWA dedicated an entire issue of its *Journal of the American Medical Women's Association* [Volume 51, numbers 1 and 2 (January/April 1996)] to "Smoking and Women's Health." Articles covered trends and effects of cigarette smoking among girls and women in the United States from 1965 to 1993, nicotine dependence in women, the prevalence and etiology of smoking among adolescent girls, smoking and reproductive health, smoking cessation techniques, international issues regarding women and tobacco, public policy and tobacco disease, tobacco litigation as a public health and cancer control strategy, the recruiting of women to cigarette smoking between 1900 and 1940, and cigarette advertising targeted to women. *See also* VIRGINIA SLIMS CIGARETTES; WOMEN, UNITED STATES

American Pharmaceutical Association (APA)

In 1971, the American Pharmaceutical Association recommended that its members stop selling tobacco products. The APA stated that tobacco sales violated the Association's code of ethics: "A pharmacy should never knowingly condone the dispensing, promoting or distributing of drugs. . . that lack therapeutic value for the patient" (*Priorities*, 1992).

References: *Priorities*, Summer 1992.

American Public Health Association (APHA)

The American Public Health Association, founded in 1872, is a nonprofit corporation, headquartered in Washington, D.C., with state affiliates. APHA has long been involved in issues concerning smoking and health; in February 1964, it served as one of the four founding agencies of The National Interagency Council on Smoking and Health. This group, which included over 30 national health organizations, dedicated itself to implementing the recommendations of the landmark 1964 surgeon general's report on smoking and health. APHA has provided leadership in activities related to the hazards of smoking. For many years, its journal has covered tobacco control activities.

American Tobacco Company

Incorporated in 1890 in New Jersey, the American Tobacco Company was founded by JAMES BUCHANAN DUKE. As the company's first president, Duke led American Tobacco to control of 80 percent of the entire tobacco industry, with the exception of cigars. For 14 years, Duke spent enormous amounts of money to enlarge his company, crush his competition, and control prices. He bought up at least 250 other tobacco companies, some of which he closed, and paid other competitors not to compete for specified amounts of time or gave them large sums of money to go out of the tobacco business permanently. By 1904, Duke's company was almost a monopoly that made 90 percent of the nation's cigarettes, 80 percent of its quid (chew tobacco), 75 percent of its pipe tobacco, and over 90 percent of its snuff; however, it made only 14 percent of the nation's cigars.

Finally, in July 1907, President Theodore Roosevelt went after Duke's American Tobacco Company (and other businessmen) because he thought the company's behavior was greedy and irresponsible. Roosevelt's attorney general sued Duke's tobacco trust for violating the Anti-Trust Act of 1890, which outlawed monopolies. Named as defendants were 28 individuals besides Duke, 65 American corporations, and two English corporations—BRITISH AMERICAN TOBACCO COMPANY and IMPERIAL (in which American Tobacco held a large minority shareholding). The suit made its way through lower courts and finally went on appeals from both the defendants and the government to the U.S. Supreme Court.

The trial began in May 1908, but it was not until May 29, 1911, that the U.S. Supreme Court handed down one of the most momentous decisions in American business history. It took Chief Justice Edward White nearly 90 minutes to read the appeal decision, which held Duke and his trust guilty of violating the anti-trust law in securing control of four-fifths of the total non-cigar manufactured tobacco industry. The Supreme Court declared:

> Indeed, the history of the combination is so replete with the doing of acts which it was the obvious purpose of the statute [the Sherman Anti-Trust Act] to forbid, so demonstrative of the existence from the beginning of a purpose to acquire dominion and control of the tobacco trade, not by the mere exertion of the ordinary right to contract and to trade, but by methods devised in order to monopolize the trade by driving their competitors out of business, which were ruthlessly carried out upon the assumption that to work upon the fears or play upon the cupidity of competitors would make success possible. (*U.S. v. American Tobacco*, 1911)

The Supreme Court ordered the trust dissolved by methods to be determined by the Circuit Court of Appeal of New York and lawful competition restored between the constituent forms. In his office, Duke responded: "In England, if a fellow had built up a whale of a business. . . he'd be knighted. Here they want to put him in jail" (Kluger, 1996).

After the break-up, the company reorganized as 14 separate companies, with one of them retaining the name of the original company. Selected to run the dismembered American Tobacco Company were PERCIVAL SMITH HILL and his son, GEORGE WASHINGTON HILL. Major cigarette brands were divided among four companies: the American Tobacco Company, R.J. REYNOLDS TOBACCO COMPANY, P. Lorillard, and LIGGETT AND MYERS TOBACCO COMPANY.

In 1995, BROWN AND WILLIAMSON TOBACCO CORPORATION bought the American Tobacco Company. *See also* BRITISH-AMERICAN TOBACCO COMPANY LTD.; DUKE, JAMES BUCHANAN; LORILLARD COMPANY INC.

References: Opinion of U.S. Supreme Court in *U.S. v. American Tobacco* (221 U.S. 105) May 29, 1911.

Richard Kluger, *Ashes to Ashes*, New York: Alfred A. Knopf, 1996, p. 51-2.

Americans for Nonsmokers Rights (ANR)

A nonprofit public interest group formed in 1976 to protect the right of nonsmokers to smoke-free air, Americans for Nonsmokers Rights pursues an action-oriented program of policy and legislation. Based in Berkeley, California, ANR's activities began with efforts to enact legislation to protect nonsmokers in the workplace and enclosed public places. From modest beginnings with the passage of a few local ordinances in the early 1980s, ANR had by 1998 promoted the enactment of more than 1,000 city and county ordinances across the United States.

In the process, ANR became a national resource on the issues of nonsmokers' rights, passive smoke, and tobacco in general. Besides aiding officials and activists nationwide, it conducted a successful national grassroots campaign to eliminate smoking on all domestic airline flights.

The American Nonsmokers' Rights Foundation, ANR's educational arm, promotes smoking prevention and education about smoking, passive smoke, and the tobacco industry. It helped produce a film on the harmful effects of passive smoking entitled *Secondhand Smoke*. The Foundation's award-winning smoking prevention program, Teens as Teachers, trains teenagers as teachers for younger children. *See also* ACTION ON SMOKING AND HEALTH (ASH); DOCTORS OUGHT TO CARE (DOC); SMOKEFREE EDUCATIONAL SERVICES; STOP TEENAGE ADDICTION TO TOBACCO (STAT)

Americans with Disabilities Act (ADA)

Under the Americans with Disabilities Act, enacted by Congress in 1990, employers with at least 15 employees, and proprietors of places of public accommodation may not discriminate against individuals disabled by tobacco smoke. *Disability* is defined as a physical impairment that substantially limits one or more of the major life activities of an individual. The term *physical impairment* includes any physical disorder, condition, cosmetic disfigurement, or anatomical loss affecting one or more of the bodily systems. In regard to a substantial limitation, the ADA cites three factors that should be considered: the nature and severity of the impairment, the duration or expected duration of the impairment, and the permanent or long-term impact resulting from the impairment. Temporarily disabling conditions do not qualify as a disability under ADA. Under federal regulations, *major life activities* include breathing, walking, working, seeing, hearing, and learning. In the case of secondhand smoke, breathing, and in some cases, working or walking are affected. The physical impairments subject to protection include severe asthma, severe tobacco-related allergies, chronic obstructive pulmonary disease, cardiovascular disease, and others.

The ADA requires employers with 15 or more employees and people who operate places where the public is invited (stores, offices, and restaurants) to make "reasonable accommodations" to the known physical limitations of an otherwise qualified individual with a disability. In cases where individuals with severe respiratory or cardiovascular diseases find their breathing impaired because of exposure to ENVIRONMENTAL TOBACCO SMOKE (ETS), they can identify themselves as disabled under the ADA and request a reasonable accommodation from their employer or in public places. If they are unable to negotiate a solution with an employer, employees can file a discrimination complaint with the U.S. Equal Employment Opportunity Commission (EEOC) or state human rights agency.

Title I of ADA covers the workplace. If a person qualified to do a job cannot do or apply for a job because of smoking in the workplace, he or she is a disabled person under the act and may ask the employer to provide a reasonable accommodation; that is, a smoke-free workplace. An employer can still claim that a smoking ban would impose an undue hardship. Under the ADA, the determination of what constitutes an undue hardship is made on a case-by-case basis.

Title III of ADA covers what are known as public accommodations. These include virtually all places where the public is invited. If a policy of permitting smoking has a discriminatory effect on someone with a tobacco smoke-related disability by effectively denying that person access to a facility's goods, services, or benefits, the owner or manager of the public accommodation must provide a reasonable modification of policies and procedures to allow access. *See also* SHIMP V. NEW JERSEY BELL

Anti-Cigarette League (ACL), Chicago

Organized in 1899 in Chicago, Illinois, by LUCY PAGE GASTON, the Anti-Cigarette League carried out its objective "To combat and discourage, by all legitimate means, the use of and traffic of cigaretts [sic]" through enacting legislation and prosecuting violators (Tate, 1995). Financial backing came largely from a group of Chicago businessmen, including Julius Rosenwald, president of Sears, Roebuck and Company; Andrew Carnegie, the steel magnate; and William C. Thorne, president of Montgomery, Ward and Company.

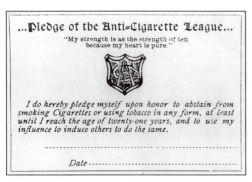

Anti-Cigarette League of Chicago pledge card.

The ACL sent recruiters around the country, distributing pledge cards to school children and soliciting donations from churches and temperance and business groups. *See also* ANTI-TOBACCO MOVEMENTS, UNITED STATES

References: Cassandra C. Tate, *The American Anticigarette movement, 1820–1930*, PhD Dissertation, Seattle: University of Washington, 1995, p. 115. (UMI Number 9609793).

Anti-Cigarette League (ACL), New York City

In 1894, Charles B. Hubbell, president of the New York Board of Education and a crusader against cigarettes in public schools, established the first Anti-Cigarette League in a New York City boys' school. Eventually, 25,000 New York schoolboys belonged to leagues established in almost all of the 63 male grammar schools.

When the boys joined a league, they signed a pledge not to smoke until they were 21. They received a diamond-shaped badge of solid silver engraved with the words "The cigarette must go." The boys took great pride in living up to their pledges. If a member was caught smoking, he turned in his badge and was barred from the league for six months. After he returned, he got his badge back and another chance to be a member.

On January 12, 1895, 200 boys, delegates from 60 male grammar schools of New York City, formed the Consolidated Anti-Cigarette League to centralize the anti-cigarette movement. *See also* ANTI-TOBACCO MOVEMENTS, UNITED STATES

Anti-Smoking Messages, 1967–1970

The FAIRNESS DOCTRINE OF THE FEDERAL COMMUNICATIONS COMMISSION (FCC) dictates that recipients of broadcast licenses have to present all sides of controversial subjects. In 1967, the FCC required all radio and television stations broadcasting cigarette commercials to donate "significant" free air time for anti-smoking messages. As a result of the FCC ruling, many health agencies and the U.S. PUBLIC HEALTH SERVICE made TV and radio spots condemning smoking. Between July 1, 1967, and December 31, 1970, these anti-smoking messages, worth millions of dollars in air time, were aired at no cost on television along with paid commercials promoting cigarette smoking.

In January 1968, networks broadcast 54 anti-cigarette commercials and five programs devoted to the problem posed by smoking. By comparison, the networks aired 501 cigarette commercials in the same month. The following three examples of anti-smoking commercials come from tapes viewed at the Museum of Broadcast Communications in Chicago, Illinois.

The AMERICAN HEART ASSOCIATION (AHA) prepared a televised message of Kokomo, Jr., a monkey in a man's suit seated at his desk reading a brochure about smoking and heart disease, where a voice said:

> This chimp is no chump. Cigarette smokers get coronary disease at a rate two to three times higher than nonsmokers. Cutting out cigarettes is one of the ways of cutting down your risk.

After the voice stopped, Kokomo, Jr., threw out a cup of cigarettes on his desk.

The U.S. Public Health Service (PHS) prepared a message showing a young person puffing and coughing in a bathroom. Then a voice said: "Remember your first cigarette?

Maybe your body was trying to tell you something?"

Another televised anti-smoking spot of the PHS said:

> Every time you light up a cigarette an alarm ought to go off in your head [alarm beeps in the background] and get louder and stronger with every puff you take. Because the awful truth is, the further down you smoke, the worse it gets. And the last part of your cigarette is a lallapalooza. That's where you get the heaviest accumulation of tars and nicotine. All the evidence shows it. Those dirty last puffs. So if you haven't stopped smoking altogether, at least stop half way.

During 1969 and 1970, three major U.S. television networks aired about 1,200 anti-smoking messages. After cigarette ads were banned from television, the networks reduced the number of anti-smoking messages. In the years 1971 and 1972, the first two years of the broadcast ban, the networks delivered 250 anti-smoking messages. In 1970, an average of 30 network spots aired each week; in 1971, an average of 10 spots.

During the years that TV showed thousands of anti-smoking messages, smoking rates dropped. In 1967, 549.3 billion cigarettes were consumed. In 1968, the second year of the anti-smoking messages, 545.6 billion cigarettes were consumed. In 1969, 528.9 billion were smoked. Government statistics showed that as many as 10 million Americans quit smoking from 1967 to 1970. In 1971, when cigarette advertising disappeared from TV, anti-smoking commercials dramatically decreased. Broadcasters no longer were required to give "significant amounts" of free time for the anti-smoking messages. In 1971, cigarette use bounced back to 555.1 billion cigarettes. *See also* TALMAN, WILLIAM

Anti-Tobacco Movements, United States

Opponents of smoking and chewing tobacco have been present in national life since the colonial period. Puritan members of the general courts of Massachusetts and Connecticut passed statutes to curb the use of tobacco. In 1634, Massachusetts declared that two or more people could not take tobacco together anywhere, publicly or privately. In mid-seventeenth-century Connecticut, the legal code classified tobacco users as common idlers.

Although a significant anti-tobacco document was published by DR. BENJAMIN RUSH in 1798 in the United States, little agitation against tobacco took place until the reform period of 1830 to 1860. During these decades, physicians and ministers like Reverend Orin Fowler, Dr. Joel Shew, REVEREND GEORGE TRASK, and DR. RUSSELL T. TRALL wrote anti-tobacco essays indicting tobacco as a deadly poison. The anti-tobacco movement was far less important than the movement against slavery or alcohol, so the crusade practically disappeared with the Civil War. During the war, however, the anti-smoking forces succeeded in their demand for taxes on domestic and imported smokes. The tax largely affected imports arriving from Europe.

By the 1880s and 1890s, anti-tobacco forces concentrated on battling cigarettes and ignored cigars, pipes, and chewing tobacco. Anti-cigarette leagues recruited Midwesterners who feared urban dwellers, cigar smokers, and users of plug and pipes. A key figure in the anti-cigarette crusade was LUCY PAGE GASTON of Illinois who lobbied to end the production and sale of cigarettes in the United States. She won the support of businessmen whose companies refused to hire individuals who smoked. They helped her finance the ANTI-CIGARETTE LEAGUE (ACL), CHICAGO.

Towards the end of the nineteenth century, the states of Iowa, North Dakota, and Tennessee enacted laws prohibiting the sale and use of cigarettes. Arkansas, Indiana, Kansas, Minnesota, Nebraska, Oklahoma, South Dakota, and Wisconsin later joined them. The anti-cigarette movement was strong in the Midwest and weakest in the East. Much of the legislation had little effect because tobacco companies found their way around the laws. In some states where the sale of cigarettes was illegal, the companies gave out free cigarettes and charged for the matches. In areas where laws were enforced, cigarettes were bootlegged; in many instances, the laws were not enforced.

American entry into World War I in 1917 boosted the sales and legitimacy of cigarettes. Not only did the U.S. government and civilian organizations send tons of free cigarettes to soldiers at the front, the civilian population took to cigarettes as well. Outdoor smoking become acceptable, and women appeared in public with cigarettes in hand. After the war, it was evident to anti-smoking crusaders that anti-cigarette laws could not be enforced. In 1921, Arkansas, Idaho, Iowa, and Tennessee repealed their laws and other states soon followed. By the end of the decade, all the state laws were overturned.

As opposition to cigarettes died down during the 1930s, special smoking rooms were provided in theaters, railroads, and steamships.

During the 1950s, mounting medical studies showed a strong statistical correlation between cigarette smoking and the incidence of lung cancer. A December 1952 article in READER'S DIGEST, titled "Cancer by the Carton," informed readers that research indicated strong links between smoking and cancer. After the story was picked up by radio and television news programs and magazines, cigarette sales declined for the first time in 21 years.

After the SURGEON'S GENERAL REPORT OF 1964 was released, anti-cigarette crusaders from all political and ideological lines coalesced around the issue of cigarette advertising, rather than on prohibiting products of the tobacco industry. The perceived failure of alcohol prohibition, the strength of the cigarette habit in 1964, and the power of the tobacco lobby worked against a repeat of the Gaston-era crusade. Television and anti-cigarette forces wanted cigarette commercials banned from television and radio. When the CIGARETTE LABELING AND ADVERTISING ACT OF 1965 passed Congress, mandating a health warning on cigarettes and nothing else, the anti-smoking coalition considered it to be a weak measure.

Legislative failures did not stop the reformers. They regrouped and planned a new assault on cigarette ads in the courts, before legislative committees, and at the FEDERAL TRADE COMMISSION (FTC) and the Federal Communications Commission (FCC). A new law signed by President Richard Nixon on April 1, 1970, strengthened the cigarette health warning and banned cigarette advertising on television and radio after January 1, 1971.

Until the mid-1970s, the concern of the tobacco control community was largely focused on how smoking harmed smokers. But after the nonsmokers' rights movement emerged in the late 1970s, anti-cigarette forces turned to eliminating smoking in all but designated areas in public facilities. Some hospitals, schools, and theaters provided "No Smoking" zones, but reformers wanted the same for restaurants, airplanes, elevators, and other public places.

During the 1980s, doctors, scientists, and Surgeon General C. EVERETT KOOP released studies that linked secondhand smoke to disease, including lung cancer, in healthy nonsmokers. As the evidence mounted, anti-tobacco reformers no longer wanted a simple separation of smokers and nonsmokers within the same air space but demanded smoke-free environments.

In 1986, the same year Surgeon General Koop released his report that said involuntary smoking is a cause of disease, experts from the medical and public health community testified before the Subcommittee on Health and the Environment, chaired by Henry Waxman (D-CA), calling for a ban on all advertising and promotion of cigarettes and smokeless tobacco products. The experts felt advertising plays an important role in promoting a deadly product and recruiting new smokers, especially children and adolescents, women, and minorities. Previously, in December 1985, the AMERICAN MEDICAL ASSOCIATION (AMA) called for a complete ban on all advertising and promotion of cigarettes and smokeless tobacco products.

While tobacco companies have said they don't intend to market to young people, numerous empirical studies have shown that campaigns like R.J. Reynolds' OLD JOE CAMEL, launched in 1988, have reached children as young as three years old and that advertising affects the behavior of children who are at an age when they are making the decision whether to smoke.

In the 1990s, teenage smoking and tobacco advertising continued to be central concerns for the public health and medical groups because nearly 9 out of 10 smokers were shown to start before they turned 18, teen smoking rates were increasing, and research showed that the earlier smokers start, the more likely they are to develop health problems later.

But some anti-tobacco activists like STANTON GLANTZ have been worried that the focus on trying to stop teenagers from smoking diverts attention away from the nation's 40 to 50 million adult smokers.

There is squabbling among the anti-smoking forces over tactics and which changes to emphasize. But tobacco critics also disagree over fundamental goals. They debate strict regulation versus prohibition of tobacco and attacking teen smoking by clamping down on youth access to tobacco products, an issue that received attention after Congress passed the 1992 SYNAR AMENDMENT that restricts nationwide the sale, distribution, and marketing of cigarettes; this issue was also addressed by the FOOD AND DRUG ADMINISTRATION (FDA) 1995 PROPOSAL FOR REGULATING TOBACCO. Some tobacco control advocates feel that reframing the goal from a smoke-free society to not wanting children and teens to smoke detracts from what they can do about issues of secondhand smoke and bans on smoking in the workplace.

One tactic to battle tobacco use by adults was pursued in 1995 by the Interfaith Center on Corporate Responsibility. It fostered shareholder pressure to get publishers to put strict controls on the content of cigarette ads. The Center proposed to a shareholders' meeting of the giant newspaper publisher Knight-Ridder Inc. that its publications limit the kinds of cigarette ads they will accept. Knight-Ridder issued a set of guidelines, which are not mandatory for its publications, that called for the elimination of cigarette ads that gave the impression that smoking led to physical beauty or sexual attractiveness. The guidelines also called for the elimination of cartoon-like ads that could be targeting kids and catchy phrases like "alive with pleasure," the slogan for Lorillard's Newport brand.

Another tactic has been used since the mid-1990s by anti-smoking litigators who pursue class-action lawsuits. In October 1997, four major tobacco companies settled the first class-action lawsuit, known as *BROIN v. PHILIP MORRIS COMPANIES INC.*, by flight attendants over the effects of smoking on non-smokers. Litigators successfully settled state medical cost reimbursement suits in Florida, Minnesota, Mississippi, and Texas. The success of such suits has been attributed to a number of factors: well-financed attorneys sharing resources and information; the absence of blameworthy plaintiffs in class actions; medical cost reimbursement cases; the unavailability to the tobacco industry of two defenses—assumption of risk and contributory negligence in the medical cost reimbursement cases; a wealth of evidence of industry wrongdoing stemming from former industry researchers and internal TOBACCO DOCUMENTS; and new facts concerning tobacco industry knowledge of the addictive and pharmacological properties of nicotine and the efforts of the industry to manipulate nicotine levels to addict smokers. *See also* ACTION ON SMOKING AND HEALTH (ASH); ADVOCACY INSTITUTE; AMERICAN CANCER SOCIETY (ACS); AMERICAN HEART ASSOCIATION (AHA); AMERICAN LUNG ASSOCIATION (ALA); AMERICAN PUBLIC HEALTH ASSOCIATION (APHA); AMERICANS FOR NON-SMOKERS RIGHTS (ANR); ANTI-CIGARETTE LEAGUE (ACL), CHICAGO; ANTI-CIGARETTE LEAGUE (ACL), NEW YORK CITY; CALIFORNIA'S PROPOSITION 99; CONNECTICUT GENERAL COURT; DOCTORS OUGHT TO CARE (DOC); SMOKEFREE EDUCATIONAL SERVICES; STOP TEENAGE ADDICTION TO TOBACCO (STAT)

Anti-Tobacco Postage Stamps

In 1980, six countries issued anti-tobacco stamps on the occasion of World Health Day to support the theme "Smoking or Health—The Choice is Yours": Argentina, Indonesia, Mali, Niger Republic, Portugal, and Tunisia. Czechoslovakia issued its second anti-tobacco stamp in 1981 (it produced its first in 1976). In 1987, Japan issued one on the occasion of the sixth world conference on smoking and health held in Tokyo. Brazil issued its anti-tobacco stamp on World Health Day, April 7, 1991; the Republic of Yemen issued one on World No-Tobacco Day, May 31, 1991; and Indonesia issued its second anti-tobacco stamp in 1991. By 1992, 43 countries had issued anti-tobacco stamps.

Arents, George, Jr. (1875–1960)

George Arents, Jr., the nephew of Lewis Ginter, began collecting books about tobacco, the family business, on the advice of his uncle. A discriminating collector, he acquired every important work dealing with tobacco as well as prints, drawings, paintings, and photographs relating to tobacco. He also collected containers and devices designed to hold or burn tobacco products as well as cigar store figures. On his death in 1960, Arents willed his collection to the New York Public Library with funds sufficient "to purchase books, manuscripts, literary material, objects and rarities of a character appropriate to [its] development and improvement" ("Tobacco Leaves," 1997–1998). Called the Arents Tobacco Collection, the materials serve scholars from many fields, including literature, history, art history, the history of the book, and the sciences.

References: "Tobacco Leaves: Selections from the Collection of George Arents, Jr." Exhibition Brochure, New York Public Library, September 20, 1997–January 3, 1998.

Argentina

Argentina is one of the major tobacco producing and exporting countries in the Western hemisphere. Both production and exportation of raw tobacco grew during the 1980s. In the early 1990s, about half the tobacco produced was exported mainly to the United States and England. In 1988, 110,000 farmers were involved in tobacco growing in some way. Production occurs almost entirely in the northern subtropical portion of the country. Three provinces, Jujuy, Salta, and Corrientes, accounted for 75 percent of production.

In response to domestic and external market trends, including the increasing numbers of women who smoke, the percentage of dark tobacco grown has declined. In the mid-1970s, 40 percent of tobacco grown was dark tobacco; in the 1980s, this figure fell to one-half that level.

Leaf tobacco is purchased by provincial farming cooperatives for export or by two multinational cigarette companies for domestic production. The cooperatives provide technical assistance to farmers. They also assist in establishing supplementary non-tobacco winter crops such as cucumbers and melons.

In the 1920s, the Argentine tobacco industry comprised approximately 30 locally owned companies and one British company. In the early 1990s, two multinational companies, Nobleza-Picardo, associated with the British-American Tobacco Company Ltd., and Messalin-Particulares, associated with Philip Morris Companies, shared the tobacco market.

The prevalence of smoking is higher among younger Argentine men and increased among women between 1971 and 1991. In the early 1990s, the mortality patterns for lung cancer and other smoking-related diseases indicated that the disease impact on the population was substantial. Yearly smoking deaths were estimated at approximately 38,000 to 49,000.

Argentina has one of the most developed tobacco prevention and control movements in the Americas. Most anti-smoking campaigns and activities originate through nongovernmental organizations such as the Argentine Union against Smoking.

Ariel

In the early 1960s, the BRITISH-AMERICAN TO-BACCO COMPANY LTD. worked on nicotine pharmacology by developing an alternative delivery system that administered one main active ingredient—nicotine—to the body free of toxins from tobacco smoke. Called Ariel, this SAFE CIGARETTE device received two patents (issued in 1966 and 1967), both of which emphasized the importance of nicotine for the smoking experience. The first patent reads as follows:

> It is a prime object of the present invention to overcome the difficulties and disadvantages heretofore encountered and to provide an improved smoking device which delivers an improved smoke stream of a controlled character and which does not contain the products of combustion. (Glantz et al., 1996)

Ariel was never brought to market. *See also* ECLIPSE; PREMIER

References: Stanton A. Glantz, John Slade, Lisa A. Bero, Peter Hanauer, Deborah E. Barnes, *The Cigarette Papers*, Berkeley: University of California Press, 1996, p. 75.

Ashes to Ashes: America's Hundred-Year Cigarette War, the Public Health, and the Unabashed Triumph of Philip Morris

Published in 1996, Richard Kluger's *Ashes to Ashes: America's Hundred-Year Cigarette War, the Public Health, and the Unabashed Triumph of Philip Morris* won the Pulitzer Prize in 1997. A definitive history of the cigarette in the United States since the late nineteenth century, Kluger's book gives a meticulous account of every phase in the tobacco industry's development. Ten years in the making, the book includes some 200 interviews with key people inside and outside the tobacco industry. Kluger describes the men who built the companies, their business strategies, marketing campaigns, and power plays as well as their attacks on anti-smoking forces in science, public health, and government. At the center of the epic story is

PHILIP MORRIS COMPANIES INC. and MARLBORO CIGARETTES, the world's number one brand.

Asia and U.S. Trade Policy

In 1984, the United States amended the Trade Act of 1974 with Section 301, which gives the United States Trade Representative (USTR), a presidential appointee, the power to impose trade sanctions against any nation whose trade policies are "unjustifiable, unreasonable, or discriminatory." The act has been used sparingly over the years because it grants the U.S. president the power to unilaterally put retaliatory tariffs on another country's goods.

The Reagan administration used Section 301 to promote U.S. tobacco interests in Asia and force Asian governments to allow the import of American cigarettes. Section 301 threats over cigarettes were justified with the argument that they provided equal access to markets in which American products could compete. If Asian countries permitted the sale of cigarettes as a legal product, then their citizens could have the opportunity to buy the cigarettes just as Americans have the opportunity to buy Japanese cars or Taiwanese computers.

Four tobacco 301 investigations were conducted from 1985 to 1990 on Japan, South Korea, Taiwan, and Thailand, countries that were largely closed to U.S. cigarette makers. These countries were controlled by national monopolies that manufactured and sold cigarettes, with little or no advertising, to adult males. Threats of trade sanctions by the United States were successfully used against these nations, which severely restricted or prohibited sale of foreign brands, to repeal "restrictive" measures including bans and tariffs on U.S. imports and advertising restrictions.

United States trade policy transformed these noncompetitive, closed markets into competitive ones with the entry of multinational tobacco companies like Philip Morris and R.J. REYNOLDS TOBACCO COMPANY, which launched huge scale cigarette marketing and advertising campaigns and promotions, in most cases unhindered by restrictions, to create a demand for cigarettes.

JAPAN, the third largest cigarette market after CHINA and the United States, had confined American tobacco companies to a tiny share through high tariffs and discriminatory distribution practices. In September 1986, the Reagan administration threatened trade sanctions on Japanese products, including computers, textiles, and auto parts. On October 3, 1986, the Japanese government announced it would suspend all tariffs on foreign cigarettes and would ease restrictions on cigarette distribution and pricing arrangements.

After an agreement between the Japanese and U.S. governments was signed opening the market, U.S. cigarette companies entered Japan with television commercials. JAPAN TO-BACCO INC., the domestic cigarette manufacturing monopoly, advertised as well in an effort to protect its market share. By the end of 1988, cigarette advertising on television had soared from fortieth place to second, and by 1990 the American market share had risen from 2 percent to 16 percent. From 1986 to 1991, smoking prevalence among Japanese females rose from 8.6 percent to 18.2 percent and 27 percent of 20- to 29-year-old women were smoking in 1993.

The Taiwanese government's tobacco monopoly, whose leading brand of cigarette was called Long Life, did not advertise. During negotiations to allow imports of U.S. cigarettes into Taiwan, the USTR insisted that the right to advertise be written into the trade agreement. In December 1986, the Taiwanese government agreed and by 1988, the Marlboro cowboy appeared on kiosks and stores throughout the country. Cigarette consumption went up as did the number of women smoking. In 1991, when the Taiwanese wanted the health warning on all cigarette packs sold in the country moved from the side of the pack to the front, the USTR protested, saying the agreement restricted the health warnings to the sides. The warning was finally allowed to be on the front, but smaller than the Taiwanese government proposed.

The South Korean government was told its textile exports were in jeopardy unless U.S. tobacco products were accepted, tariffs reduced on imported cigarettes, the number of retail outlets selling exports increased, and advertising permitted. The USTR insisted that the law be changed to allow American cigarette companies to advertise. When South Korea signed an agreement opening its market in 1988, it was forced to permit magazine ads, free samples, and the sponsorship of sporting events. To compete with cigarettes like VIRGINIA SLIMS, the Korean tobacco monopoly introduced its own women's brands. Between 1988 and 1989, the smoking rate for male teenagers rose from 18 percent to 30 percent and the rate for female teenagers rose from 2 to 9 percent.

When negotiations began in Thailand in 1989, the government defeated the USTR by turning the trade dispute into a health matter. The Thai campaign included ads from an anti-smoking organization that suggested if American trade policy was successful more Asians would die from smoking than died in World War II, the Korean War, and the Vietnam War combined.

Thailand proposed to submit the dispute with the U.S. government to the General Agreement on Tariffs and Trade (GATT), the international organization that oversees trade between member nations. In 1990, GATT ruled that Thailand had to open its market to foreign cigarettes, but recommended that it keep restrictions on advertising.

By the time of the GATT ruling, Thailand had enacted the most stringent regulations in the world, including a ban on advertising and promotions and distribution of samples, bans on reduction of price as a promotional aid, and bans on cigarette displays of any sort in retail shops. American tobacco companies were not able to mount their usual campaigns.

In 1992, after the United States threatened retaliatory tariffs on Chinese exports under Section 301, China signed a Memorandum of Understanding. It required China to lift all import licensing requirements for cigarettes, cigars, tobacco, and cigarette filters by December 1994. The agreement also required China to lift all scientifically unjustified health standards related to tobacco.

During the Clinton administration, which believed health-based regulations are legitimate, U.S. trade policy shifted. The USTR announced it would no longer oppose countries that wanted to restrict cigarette advertising or enact other health measures, even if those measures violated provisions of trade agreements with the United States. *See also* GLOBAL TOBACCO USE

ASSIST Program. *See* AMERICAN CANCER SOCIETY (ACS)

Auction Warehouse

The auction is the place where the sale of tobacco to the highest bidder is conducted. The first auction, of HOGSHEAD tobacco, was conducted before 1810 in Lynchburg, Virginia. Hogsheads were opened and the contents auctioned off. The heavy volume soon made opening hogsheads too time consuming and samples of loose leaf were accepted for bidding. In 1842, the first loose-leaf auction was held in RICHMOND, VIRGINIA.

After the Civil War, the practice of auctioning tobacco spread throughout Virginia, Kentucky, and Tennessee. Today, the loose-leaf auction is the dominant form of sale.

Auerbach, Oscar (1905–1997)

A landmark study about the effects of cigarette smoking on the lungs conducted by Dr. Oscar Auerbach provided much of the scientific basis for the 1964 surgeon general's report on cancer. The pioneering research by Dr. Auerbach, a pathologist at the Veterans Administration Hospital in East Orange, New Jersey, who was an expert on smoking and cancer, was financed by the AMERICAN CANCER SOCIETY (ACS) and the Veterans Administration.

On February 5, 1970, the ACS's report "Effects of Cigarette Smoking on Dogs" was made public. This study on smoking and health produced two important findings. First, lung cancer can be induced in test animals by cigarette smoking, and, second, filters can reduce the cancer-causing qualities of cigarette smoke by reducing tar and nicotine. The study found that filters, however,

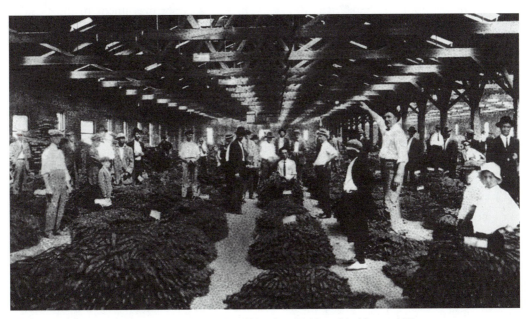

Piles of tobacco leaves in an auction warehouse. *North Carolina Division of Archives and History.*

do not make cigarettes safe, only less harmful.

Auerbach took 94 pure-bred, healthy young male beagle dogs, opened a hole in their windpipes and inserted a tube leading to a cigarette holder. Three dogs died before the study started. Eight dogs were used as controls and did not have tobacco smoke introduced into their lungs. The others were trained to smoke by starting on one filter-tip cigarette a day. According to DR. EDWARD CUYLER HAMMOND, an ACS vice president, at first they resisted but "after they became habituated, . . . then it was hard to keep them away from the stuff" (Kluger, 1996). The cigarettes were specially picked, a brand using filter tips that remove 40 percent of the tar and 37 percent of the nicotine. The researchers purchased 480,000 cigarettes of the unnamed brand and removed the filters from some.

The dogs were divided into four groups. One group smoked only filter-tipped cigarettes. Another was the "heavy smokers" group on nine cigarettes a day. The third was "lighter smokers" on about 4½ cigarettes a day. A fourth category was made up of the 38 heaviest dogs, which were put on the "heavy smoker" ration of nine cigarettes a day for as long as they lived. A dozen of them (31.6 percent) died during the study and two of them when autopsied were found to have lung cancer. In the other group of heavy smoking dogs, half also died during the study. The deaths were mostly due to lung or heart ailments that included emphysema, fibrosis, and corpulmonale, a heart disease that starts with lung problems and includes an unusual enlargement of the right side of the heart. Hammond reported these were all rare causes of deaths in dogs. He also said the lungs of the smoking dogs showed the same type of changes found in the lungs of humans who smoke—"the progressive destruction of lung tissue" in a way that rarely occurs in nonsmokers (Kluger, 1996). Ten cases of lung cancer were found later in this group. None of the control dogs died, Hammond reported, and only two light-smoking and two filter-smoking dogs (16.7 percent) died.

Hammond emphasized that the numbers were not large enough to make a big point of the deaths.

At the end of 875 days, all the remaining dogs, except those in the special "largest dog" groups, were killed. Their lungs were removed, given coded identifications and shuffled so that Dr. Auerbach did not know which group of specimens he was studying. From these studies of pathological slides of the lungs of the dogs came the most significant part of the report. Dr. Auerbach noted tumors that indicated "progressive changes that went from the benign to the malignant." He also saw the giant nuclear structure that characterizes cancer cells and the spreading of the cancer throughout the lung. The key sign of cancer is invasive behavior, the aggressive behavior of cells breaking through natural boundaries and membranes. This occurred in 12 of the heavy-smoking dogs. In addition, Dr. Auerbach reported finding "early invasive squamous (sheet) cell" cancer in the bronchial tubes of two dogs that smoked filtered cigarettes, exactly like those in humans (Kluger, 1996).

The American Cancer Society said the Auerbach findings "effectively refute contentions by cigarette manufacturing interests that there was no cigarette-cancer link" (Burkhart, 1997).

References: Ford Burkhart, "Oscar Auerbach, 92, Dies: Linked Smoking to Cancer," *New York Times,* January 16, 1997, p.25, sectionD.

Richard Kluger, *Ashes to Ashes,* New York: Alfred A. Knopf, 1996, p. 351.

Austin v. Tennessee (1898)

The most famous Supreme Court case involving an anti-cigarette state law, *Austin v. Tennessee,* concerned Tennessee's attempt to keep from its territory an object that Congress had permitted to be manufactured and one from which it derived considerable revenue. The defendant, William B. Austin, had violated the statute by buying cigarettes from the North Carolina factory of the AMERICAN TOBACCO COMPANY and shipping them to Austin's place of business in packages containing 10 cigarettes each. These packages, considered "original packages," were placed in open baskets for delivery and sale in Tennessee.

Cases that dealt with infringement of state law on the exclusive power of Congress to regulate commerce between the states focused on whether cigarettes imported into a state were still in their "original package," the package in which they were placed at the point of origin, or whether they had left their "original packages" and had mingled with the mass of property within a state. The interstate commerce clause of the Constitution prevented undue state restrictions on the importation of goods into the state that were still within their original package. The term "original package" referred to the container in which the cigarettes had been placed for shipping.

The Supreme Court held that the 10-cigarette boxes that Austin imported without a shipping container were designed to bypass the limits of the "original package" rule and to sneak cigarettes into Tennessee. The Supreme Court held that Tennessee could ban cigarette traffic within its borders—as long as the cigarettes had left their "original packages, " which, newly defined, meant large shipping containers. Cigarettes could pass through the state but could not be mingled with the "mass of property" in the state.

B

Baltimore, Maryland

In 1880, Baltimore, Maryland, matched RICHMOND, VIRGINIA, in cigarette output and was the nation's sixth largest cigar-making center. During the 1890s, Maryland was the leading state in smoking tobacco output, capturing about 15 percent of the pipe tobacco market, with Baltimore firms Gail and Ax and Marburg and Felgner as the big producers.

Baltimore's output ranged from plug cuts to long cuts to granulateds and "German smoking," a coarse, heavy product. As a natural tobacco market, the port of Baltimore received leaf from every part of the country and offered a complete selection of smoking tobaccos.

In 1994, Baltimore became the second city in the United States to ban tobacco billboards throughout the city except in heavily industrialized areas and near stadiums and sports parks. *See also* BALTIMORE, MARYLAND, AND BILLBOARDS

Baltimore Billboard Ordinance

In March 1994, Baltimore, Maryland, became the first city in the United States to ban outdoor tobacco ads on billboards, on the sides of buildings, and on freestanding signboards in certain parts of the city, namely, "neighborhoods in which children would typically be found such as the areas in which they live, attend schools and recreate" (Kelder, 1994). The move followed a similar measure governing advertising for alcoholic beverages, including beer and wine. The ban arose from an effort by a coalition of community groups that argued the tobacco and alcohol ads were directed at the young in poor and mostly black neighborhoods.

The ban exempted heavily industrialized areas and zones near stadiums and sports parks where children are not normally found. While cities such as Boston, San Francisco, and Denver have voted to keep tobacco ads off public transportation and other city-owned property, the Baltimore City Council ordinance restricted ads on privately owned space. Exempted from the bans were billboards on public transportation, (although the Maryland governor signed an executive order banning tobacco and alcohol ads on buses), along interstate highways, in sports stadiums, and on taxicabs.

Anheuser-Busch, the world's largest brewery, and Penn Advertising of Baltimore, a company that owned most of Baltimore's billboards, challenged the ban, arguing it violated their First Amendment right to commercial speech.

On August 11, 1994, a federal court in Maryland upheld the constitutionality of the city's ordinance banning cigarette advertising in certain designated zones throughout the city, the first federal court case addressing a First Amendment challenge to a ban on cigarette billboard advertising. The plaintiff argued that the ordinance violated the First

Amendment and was preempted by the federal CIGARETTE LABELING AND ADVERTISING ACT OF 1965. The city argued that the ban was based on the city's interest in preventing the illegal purchase of cigarettes by minors. The federal court in Maryland agreed that this interest was substantial and that the ordinance directly furthered this interest. The court also felt that it was reasonable to assume that if advertising increases consumption among the general public, it also increases consumption by minors.

The U.S. Court of Appeals for the Fourth Circuit in Richmond, Virginia, upheld the ordinance in 1995. Then, in 1996, the U.S. Supreme Court overruled that decision. The justices had struck down a restriction on liquor ads in Rhode Island and said the Baltimore case needed to be reconsidered in light of that ruling. But in November 1996, the Richmond appeals court again upheld the Baltimore ordinance. On April 28, 1997, the United States Supreme Court let stand Baltimore's ban on tobacco billboard advertising without hearing the case. *See also* CINCINNATI, OHIO

References: Graham Kelder, "Ban on Cigarette Billboard Advertising Ruled Constitutional," *Tobacco on Trial*, October 1994, p. 12.

Banzhaf, John, III. *See* ACTION ON SMOKING AND HEALTH (ASH)

Barbour, Haley (1947–)

Tobacco lobbyist Haley Barbour, a former Republican National Committee chairman, put a $50-billion tax credit for the tobacco industry into a new tax bill. Designed to offset the costs arising from the tobacco settlement of June 1997, the tax bill included a 15¢ rise per pack in federal taxes (then at 24¢). Over 25 years, this new tax would add up to $50 billion. The Republican leadership in Congress, Senator Trent Lott of Mississippi and Representative Newt Gingrich of Georgia, supported the provision. In September 1997, an amendment ro repeal the $50-billion credit, proposed by Democrat Richard Durbin of Illinois, was passed overwhelmingly by Congress. *See also* TOBACCO SETTLEMENT—JUNE 1997

Barn

The tobacco barn, the building in which tobacco leaf is cured, usually measures 16, 21, or 25 feet square. This size permits the hang-

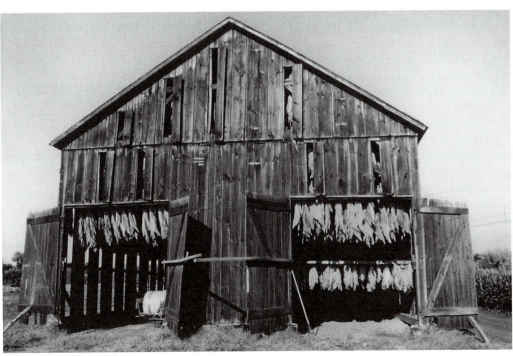

Tobacco barn. ©*Doris Friedman.*

ing of four, five, or six rows of tobacco leaves. The smallest barn holds up to 50,000 leaves, the product of 30 acres. Cigar wrapper leaf hangs in slatted barns. *See also* BRIGHT TOBACCO LEAF

Barrett, Don (1945–)

A Mississippi attorney who won a 1990 product liability case without damages against the tobacco industry, Don Barrett played a key role in setting in motion the Liggett Group's settlement with 22 states. A graduate of the University of Mississippi Law School class of 1969, Barrett represented NATHAN HORTON, a smoker with lung cancer who sued the AMERICAN TOBACCO COMPANY. After Horton died in January 1987, his wife, Ella, took up the case on his behalf.

The first trial ended in a mistrial. In the retrial in 1990, the jury decided that cigarette smoking caused Nathan Horton's lung cancer but refused to award damages, saying both the company and Horton were at fault. Both Barrett and the tobacco company lawyers claimed victory.

In 1993, Barrett, along with RICHARD F. SCRUGGS, represented Jeannette Wilks who sued the American Tobacco Company on behalf of her father, Anderson Smith, who died in 1986 after smoking heavily for 45 years. Since Smith was diagnosed as a paranoid schizophrenic who began smoking while hospitalized, Barrett and Scruggs felt he did not have the ability to make an informed decision. This defense, they hoped, would get around the tobacco company's presumption of risk defense. When the judge ruled that the tobacco company could not use that defense, the company argued successfully that it was irrelevant that Smith was mentally retarded. Barrett and Scruggs lost the case.

In 1993, Barrett was part of a team of lawyers that developed the MISSISSIPPI MEDICAID CASE, and in 1994 he joined the Castano lawsuit, the world's largest class action on behalf of all nicotine-addicted smokers, potentially tens of millions of Americans.

In early 1994, MERRELL WILLIAMS, who had stolen Brown and Williamson documents, needed a job and contacted Barrett because he remembered how the attorney handled the Nathan Horton case. Barrett, again with the help of Richard F. Scruggs, arranged a paralegal job for him. Williams also turned over his documents to Scruggs. At an executive committee meeting of the Castano group, Barrett shared some of the sensitive documents with the group of lawyers, which quickly distributed them to Henry Waxman's subcommittee on Health and the Environment of the House Energy and Commerce Committee in Washington and to the media. Barrett also sent a copy of the documents to STANTON GLANTZ under the name "Mr. Butts."

In an accidental meeting with Marc Kasowitz, personal lawyer of BENNETT LeBow, a financier with a controlling interest in LIGGETT AND MYERS TOBACCO COMPANY, Barrett helped set in motion Liggett's settlement with 22 states. *See also* CASTANO V. AMERICAN TOBACCO COMPANY

Basibali

Basibali is one of the two main types of TURKISH TOBACCO. The plant is larger than BASMA, the other type, and has coarser leaves that are attached to the stalk with a short stem.

Basma

One of the two main types of TURKISH TOBACCO, the Basma plant is smaller than the BASIBALI, the other type, measuring about two to three feet tall. Its leaves, 2 to 10 inches long, do not have stems but grow on the stalk of the plant. Generally, eight rows of three leaves grow on each mature stalk.

BAT Industries PLC

BAT Industries PLC (formerly BRITISH-AMERICAN TOBACCO COMPANY LTD.), headquartered in London, England, is the second largest private cigarette manufacturer in the world. Its major tobacco brands are Capri, GPC,

Kool, LUCKY STRIKE, and Misty. Its chief executive officer is Martin Broughton.

BAT Industries is the parent company of many cigarette manufacturers throughout the world including Brown and Williamson Tobacco Corporation of the United States, BAT Cigarettenfabriken of Germany, Souza Cruz of Brazil, and British-American Tobacco, the latter of which produces cigarettes in more than 45 countries for domestic and export markets in Europe, Australia, Latin America, Asia, and Africa. BAT Industries is associated with Imasco in Canada, which is the parent company for IMPERIAL TOBACCO COMPANY OF GREAT BRITAIN AND IRELAND. In 1994, BAT bought the AMERICAN TOBACCO COMPANY, makers of Lucky Strike cigarettes.

BAT is also the parent company of several insurance and financial services including Farmers Group of the United States and Eagle Star and Allied Dunbar, both of the United Kingdom.

BAT established research facilities in England, Germany, and Switzerland to study the health effects of smoking.

Beagles and Cigarette Testing. *See* AUERBACH, OSCAR

Bernays, Edward L. (1891–1995)

Born in Vienna, Austria, Edward Bernays, the nephew of Sigmund Freud, has been called the father of modern public relations. He put his talent as a public relations counselor to use when he was solicited in 1928 by GEORGE WASHINGTON HILL, president of the AMERICAN TOBACCO COMPANY, to plan a marketing strategy to attract more women to cigarettes in general and LUCKY STRIKE CIGARETTES in particular. Bernays used a number of tools, including advertising, the media, public relations, and psychoanalysis to undermine the traditional social and cultural prohibitions against women smoking. Bernays and Hill developed the "Reach for a Lucky instead of a Sweet" advertising campaign that suggested to women that smoking Lucky cigarettes would help them slim down.

In 1929, as Hill sought even more aggressive ways to change the meaning of women's smoking and to publicly attract this growing market, Bernays set out to identify and destroy the taboos associated with public smoking by women. He got advice from a noted psychoanalyst, Dr. A.A. Brill, who explained that "Some women regard cigarettes as symbols of freedom. . . .Cigarettes, which are equated with men, become torches of freedom" (Bernays, 1965). Using the "torches of freedom" as a symbol, Bernays recruited 10 debutantes to march down Fifth Avenue puffing Lucky cigarettes during the 1929 New York City Easter parade. Newspapers around the country reported the event, and soon reports of women smoking in the streets came from cities and towns across the nation. Bernays wrote that he learned age-old customs "could be broken down by a dramatic appeal, disseminated by the network of media" (Bernays, 1965). He and Hill had successfully promoted the cigarette as the symbol of the independent feminist and glamorous flapper.

In 1934, Bernays again got involved in the effort to promote smoking among women. Hill, concerned that women did not like the forest-green color of the Lucky Strike package because it clashed with their wardrobe, asked the publicist to make green a fashionable color. Bernays developed a far-reaching strategy that centered on making green the fashion color of the 1934 season. He staged a Green Ball and convinced Paris dress makers to make green gowns for the event. He convinced textile manufacturers to sponsor a Green Fashions Fall luncheon for fashion editors. The menu featured green beans, asparagus salad, pistachio mousse glacé, and creme de menthe. He invited artists to talk about the use of green in the works of the great masters, and a symposia of psychologists discussed the implications of the color green in the area of mental health. He wrote interior decorators, art groups, department stores, and club women on green paper describing the sudden "dominance" of green. He talked department stores into featuring green dresses and suits in window displays. He even persuaded an important gallery to hold a "Green Exhibition" of paintings. Within six months, he made green the hot new color. Lucky Strikes sales did not climb during the Depression years, but they did not drop either. Bernays later wrote: "I had wondered at the alacrity with which scientists, academicians and professional men participated in events of this kind. I learned they welcomed the opportunity to discuss their favorite subject and enjoyed the resultant publicity" (Bernays, 1965).

At the end of his life, Bernays became active in the anti-smoking movement. When a reporter asked him if he felt responsible for the epidemic of diseases attributed to smoking cigarettes, he said the risks of smoking were poorly understood at the time he promoted their use. *See also* WOMEN, UNITED STATES

References: Edward L. Bernays, *Biography of an Idea: Memoir of Public Relations Counsel Edward L. Bernays*, New York: Simon and Schuster, 1965, p.391.

Bible, Geoffrey (1938–)

Chairman and chief executive officer of PHILIP MORRIS COMPANIES INC., the world's largest tobacco company, Australian-born Geoffrey Bible spent most of his career in Europe before replacing CEO Michael Miles in 1994. In 1968, he joined Philip Morris's overseas unit as manager of finance and director of planning. Two years later, he left the company to manage a Geneva office of a brokerage company. He returned to the tobacco company in 1976 as vice president of Philip Morris International's finance and strategic development.

In 1981, Bible managed the company's business in Australia where he successfully competed with Rothmans, a South African cigarette company. He put 30, rather than the standard 20, cigarettes in a pack of Peter Jacksons, a Philip Morris brand, without raising the price. After Peter Jackson's market share doubled and Philip Morris's overall sales in Australia skyrocketed, so did Bible's career with the company.

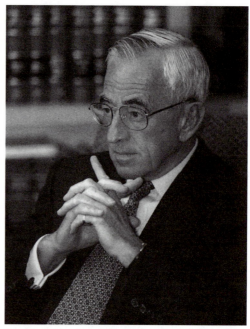

Geoffrey Bible, chairman of Philip Morris, is shown here as he is about to be deposed in West Palm Beach, Florida, in August 1997 as part of the state of Florida's lawsuit against cigarette manufacturers. *AP/Wide World Photos.*

In 1983, Bible was promoted to executive vice president and four years later he was made head of Philip Morris's international tobacco operations. In that office, he negotiated with foreign ministers to get favorable long-term tax and royalty incentives for the tobacco company. After he built a large new plant in Turkey, Philip Morris sales in that country surpassed the company's sales in France and England combined. In 1989, after communism collapsed in Eastern Europe, Bible poured cigarettes into the region and into the Soviet Union, where he spent hundreds of millions of dollars marketing and advertising Philip Morris brands.

After he became chief executive officer of Philip Morris Companies Inc. in 1994, Bible built profits as a whole, unlike his predecessor, Miles, who wanted to split the company into separate food and tobacco companies to enable shareholders to invest in Kraft without having to deal with the prospective costs of tobacco litigation. He also dumped the slow-growing, less profitable businesses, like baked goods, and concentrated on high-margin products like tobacco, cheese, coffee, and candy. By the end of 1996, Bible's successful plan and shrewd marketing decisions made Philip Morris, now a diversified corporation, the world's largest selling cigarette manufacturer. In 1997, Philip Morris had sales of $72 billion, $40 billion of which came from tobacco (two-thirds of which came from international sales).

At the same time Bible was building up Philip Morris, between 1994 and 1997, he and the other top executives of the largest U.S. tobacco companies were besieged by a string of lawsuits by sick smokers, leaks of confidential records, testimony by whistle blowers, lawsuits by ambitious state attorneys general, proposed regulations by the activist FOOD AND DRUG ADMINISTRATION (FDA), and the outspoken words of anti-tobacco president Bill Clinton.

In August 1997, in a pretrial deposition in preparation for the trial of the state of Florida's lawsuit against the major tobacco companies, Bible testified about nicotine when questioned by RONALD MOTLEY, a lawyer representing the state of Florida. Bible said about 100,000 Americans "might have" died from smoking-related diseases. He also said that cigarettes were "certainly not pharmacologically addictive," but people might get hooked in a "behavioral" way ("Philip Morris Chief Admits Smoking Deaths," 1997).

In January 1998, Bible and four other executives of the nation's largest tobacco companies appeared under oath before the House Commerce Committee and testified that nicotine was additive. Bible said he regretted the years of conflict that had existed between the tobacco industry and anti-smoking advocates. He also said that the landmark national tobacco settlement he and the other top tobacco executives signed with 40 state attorneys general in June 1997 offered a chance to change that relationship. (However, the 1997 settlement subsequently collapsed). *See also* PHILIP MORRIS INTERNATIONAL INC.; TOBACCO SETTLEMENT—JUNE 1997; TOBACCO SETTLEMENT—NOVEMBER 1998; WAXMAN HEARINGS

References: "Philip Morris Chief Admits Smoking Deaths," *New York Times*, August 22, 1997, p. A 18.

Bidi

Nearly as long as a regular cigarette, but half as thick, bidis resemble CLOVE CIGARETTES. They contain less tobacco than regular cigarettes, but the unprocessed tobacco is richer in NICOTINE. Bidis, popular in India for centuries, have candy-like flavors and aromas that make them popular with teens. Most bidis lack health warnings.

Bill of Rights Tour

In 1990, PHILIP MORRIS COMPANIES INC., paid $600,000 to the National Archives (the keeper of the nation's most treasured historic documents) to sponsor a national tour of the Bill of Rights (the first 10 amendments to the U.S. Constitution) on its 200th anniversary. The tobacco company distributed more than two million copies of the document as part of the Bicentennial celebration of the Bill of Rights, which concluded on December 16, 1991, the 200th anniversary of the document. Philip Morris also sent a traveling exhibit with one of the original copies of the Bill of Rights to all 50 states. As a result of the campaign, Philip Morris's corporation name appeared on television advertising for the first time since 1971 when the cigarette ad ban went into effect.

The tour was designed to show Philip Morris was committed to free speech, a right guaranteed by the First Amendment. Along the tour stops, protestors expressed their outrage that Philip Morris implied indirectly that there is a constitutional right to smoke. "Nicotinia," a sculpture designed by Washington State DOCTORS OUGHT TO CARE (DOC), also followed the tour each step of the way. A 15-foot replica of the Statue of Liberty holding a cigarette (in place of a torch), "Nicotina" was wrapped in chains of addiction. At the base of the statue, an electronic "Death Clock" ticked off how many tobacco deaths occurred by each stop of the tour. *See also* entries under PHILIP MORRIS

Billboards

Cigarettes were the most heavily advertised product on billboards (with alcoholic beverages second). Billboards were often located near elementary schools, churches, parks, playgrounds, sports stadiums, shopping centers, and homes.

In 1974, ACTION ON SMOKING AND HEALTH (ASH), Dr. Douglas A. Campbell, the Inter-Agency Council of D.C., and the Seventh Day Adventist Temperance Department petitioned the FEDERAL TRADE COMMISSION (FTC) to establish rules regulating the advertising of cigarettes on billboards. In their petition, the petitioners described "The Unique Harm of Cigarette Billboards":

> There are three basic reasons why cigarette billboards are more harmful than other cigarette ads. First of all billboards are difficult to ignore, since they are thrust upon the viewer. Secondly, young children will see the ads and will be unable to understand the severity of the health hazard created by smoking. Both of these reasons were given for the Congressionally mandated ban on television and radio cigarette ads. Finally, eliminating cigarette billboards would remove some of the visible pollution from the sides of our highways in furtherance of the goals of the Highway Beautification Act of 1965.
>
> People do not choose to look at billboards as they choose to read magazines or newspapers. Billboards are intentionally placed on the sides of roadways and in our cities in order to attract the eyes and minds of people who are looking for something else, a street address, scenery. These advertisements often have a short verbal message or a picture and seek to influence their audience at the first glance. Turning away from the billboard does not remove the effects of the advertisement, since the damage may have already been done.
>
> Children are particularly susceptible to the ill effects of cigarette advertisements. Even before they can read, young children enjoy looking out of car windows at the new world around them. They are likely to be attracted and influenced by a cowboy smoking a cigarette, or by a huge, larger than life sized, adult smoking cigarettes. Our hope of reducing the amount of cigarettes consumed rests clearly on the possibility of preventing young people from getting hooked on this harmful and often deadly habit.

Numerous studies documented that kids in low-income neighborhoods saw more billboards with tobacco ads than kids in higher-income neighborhoods.

- **1986 study in San Francisco, California.** A Department of Planning survey found that 62 percent of the billboards in African-American neighborhoods and 42 percent in Latino neighborhoods advertised cigarettes and alcoholic beverages compared to only 36 percent citywide.
- **1987 study in St. Louis, Missouri.** A city study found that 53.9 percent of all billboards advertised tobacco and alcohol. It found that there were four times more tobacco and alcohol ads in African-American neighborhoods than in white neighborhoods.
- **1988 study in Philadelphia, Pennsylvania.** The *Philadelphia Inquirer* surveyed billboards along a 19-block stretch of Ridge Avenue, which passes through one of the poorest neighborhoods in the city. Of 73 billboards, 56 advertised tobacco and alcohol.
- **1989 study in New Orleans, Louisiana.** The New Orleans Planning Commission released a study that found 515 billboards in a predominantly black city council district compared to only 138 in a nearby predominantly white district. Cigarettes were advertised on 58 percent of all the billboards in New Orleans.
- **1989 study in Detroit, Michigan.** The *Detroit Free Press* surveyed nearly 1,000 billboards on 10 major roads and freeways linking the city to the suburbs. It found 48 percent of the billboards advertised tobacco and alcohol, while just beyond the city's borders only 24.7 percent did so.

Under the Tobacco Settlement of November 1998, all cigarette billboards had to be removed by April 23, 1999. The agreement allows states to take over billboard leases that have been held by tobacco companies and put anti-smoking ads on them at the companies expense until the lease expires. *See also* BALTIMORE BILLBOARD ORDINANCE; CINCINNATI, OHIO; TOBACCO SETTLEMENT—NOVEMBER 1998

Binder

A binder is a single leaf of tobacco wound around the filler of the cigar to hold it together. Most binder leaves are raised in Wisconsin, Pennsylvania, New York, and the Connecticut Valley. *See also* CIGAR; CONNECTICUT TOBACCO; LANCASTER COUNTY, PENNSYLVANIA

Black Cat

A brand launched in 1904 by the British tobacco company Carreras and Marcianus, Black Cat was heavily advertised with a feline trademark. The name and symbol came from a cat kept at the original Wardour Street offices of the firm. Smokers referred so constantly to the "Black Cat shop" that the son of the founder put a picture of the animal on some labels. A national Black Cat Day was staged in 1913 when the front page of the *Daily Mail* was used to encourage the nation to walk the streets with their cigarette packs, in hopes the Black Cat man would approach them with the question: "Are you a Black Cat smoker?" Thousands of gold sovereigns were handed out to those who were. Black Cat went into World War I with advertisements showing the cat handing out cigarettes to French soldiers at Verdun. *See also* WORLD WAR I

Black Elk (c. 1862–1950)

Black Elk, sacred practitioner of the Oglala Lakota religion, shared his ancient stories of the Sacred Pipe with Joseph Epes Brown in the fall of 1947. Published in 1953 by the University of Oklahoma Press, *The Sacred Pipe* contains Black Elk's explanation of the meaning of the Sacred Pipe, beginning with White Buffalo Cow Woman who brought it to the Lakota people and invoked them to use it in seven rites. With the Pipe, which is like a portable altar, the Lakotas send their voices to the Great Spirit in prayer. Black Elk believed that his people would live as long as the rites were known and the Sacred Pipe was used. Without the Pipe, his people would be without a center and would perish. *See also* NATIVE AMERICANS; PIPE SMOKING AND NATIVE AMERICANS

Black Shank

One of the most destructive tobacco diseases, blank shank is a soil fungus that attacks the plant at any stage of growth. Discoloration of the affected stalk and roots is followed by the wilting and death of the plant. *See also* BLUE MOLD

Blackwell, William T. (1839–1903)

Before his death in 1869, JOHN RUFFIN GREEN, the originator of BULL DURHAM SMOKING TOBACCO, took into partnership William T. Blackwell, a merchant and tobacco peddler. Blackwell and Julian Shakespeare Carr, who was taken into partnership in 1870, developed modern methods of mass production and distribution. Their Bull Durham factory in North Carolina, which became the largest smoking-tobacco factory in the world, was equipped with the latest machinery for shredding tobacco leaf, making and labeling bags, and packing the granulated mixture into bags.

Carr, who reportedly said, "Yes, sir, as long as I have a dollar to spare, I will invest it in advertising" and Blackwell created the first great advertising campaign for their Bull Durham product (Robert, 1967). Sign painters pictured the bull all over the country and even in Europe and Asia; some displays were as large as 80 by 100 feet.

Blackwell and Carr defended their brand and trademark in historic litigation that restrained imitators of the bull. The case involved judicial comparison of Blackwell's Genuine Durham Smoking Tobacco with its full-view bull and a label of a beast's head by Wesley A. Wright on his Original Durham Smoking Tobacco. In 1875, in *William T. Blackwell v. Wesley A. Wright,* the state supreme court ruled that there had been no infringement on Blackwell's rights, but he and

Carr persisted and were successful in subsequent state litigation.

In the 1880s, the firm changed from a partnership to a corporation. Blackwell then left the company, but Carr remained.

References: Joseph C. Robert, *The Story of Tobacco in America*, Chapel Hill: The University of North Carolina Press, 1949, 1967, p. 124.

Bloch, Michele Helene (1954–)

A health policy consultant and physician, Michele Helene Bloch is a researcher and teacher of effective tobacco control strategies, focusing on women and girls. She developed and directed the first national network of health and women's organizations dedicated to reducing the prevalence of smoking among women and girls.

Trained in anatomic pathology at Washington University School of Medicine in St. Louis, Missouri, Dr. Bloch has taught and supervised groups of medical students in pathology laboratories. She was affiliated with the ADVOCACY INSTITUTE in Washington, D.C. from 1988 to 1992, working on women's programs and smoking control advocacy. Dr. Bloch has published articles on women and smoking, the tobacco industry, and tobacco control advocacy.

Blue Mold

Blue mold is a fungus disease that causes great destruction in tobacco seedbeds. It first appears as a circular patch of yellow on the leaves and may reveal on the underside a fungus growth of a pale white or violet color.

Blum, Alan (1948–)

An associate professor at Baylor College of Medicine in Houston, Texas, Dr. Alan Blum founded DOCTORS OUGHT TO CARE (DOC), a 71-chapter national tobacco control organization headquartered in Houston. Blum has given at least 1,500 lectures on the dangers of smoking in the United States. He has pleaded with government agencies not to allow cigarette advertising at sports events. *See also* ACTION ON SMOKING AND HEALTH (ASH); AMERICANS FOR NONSMOKERS RIGHTS (ANR); ANTI-TOBACCO MOVEMENTS, UNITED STATES; SMOKEFREE EDUCATIONAL SERVICES; STOP TEENAGE ADDICTION TO TOBACCO (STAT)

Bonsack, James Albert. *See* BONSACK MACHINE

Bonsack Machine

On March 8, 1881, James Albert Bonsack (1859–1924), a mechanic from Lynchburg, Virginia, patented a design for a cigarette-rolling machine (it was registered in 1880), the first practical machine for shaping, rolling, and cutting cigarettes. His invention poured a flow of tobacco through a feeder device onto a thin strip of paper rolled into a single, continuous tube. As it emerged from the machine, a rotary cutting knife cut it into equal lengths. The Bonsack machine had some technical problems. The flow of shredded tobacco towards the rollers often stalled and slowed production. After mechanic William O'Brien fixed the problems that slowed down the production of cigarettes, the machines were soon spitting out 200 cigarettes a minute.

John F. Allen and LEWIS GINTER, Richmond, Virginia, businessmen who owned a factory making hand-rolled cigarettes, supplied a national and international market. Believing the demand for cigarettes outstripped the capabilities of the female hand rollers, they sponsored a contest for a practical cigarette-producing machine. After a short trial run using the Bonsack machine, the men rejected it because they believed people would not buy mass-produced cigarettes.

Cigarette manufacturer JAMES BUCHANAN DUKE of Durham, North Carolina, thought otherwise and acquired exclusive rights to the use of the Bonsack machine. The Dukes, the first to use the machine on a large scale, set up Bonsack machines in their Durham, North Carolina, factory, W. Duke, Sons and Company. They labeled their Pin Head brand with "These cigarettes are manufactured on the Bonsack Cigarette Machine." On April 30, 1884, a day now called the "birthday" of the

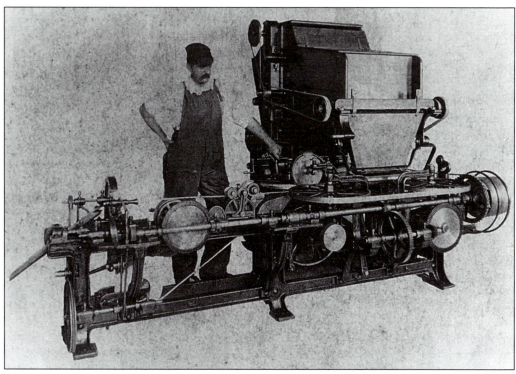

The Bonsack machine for the manufacture of cigarettes. *North Carolina Division of Archives and History.*

modern cigarette, Duke's Bonsack machine operated for a full 10-hour day turning out 120,000 cigarettes. It would have taken 40 hand rollers rolling five cigarettes a minute for 10 hours to make that many cigarettes. By the end of 1884, 14 Bonsack machines were in use, seven in the United States and seven in Europe. *See also* ALLEN AND GINTER; CIGARETTE-MAKING MACHINES

Brazil

Brazil is the world's third largest producer of tobacco, surpassed only by China and the United States, and the world's second largest exporter of tobacco, surpassed only by the United States. The cultural and economic importance of tobacco in Brazil is reflected by the image of a sheaf of tobacco, along with a coffee branch, on the official Seal of the Republic.

Approximately 160,000 farms, employing full- or part-time approximately 600,000 farmers, grew tobacco in the late 1980s. Tobacco is Brazil's third largest export product, behind coffee and soybeans. Most tobacco production occurs in the southern states of Rio Grande do Sul, Santa Catarina, and Paraná, where light tobacco for manufacturing cigarettes is the predominant type grown. The northeastern states of Alagoas and Bahia produce dark tobacco used in Brazil for cigars and pipes.

In 1988, 219 factories were involved in tobacco processing, including 99 for leaf tobacco, 107 for twist tobacco, and 13 for cigar and cigarette manufacturing.

Brazil has been a producer and exporter of tobacco since its colonization in the 1500s. Some of the earliest writings on Brazil note the region's tobacco culture. In 1555, several members of de Villegagnon's colonizing expedition gave their impressions of the use by Brazilians of the tobacco leaf. Jean de Léry recalled that

> You will never see the Brazilians when they do not each have a tube of this plant hung around their necks. All the time and even in talking to you it helps keep them in countenance. . . . I will say that, having myself tried the smoke of *petun*, I have found that

it refreshes and keeps one from feeling hungry. (Heimann, 1960)

Four companies, one a private national company called Sudan and three linked to multinational firms—Souza Cruz Do Sol, a subsidiary of the BRITISH-AMERICAN TOBACCO COMPANY LTD., Philip Morris, and R.J. REYNOLDS TOBACCO COMPANY—controlled cigarette production in Brazil during the 1970s and 1980s.

The tobacco industry in Santa Cruz Do Sul has grown considerably. In 1997, multinational tobacco companies like BAT INDUSTRIES PLC, Philip Morris, and Universal Leaf Tobacco made up 70 percent of the economy. The industry serves as banker and agrarian extension agent for 160,000 small farmers, providing them with seed, fertilizer, and technical assistance. The industry is also financing the local university library and providing teaching materials to schools.

The impact of prolonged exposure to tobacco is evident in mortality patterns of the Brazilian population. At least 32,400 deaths annually have been attributed to smoking. The prevalence of smoking among Brazilian men was nearly 50 percent between 1971 and the late 1980s. The prevalence of smoking among women has increased substantially, and the rate of smoking among urban women has approached that of men. *See also* PHILIP MORRIS INTERNATIONAL INC.

References: Robert K. Heimann, *Tobacco and Americans*, New York: McGraw-Hill Book Company, 1960, p. 19.

Brean, Herbert (1907–1973)

In his 1951 book, *How to Stop Smoking,* Herbert Brean argued that smoking wasted time. He figured it took slightly longer than one minute to remove a cigarette from the pack, light it, place it in an ashtray as it burned, pick it up and lay it down, until the cigarette is smoked. At the rate of 30 cigarettes a day, he calculated a person wasted 30 minutes a day, 3½ hours a week, 14 hours a month, and 168 hours a year, for a total of a week a year. Brean's book sold three-quarters of a million copies. *See also* SMOKING CESSATION

Bright Tobacco

Bright tobacco leaf is a term commonly indicating FLUE-CURED TOBACCOS used chiefly in making cigarettes. During the first half of the nineteenth century, farmers experimented with new soils, cross-breeding, and curing methods to produce a tobacco of milder flavor. Although some light-bodied, yellow leaf was obtained in curing barns, growers could not systematically repeat its production.

An accident in 1839 in a curing barn on the Caswell County, North Carolina, farm of four tobacco planters—Abisha, Elias, Thomas, and William Slade—led to a breakthrough. In late summer, a slave named Stephen fell asleep while curing tobacco leaves near the direct heat of open wood fires, the general method of curing leaf at the time. When he awakened, he threw hot charcoal on the dying barn-floor fires. The heat came up fast and caused the drying leaves to become a bright yellow color never before obtained for cured tobacco.

In 1860, the Census Bureau called Bright tobacco "one of the most abnormal developments in agriculture that the world has ever known" (Robert, 1967). Other growers adopted the "Slade formula," raising the heat from charcoal fires to a high degree after the leaves hanging in the barn were partially cured. (Over 20 years later, charcoal was displaced by flue curing.) Later it was discovered that thin, starved soil, seed of high quality, other natural factors, barn management, and intense heat were required to control the coloring of the leaf, which could be cured to a golden shade. By the 1850s, Bright leaf was the type generally produced in the border districts of North Carolina and Virginia.

Today, Bright, also called flue-cured, tobacco is the principal type used in the United Kingdom and North America, forming almost the whole content of cigarettes and a large part of the ingredients of pipe tobacco. Produced in Florida, Georgia, North and South Carolina, and Virginia, as well as in Rhodesia, Canada, India, Zambia, and Malawi, Bright leaf ranges from light-lemon to dark-mahogany in color.

References: Joseph C. Robert, *The Story of Tobacco in America,* Chapel Hill: The University of North Carolina Press, 1949, 1967, p. 183.

Brissot, Jean Pierre (1754–1793)

Jean Pierre Brissot, born in Chartres, France, wrote a description of tobacco as paper currency. In 1788, he traveled to the United States as an agent for a syndicate that wished to speculate in American lands. His work, *Nouveau Voyage dan les États-Unis de l'Amérique septentrionale* (1791), was so popular it was translated into German, English, and Swedish. In the following excerpt, Brissot discussed the problems incurred by the scarcity of coin and the circulation of tobacco money.

> I will not enlarge further on the subject of tobacco, which many authors have explained; but I will give some description of that kind of paper currency called tobacco money, the use of which proves that nations need not have so much concern as they usually do about the absence of specie. In a free and fertile country the constant produce of the land may give a fixed value to any kind of representation of property.
>
> The state has public warehouses, where the tobacco is deposited. Inspectors in charge test the quality of the tobacco which, if merchantable, is accepted, and the proprietor is given a note for the quantity deposited. The note circulates freely in the state, varying in value with the known price of tobacco. The price is different according to the place of inspection. The tobacco travels to one place or the other, according to its quality, and if it is refused at all places it is exported to the islands or consumed in the country. There are two cuttings a year of this crop, of which the first only is presented for inspection; the second is consumed in the country or smuggled to the islands.
>
> As Virginia produces about 80,000 hogsheads, there circulates in the state about £800,000 in these notes; this is the reason why the Virginians do not need a great quantity of specie or of copper coin. The rapid circulation of this tobacco money takes their place.
>
> The scarcity of small money, however, subjects the people to great inconveniences, and gives rise to the pernicious practice of cutting pieces of silver coin into halves and quarters, a source of many little knaveries. Someone cuts a dollar into three pieces, keeps the middle piece, and passes the other two for half dollars. The person who receives these without weighing loses the difference, and the one who takes them by weight makes a fraudulent profit by passing the pieces again at their pretended value; and so the cheat goes round. But notwithstanding this pitiful recours of cutting the silver, there is still a shortage of small change and society suffers thereby. It is calculated that in the towns the small expenses of a family are doubled on account of this difficulty. This circumstance reflects a striking want of order in the government and increases the misery of the poor.

British-American Tobacco Company Ltd.

The British-American Tobacco Company Ltd. (BATCo or simply BAT) was formed in 1902 by a historic agreement between Imperial Tobacco and James Buchanan Duke's AMERICAN TOBACCO COMPANY. American Tobacco withdrew from the British market and Imperial agreed not to enter the American market, each company agreeing not to compete for the other's domestic market. They also assigned brand rights to each other for home sales. In 1911, after the U.S. Supreme Court declared Duke's American Tobacco Company to be an illegal monopoly, he was forced to sell his majority shareholding in BAT and cancel the trans-Atlantic agreement. BAT was then free to conduct business all over the world.

In 1927, BAT bought BROWN AND WILLIAMSON TOBACCO COMPANY, a small snuff and plug firm located in Winston-Salem, North Carolina. It introduced machine-made cigarettes to the firm's sales lists, notably a coupon brand called Sir Walter Raleigh, followed later by mentholated Kool and filter-tipped Viceroy. In 1976, BAT merged with Tobacco Securities Trust to form BAT INDUSTRIES PLC. *See also* DUKE, JAMES BUCHANAN; RALEIGH CIGARETTE; VICEROY CIGARETTES

Broadcast Ban on Cigarette Advertising

In 1969, six of the seven commissioners of the Federal Communications Commission (FCC) announced their intention to ban cigarette advertising on radio and television. The powerful influence of tobacco advertising reaching large numbers of children and teens concerned them.

The advertising community was divided over cigarette advertising. "I think a lot of people in advertising don't like to work on cigarette accounts," said William B. Lewis, who left an ad agency and joined the AMERICAN CANCER SOCIETY (ACS). "A broadcast ban would be unfair, un-American, and undemocratic," said Mary Wells, who worked on the Benson and Hedges account.

In April 1970, President Richard Nixon signed the Public Health Cigarette Smoking Act of 1969. The law banned cigarette advertising on television and radio as of midnight January 1, 1971. Congress gave tobacco companies an extra day to air their commercials during New Year's Day football bowl games. All the cigarette makers spent heavily on their final TV fling. Philip Morris, maker of Marlboro, poured $1.2 million into commercials that aired between 11:30 P.M. and midnight on all three networks. *See also* ADVERTISING AND CIGARETTES AND TOBACCO; ADVERTISING AND CIGARS; ANTI-SMOKING MESSAGES, 1967–1970

Broadleaf Tobacco

A descendant of the native tobacco raised in New England before the colonists adopted it for cultivation, broadleaf is produced in the Connecticut Valley and sold as sorted and unsorted tobacco. The entire crop is used in manufacturing cigars. Broadleaf is commonly used as a BINDER in domestic Havana cigars. *See also* CIGAR; CONNECTICUT TOBACCO

Broin v. Philip Morris Companies Inc.

In October 1997, four major tobacco companies settled the first class-action lawsuit filed against them. Known as *Broin v. Philip Morris Companies Inc.*, flight attendants sued over the effects of smoking on nonsmokers. PHILIP MORRIS COMPANIES INC., R.J. REYNOLDS TOBACCO COMPANY, the LORILLARD COMPANY INC., and the BROWN AND WILLIAMSON TOBACCO CORPORATION agreed to spend $300 million for the study of tobacco-related diseases.

In settling with an estimated 60,000 former and current flight attendants and their survivors, who received no money, the tobacco industry did not admit the connection between secondhand smoke and illness. The plaintiffs' lawyers, Stanley and Susan Rosenblatt, who filed the lawsuit on October 31, 1991, accusing the tobacco companies of "fraud, lies and misrepresentation," received $49 million in legal fees and expenses.

The trial took place in Dade County Circuit Court in Miami, Florida. The flight attendants and their survivors claimed that secondhand smoke emitted from passengers' cigarettes in airplanes caused the attendants to become ill with cancer and other illnesses. The plaintiffs sought $5 billion in compensatory and punitive damages.

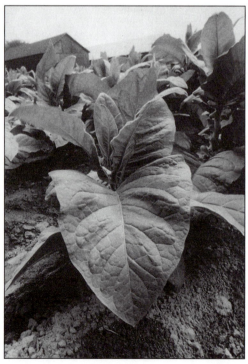

Broadleaf tobacco. ©*Doris Friedman.*

The lead plaintiff, Norma Broin (1955–), a flight attendant for American Airlines who never smoked but developed lung cancer, and the other plaintiffs in the class action could seek only compensatory, not punitive damages in individual trials. A research institute, named after Norma Broin, would be established by the tobacco companies, who agreed to pay $300 million over three years, beginning in April 1998. The companies also agreed to waive the statute of limitations on any lawsuits filed by flight attendants within a year after final approval of the settlement and to support federal smoking bans on international flights. In any suits brought by individual flight attendants, the four cigarette makers agreed to assume the burden of proving secondhand smoke did not cause emphysema, lung cancer, chronic obstructive pulmonary disease, chronic bronchitis, and chronic sinusitis. *See also* CASTANO V. AMERICAN TOBACCO COMPANY; ENGLE V. R.J. REYNOLDS ET AL.; TOBACCO LITIGATION: FIRST, SECOND, AND THIRD WAVES

Brooke Group Ltd. Inc.

The Brooke Group Ltd. Inc., founded in 1990, has been the parent organization of the Liggett Group, its tobacco unit, since 1986. Until November 1998, Brooke's major cigarette brands were Chesterfield, Eve, Lark, and L and M. At that time, Philip Morris bought Chesterfield, Lark, and L and M. The tobacco company had owned the international rights to these three brands for about two decades. Besides cigarettes, Brooke owns real estate and finance businesses.

BENNETT LEBOW, the chief executive officer of the Brooke Group Ltd., broke rank with other large tobacco companies and became the first tobacco company CEO to settle, unilaterally, out of court, a lawsuit with class-action lawyers and five states in March 1996. *See also* LIGGETT AND MYERS TOBACCO COMPANY

Brown and Williamson Tobacco Corporation

Brown and Williamson Tobacco Corporation, the nation's third-largest tobacco company, began in 1906 when merchants Robert Williamson and George Brown formed a small snuff and plug firm located in Winston-Salem, North Carolina. After the company was purchased in 1927 by the BRITISH-AMERICAN TOBACCO COMPANY LTD., its name changed to the Brown and Williamson Tobacco Corporation. The company, headquartered in Louisville, Kentucky, introduced specialty brands and pioneered both filter and menthol cigarettes. It also revived coupons in newly packaged RALEIGH CIGARETTES. Since 1995, Nick Brookes has been the chief executive officer.

In the United States, Brown and Williamson Tobacco Corporation, now a wholly owned subsidiary of BAT INDUSTRIES PLC, a British tobacco company, makes cigarette brands, including Barclay, Belair, Capri, Fact, Kool, Misty, Raleigh, Richland, VICEROY, and GPC generic cigarettes. In 1994, LUCKY STRIKES were added to the roster when Brown and Williamson bought the AMERICAN TOBACCO COMPANY.

Brown and Williamson Tobacco Corporation—Merrell Williams Documents

MERRELL WILLIAMS, a Louisiana-born paralegal, stole BROWN AND WILLIAMSON TOBACCO CORPORATION documents from the law firm of Wyatt, Tarrant, and Combs, the largest law firm in Kentucky. At the end of 1987, Williams worked on a project that involved sorting Brown and Williamson Tobacco Corporation archive documents on product promotion and smoking and health going back to the 1950s. There were also memos and letters from other tobacco companies, and many of the documents concerned contacts with Brown and Williamson's London-based parent, BAT INDUSTRIES PLC.

Williams, who had signed a confidentiality agreement, learned that the tobacco companies had done research about the effects of nicotine and cancer-causing agents in tobacco smoke, but had not made the research public. He felt he had uncovered a widespread cover-up of the harmful effects of smoking, which included the participation of company lawyers. Williams began photocopying and stealing the more than 4,000 pages of documents. In February 1992, Williams was told the project at Wyatt was being cut back and his job was ended.

In March 1993, Williams, a smoker, underwent major heart surgery. He turned his bypass surgery into a personal injury case with Brown and Williamson as defendants. He claimed his heart condition had been caused by the stress of reviewing the documents as well as a lifetime of smoking the company's cigarettes. The Wyatt firm filed a civil suit in the circuit court for Jefferson County, Kentucky, accusing Williams of stealing company documents and breaching his confidentiality agreement.

Despite a court order not to discuss or disseminate any of the information in the documents, Williams hid the stolen documents in Florida for safe keeping until he made a deal with attorneys DON BARRETT and RICHARD F. SCRUGGS to transfer the papers to Mississippi. Williams eventually signed the documents over to Attorney General MICHAEL C. MOORE of Mississippi. Since the papers were stolen property, inadmissible in court, and shielded by attorney-client privilege, the Mississippi attorneys could not use them in the MISSISSIPPI MEDICAID CASE against the tobacco companies. Scruggs and the other lawyers copied the documents and disseminated them anonymously so they would be put in the public domain. Within days, the stolen documents were on the desk of California Democratic Congressman Henry Waxman, one of tobacco's biggest opponents. On May 7, 1994, the *New York Times* published a front-page story titled "Tobacco Company Was Silent on Hazards," the first of several high-profile stories based on the stolen documents.

On May 12, 1994, Professor Stanton Glantz of the University of California, San Francisco, received an unsolicited box of Brown and Williamson tobacco company documents (Merrell Williams's stolen documents) from a return address marked "Mr. Butts." Dated from the early 1950s to the early 1980s, many of the documents, labeled "confidential" or "privileged," contained internal discussions of the tobacco industry's public relations and legal strategies over the years.

In district and state courts, Brown and Williamson tried unsuccessfully to have the "Mr. Butts" documents suppressed, and demands that the University of California return the documents were denied. Courts noted that much, if not all, of the information in the documents had already been made available to the news media through leaks. Eventually, all of the Brown and Williamson documents were declared to be in the public domain, either by Congress or by the courts. On July 1, 1995, at 12:01 A.M. Pacific Standard time, the University of California San Francisco Library and Center for Knowledge Management posted the documents on the Internet making the papers available to the world. The library also made a CD-ROM. President Bill Clinton, who read the papers, used them as part of his decision-making process to ask the federal FOOD AND DRUG ADMINISTRATION (FDA) to propose regulations of nicotine as an addictive drug and cigarettes and smokeless tobacco products as drug delivery devices.

Brynner, Yul (1915–1985)

The morning after his death from lung cancer, ABC-TV's "Good Morning America (GMA)" rebroadcast an interview with Yul Brynner in which the actor delivered a strong anti-smoking message. Convinced that his five-pack-a-day smoking habit caused his lung cancer, Brynner shot extra footage during his GMA interview to be used after his death. The spot, produced by McCaffrey and McCall advertising agency, showed Brynner looking into the camera and saying, "Now that I'm gone, I tell you: Don't smoke. Whatever you do, don't smoke" ("Yul Brynner Speaks Out," 1986). *See also* ANTI-SMOKING MESSAGES, 1967-1970

References: "Yul Brynner Speaks Out on Smoking," *Smoking and Health Report*, vol. 3, no. 3 (April 1986), p. 8.

Buckley, Christopher (1952–)

Educated at Yale University and editor of *Esquire* at the age of 24, Christopher Buckley wrote speeches for Vice President George Bush from 1981 to 1983. An editor of *Forbes FYI* magazine, Buckley wrote *Thank You for Smoking* (1994), a satiric novel about the trials and tribulations of fictional Nick Naylor, tobacco lobbyist and chief spokesman for the industry-sponsored Academy of Tobacco Studies, who derives solace from a sign above his desk that reads: "Smoking is the nation's leading cause of statistics."

In the following excerpt from *Thank You for Smoking*, Naylor, a master of media manipulation, gives a speech at a "Clean Lungs 2000" conference of 2,500 health professionals, despite knowing that "the Clean Lungs 2000 leadership had fought like Marines on Mount Suribachi to keep him out of the conference." Naylor, who eventually finds himself under attack during the question-and-answer period, argues that the anti-smoking movement risks American freedom and then equates the modern American anti-smoking movement with the anti-tobacco hysteria during the reign of MURAD IV, the Turkish sultan who went to extremes to stop his subjects from smoking.

> But then it happened, during the Q and A. Some woman about halfway back got up, said that Nick "seemed like a nice young man," prompting guffaws; said she wanted "to share a recent experience" with him. Nick braced. For him, no "shared experience" with anyone in this crowd could possibly bode well. She launched into a graphic account of a dear departed's "courageous battle" with lung cancer. Then, more in sadness than in anger, she asked Nick, "How can you sleep at night?"
>
> No stranger to these occasions, Nick nodded sympathetically as Uncle Harry's heroic last hours were luridly recounted. "I appreciate your sharing that with us all, ma'am, and I think I speak for all of us in this room when I say that we regret your tragic loss, but I think the issue here before us today is whether we as Americans want to abide by such documents as the Declaration of Independence, the Constitution, and the Bill of Rights. If the answer is yes, then I think our course is clear. And I think your uncle, who was I'm sure a very *fine* man, were he here today, might just agree that if we go tampering with the bedrock principles that our Founding Fathers laid down, many of whom, you'll recall, were themselves tobacco farmers, just for the sake of indulging a lot of frankly unscientific speculation, then we're placing at risk not only our own freedom, but those of our children, and our children's children."
>
> It was crucial not to pause here to let the stunning nonsequitor embed itself in their neural processors. "Anti-tobacco hysteria is not exactly new. You remember, of course, Murad the Fourth, the Turkish sultan." Of course no one had the faintest notion who on earth Murad the Fourth was, but people like a little intellectual flattery. "Murad, remember, got it into his head that people shouldn't smoke, so he outlawed it, and he would go out at night dressed up like a regular Turk and wander the streets of Istanbul pretending to have a nicotine fit and begging people to sell him some tobacco. And if someone took pity on him and gave him something to smoke —*whammo!*—Murad would behead him on the spot. And leave he body right there in the street to rot. WARNING: SELLING TOBACCO TO MURAD IV CAN BE DANGEROUS TO YOUR HEALTH." Nick moved quickly to the kill: "Myself, I'd like to think that we as a nation have progressed beyond the days of summary executions for the crime of pursuing our own definition of happiness." Thus, having compared the modern American anti-smoking movement to the depredations of a bloodthirsty seventeenth-century Ottoman, Nick could depart, satisfied that he had temporarily beaten back the horde a few inches. Not a lot of ground, but in this war, it was practically a major victory. (Buckley, 1994)

References: Christopher Buckley, *Thank You for Smoking*, New York: Random House, 1994, p. 5.

Bull Durham Smoking Tobacco

Bull Durham smoking tobacco was first manufactured in the 1860s by JOHN RUFFIN GREEN of Durham's Station, North Carolina, and after 1870 by WILLIAM T. BLACKWELL and Julian Shakespeare Carr who created the world-famous trademark of the Durham bull. By the 1870s, Bull Durham was the nation's leading brand thanks to newspaper advertising and efficient distribution. The Durham bull was advertised all over the U.S. and Europe. Celebrities like Lord Tennyson, Rudyard Kipling, Thomas Carlyle, James Russell Lowell, and Will Rogers endorsed it.

Bull Durham was also the tobacco product that pushed JAMES BUCHANAN DUKE out of the chewing tobacco business and into the cigarette business. Duke wrote: "My company is up against a stone wall. It can't compete with Bull Durham. Something has to be done and . . . quick. I am going into the cigarette business" (*"Sold American,"* 1954).

References: *"Sold American!" The First Fifty Years*, The American Tobacco Company, 1954, p. 19.

Burbank, Luther (1849–1926)

For more than 50 years, horticulturist Luther Burbank made his home in Santa Rosa, California, where he conducted plant-breeding experiments that brought him world renown. In his working career, he introduced more than 800 new varieties of plants—including more than 200 varieties of fruits, many vegetables, nuts and grains, and hundreds of ornamental flowers, making him the best known plant breeder in the U.S. His methods and results were described in his book *How Plants are Trained to Work for Man* (1921) and in numerous biographies. In his book, Burbank also warned people about the dangers of smoking tobacco.

> You have seen pictures of military cemeteries near great battlefields. Upon every headstone is chiseled the inscription: "Killed in Action." If one knew nothing about war, these headstones would be sufficient to impress upon him that war is deadly, that it kills. How much would you know about tobacco if upon the headstone of everyone killed by it were inscribed, "Killed by Tobacco?" You would know a lot more about it than you do know, but you would not know it all, because tobacco does more than kill. It half kills. It has its victims in the cemeteries and in the streets. It is bad enough to be dead, but it is a question if it is not sometimes worse to be half dead—to be nervous, irritable, unable to sleep well, with efficiency cut in two and vitality ready to snap at the first great strain.
>
> Let me tell you how tobacco kills. Smokers do not all drop dead around cigar lighters in tobacco stores. They go away and years later die of something else. From the tobacco trusts' point of view, that is one of the finest things about tobacco. The victims do not die on the premises. They go away and, when they die, the doctors certify that they died of something else—pneumonia, heart disease, typhoid fever, or what not. In other words, tobacco kills indirectly and escapes the blame.
>
> Nicotine, after you have used it awhile, puts you in a position to be 'bumped off' by the first thing that hits you. If you saw some men undermine a building until it was ready to topple into the street, and then saw a woman hit the building with a baby carriage and make it topple, you would not say the women wrecked the building, would you? Yet when a smoker dies of pneumonia, the doctor's health certificate gives pneumonia, and not tobacco, as the cause of death.
>
> What a shock people would get if they went through cemeteries and saw tombstones declaring the fact that this man died of typhoid, made fatal by a tobacco weakened heart, and that man succumbed to nervous prostration because tobacco had shot his nerves to pieces, and another gave up the ghost because tobacco had ruined his stomach.

Bureau of Alcohol, Tobacco, and Firearms (ATF)

Over the years, the Bureau of Alcohol, Tobacco, and Firearms (ATF), a law enforcement organization within the United States

Department of the Treasury, has been charged by Congress with unique responsibilities for reducing violent crime, collecting revenue, and protecting the public. ATF enforces federal laws and regulations relating to tobacco, alcohol, firearms, explosives, and arson. The common thread in ATF's responsibilities over these varied products is they all are legal commodities produced by a highly regulated industry and are also controversial products that have been traditionally susceptible to criminal diversion and misuse or abuse.

The goals of the ATF tobacco programs are to ensure the collection of tobacco excise taxes and to qualify applicants for permits to manufacture tobacco products or operate tobacco export warehouses. Tobacco inspections verify an applicant's qualification information, check the security of the premises, and ensure tax compliance. ATF special agents investigate trafficking of contraband tobacco products in violation of federal law and sections of the Internal Revenue Code.

In 1978, Congress passed the Contraband Cigarette Trafficking Act, giving ATF the authority to investigate interstate diversion of cigarettes in avoidance of paying state tax by prohibiting the shipment, transportation, or possession of more than 60,000 cigarettes (which is equal to 3,000 packs or 300 cartons) not bearing a tax stamp of evidence of tax payment in states that require such evidence. The problem of cigarette smuggling has evolved into large commercial operations resulting in cigarettes ending up on retail shelves or distributed by organized crime.

In recent years, some foreign governments and certain state governments have imposed a higher excise tax on tobacco products, thus creating a lucrative black market. Diversion involves products for both export and domestic consumption from a manufacturer to individuals acting as brokers or wholesalers. Rather than shipping the product to the destination stated on required federal records, the product is diverted and sold illegally. Some wholesalers have been found to be sources of supply, with retailers becoming increasingly active in these illegal sales. Unlike tobacco manufacturers, tobacco wholesalers and retailers are not statutorily required to hold permits and licenses issued by ATF.

For example, due to extremely high Canadian taxes on tobacco, significant quantities of U.S. manufactured tobacco products were smuggled into Canada. In addition, large amounts of Canadian manufactured tobacco products were "exported" into the United States and then smuggled back into Canada. As a result of this smuggling, Canada lost billions of dollars in tax revenues.

There has also been a significant increase in trafficking in cigarettes from states with low taxes on tobacco to states with high taxes. In a 1997 survey that ATF conducted on behalf of the House Appropriations Committee, the agency received estimates from several states on revenue they had lost. Michigan estimated losing approximately $75 million a year to cigarette diversion. Washington State estimated losing around $63 million per year from cigarettes diverted from low tax states. California estimated its annual loss to be approximately $30 million a year.

During the 1990s, tobacco crimes grew larger and more complex and extended to both interstate and international investigations. Although limited resources hamper ATF, the agency has increased its tobacco investigations over 300 percent since 1992. ATF's largest contraband cigarette trafficking investigation involved the trafficking of cigarettes from the Flathead Indian Reservation in Montana to Washington State. In this case, nine people were involved in racketeering. ATF has also investigated a smuggling ring on the St. Regis/Akwesasne Mohawk Indian Reservation. In addition to illegal trafficking by traditional organized crime groups and some NATIVE AMERICANS, ATF has also uncovered involvement in cigarette smuggling by Russian, Middle Eastern, and Asian organized crime groups.

On the international level, ATF maintains an ongoing liaison with foreign law and revenue enforcement authorities, such as the Royal Canadian Mounted Police and Revenue Canada. The Bureau also works with criminal investigators and tax officials in Eastern European countries to develop and implement criminal and regulatory enforcement schemes involving cigarettes. *See also* CANADA

Burley Tobacco

Since the 1860s, Burley, a new type of tobacco, grown in naturally fertile limestone soil, cured by air, and heavier bodied than BRIGHT TOBACCO, reached its highest state of development in the bluegrass region of Kentucky, eastern Tennessee, and southern Ohio. It's also grown in Virginia, North Carolina, Missouri, West Virginia, and Indiana as well as in Canada, India, and Malawi. Virginia manufacturers formerly used great quantities of the leaf in chewing (plug) and smoking tobaccos. Now Burley is widely grown in the United States for cigarettes and pipe mixtures. Its leaves are reddish-brown from air curing.

Burney, Leroy (1906–1998)

Surgeon general of the United States Public Health Service from 1956 to 1961, Dr. Leroy E. Burney was believed to be one of the first federal officials to identify smoking as a cause of lung cancer. Dr. Burney, who received his medical degree from Indiana University in 1930, also earned a degree in public health from Johns Hopkins Hospital. He joined the Public Health Service in 1932, was Indiana state health officer from 1945 to 1954, and became the eighth surgeon general in 1956.

On July 12, 1957, Dr. Burney issued a statement at a televised press conference saying that prolonged cigarette smoking was a causative factor in the etiology of lung cancer. This was the first time the Public Health Service took a position on the controversial subject. The statement was based on research conducted principally in Great Britain by Dr. RICHARD DOLL and Dr. A. BRADFORD HILL and in the United States by EDWARD CUYLER HAMMOND and DANIEL HORN as well as by others over many years. In 1959, as the result of additional evidence, Dr. Burney stated in an article he authored in the *Journal of the American Medical Association (JAMA)* that the "weight of evidence at present implicates

smoking as the principal etiological factor" in the increased incidence of lung cancer. He felt "stopping cigarette smoking even after long exposure is beneficial" (Kluger, 1996).

References: Richard Kluger, *Ashes to Ashes*, New York: Alfred A. Knopf, 1996, p. 202.

Burns, David (1947–)

A Harvard-educated medical school professor in pulmonary and critical care medicine at the University of California at San Diego, Dr. David Burns drafted the 1975 surgeon general's report on the risks of smoking. In 1979, along with Donald Shopland, Dr. Burns worked on the 1979 surgeon general's report, the 15th anniversary of the original one, and set a new standard for accuracy and comprehensiveness. He has been involved as a scientific editor of the surgeon general's reports on other topics since 1980.

Dr. Burns was also senior editor of a 1997 National Cancer Institute monograph that concluded that despite the introduction of lower-tar cigarettes, they have not brought any reduction in the mortality risks of smoking. Indeed, studies show that the risk of death from lung cancer, heart disease, and other smoking-related causes has risen since the 1950s. According to Dr. Burns, the research shows that smokers today are smoking each cigarette more intensely than smokers did forty years ago, with larger puffs and deeper patterns of inhalation. But he said it was not clear to what degree such changes in smoking habits caused the higher mortality risks.

Besides working as a frequent consultant to the federal government, Dr. Burns has done volunteer work as an adviser and public witness for campaigns to ban smoking in public places.

Butler, Bur (1934–1994)

Nonsmoker Bur Butler, an owner of a Laurel, Mississippi, barbershop, died of lung cancer. When Butler went to the doctor in 1992, the doctor asked him how many packs a day he smoked because he had smoker lungs. Butler's entire exposure to tobacco smoke was from 30 years of secondhand smoke by his customers. Butler, represented by RON MOTLEY, filed a lawsuit against virtually the entire tobacco industry claiming it engaged in a conspiracy to mislead him and the general public about the dangers of smoking. He died on May 7, 1994, and his claim was continued by his wife.

On June 2, 1999, a jury ruled that the tobacco industry was not liable for the cancer that killed Butler. Tobacco company lawyers said Mr. Butler had a family history of cancer and that he also had been exposed to asbestos in talcum powder and methylene chloride in hair spray used in his barber shop.

Byrd, William, II (1674–1744)

The most noted representative of colonial Virginia tobacco planters, William Byrd II of Westover was admitted to the English bar and the Royal Society and became the agent for the colony of Virginia in England. He was also a member of the Virginia House of Burgesses. Byrd read widely and built up a library of 3,600 volumes, one of the largest in the colonies. A writer himself, he penned a pamphlet entitled *A Discourse Concerning the Plague, with Some Preservatives against It. By a Lover of Mankind* (1721). In it, Byrd argued that the generous use of tobacco was an excellent preventive and he advocated nicotine therapy: "In *England* it [the plague] us'd formerly to make a visit about once in twenty or thirty years: but since the universal use of Tobacco, it has now been kept off above fifty-four years." Byrd suggested people "shou'd wear it about our clothes, and about our coaches. We should hand bundles of it round our beds, and in the apartments wherein we most converse" (Robert, 1967). By the time Byrd died in 1744, he held 179,000 acres in Virginia.

References: Joseph C. Robert, *The Story of Tobacco in America*, Chapel Hill: The University of North Carolina Press, 1949, 1967, p. 22.

C

Cabral, Pedro Alvarez (c. 1460–1526)

Pedro Alvarez Cabral, a Portuguese navigator, was sent by King Emanuel I of Portugal to establish trade with the East Indies. For some unknown reason, he took a westward course and, blown by wind and current, accidentally reached the coast of BRAZIL in April 1500. His account of tobacco was published in 1571 in a work about the people of Brazil by Lisbon historian Damiâo de Goes, who cultivated the plant in the royal gardens.

> They have many odoriferous and medicinal herbs different from ours; among them is one we call fumo which some call Betum and I will call the holy herb, because of its powerful virtue in wonderful ways, of which I have had experience, principally in desperate cases: for ulcerated abscesses, fistulas, sores, inveterate polyps and many other ailments. (Heimann, 1960)

Cabral also observed the tobacco rites among the Tupinambas of Brazil.

> They [the shamans] carry a calabash made like the head of a man, with mouth, nostrils, eyes and hair, placed on the top of an arrow, within which they make smoke with dried leaves of the plant betum, and the smoke which is in the head they inhale to such an extent that they are drunk. (Heimann, 1960)

References: Robert K. Heimann, *Tobacco and Americans*, New York: McGraw-Hill Book Company, 1960, p. 9.

Califano, Joseph A. (1931–)

After leaving the White House as President Lyndon Johnson's staff assistant for domestic affairs in January 1969, Joseph Califano was named secretary of Health, Education, and Welfare (HEW) by President Jimmy Carter in December 1976. He held the position for 30 months until he resigned in July 1979. In excerpts from his 1981 book *Governing America*, Califano explained the political controversy that erupted over his anti-smoking policies, which led to his resignation.

In July 1977, Califano and Dr. Julius Richmond, the surgeon general and the assistant secretary for health, decided to issue a new surgeon general's report on smoking in January 1979 to celebrate the 15th anniversary of the original report on smoking issued by Dr. Luther Terry in 1964. Califano asked his staff to gather the facts on smoking and health. He learned that 75 percent of the adults who smoke cigarettes were addicted before they were 21 years old and virtually all cigarette smokers were addicted before they were 25. The number of teenage smokers had increased from 3 million to 4.5 million between 1968 and 1974 and over that period the percentage of teen-age girls who smoked had doubled. He learned the tobacco companies spent about $1 billion of tax deductible money annually to advertise the pleasures of smoking cigarettes. Nonetheless, 90 percent of adult smokers wanted to quit and virtually all of them at some time or other have tried.

Califano and Surgeon General Richmond mounted a highly visible anti-smoking campaign consisting of a massive public education drive and a drive to encourage laws to prohibit or restrict smoking in public places. Both were aimed at the latent desire in adults to action and at encouraging the young not to smoke in the first place.

Califano planned a speech to announce the anti-smoking program. However, White House health aide Dr. Peter Bourne urged him not to mount a major anti-smoking campaign. In an unprecedented press conference, TOBACCO INSTITUTE spokesmen HORACE KORNEGAY, a former North Carolina congressman, and William Dwyer denounced Califano for not giving the Institute an advance text.

Califano's speech called smoking "slow motion suicide" (a phrase of his speech writer, Ervin Duggan), and designated it "Public Health Enemy Number One." The Tobacco Institute cast him as a zealot.

Califano's speech was to be delivered before the Interagency Council on Smoking and Health in a small room in the Shoreham Hotel in Washington. The secretary and his aides had not anticipated a large group, but the Tobacco Institute's denouncement of the speech brought attention to the event and every foot of floor space was taken.

The theory of the public campaign announced in the speech was that a choice is free only if it is informed, a decision genuinely voluntary only if it is based on all the relevant information. The campaign sought to offset the billions of dollars for seductive advertising spent each year by the tobacco companies. By marshaling limited federal resources, Califano believed HEW could mount an effective public education campaign through the media if it were newsworthy and interesting, and deployed such state and local resources as teachers, doctors, nurses, and relatives of victims of lung cancer, emphysema, and heart disease.

When Califano became HEW secretary in 1976, the anti-smoking program was in a small office in Atlanta and its annual budget of $750,000 barely supported a passive NATIONAL CLEARINGHOUSE ON SMOKING AND HEALTH. He formed an OFFICE OF SMOKING AND HEALTH in Washington and named John Pinney, who had headed he National Council on Alcoholism in Washington, to direct it. At Califano's recommendation, Congress more than doubled the research and education budget for HEW's anti-smoking effort-from $19.1 million to $51.5 million.

The political fallout from the anti-smoking effort was intense. The tobacco industry financed bumper stickers announcing "Califano is Dangerous to My Health," and there were highway billboards saying, "California Blows Smoke." The White House staff, which judged the program politically dangerous, charged that he mounted the campaign without getting "political clearance" or "thinking through the political details."

On May 1, 1978, in a private meeting with Califano in the Oval Office, President Jimmy Carter made it clear that the anti-smoking program was to be a HEW/Califano effort. But he expressed no objection to Califano's energetic pursuit of the program, possibly because, as he said in January 1978: "My own father did smoke four or five packs a day and he died with lung cancer, perhaps because of cigarette smoking" (Califano, 1981).

In early August 1978, Carter visited a tobacco warehouse in Wilson, North Carolina, and spoke at a Democratic Party rally where he kidded the audience about Secretary Califano: "I had planned today to bring Joe Califano with me, but he decided not to come. He discovered that not only is North Carolina the number-one tobacco-producing state, but that you produce more bricks than anyone in the nation as well." The crowd responded with applause mixed with laughter. The president continued: "Joe Califano did encourage me to come though. He said it was time for the White House staff to start smoking something regular," an allusion to rumors of pot smoking by some members of the president's staff. The president then told the audience his family had grown tobacco in

North Carolina before moving to Georgia to grow peanuts. The health program the president described, however, was not HEW's. As he put it, a research plan would be conducted "to make the smoking of tobacco even more safe than it is today" (Califano, 1981).

When Surgeon General Richmond and Califano walked into a press conference on the morning of January 11, 1979, to release the surgeon general's report that concluded the case against cigarette smoking was "overwhelming," the HEW auditorium was filled with reporters. The evening television coverage was extensive, local television coverage was enormous, and so was the play in newspapers.

Califano later wrote in his 1981 book *Governing America* that the anti-smoking campaign generated more political opposition than any other effort he undertook at HEW. House Speaker Tip O'Neill told him in late 1978: "You're driving the tobacco people crazy. These guys are vicious. They're out to destroy you." In April 1979, Ted Kennedy told him: "You've got to get out of the Cabinet before the election. The president can't run in North Carolina with you at HEW. He's going to have to get rid of you" (Califano, 1981).

The anti-smoking campaign had an impact. Its success was measured by a decline in per capita cigarette consumption in the United States in 1979 to its lowest level in 22 years and a decline in the consumption of tobacco that same year to the lowest in 46 years. In the two weeks following the release of the surgeon general's report, more Americans tried to quit smoking than in any other two-week period since the release of the first report in 1964.

References: Joseph A. Califano, *Governing America*, New York: Simon and Schuster, 1981, pp. 190, 193, 196.

California's Clean Indoor Air Act of 1978

This act was the first attempt in the nation to pass a statewide clean indoor air law through the initiative process. Proposition 5, as it was called, would have required smoking and no-smoking sections in workplaces, public places, and restaurants. In November 1978, voters turned down Proposition 5. Acting through a campaign committee known as Californians for Common Sense, which tried to minimize its industry connections, the major tobacco companies played a role in defeating the measure.

California's Proposition 99

In a 1988 referendum, California voters approved a 25¢ increase in the state tax on a pack of cigarettes to finance a statewide anti-tobacco program. The proceeds were designated to finance anti-smoking advertising and school education and to provide grants to cities to develop anti-smoking policies.

The toll of smoking in California had long been a major concern of public health and medical communities as well as of voluntary organizations such as the AMERICAN LUNG ASSOCIATION (ALA), the AMERICAN CANCER SOCIETY (ACS), and the AMERICAN HEART ASSOCIATION (AHA). For many years, this constituency sought legislation to establish a tobacco tax that would provide significant funding for a statewide health education program to reduce tobacco use.

In 1988, this constituency mounted a grassroots movement to place an initiative, called Proposition 99, on the November ballot. The Coalition for a Healthy California raised $1 million to support the effort. Despite the $22 million counterattack by the tobacco industry, which included a massive media campaign, voters passed the initiative by a margin of 58 percent to 42 percent.

Proposition 99 established a new tax on tobacco in California, effective January 1, 1989, and set aside 20 percent of revenues from the new tax (more than $100 million a year) in a Health Education Account to support a comprehensive statewide tobacco control program. Since October 1989, yearly appropriations from this account have been made to the California Department of Health Services and the California Department of Education to foster and coordinate the program. The state health department funded 61 local coalitions supported by local health departments, 10 regional coalitions staffed by administrative agencies, and four ethnic networks. Proposition 99 legislation charged the program with reducing tobacco use, especially among high-risk persons and groups, and established a 75-percent reduction in tobacco use by the year 2000 as the program's goal.

Because tobacco use went down 30 percent in California after the approval of the initiative and the smoking rate among teenagers leveled, the reduced sale of cigarettes led to a drop in tax revenues from $900 million in 1989 to less than $600 million in 1994. The state's anti-smoking campaign had less money to spend. In 1991, cigarette consumption rates rose when the state halted its anti-smoking ads.

Massachusetts and Michigan followed the California model, enacting new tobacco taxes with some of the funds earmarked for anti-tobacco education efforts. The AMERICAN MEDICAL ASSOCIATION (AMA) teamed up with the Robert Wood Johnson Foundation to finance anti-smoking programs in 19 states, with the goal of duplicating the success of California's program in each state.

Calumet

The calumet was an important ceremonial pipe used by NATIVE AMERICANS. The word is said to be derived from the Latin word "calamus" or reed. Although the form of the calumet differed in various areas, the pipe was almost universally used in religious ceremonies and as a "pipe of peace." *See also* PIPE SMOKING AND NATIVE AMERICANS

Camel Cigarettes

In 1913, the R.J. REYNOLDS TOBACCO COMPANY, headquartered in Winston-Salem, North Carolina, introduced Camels, the first "modern" blended cigarette, containing "Turkish and domestic tobaccos" (flue-cured tobacco, seasoned with Turkish and sweetened burley). The name "Camel" was picked to suggest the Middle Eastern origin of the leaf. Just as the package designers were looking around for a model of a camel to copy,

Barnum and Bailey's circus came to town. Reynolds sent an employee to photograph "Old Joe," an Arabian dromedary (one-humped camel), one of the stars of the circus. The package designer used the photo to make a drawing of OLD JOE CAMEL for the cigarette pack. The same image still appears on Camel cigarettes and advertisements today. The artist added the pyramids and palm trees for a special effect.

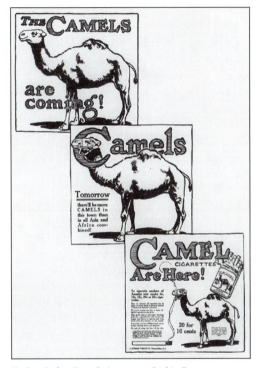

Early ads for Camel cigarettes. *Corbis-Bettmann.*

Reynolds introduced Camel in Cleveland, Ohio. On October 21, 1913, the N.W. Ayer advertising agency, hired by RICHARD JOSHUA REYNOLDS, launched the first national cigarette advertising campaign in the nation which "revolutionized the cigarette industry." Because Reynolds felt Camel had the potential to be the nation's best-selling brand, he invested millions in advertising, unprecedented amounts to wager on a single brand. In one city, an ad announced: "Camels! Tomorrow there will be more Camels in this town than in all Asia and Africa combined!" The effort and money worked. In 1919, two of every five cigarettes sold were Camels, making them the number-one selling cigarette.

The ad campaign was built around the theme that Camels did not offer premiums like other cigarette companies because the tobaccos used in the Camel blend were too costly to permit anything except the product itself. On the back of the pack, Reynolds warned smokers: "Don't look for premiums or coupons, as the cost of the tobaccos blended in CAMEL Cigarettes prohibits the use of them." *See also* FEDERAL TRADE COMMISSION (FTC) AND JOE CAMEL ADVERTISING

Campaign for Tobacco-Free Kids. *See* NATIONAL CENTER FOR TOBACCO-FREE KIDS

Canada

The cultivation of tobacco in Canada has a long history. It was well established by native people when the first European settlers arrived in New France (later Québec) in the 1600s. The French colonists began trading tobacco as early as 1652, but cultivation was not extensive until 1735 when the French government first encouraged production.

The early tobacco crops were air cured and grown mostly in Québec. Production in 1870 was 724,000 kg; this increased more than tenfold to 7,938,000 kg in 1910, when production turned to flue curing tobacco and Ontario became the primary producing area. In 1989, Ontario produced 88 percent of the tobacco grown in Canada. Other production areas are Québec and Prince Edward Island. In 1989, there were 1,441 tobacco farmers representing about 4 percent of the farming population.

Historically, the federal and provincial departments of agriculture have encouraged tobacco cultivation and carried out research in attempts to improve crop yields. In 1986, the Ontario Ministry of Agriculture and Food established the Tobacco Planning Advisory Committee to strengthen the province's tobacco industry and help it cope with declining demand. In addition to the Canadian and Ontario governments, Committee membership includes domestic manufacturers of tobacco products, leaf dealers, and the Ontario Flue-cured Tobacco Growers Marketing Board, an organization of growers who practice supply management aimed at stabilizing prices.

A relatively new government activity is the Tobacco Diversification Plan, a program of the federal Department of Agriculture that assists in the orderly downsizing of the Canadian tobacco industry by providing incentives to farmers to cease tobacco production and develop alternative crops for tobacco lands. Another goal of the program is to improve the economic viability of those farmers who choose to continue in tobacco production. One component of the program, the Tobacco Transition Adjustment Initiative, has assisted significant numbers of farmers to stop producing tobacco. The other component of the program, the Alternative Enterprise Initiative, has had less success because some tobacco farmers have been unwilling to leave a well-established, high-income crop for riskier lower-income crops.

The tobacco industry began around 1932 and Simcoe, Ontario, has been the marketing center for tobacco used in the production of Canadian cigarettes. Tobacco is of relatively minor and declining importance as an agricultural commodity, although in the early 1990s, it was the third-largest cash crop in Ontario.

In the early 1990s, three foreign-controlled tobacco companies manufactured tobacco products in Canada: Imperial Tobacco, Rothmans/Benson and Hedges, and RJR-MacDonald.

Canada's smoking industry agreed to withdraw tobacco ads from radio and television in the 1970s, but challenged the TOBACCO PRODUCTS CONTROL ACT OF 1988 passed by the Canadian government. That law prohibited advertising in all forms and restricted the use of brand names in sponsorship of sports or cultural events and the display of tobacco trademarks on non-tobacco products. In 1991, Canada's ban on tobacco advertising was overturned in a Québec Superior Court ruling that said the law was unconstitutional because it violated the right to free speech. That ruling was overturned by a Québec appeals court, and on September 21, 1995, the

Supreme Court struck down key sections of the 1988 law.

The major significance of the tobacco industry in Canada has been the tax revenues it produced for the federal and provincial governments from cigarette sales. But the high rate of taxation on domestically manufactured cigarettes and fine-cut tobacco, 77 percent of the total price, provided considerable temptation to smuggle tobacco into Canada. Several regions of Canada where smuggling occurred fairly consistently included an Indian reserve straddling the Canada-United States border and a region between the French islands of St. Pierre et Miquelon and neighboring Newfoundland. In 1990, Peat Marwick Thorne estimated that overall, 70 percent of the smuggled cigarettes were manufactured in Canada, exported legally, and reimported illegally.

In February 1994, the Canadian government, in a move to combat smuggling of low-priced cigarettes from the United States, lowered cigarette taxes by more than 50 percent. In November 1996, cigarette taxes rose sharply again in Ontario and Québec, Canada's two most populous provinces.

Since 1965, the Department of National Health and Welfare has monitored tobacco use in Canada through regular population surveys. In 1996, health minister David Dingwall said about 7 million of Canada's 30 million people smoked. Projections of the prevalence of smoking to 2010 based on 15 years of consistent trends suggest that smoking will be more common among women then men. Consistent differences among ethnic groups in Canada are evident. French speakers are more likely to be smokers than English speakers, who in turn have a higher prevalence of smoking than speakers of other languages.

Since the 1960s, deaths in Canada attributable to smoking have been documented. This information has contributed to the public debate about prohibitions on advertising, selling, and consuming tobacco. In 1996, smoking was responsible for an estimated 40,000 deaths.

Canada enjoys one of the most comprehensive national tobacco-use prevention and control programs in the world; it involves three levels of the government and several different departments and agencies at each level. Before it was struck down, advertising was governed by the federal Tobacco Products Control Act; purchasing was affected by federal and provincial taxation policies and municipal restrictions on vendors and machines; and consumption was restricted by the Non-smokers' Health Act, passed in 1988 by Parliament, as well as by provincial statutes and municipal by-laws.

The Non-Smokers Health Act provided a smoke-free environment for all workplaces under federal jurisdiction. Amended after 1990, the law covered not only the federal public service, but also Crown corporations and federally regulated industries such as banking, insurance, trucking, and broadcasting.

Federal and provincial governments offer incentives to tobacco growers to cease production, and they provide the public with health education materials and information about smoking cessation programs. All of these activities are included under the National Strategy to Reduce Tobacco Use, a framework developed in May 1985, and subscribed to by a broad spectrum of government and national health agencies. The National Strategy is committed to the protection of nonsmokers, the prevention of smoking, and cessation by current smokers. The strategy provides access to information and message promotion directed at the general public, and indicates availability of services/programs for high-risk groups.

The National Clearinghouse on Tobacco and Health was established in 1989. It has compiled an extensive directory of Canadian agencies, peer-assisted learning, community self-help groups, and individuals involved in the creation of a tobacco-free society and distributes information on smoking cessation programs and other select issues.

A close working relationship exists in Canada among the federal government, provincial health departments, and voluntary groups. Two umbrella organizations, the Canadian Council on Smoking and Health and the Ontario Interagency Council on Smoking and Health, have member agencies from the government and voluntary sector. Non-governmental bodies, including the Canadian Cancer Society, Canadian Lung Association, and Canadian Medical Association, pressure the government to reinforce its anti-tobacco message. *See also* BUREAU OF ALCOHOL, TOBACCO, AND FIREARMS (ATF); CARTIER, JACQUES

Candy Cigarettes

During the 1960s, at least five U.S. candy manufacturers made candy cigarettes in packages that had the exact spelling or nearly the same spellings of popular brand names like CAMEL, LUCKY STRIKE, L and M, MARLBORO, PALL MALL, Salem, Winston, CHESTERFIELD, Oasis, Lark, and VICEROY. In 1967, the Federal Trade Commission (FTC) complained to the tobacco industry that cigarette companies permitted the sale of candy and bubble gum in packages that looked just like real cigarette brands. The FTC said that this amounted to "an indirect form of advertising aimed at children." The AMERICAN TOBACCO COMPANY said it always denied requests by candy makers to use its cigarette trademarks and package designs. The company would not say whether it had done anything about the use of the Lucky Strike and Pall Mall names by Philadelphia Chewing Gum Corporation. It is illegal to use a registered trademark without permission.

Candy makers did not seem concerned about using tobacco company trademarks without their permission. One candy maker said no tobacco company had ever taken action against it for using real cigarette trademarks on candy cigarette boxes. Another candy company said, "The [tobacco] companies don't object. That's the point. We've been doing it for many years. They don't care" (*Preventing Tobacco Use*, 1994).

In the 1980s and 1990s, candy cigarettes—sugar, chocolate, and bubble gum varieties—were still popular. Candy cigarettes were often displayed alongside real cigarettes in airport shops, pharmacies, and supermarkets. One candy cigarette actually blew smoke—confectioner's sugar. Another, the "Tricky Squirt Cigarette," was printed with a Marlboro look-alike logo. In the spot normally occupied by the health warning, this statement appeared: "Remarks: In case this trick hurts your victims, please offer them a real cigarette to soothe their nerves."

References: *Preventing Tobacco Use Among Young People*, U.S. Surgeon General's Report, 1994, p. 170.

Carbon Monoxide

Carbon monoxide is a gas that results when materials are burned. Carbon monoxide production is increased by restricting the oxygen supply, as is the case inside a cigarette. Carbon monoxide easily passes from the tiny air holes in the lungs into the bloodstream. There it combines with hemoglobin, that part of the blood that normally carries carbon dioxide out of the body and oxygen back into the body. When the hemoglobin is bound up by carbon monoxide, a shortage of oxygen may result. High levels of carbon monoxide can starve the body of oxygen. When the heart detects insufficient levels of oxygen, it may flutter. In extreme cases, heart attacks may result.

Each cigarette causes a brief boost in the carbon monoxide level, which lasts for a few minutes. Then the level declines until the next cigarette is smoked. However, each cigarette adds slightly to the person's overall carbon monoxide level. *See also* NICOTINE; TAR

Cárdenas, Juan de

Juan de Cárdenas, a practicing Mexican physician, wrote that the smoking of cigarettes, cigars, and pipes was common among the white men in Mexico by the late sixteenth century. He observed that

some are accustomed to take it [tobacco] in small clay or silver pipes or those of hard wood. Others wrap the tobacco in a corn husk or in paper or in a tube of cane. . . . The smoke which is taken in clay, silver, or wood pipes is stronger, because only the plant is smoked and no other thing outside of it; whereas smoked in a leaf, in paper or in a reed the smoke is weaker, since it is not only the tobacco which is smoked but also the leaf or the reed in which is it contained. . . . (Heimann, 1960)

Cárdenas also noted that "soldiers subject to privations, keep off cold, hunger and thirst by smoking; all the inhabitants of the hot countries of the Indies alleviate their discomforts by the smoke of this blessed and medicinal plant" (Heimann, 1960).

References: Robert K. Heimann, *Tobacco and Americans*, New York: McGraw-Hill Book Company, 1960, p. 15.

Carlson, Regina (1942–)

A pioneer in the nonsmokers' advocacy movement, Regina Carlson cofounded in 1974 the NEW JERSEY GROUP AGAINST SMOKING POLLUTION (GASP). Before becoming executive director, she was the organization's legislative coordinator and president. Carlson works with citizens, legislators, and businesses to secure smoke-free air for nonsmokers, to ensure tobacco-free lives for children, and to confront the tobacco industry.

The author of an AMERICAN LUNG ASSOCIATION (ALA) report (1979) on smoke-free workplaces, Carlson has advised thousands of employers, including Mobil Oil, RCA, American Hoechst International, A-P-A Transport, the Prudential Insurance Company, Hoffmann-LaRoche, Northwestern Bell, AT&T, and Johnson and Johnson. Her smoke-free environmental manuals have been published by New Jersey GASP, the New Jersey Department of Health, the American Lung Association (ALA), and the AMERICAN CANCER SOCIETY (ACS). In addition to hundreds of media interviews, her articles about smoke-free environments have appeared in newspapers and scholarly publications. In 1997, Carlson authored *Smokefree Air Everywhere: Why and How for Decision Makers in Workplaces and Public Places,* her fourth smoke-free policy guide.

Carlson's work has won her countless honors and recognition. In 1989, the ADVOCACY INSTITUTE (AI)gave her its "Sparkplug" Award for igniting the energy of others. In 1996, she was named a New Jersey Woman of Achievement by Douglass College, Rutgers University, and the New Jersey State Federation of Women's Clubs. In 1998, the Academy of Medicine of New Jersey gave her its Citizen Award, the highest award it bestows on non-physicians.

Carmen

Carmen, an opera by Georges Bizet, opened at the Opéra Comique in Paris on March 3, 1875. Bizet, who had never been to Spain or Cuba, featured Carmen, a worker in a tobacco factory, and singers smoking on stage. The opera associated cigarettes with unsavory lower-class individuals.

Carr, Julian Shakespeare. *See* BLACKWELL, WILLIAM T.

Carreras and Marcianus Company

Founded by José Joaquim Carreras, an expert in tobacco blending and cigar making, the British Carreras and Marcianus Company pioneered coupon use. As far back as 1905, the company had a promotion in which stamp albums and foreign stamps were given away in return for vouchers placed in packs of cigarettes. *See also* BLACK CAT

Carter, Grady (1945–)

A retired air traffic controller, Grady Carter lost the upper lobe of his left lung to cancer after smoking for 40 years, and was awarded $750,000 by a state circuit court jury in Jacksonville, Florida. This was the second time the tobacco industry had been ordered to pay damages in a liability case. The monetary award was to reimburse Carter for medical and related expenses.

After a three-week trial, on August 9, 1996, the jury found that LUCKY STRIKE CIGARETTES, the cigarettes Carter mainly smoked, were a defective product and that BROWN AND WILLIAMSON TOBACCO CORPORATION, their maker, had been negligent in not informing the public about their danger earlier. The only other monetary award against a tobacco company in a liability case was won in 1988 by the family of ROSE CIPOLLONE, but it was reversed on appeal. So, too, was the Carter award. In June 1998, the First District Court of Appeals in Tallahassee, Florida, struck down the jury verdict against Brown and Williamson, ruling that the lawsuit was filed two days too late (Florida's four-year statute of limitations had expired). The court also found that certain documents were improperly admitted as evidence against Brown and Williamson and that a 1969 federal law bars lawsuits from claiming the wording of cigarette warning labels is inadequate.

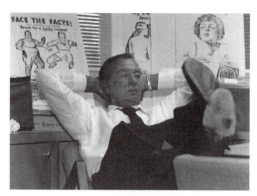

Grady Carter won $750,000 in damages from the tobacco industry. *The Florida Times-Union.*

Carter started smoking unfiltered Lucky Strikes when he was 17 years old. He ignored requests from his family to stop and turned down the Federal Aviation Administration's offer to send him to no-smoking classes. He tried to quit several times but continued to crave cigarettes; he finally quit when he was diagnosed with cancer in 1991. Because he loved to smoke, Carter did not solely blame the tobacco company for his illness. But after he saw the April 14, 1994, evening news during which seven tobacco executives from the major tobacco companies swore to Congress that nicotine was not addictive, he felt he had to take action. Carter felt that the companies withheld evidence that might have helped him quit.

Carter, represented by NORWOOD "WOODY" WILNER of Jacksonville, sued Brown and Williamson Tobacco Corporation. During the trial, Wilner won the court's approval to admit into evidence internal documents stolen by former law-firm paralegal Merrell

Williams from Brown and Williamson's files. This was the first time the Williams documents were used as evidence. *See also* BROWN AND WILLIAMSON TOBACCO CORPORATION— MERRELL WILLIAMS DOCUMENTS; MADDOX, ROLAND

Carter, Robert (1663–1732)

Robert Carter, a tobacco planter in colonial Virginia who was also known as King Carter, had holdings exceeding 300,000 acres. He dominated the Virginia political scene, and held virtually every colonial office at one time or the other. His position in Virginia society was such that services at the church he attended did not begin until he arrived. *See also* BYRD, WILLIAM, II

Cartier, Jacques (1491–1557)

French sailor and explorer Jacques Cartier made three voyages to Canada. When he explored the St. Lawrence River in 1535, Cartier reported that

> The Indians have a certain herb, of which they lay up a store every Summer, having first dried it in the sun. They always carry some of it in a small bag hanging around their necks. In this bag they also keep a hollow tube of wood or stone. Before using the herb they pound it to a powder, which they cram into one end of the tube and plug it with red-hot charcoal. Then they suck themselves so full of smoke that it oozes from their mouths like smoke from the flue of a chimney. They say the habit is most wholesome. ("*Sold American,*" 1954)

Cartier observed the native people smoking NICOTIANA RUSTICA, which "bit our tongues like pepper," not the mild NICOTIANA TABACUM from Central and South America that supplanted the strong, native variety decades later.

References: "*Sold American!*" *The First Fifty Years,* The American Tobacco Company, 1954, p. 9.

Castano, Peter (1950–1993)

The death of Peter Castano, a Louisiana criminal defense attorney whose death certificate said he died from lung cancer due to smoking, led to a lawsuit that became the first and largest federal class action in the cigarette industry. Castano, already a heavy smoker in his teens, tried to quit smoking numerous times. At Castano's funeral, his wife asked WENDELL GAUTHIER to sue the tobacco industry for the family. Believing the odds of success were low, he did not immediately accept. Gauthier later agreed to take the case, arguing that addiction, a new legal issue, caused his friend's death. *See also* CASTANO V. AMERICAN TOBACCO COMPANY

Castano v. American Tobacco Company

On March 24, 1994, Dianne Castano and three other plaintiffs filed a suit against various tobacco companies in U.S. District Court in New Orleans, Louisiana. *Castano v. American Tobacco Company* eventually evolved into the largest class action in U.S. judicial history. There were eight named defendants: PHILIP MORRIS COMPANIES INC., R.J. REYNOLDS COMPANY, BROWN AND WILLIAMSON TOBACCO CORPORATION and the AMERICAN TOBACCO COMPANY, LORILLARD COMPANY INC., LIGGETT AND MYERS TOBACCO COMPANY, the UNITED STATES TOBACCO COMPANY, BATUS Inc. (onetime owner of Brown and Williamson), and the TOBACCO INSTITUTE. (In March 1996, Liggett settled with the *Castano* plaintiffs.)

The 14-page lawsuit charged that the companies engaged in fraud by misrepresenting that tobacco is non-addictive, were negligent in not accurately describing their products, violated consumer protection statutes, breached an express warranty that their products were not addictive and an implied warranty that their products were fit for consumption, and caused intentional emotional distress for those who smoked their cigarettes. The suit asked for compensatory and punitive damages, plus funds to treat smoking-related diseases.

Diane Castano was the widow of PETER CASTANO, a New Orleans lawyer who died in 1993 at the age of 43. She wanted to sue the tobacco companies and asked WENDELL GAUTHIER, a close friend of Peter Castano

since law school, to take the case. He agreed and recruited Louisiana colleagues, many of them friends of Castano, and celebrity and famous trial lawyers, after research bolstered his theory that addiction, not failure to warn of the health dangers of smoking, should be the new legal issue.

Gauthier's idea was to create a class of more than 50 million smokers nationwide who would sue the tobacco companies for the costs of medical monitoring to pay for checkups of addicted smokers and smoking cessation programs, compensation for being addicted, and punitive damages. He contended that smokers were not forewarned that smoking was habit forming and nothing on cigarette packs spelled out that cigarettes were addictive. Although the lawsuit carried Castano's name and three other plaintiffs who smoked, it was in actuality the world's largest class action on behalf of all nicotine-addicted smokers. Gauthier eventually lined up 65 of the nation's top lawyers to take part in the case.

Judge OKLA B. JONES II of the New Orleans District Court certified the suit for trial on February 17, 1995. The ruling formally granted class-action status to the 1994 lawsuit filed by three smokers and Castano's widow and gave plaintiffs a broad boundary line for their class. The judge defined the class in *Castano* as:

> (a) All nicotine-dependent persons in the United States, its territories, possessions and the Commonwealth of Puerto Rico, who have purchased and smoked cigarettes manufactured by the defendants; (b) the estates, representatives, and administrators of these nicotine-dependent cigarette smokers; and (c) the spouses, children, relatives and "significant others" of these nicotine-dependent cigarette smokers as their heirs or survivors. (Scheg, 1996)

Jones was bound by Rule 23 of the Federal Rules of Civil Procedure. A class action must have too many plaintiffs to conduct individual trials, the claim must be typical of the class as a whole, and the representatives of the class must be able to safeguard adequately the interests of the class. Rule 23 also requires that questions of law common to members of the class "predominate" over questions affecting individual members. In other words, if members of the class come from different states that have different tort laws, (law of personal property damages as opposed to contractual or statutory damages) class action may not be an appropriate form for seeking justice. The class approach must also be "superior" to other methods available for adjudicating the claims.

Judge Jones split the lawsuit into two parts. The first would be a single trial of the claim that nicotine was addictive and that tobacco companies fraudulently failed to inform smokers of this fact. The second series of trials would assess potential damages, but the judge would decide how to manage the second trials if the first trial was won. As the lawyers prepared their appeal arguments, Judge Jones died suddenly from leukemia in January 1996.

In July 1995, the U.S. Court of Appeals for the Fifth Circuit agreed to review the case after the tobacco companies appealed Judge Jones' February 1995 ruling. On May 23, 1996, three judges, randomly selected from the 21 judges serving on the Fifth Circuit Court of Appeals, unanimously dismissed or decertified the *Castano* class action. In a 36-page opinion, three judges agreed that variations in state laws were too great and adversely affected the conditions of "predominance" and "superiority." They agreed with Kenneth Starr, tobacco industry counsel, that nicotine addiction as a cause of action needed to be tested in state courts before creating a national claim. *See also* Broin v. Philip Morris Companies Inc.; Engle v. R.J. Reynolds; LeBow, Bennett; Tobacco Litigation: First, Second, and Third Waves

References: Kathleen E. Scheg, "Public Policy: Effective Treatment for Tobacco Disease," *Journal of the American Medical Women's Association*, vol. 51, nos. 1 & 2 (January/April 1996), p. 60.

Catlin, George (1796–1872)

American artist, traveler, and author George Catlin devoted himself to capturing in verbal and visual pictures every facet of the lives of Native Americans living in the Plains region. He left behind descriptions of pipes, PIPESTONE, and the sacred quarry from which native pipe carvers got their material for pipe bowls. In *Letters and Notes on the Manners, Customs, and Conditions of the North American Indians Written During Eight Years' Travel (1832–1839) amongst the Wildest Tribes of Indians of North America,* published in London in 1844, Catlin, who was a keen observer, described the pipe of Mah-to-toh-pa, a Mandan, one of the numerous men who sat for a portrait.

> His pipe was ingeniously carved out of red steatite, the stem of which was 3 feet long and 2 inches wide, made from the stalk of a young ash: about half its length was wound with delicate braids of the porcupine, so ingeniously wrought as to represent figures of men and animals upon it. It was also ornamented with the skins and beaks of woodpeckers' heads, and the hair of the white buffalo's tail. The lower half of the stem was painted red, and on its edges it bore the notches he had recorded for the snows (years) of his life. (p. 147)

Catlin was the first to describe in detail the pipestone quarry, in the valley of a head-stream of the Mississippi 400 miles west of the present-day city of Minneapolis, Minnesota, from which all the Plains Indians got the material for their pipe bowls. As a result, this material, a deep, rich red that takes on a beautiful polish, is usually called catlinite. He ventured to explain that the stone was different from any known mineral compound ever discovered in any part of Europe or other parts of the American continent. Indeed, he "challenged the world to produce anything like it, except it be from the same locality" (p. 167).

Within the sacred quarry, Catlin explained that a truce was to be observed.

> The Great Spirit at an ancient period, here called the Indian nations together, and standing on the precipice of the red pipe stone rock, broke from its wall a piece, and made a huge pipe by turning it in his hand, which he smoked over them, and to the North, the South, the East, and the West,

and told them that this stone was red—that it was their flesh—that they must use it for their pipes of peace—that it belonged to them all, and that the war-club and scalping knife must not be raised on its ground. (p. 164)

When Catlin visited the quarry, there was a complaint that the truce had been broken, that the Dakotas had seized the quarry for themselves, and that many tribes could not obtain the ritual stone.

It will be seen by some of the traditions inserted in this Letter, from my notes taken on the Upper Missouri four years since, that those tribes have visited this place freely in former times; and that it has once been held and owned in common, as neutral ground, amongst the different tribes who met here to renew their pipes, under some superstition which stayed the tomahawk of natural foes, always raised in deadly hate and vengeance in other places. It will be seen also, that within a few years past . . . . the Sioux have laid entire claim to this quarry; and as it is in the centre of their country, and they are more powerful than any other tribe, they are able successfully to prevent any access to it. (p. 167)

See also NATIVE AMERICANS; PIPE SMOKING AND NATIVE AMERICANS

Centers for Disease Control and Prevention (CDC)

Part of the U.S. PUBLIC HEALTH SERVICE of the U.S. DEPARTMENT OF HEALTH AND HUMAN SERVICES, the Centers for Disease Control and Prevention (CDC) have a mission to promote health and the quality of life by preventing and controlling disease, injury, and disability. Headquartered in Atlanta, Georgia, the CDC's OFFICE ON SMOKING AND HEALTH, a division of the CDC's National Center for Chronic Disease Prevention and Health Promotion, targets tobacco-related diseases.

With estimated fiscal year appropriations of approximately $74 million, the CDC provides national leadership for a comprehensive, broad-based approach to preventing and controlling tobacco use. Through collaboration with the states; with national, profes-

sional, and voluntary organizations; with academic institutions; and with other federal agencies, the CDC leads and coordinates strategic efforts to prevent tobacco use among young people, promote smoking cessation, and reduce exposure to environmental tobacco smoke. Designed to reach multiple populations, these activities target high-risk groups, such as young people, racial and ethnic minority groups, blue-collar workers, persons with low income, and women. The CDC supports and actively collaborates with a variety of national organizations (for example, the National Association for African-Americans for Positive Imagery) to ensure the participation of diverse community groups, coalitions, and community leaders in tobacco control efforts.

The CDC strengthens and expands the scientific foundation for tobacco-use prevention and control by examining trends, patterns, health effects, and the economic costs associated with tobacco use. Its programs include the following:

- The Surgeon General's Reports 1964–1998 on the health consequences of tobacco use have documented comprehensive, scientific findings on cigarette smoking and smokeless tobacco use. Recent reports have addressed tobacco use among adolescents and special populations.
- The CDC's *Morbidity and Mortality Weekly Report (MMWR)* and *MMWR Surveillance Summaries,* published by its Epidemiology Program Office, serve as major outlets for surveillance data and research findings on tobacco use. Topics include the enactment and status of state laws on tobacco use and trends in smoking initiation and prevalence among young people.
- The CDC's State Tobacco Activities Tracking and Evaluation (STATE) system is a state-based comprehensive surveillance system that tracks legislative, programmatic, and epidemiologic data that will be used for reporting on current status and trends of tobacco use. The system will answer state-spe-

TABLE 1. Total and per capita yearly consumption* of manufactured cigarettes and percentage changes in per capita consumption — United States, 1900–1994

Year	Total cigarettes (billions)	Cigarettes per capita[†]	Percentage changes in per capita consumption from previous year
1900	2.5	54	
1901	2.5	53	- 1.9
1902	2.8	60	+13.2
1903	3.1	64	+ 6.7
1904	3.3	66	+ 3.1
1905	3.6	70	+ 6.1
1906	4.5	86	+22.9
1907	5.3	99	+15.1
1908	5.7	105	+ 6.1
1909	7.0	125	+19.0
1910	8.6	151	+20.8
1911	10.1	173	+14.6
1912	13.2	223	+28.9
1913	15.8	260	+16.6
1914	16.5	267	+ 2.7
1915	17.9	285	+ 6.7
1916	25.2	395	+38.6
1917	35.7	551	+39.5
1918	45.6	697	+26.5
1919	48.0	727	+ 4.3
1920	44.6	665	- 8.5
1921	50.7	742	+11.6
1922	53.4	770	+ 3.8
1923	64.4	911	+18.3
1924	71.0	982	+ 7.8
1925	79.8	1,085	+10.5
1926	89.1	1,191	+ 9.8
1927	97.5	1,279	+ 7.4
1928	106.0	1,366	+ 6.8
1929	118.6	1,504	+10.1
1930	119.3	1,485	- 1.3
1931	114.0	1,399	- 5.8
1932	102.8	1,245	-11.0
1933	111.6	1,334	+ 7.1
1934	125.7	1,483	+11.2
1935	134.4	1,564	+ 5.5
1936	152.7	1,754	+12.1
1937	162.8	1,847	+ 5.3
1938	163.4	1,830	- 0.9
1939	172.1	1,900	+ 3.8
1940	181.9	1,976	+ 4.0
1941	208.9	2,236	+13.2
1942	245.0	2,585	+15.6
1943	284.3	2,956	+14.4
1944	296.3	3,039	+ 2.8
1945	340.6	3,449	+13.5
1946	344.3	3,446	- 0.1
1947	345.4	3,416	- 0.9
1948	358.9	3,505	+ 2.6
1949	360.9	3,480	- 0.7
1950	369.8	3,552	+ 2.1
1951	397.1	3,744	+ 5.4
1952	416.0	3,886	+ 3.8
1953	408.2	3,778	- 2.8
1954	387.0	3,546	- 6.1

TABLE 1. Total and per capita yearly consumption* of manufactured cigarettes and percentage changes in per capita consumption — United States, 1900–1994 — Continued

Year	Total cigarettes (billions)	Cigarettes per capita[†]	Percentage changes in per capita consumption from previous year
1955	396.4	3,597	+ 1.4
1956	406.5	3,650	+ 1.5
1957	422.5	3,755	+ 2.9
1958	448.9	3,953	+ 5.3
1959	467.5	4,073	+ 3.0
1960	484.4	4,171	+ 2.4
1961	502.5	4,266	+ 2.3
1962	508.4	4,266	0.0
1963	523.9	4,345	+ 1.9
1964	511.3	4,194	- 3.5
1965	528.8	4,258	+ 1.5
1966	541.3	4,287	+ 0.7
1967	549.3	4,280	- 0.2
1968	545.6	4,186	- 2.2
1969	528.9	3,993	- 4.6
1970	536.5	3,985	- 0.2
1971	555.1	4,037	+ 1.3
1972	566.8	4,043	+ 0.1
1973	589.7	4,148	+ 2.6
1974	599.0	4,141	- 0.2
1975	607.2	4,122	- 0.5
1976	613.5	4,091	- 0.8
1977	617.0	4,043	- 1.2
1978	616.0	3,970	- 1.8
1979	621.5	3,861	- 2.7
1980	631.5	3,849	- 0.3
1981	640.0	3,836	- 0.3
1982	634.0	3,739	- 2.5
1983	600.0	3,488	- 6.7
1984	600.4	3,446	- 1.2
1985	594.0	3,370	- 2.2
1986	583.8	3,274	- 2.8
1987	575.0	3,197	- 2.4
1988	562.5	3,096	- 3.3
1989	540.0	2,926	- 5.5
1990	525.0	2,817	- 3.7
1991	510.0	2,713	- 3.7
1992	500.0	2,640	- 2.7
1993[§]	485.0	2,539	- 3.8
1994[¶]	480.0	2,493	- 1.8

*U.S. military forces overseas are included in the estimated total consumption for the periods 1917–1919 and 1940–1994 and in the estimated per capita consumption for 1930–1994.
[†] Among persons ≥18 years of age.
[§] Subject to revision.
[¶] Estimated, based on projection for entire year.

Sources: References 17–19.

A page from the CDC publication *Morbidity and Mortality Weekly (MMWR)*.

cific queries and generate reports on topic areas of particular interest to individual states. In 1999, information from the STATE system became available to states via the Internet. The CDC is collaborating with the World Health Organization (WHO) to create a similar system to support international efforts to reduce tobacco use.

- The CDC responds to a diverse audience, including personal inquiries and automatic voice-operated facsimile requests, through a variety of channels, including brochures, fact sheets, articles, and video products—many available through a toll-free dissemination service. In addition, the CDC provides the public with ready access to tobacco use prevention information through a Web site on the Internet. The CDC Web site provides access to the surgeon general's reports, government research on nicotine dependence, secondhand smoke, and tobacco advertising, educational materials on SMOK-

ING CESSATION, and statistical data on prevalence of smoking among youth and adults, among other things.

- Through the Media Campaign Resource Center, the CDC develops, obtains, and distributes high-quality materials to help states and local programs conduct counter-advertising media campaigns to prevent tobacco use. Materials available include television, radio, magazine, newspaper, and billboard advertisements. The resource center also provides direct technical assistance in conducting counter-advertising campaigns.

- Through an agreement with the World Health Organization, the CDC serves as the only WHO Collaborating Center for Smoking and Health in the United States and as the catalyst for communication between all nine international WHO Collaborating Centers and the six WHO Regional Offices. The CDC prepares and implements international and regional studies as well as epidemiologic research, and provides health education and other assistance to help international organizations and other countries reduce tobacco use.

Beginning in 1999, the CDC is supporting comprehensive programs for preventing and controlling tobacco use in all 50 states, the District of Columbia, and eight territories (American Samoa, the Commonwealth of Puerto Rico, the Virgin Islands, the Federated States of Micronesia, Guam, the Northern Mariana Islands, the Republic of the Marshall Islands, and the Republic of Palau).

Chaber, Madelyn (1950–)

In February 1999, attorney Madelyn Chaber won a $51.5-million award against PHILIP MORRIS COMPANIES INC. in a lawsuit in San Francisco, California, in which she represented PATRICIA HENLEY, a former smoker with inoperable lung cancer. The amount was triple what Chaber had sought from the San Francisco Superior Court jury. Chaber, a former New York elementary school teacher who lost her job during a citywide teachers strike in 1975, credited the teaching profession for her presentation style and her ability to communicate ideas.

After losing her job, she took the law boards, earned a top score, and began her new career in law. As a new attorney, she was involved in asbestos litigation in San Francisco. She joined a plaintiffs' firm that handled lawsuits that blamed the material for a variety of pulmonary diseases, including asbestosis, a hardening of the lungs, and mesothelioma, a form of lung cancer.

In 1988, Chaber won a $2.7-million verdict for the widow of a San Francisco pipe fitter exposed to asbestos who died of mesothelioma. In 1994, she handled her first tobacco case, a lawsuit against LORILLARD COMPANY INC. on behalf of MILTON HOROWITZ, a California clinical psychologist with mesothelioma. She won a $2 million verdict in 1995, shortly before Mr. Horowitz died.

A partner in the law firm of Wartnick, Chaber, Harowitz, Smith and Tigerman, Chaber, a former smoker, provided the jury with more than 1,000 Philip Morris documents pulled from the company's files and made public during the MINNESOTA MEDICAID CASE.

Cherner, Joe (1958–)

Joe Cherner is a New York bond trader turned health activist and the 1988 "Man of the Year" at Kidder Peabody and Co., where he served as senior vice president. He took a public service leave of absence to devote time and energy to public health causes.

In 1988, he founded (with $100,000 of his own money) and became president of SMOKEFREE EDUCATIONAL SERVICES, a nonprofit organiztion headquartered in New York City. Along with others, Cherner successfully crusaded for health legislation to ban the distribution of free sample cigarettes and all vending machine sales of cigarettes. He also successfully crusaded for a ban on smoking in restaurants.

In 1988, Cherner organized a contest for New York City school kids, the largest counter-advertising contest ever conducted. Nearly $70,000 worth of bonds were awarded to 21 school children for their winning posters, videos, and audio anti-smoking advertisements. He visited schools to promote the contest, accompanied by anti-smoking celebrities such as Dr. C. EVERETT KOOP; Ron Darling, the New York Mets baseball pitcher whose father took a battery-operated fan into restaurants with him to blow away smoke; and PATRICK REYNOLDS, who told classes about seeing his grandfather, RICHARD JOSHUA REYNOLDS, disabled by emphysema.

During the 1990s, Cherner photographed Newport employees distributing cigarettes to minors and showed the photos to members of the city council, the state legislature, and the governor. He also brought cancer victims to cigarette company shareholders' meetings; sold stickers printed with anti-smoking slogans that supporters plastered over cigarette ads on subway cars and buses; and invited children to show up at City Hall hearings with illegally purchased cigarettes. In 1993, he crusaded against a billboard in Shea Stadium for MARLBORO CIGARETTES that frequently appeared on television when games were broadcast. In 1997, Cherner created parodies of cigarette ads ("Virginia Slime") that were displayed on the roofs of some New York City taxis. *See also* ACTION ON SMOKING AND HEALTH (ASH), AMERICANS FOR NONSMOKERS RIGHTS (ANR); DOCTORS OUGHT TO CARE (DOC); STOP TEENAGE ADDICTION TO TOBACCO (STAT)

The Cherokee Tobacco (1871)

A Supreme Court case entitled *Two Hundred and Seven Half-Pound Papers of Smoking Tobacco, etc., Elias Boudinot et al., Claimant Plaintiffs in error v. United States* (78 U.S. 616 [1871]), also know as *The Cherokee Tobacco,* ruled that the Cherokees had to pay taxes on tobacco manufactured in the Cherokee Nation despite treaty rights previously guaranteed to the Cherokee by the federal government exempting the tribe from such taxation.

The case involved Elias C. Boudinot and his uncle, Cherokees who negotiated a business deal with tobacco-factory owners in Missouri before moving their operation into Cherokee Nation territory to take advantage of its tax-exempt status. The men refused to pay taxes required by the Internal Revenue Act of 1868 on tobacco manufactured in the Cherokee Nation. Section 107 of this law said that the internal revenue laws imposing taxes on liquor and tobacco products were to be "construed to extend to such articles produced anywhere within the exterior boundaries of the United States, whether the same shall be within a collection district or not." Boudinot and his uncle claimed the Cherokee treaty of 1866 exempted them from such taxation. Article 10 of the treaty stated that Cherokee citizens had the right to sell any product or merchandise without having to pay "any tax thereon which is now or may be levied by the United States" (Kappler, 1904). In essence, when a treaty between two sovereign nations (the United States and the Cherokee Nation) conflicted with a domestic revenue law, the treaty lost.

Justice Noah Swayne wrote the decision in the case for a deeply divided Supreme Court (a 4-to-2 decision with three justices not involved in the decision) that decided against the Cherokees on the grounds that a law of Congress can supersede the provisions of a treaty. He said the 1868 Revenue Act extended over the Indian territories "only as to liquors and tobacco. In all other respects the Indians in those territories are exempt" (Wilkins, 1997, p. 57). Swayne further explained that

> Revenue is indispensable to meet the public necessities. Is it unreasonable that this small portion of it shall rest upon these Indians? The [fraud] that might otherwise be perpetuated there by others, under the guise of Indian names and simulated Indian ownership, is also a consideration. . . . (Wilkins, 1997, pp. 59–60)

Regarding the 1868 Revenue Act, Justice Swayne said that

> This consideration [of "illicit gain"] doubtless had great weight with those by whom the law was framed. The language of the section is as clear and explicit as could be employed. It embraces indisputably the Indian territories. Congress not having thought proper to exclude them it is not to this court to make the exception. If the exemption had been intended it would doubtless have been expressed. (Wilkins, 1997, p. 58)

Felix S. Cohen, an authority in the area of American Indian law, suggested in his legendary work, *Handbook of Federal Indian Law,* that *The Cherokee Tobacco* was implicity overruled in the 1912 case *Choate v. Trapp* (224 U.S. 665, 673 [1912]).

References: Charles Kappler, comp., *Indian Affairs: Laws and Treaties*, Washington, DC: U.S. Government Printing Office, 1904.

David E. Wilkins, *American Indian Sovereignty and the U.S. Supreme Court*, Austin: University of Texas Press, 1997, p. 57–60.

Cheroot

A cheroot is a CIGAR of simple construction and usually small in size, open at both ends, and made from cheap domestic tobaccos not commonly used in standard cigars. Cheroots are frequently made without a binder.

Chesterfield Cigarettes

Made by LIGGETT AND MYERS TOBACCO COMPANY, Chesterfields revolutionized cigarette advertising in 1926 with an ad showing a woman asking that a man blow cigarette smoke in her direction. A storm of protest rose against the advertisement, but other tobacco companies soon followed suit.

James Buchanan Duke's tobacco trust was broken up in 1911, and the Chesterfield brand appeared for the first time in 1912, along with "a painted flower satin insert for the consumer . . . unquestionably the most attractive satin insert ever used." By 1915, Chesterfield cigarettes were promoted in a modern package of 20s rather than in the earlier slide-and-shell package of 10s.

When Chesterfield cigarettes were first introduced, they had limited success because of their English name and Turkish tobaccos. After Liggett and Myers advertised Chesterfields as "a balanced blend of the finest aromatic Turkish tobacco and the choicest of several American varieties," the brand did well. The company played down its BURLEY TOBACCO base in its advertising copy: "The Chesterfield blend contains the most famous Turkish tobaccos—Samsoun for richness, Cavella for aroma, Smyrna for sweetness, Xanthi for fragrance, combined with the best domestic leaf." Most of the tobacco was Burley and Bright.

As the result of a 1997 settlement between Bennett LeBow's Liggett and Myers and 22 states, Chesterfield packs included a warning (in addition to the traditional surgeon general's warning) that said: "Warning: Smoking is Addictive."

Shortly after the tobacco settlement of November 1998 in which the attorneys general of 46 states accepted a $206 billion plan to settle state lawsuits against cigarette makers, PHILIP MORRIS COMPANIES INC. announced a deal to buy Chesterfield from the Liggett Group, along with two other of its brands. *See also* BRIGHT TOBACCO LEAF; DUKE, JAMES BUCHANAN; LEBOW, BENNETT; TOBACCO SETTLEMENT—NOVEMBER 1998

Chewing Tobacco

While the PIPE was the prevailing form of tobacco consumption throughout most of the colonial period, the chief method of tobacco consumption by all classes during the first half of the nineteenth century was chewing—the only tobacco custom that did not originate in conscious imitation of European habits. One British journal referred to chewing as "the peculiarly disgusting American form of tobacco vice" (Robert, 1967). It led other modes of tobacco consumption until well past the middle of the nineteenth century when cigar smoking became popular.

At the end of the nineteenth century, there were only 10 sizeable manufacturers of plug,

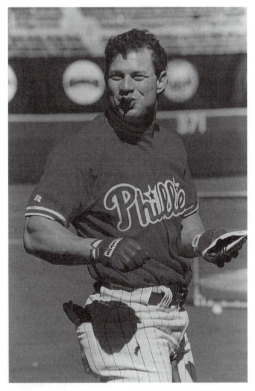

Lenny Dykstra, then centerfielder for the Phildelphia Phillies, enjoys a mouthful of chewing tobacco in this photo from October 1993. *AP/Wide World Photos.*

or chewing tobacco: LIGGETT AND MYERS TOBACCO COMPANY, Drummond, and Butler in St. Louis, Missouri; Finder and the National Tobacco Works in Louisville, Kentucky; Sorg in Middletown, Ohio; Scotten in Detroit, Michigan; LORILLARD COMPANY INC. in Jersey City, New Jersey; and Reynolds and Hanes in Winston, North Carolina. They did 60 percent of the nation's plug manufacture.

The term "chewing tobacco" covered several kinds of product. "Flat plug" meant compressed rectangular cakes of BRIGHT TOBACCO LEAF, sweetened lightly or not at all. "Navy" also referred to flat, rectangular cakes but made from BURLEY TOBACCO LEAF and highly flavored. The cakes averaged a pound in weight, 3 by 16 inches in size, and about 1 inch thick. They were scored so retailers could cut and sell small slices for chews. "Twist" accounted for about one-twentieth of plug volume and was a tobacco rope braided by hand and then compressed. "Fine cut chewing" resembled long cut smoking tobacco because it comprised shredded stripped leaf and was not compressed. It was made specifically for chewing.

The plug wars of 1890–1910 represented the high-water mark of tobacco manufacturing west of the Appalachians. During those years, Missouri, Kentucky, and Ohio kept 60 percent or more of the plug market. Towards the end of that period, only one eastern town, Winston, North Carolina, held an important concentration of plug volume. By 1912, the Reynolds Company and its subsidiaries turned out about a quarter of the nation's plug total.

References: Joseph C. Robert, *The Story of Tobacco in America*, Chapel Hill: The University of North Carolina Press, 1949, 1967, p. 102.

Children and Teens, United States

Adolescence is the time of life when most tobacco users begin, develop, and establish their behavior. Nearly all first use of tobacco occurs before high school graduation. Young people who begin smoking at an earlier age are more likely than later starters to develop long-term nicotine addiction. The 1988 Surgeon General's Report found that nicotine in tobacco is as addictive as heroin or cocaine, and most adolescent smokers who smoke regularly report that they want to quit but are unable to do so. Those who try to quit smoking report withdrawal symptoms similar to those of adults. If the behavior persists through adulthood, it increases the risk of long-term, severe health consequences. But young smokers are also susceptible to significant health problems, including decreased physical fitness, respiratory illnesses, early development of artery disease, and reduced lung development, which may decrease the normal level of lung function.

Despite three decades of explicit health warnings, large numbers of young people continue to start using tobacco. It is estimated that 3,000 young people try their first cigarette per day. According to the 1994 Surgeon General's Report, the first to focus on the problem of tobacco use among young people, three million adolescents smoke cigarettes and over one million adolescent males use smokeless tobacco. Overall, about one-third of high school-aged adolescents smoke or use smokeless tobacco. Smoking among U.S. adolescents declined sharply in the 1970s, but the decline slowed significantly in the 1980s. Then smoking suddenly began to rise in 1988, when, according to the CENTERS FOR DISEASE CONTROL AND PREVENTION (CDC), 700,000 teens under the age of 18 became daily smokers. Less than a decade later, in 1996, the number of teens who became daily smokers, two-thirds of whom were under 18, had risen to 1.2 million.

Although current smoking prevalence among female adolescents began exceeding that among males by the middle to late 1970s, both sexes are now equally likely to smoke. Males are significantly more likely than females to use smokeless tobacco. Nationally, white adolescents are more likely to use all forms of tobacco than are African Americans and Hispanics.

Socio-demographic, environmental, behavioral, and personal factors can encourage the onset of tobacco use. Young people from single-parent homes or families with lower socio-economic status are at increased risk of starting to use tobacco. Peer influence appears to be a more potent factor than parental tobacco use. Young people often try cigarettes or smokeless tobacco with friends, and the peer group may provide expectations, reinforcement, and cues for experimentation. Another strong influence is the way young people perceive their social environment. Adolescents consistently overestimate the number of young people and adults who smoke. Those with the highest estimates are more likely to become smokers, and those who perceive that cigarettes are easily accessible and generally available are more likely to begin smoking.

Adolescents are vulnerable to a range of hazardous behaviors and activities, including tobacco use, during periods of transitions to physical maturity, to a coherent sense of self, and to emotional independence. When adolescents report that smoking serves positive functions for bonding with peers, being independent, and having a positive social image, they are at increased risk for smoking.

Young people face other enormous pressures to smoke. The tobacco industry spends an annual budget of nearly $4 billion to advertise and promote cigarettes, and children and adolescents are exposed to cigarette advertising and promotional activities. Cigarette advertising in the print media persists, portraying the attractiveness of smoking. Human models or cartoon characters display images of youthful activities, adventure and risk taking, good looks, popularity, sexual attraction, independence, affluence, thinness, and health. Cigarette ads appear in many publications teenagers read, particularly those featuring sports celebrities and attractive lifestyles. Ads appear to stimulate some adolescents who have relatively low self-images to adopt smoking as a way to improve their own self-image. Cigarette ads also appear to affect adolescents' perceptions of the pervasiveness of smoking.

While tobacco companies say they don't intend to market to young people, awareness of tobacco products and messages is high among even the youngest children. Numerous empirical studies show that campaigns like R.J. Reynolds' "Old Joe" campaign are reaching children as young as three years old.

One study by Dr. PAUL FISCHER published in the *Journal of the American Medical Association (JAMA)* showed that 30 percent of three-year-olds and 91 percent of six-year-olds could identify "OLD JOE CAMEL" as a symbol for smoking. After the Joe Camel campaign was introduced, Camel's market share among under-age smokers jumped from 0.5 percent to 32.8 percent in three years.

THE CENTERS FOR DISEASE CONTROL AND PREVENTION (CDC) reported in 1992 and 1994 that 86 percent of the under-age smokers ages 12 to 18 who purchase their own cigarettes purchase one of the three most heavily advertised brands: MARLBORO, CAMEL, and Newport. A 1995 study of teens by cancer researchers at the University of California at San Diego published in the October issue of the *Journal of the National Cancer Institute* concluded that advertising, not peer pressure or the example of a family member smoking, was most persuasive in influencing children under 18 to start smoking. A 1996 study by Richard Pollay of the University of British Columbia, who did a 20-year tracking of cigarette advertising, found that teens are three times as likely as adults to respond to cigarette ads and that 79 percent of teens smoke brands heavily advertised.

There has been a continuing shift from advertising to promotion, largely because radio and television have been barred since 1971 from using cigarette advertising. Promotional activities have included sponsorship of car races, rodeos, and other sporting events and public entertainment, outdoor BILLBOARDS, point-of-purchase displays, and the distribution of specialty items (T-shirts, hats, lighters, gym bags), with no health warnings, that appeal to the young. Current research suggests that pervasive tobacco promotions create the perception that more people smoke than actually do and provide conduits between actual self-image and ideal self-image.

Despite laws in all 50 states and the District of Columbia banning the sale of tobacco products to persons under the age of 18, children can easily buy these products. Vending machines are a primary source of tobacco products for young smokers. The 1994 Surgeon General's Report found that young people were able to buy cigarettes in vending machines an average of 88 percent of the time. Young people can get tobacco products through mail-order sales that only require consumers to provide a birth date, that can be easily falsified, or check a box to verify age. Self-service displays also allow children to easily obtain tobacco products. Children also get free samples that are given away on street corners, at shopping malls, and sporting events even though an industry code prohibits distribution to anyone under 21. The tobacco settlement of November 1998 restricts some of the tobacco advertising that appeals to children and teens. *See also* OLD JOE CAMEL; PIERCE, JOHN P.; TOBACCO SETTLEMENT—NOVEMBER 1998

China

Scholars believe that the Portuguese, who landed at Macao and founded a small colony in Canton, introduced tobacco into south and southwest China in the sixteenth century. Trade with the Spanish-held Philippines provided a steady source of supply and the plant gradually became accepted throughout the interior of the country. Northern and northeast China received tobacco from Japan during the wars surrounding the temporary annexation of Korea by Japan. From there, it spread to Manchuria in central China, and the Manchu spread it farther.

Around 1600, tobacco was heralded as a medicine for colds, malaria, and cholera. The first account of tobacco in China was written by physician Chang Kiai-pin, who studied the physiological effects of smoking and recommended its remedial uses. In general, the medical profession was favorable, though some denounced its deleterious effects. It became known as "the kindly plant," "smoke that revives the spirit," and "pill of five elements." Its use spread quickly among all ages and classes, in the northern as well as southern provinces, and it was especially popular among the Manchu soldiers. During the reign of the Ming Emperor Wan-Li (1573–1620), the habit of smoking became as much an institution as tea drinking.

Despite tobacco's popularity, Chinese rulers began to prohibit its use. In 1638, a decree was issued threatening decapitation of anyone found guilty of trafficking in tobacco from the "outer barbarians." The decree was ineffective and illicit use continued and expanded. Tobacco became popular as an intoxicant, to reduce hunger, and to aid digestion. The order was finally rescinded because it was thought to cure colds in the army. Its cultivation and sale were permitted in return for payment of a tax. In 1641, Tsung Cheng, the last ruler of the Ming dynasty, issued an edict prohibiting smoking tobacco, but his efforts failed because princes and high officers continued to smoke privately. The emperor blamed his failures on the continued use of tobacco within court circles. In 1644, after conquering Peking, the Manchu revoked all existing tobacco prohibitions and smoking became the court vogue. Encouraged by the court example, the Chinese became great smokers and the most active propagators of tobacco and smoking all over

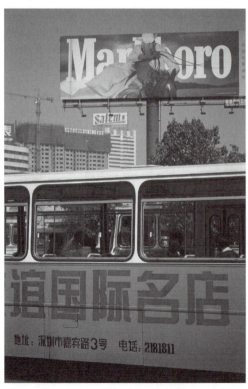

A bus passes a billboard advertising Marlboro cigarettes in Shenzen, China. *Corbis/Macduff Everton.*

Asia, playing the same role as the English in Europe.

About 1650, SNUFF was introduced by the Jesuits and was used therapeutically. At first, snuff use remained restricted to aristocratic circles. Because of its exotic character and foreign source, it was regarded with suspicion. By 1700, snuff taking reached its height of popularity. It was imported from France until the growing demand caused the Chinese to open their own factories in Canton and Peking.

In 1694, tobacco cultivation appeared on Taiwan. Since then, *NICOTIANA TABACUM* has been grown in nearly all provinces of China in all types of soil and climatic conditions.

By the 1990s, China had became the largest producer of tobacco in the world, producing four times as much as the next largest producer, the United States. The government monopoly, the China National Tobacco Corporation (CNTC) dominates the market. CNTC employed 10 million farmers growing tobacco leaf, over half-a-million workers in the industry, and three million retailers.

In 1993, CNTC sold 1,700 billion cigarettes, which amounts to 31 percent of the global market or about the same market as the three largest multi-national tobacco companies combined.

In 1996, China collected more than the equivalent of $U.S.10 billion in tobacco taxes. Tobacco is the largest industrial tax source in China.

China, Tobacco, and Health

In the late 1990s, China, the world's largest consumer of cigarettes, surpassed the United States as the country with the largest number of deaths from smoking—around three-quarters of a million deaths, mostly men. This figure derives from research undertaken by researchers from China and the United Kingdom, led by Professor Liu Boqi of the Chinese Academy of Medical Sciences. He investigated the smoking habits of one million Chinese people in 99 rural and urban areas who died between 1986 and 1988. Results from this study, the largest ever conducted on smoking deaths, as well as other studies led by Professor Niu Shiru and Dr. Yang Gonghuan, both of the Chinese Academy of Preventive Medicine, showed that the Chinese face a huge task in curbing tobacco use.

According to research findings, smoking kills 2,000 people in China every day. Because cigarette-related diseases can take decades to develop, the late 1990s rise in cigarette consumption won't show up in the mortality tables until well into the twenty-first century. Epidemiologists in China and at the CENTERS FOR DISEASE CONTROL AND PREVENTION (CDC) in Atlanta, Georgia, who say lung cancer rates are increasing 4.5 percent a year, estimate that by 2020 around two million Chinese will die of smoking-related illnesses each year.

One in three cigarettes smoked in the world in the late 1990s were smoked in China. A tobacco analyst at Salomon Smith Barney estimated in 1998 that more than 300 million Chinese smokers account for more than one and three-quarter trillion of the five trillion cigarettes sold annually in the world, roughly one-third of the world's total, or about the same number as in all developed countries combined. According to a 1996 national survey, 63 percent of Chinese men smoked, compared to only 4 percent of Chinese women. In 1984, when the first national survey was conducted, men smoked an average of 13 cigarettes a day. In 1996, this figure increased to 15 cigarettes a day.

In China, tobacco control measures began tentatively in 1979 and increased after 1987. The Chinese Association on Smoking and Health (CASH) was established in 1990 as the central coordinating organization on tobacco control, and provincial associations have been established in more than half the provinces. During the 1990s, the Chinese government began to take steps to counter smoking. Chinese government leaders adopted a number of laws and regulations designed to promote smoking control efforts. A 1994 law banned tobacco advertising in the electronic and print media. Tobacco smoking was banned in many public places like schools, hospitals, and government offices. From May 1997, smoking was prohibited on railway carriages, taxis, buses, subways; at airports and train stations; and on all flights of China's airlines. By the end of 1997, 300 Chinese cities had regulations banning smoking in public places. Finally, China hosted the 1997 World Conference on Tobacco or Health, which gave considerable impetus to the country's tobacco control movement. Nevertheless, smoking continues to be widespread and enforcement uneven. *See also* CHINA; GLOBAL TOBACCO USE

Churchill, Winston (1874–1965)

Winston Churchill, arguably the most famous cigar-smoking politician and one of history's greatest statesmen, discovered cigars while garrisoned in Cuba in 1895. He smoked at least 10 cigars a day, roughly 3,000 per year, amounting to over a quarter of a million over his lifetime. Churchill's favorite brands were Romeo y Julieta and the now-defunct La Aroma de Cuba. A number of regular suppliers in Havana kept him well stocked with cigars throughout his life. At Chartwell Manor, his country home in Kent, England, Churchill stocked between 3,000 and 4,000 cigars in a room near his study. He kept the cigars in boxes with labels reading "large" and "small," "wrapped" and "naked," to distinguish their sizes and whether or not they were wrapped in cellophane.

It is reported that Churchill was careless with the lit end of his cigars and frequently dropped ash on himself. As recorded by Phyllis Moir, one of Churchill's private secretaries, in her memoir *I Was Winston Churchill's Private Secretary*, an image that remained in her mind after leaving his employment was when Churchill "sunk deep in the depths of a huge armchair, a little mound of silver-gray cigar ash piled on his well rounded midriff" (Welsh, 1995, p. 4). Not only did he drop ash on himself, he had a tendency to burn his clothes.

According to Roy Howells, one of Churchill's valets who wrote a book *Simply Churchill*, "Sir Winston's suits were constantly going in for repair because of holes caused by cigar burns. He used to burn his

suit that way when he became too engrossed in reading; the cigar would droop slightly and catch the lapel" (Welsh, 1995, p.4). The problem was so great that, according to Edmund Murray, Churchill's bodyguard for a time, Clementine, Churchill's wife, designed a bib for him to wear in bed to help prevent him from burning his silk pajamas.

In an essay titled "A Second Choice" from his book, *Thoughts and Adventures,* Churchill wrote:

> I remember my father in his most sparkling mood, his eye gleaming through the haze of a cigarette, saying, "Why begin? If you want to have an eye that is true [but] a hand that does not quiver... don't smoke! But consider! How can I tell that the soothing influence of tobacco upon my nervous system may not have enabled me to comport myself with calm and courtesy in some awkward personal encounter or negotiation, or carried me serenely through some critical hours of anxious waiting? How can I tell that my temper would have been as sweet or my companionship as agreeable if I had abjured from my youth the goddess Nicotine?" (Welsh, 1995, pp. 9–10)

Churchill preferred his nicotine through cigars; he disliked cigarettes. Once when Howells, his valet, declined to join Churchill for a cigar, explaining that he only smoked cigarettes, Churchill said: "Too many of those will kill you" (Welsh, 1995, p. 10).

Once during the war Churchill was required to take his first high-altitude airplane flight in an unpressurized cabin. According to his renowned biographer Martin Gilbert, when the prime minister went to the airfield to be outfitted with a flight suit and oxygen mask, he requested a special mask designed to accommodate his cigar smoking; the next day he was puffing away 15,000 feet above the earth.

During WORLD WAR II, as Churchill steered Great Britain through its "darkest hours," Cuban cigar companies sent 5,000 cigars each year to keep him well-stocked in case German U-boats caused shipping interruptions. After the war, there was a proposal to build a gigantic statue of the statesman with cigar in hand on the Cliffs of Dover; his

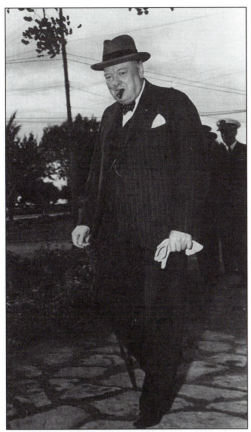

British Prime Minister Winston Churchill with his ever-present cigar. *Library of Congress.*

glowing cigar ash was to be a revolving light-house beacon for ships at sea. Though the monument was never built, England is populated with smaller statues of Churchill, and he appears in a stained glass window in the parish church at Cransley. The cigar, of course, is ever present.

The public was well aware of Churchill's cigar passion, and went so far as to use it against him. During the electoral campaign of June 1945, Labor party opponents criticized him for smoking expensive cigars while the common folk endured the rationing of cigarettes. In 1947, a Labor member of the House of Lords, Lord Chorley, suggested that Churchill be deprived of cigars for two years as punishment for his attacks on Labor leaders. Though Labor held the majority, when put to a vote the proposal was defeated.

Phyllis Moir recalled that Churchill always traveled with several boxes of long, very strong-smelling, and very expensive Havana cigars. Although Sir Winston smoked many kinds of cigars, his favorite was a seven-incher with a 48-ring gauge. The Romeo y Julieta factory in Havana immortalized that size by naming it the Churchill. "He smoked about 15 cigars a day but seldom smoked one to the end. He threw them away after he had got the best out of them. I very rarely saw him without one. Hostesses invariably complained that wherever he went he left behind him a trail of cigar ash on their valuable carpets" (Conrad, 1996, p. 34).

Phyllis Moir boasted of Churchill's health in spite of his high intake of champagne, brandy, and cigars. "He is blessed with a positively Herculean constitution. In spite of the terrific pace at which he has lived he can proudly state that now in his sixties he is in excellent physical condition" (Conrad, 1996, p. 34). Viscount Montgomery (the wartime general known as "Monty") once boasted: "I do not drink. I do not smoke. I sleep a great deal. That is why I am in one-hundred-per-cent form." Churchill, who found Monty's vanity often hard to accept, retorted, "I drink a great deal. I sleep little, and I smoke cigar after cigar. That is why I am in two-hundred-per-cent form" (Conrad, 1996, p. 35). And he lived to the age of 90.

In July 1998, three cigar items (an ash-tray, gold single cigar case, and Don Joaquin cigar box) owned by Churchill were auctioned in London. A silver ashtray, equipped with its own suitcase, was particularly beloved by the prime minister. According to his long-time valet, Roy Howells, "On the Riviera (where Churchill spent the last years of his life), it was ceremoniously handed over to the head waiter of his private dining room each day before lunch, and then returned with great decorum after dinner" (Welsh, 1995, p. 4).

References: Barnaby Conrad III, *The Cigar*, San Francisco: Chronicle Books 1996, p. 34–35.

Peter Welsh, "A Gentleman of History," *Cigar Aficionado (online) Library Archives*, Autumn 1995, pp. 4, 9–10.

Cigar

A cigar is any tubular construction of tobacco leaf in which the filler, or body, is wrapped in tobacco leaf. Cigars have three parts: the filler blended from two or more types of leaf, the inner binder, and the outer wrapper. These must be selected and put together by hand even where the actual rolling is done by machine, since the cigar is a custom-made item.

The filler is the biggest mass of a cigar. In the case of hand-made cigars, usually it consists of strips of tobacco cut to the length of a cigar, known as long leaf. Short leaf indicates smaller cut-up pieces normally used for machine-made cigars. Since long leaf is more expensive, it is kept for premium cigars. There are three different kinds of leaf used for filler blends: leaves with little oil, but full flavored; leaves with less oil or gum, little body, without juice, and less flavorful; and the least gummy or oily grade of tobacco, with little flavor. Filler consists of a blend of two to four different styles of leaves. The blends provide variation in tastes and aromas. Less expensive cigars often use "scrap" filler, the leftovers from all the above types.

The binder encloses the filler and gives the cigar its proper shape and size. Leaves used for this purpose usually have the tensile strength to hold the cigar together. In many cases, the binder is chosen for its physical properties rather than its smoking qualities.

The wrapper's quality is crucial in any cigar. A good wrapper, which is smooth, silky, and oily, has flavor and steady-burning qualities. Wrappers must be elastic and without coarse veins. Wrappers of non-Cuban cigars come from Cameroon, Connecticut, Costa Rica, Ecuador, Honduras, Mexico, Nicaragua, and Sumatra.

From the earliest times, CUBA has been renowned for growing fine cigar leaf and superior cigars are synonymous with Cuba. "Genuine Havanas," are hand-made in Cuba entirely of HAVANA tobacco leaf. Since the 1962 U.S. embargo on Cuban tobacco, cigar leaf has been grown in Honduras and the Dominican Republic.

The tobacco leaf for the majority of U.S. cigars has been produced in the United States. The better grades of domestic cigars include some proportion of Cuban leaf. The term "clear Havana" refers to cigars made in

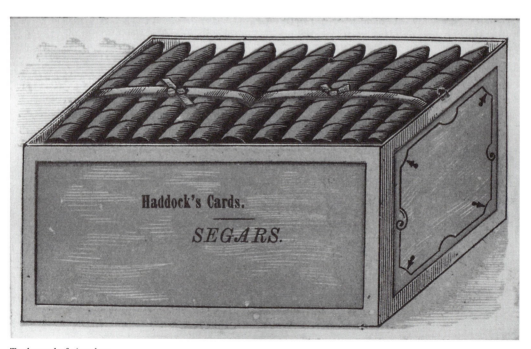

Trade card of cigar box.

the United States but using Cuban leaf for filler, binder, and wrapper.

In the United States, the bulk of cigar tobacco is grown in Massachusetts, Connecticut, New York, Pennsylvania, Wisconsin, Ohio, Florida, and Georgia. The finest grades of domestic wrapper leaf are raised in the Connecticut Valley and in a few counties of western Florida and southern Georgia. Tobacco leaf for cigar binder is grown in the Connecticut Valley, Wisconsin, Florida, and Georgia. Leaf for grades of filler ("short filler" or "scrap") is grown in New York, Pennsylvania, and Ohio.

With the exception of wrapper types, cigars use AIR-CURED TOBACCO. *See also* CIGAR MANUFACTURING, UNITED STATES; CIGAR SIZE AND SHAPE; CIGAR WRAPPER; CONNECTICUT TOBACCO; CUBAN TOBACCO HISTORY; LANCASTER COUNTY, PENNSYLVANIA

Cigar Act. *See* CIGAR REGULATION

Cigar Aficionado

Launched in 1992 by publisher Marvin R. Shanken, *Cigar Aficionado* is an over-sized glossy magazine that celebrates the pleasures of cigar smoking by chronicling the people, places, accessories, and collectibles that makes cigars a unique cultural phenomenon. One of the most successful magazine start-ups of the 1990s, the magazine's readership went from 40,000 the first year to over 400,000 in 1997.

The magazine contains interviews with celebrities, sports stars, and other cigar smokers; exclusive ratings and tasting notes on the finest cigars; and descriptions of cigar accessories such as lighters and humidors. Celebrities, both men and women, appear on the covers with cigars in hand. Feature stories profile the prominent people illustrated on the cover. Past issues have pictured Fidel Castro, Bill Cosby, Danny DeVito, Matt Dillon, Linda Evangelista, Wayne Gretsky, Demi Moore, Jack Nicholson, Claudia Schiffer, Arnold Schwarzenegger, and Tom Selleck. Each issue of the magazine includes advertising for cigars, upscale clothing, luxury cars, expensive watches, jewelry, premium liquor, casinos and other resorts, and perfume.

Cigar Aficionado has launched a line of clothing and accessories named for the magazine as well as a fragrance for men. *See also* ADVERTISING AND CIGARS; CIGAR RESURGENCE; *SMOKE: CIGARS, PIPES, AND LIFE'S OTHER BURNING DESIRES*

The Cigar and Health

Part of the resurgence of cigars in the 1990s is attributed to the widespread but mistaken belief that cigars are less dangerous than cigarettes. Cigars are not required to carry labels with health warnings, except in California and Massachusetts. Cigar makers are not required to disclose product ingredients and are allowed to advertise large cigars and cigarillos on television and radio, unlike cigarettes and smokeless tobacco.

But health experts argue that cigar smoking is just as unhealthy as cigarette smoking. While cigarette smoke is deeply inhaled, cigar smoke generally is not inhaled but held in the mouth. Because less cigar smoke reaches the lungs, smoking cigars carries less risk of lung cancer than smoking cigarettes. However, cigar smoke does damage other sites. The FEDERAL TRADE COMMISSION has recommended that Congress impose health warning labels on cigars and a ban on television and radio advertising.

The National Cancer Institute's 1998 232-page report on cigars and health states that "cigar smoke is tobacco smoke" and many of its 4,000 different compounds are poisonous or carcinogenic. Most of the chemicals end up in the mouth and throat, so cigar smokers die from tumors of the lip, mouth, pharynx, larynx, and esophagus at rates comparable to cigarette smokers.

The report analyzed years of medical and survey data on cigar smokers to suggest the following consequences:

- People who smoke just cigars have a significantly higher risk of smoking-related death than those who never smoked, although the risk is not as great as that for cigarette smokers.

- The mortality risk from cancers of the mouth and esophagus is about the same for cigar smokers as for cigarette smokers.
- Strong evidence indicates that cigar smoking is related to pancreatic cancer.
- Sidestream smoke from cigars is more dangerous than that from cigarettes. Cigar smoke emits 30 times more carbon monoxide, 20 times more ammonia, as much as 90 times more of the highly carcinogenic nitrosamines specific to tobacco, and up to 10 times more cadmium and methylethylnitrosamine (both cancer-causing agents).

The Kaiser HMO released a large study in early 1998 that linked cigar smoking and specific cancers. It compared 1,810 cigar smokers with 22,654 nonsmoking men. In that study, cigar smokers were twice as likely to develop cancers of the lung, mouth, and pharynx.

The Cigar and Presidents

For almost two centuries, cigars in the White House have been a tradition. At least 16 of the 42 presidents have smoked them.

- John Adams, the second president liked fine cigars.
- James Madison, the fourth president, avidly smoked cigars until his death at 85. His wife, Dolly, sniffed SNUFF.
- JOHN QUINCY ADAMS, the sixth president and son of the second, also liked fine cigars.
- Andrew Jackson, the seventh president, and his wife smoked cigars together.
- Zachary Taylor, the 12th president, smoked alone or with male friends because his wife was bothered by his cigars.
- Ulysses S. Grant, the 18th president, is so closely associated with cigars that he is almost always illustrated, photographed, sculpted, or caricatured with one. He smoked at least 10 cigars per day; on some days as many as 20.

When he ran for president on the Republican ticket, the cigar was such a well-known aspect of his person that the 1868 campaign song was "A Smokin' His Cigar."
- Chester Arthur, the 21st president, who gave lavish, midnight suppers, enjoyed champagne and expensive cigars after a meal.
- Benjamin Harrison, the 23rd president, had cigars shipped to him by a tobacconist from his hometown of Indianapolis, Indiana.
- William McKinley, the 25th president, did not smoke in public nor permit himself to be photographed with a cigar, but in private he was nearly obsessive about smoking. In the White House, one never saw him without a cigar in his mouth except at meals or when he slept. He smoked his favorite imported Garcias with men in his office. He held an unlit cigar in his mouth when his wife was around since she did not like smoke.
- William Howard Taft, the 27th president, began as a cigar smoker, but dropped them at the end of his term.
- Warren Harding, the 29th president, was so careful about the aroma of his tobacco that he brought his cigar humidor with him to the White House from his home in Ohio. Harding was never photographed smoking cigarettes, but he appeared on the golf course and in informal settings with his cigar.
- Calvin Coolidge, the 30th president, smoked cigars. Whenever people offered him a cigar, he examined its size and shape, sniffed its aroma, and then produced an enormous 12-inch super corona from his own pocket. Coolidge invited congressmen for an 8:00 A.M. White House breakfast. After the plates were cleared, and cigars were passed around, the president raised the issue of the day. Coolidge smoked good quality Havana cigars that were given to him.

- Herbert Hoover, the 31st president, smoked good brands of cigars. He liked them big and strong.
- John Kennedy, the 35th president, liked cigars as a young man. He smoked the thin, petit corona size. In 1962, Kennedy signed the trade embargo that banned Cuban cigars from the United States. Before he did, he told Pierre Salinger, his cigar-smoking press secretary, that he needed about 1,000 cigars. Salinger rounded up 1,100. The president told him: "Now that I have enough cigars to last awhile, I can sign this [the decree]!" (Conrad, 1996)
- Richard Nixon, the 37th president, enjoyed ritual cigar smoking as a statesman-like gesture with other leaders. His was the last presidency during which cigars were offered to men after dinner in the Green Room.
- Bill Clinton, the 42nd president, smokes cigars on the golf course.

References: Barnaby Conrad III, *The Cigar*, San Francisco: Chronicle Books, 1996, p. 41.

Cigar Association of America (CAA)

Founded in 1937, the Cigar Association of America is a national trade association, headquartered in Washington, D.C., representing manufacturers (machine and hand-made), importers, and major suppliers to the industry. The association's activities focus on collecting and disseminating statistics to the industry, including imports, exports, and production, and serving as an information clearinghouse for the cigar industry.

Cigar Bands

The paper band that encircles the cigar most likely was invented in the 1830s by Gustave Bock, factory owner and immigrant from the Netherlands. In the 1830s, he ordered paper rings with his signature to be placed on exported cigars to distinguish them from other, especially counterfeit, brands. Another story, however, explains that the origin of the band has to do with Catherine the Great of Russia

(1729–1796), who ordered cigars wrapped in silk to protect her fingers from cigar stains. Some believe that cigar smokers adopted silk cigar rings in imitation of the queen. Another story explains that cigar bands protected the white gloves of nineteenth-century English dandies who held cigars by the band. The story that suggests bands hold poorly made cigars together is dismissed by the fact that bands usually do not constrict the cigars and by Cuban tradition that bands are to be removed before smoking.

By 1855, virtually all Cuban cigar makers banded their exports, registered their bands with the government, and advised consumers to insist on buying banded cigars. By 1900, when brand competition was fierce, at least two billion bands were sold in the United States alone. Even inexpensive cigars wore full-color bands. Today, the bands of non-Cuban cigars often include the date of origin

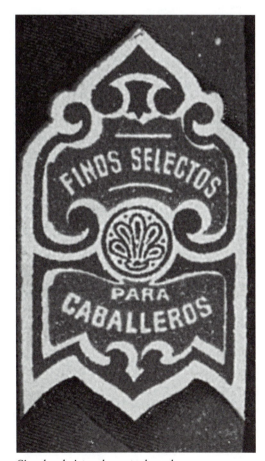

Cigar band pictured on a trade card.

71

of the brand in the space where the Cuban version has the word "Havana."

Traditionally, bands were put on by hand, usually by women, and secured with a dab of plant-based glue, which workers applied with the tips of their third fingers. Great skill was required because bands had to be put on at the same height on each cigar and the glue could not ooze out from under the bands or the wrappers would be damaged.

At the turn of the century, some tobacco companies, like the American Cigar Company, offered premiums in exchange for bands. In the company's 1904 catalog, 50 bands "bought" a set of children's silverware, 600 bands earned a year's subscription to *Scientific Monthly*, and 179,950 bands fetched a baby grand piano delivered to the door. Turn-of-the-century children literally searched in gutters for the 150 bands it took to get a baseball glove at a local redemption center.

By the 1920s and 1930s, when thousands of cigar companies went out of business, the variety of cigar brands dropped dramatically, along with interest in cigar bands. Although the hobby of band collecting is almost dead in the United States, it thrives in Europe and Australia where there are active band-collecting clubs.

Debates still continue about whether or not the cigar band should be removed or remain on the cigar while smoking it. Opinions also differ about the etiquette regarding its removal. In the end, removal is a matter of choice, although tradition dictates removal and the British consider it bad form to advertise the brand one is smoking.

In Cuban novelist Guillermo Cabrera Infante's book *Holy Smoke* (1985), a celebration of the cigar, he writes: "The band, though placed around a cigar last, must always come off first, no matter what bogus connoisseurs might tell you." A few lines later, he adds: "On the other hand you can leave the band if you want to advertise what you smoke, [but] on the other hand, if you don't want to appear too nouveau riche, you can strike off the band—and throw it away."

The Cigar in Comic Strips

Comic strip characters have been chomping on cigars since the end of the nineteenth century. A symbol employed by comic-strip artists, the cigar has served as an emblem of the plutocrat, politician, and boss, or in the words of Jeff MacNelly—creator of P. Martin Shoemaker, a bird that puffs on a cigar while typing his newspaper column—"worldly gruffness."

In "The Katzenjammer Kids," a strip created by Rudolph Dirks in 1897 and still in circulation today, a cigar juts from the jaws of Der Captain. Flip, the companion of Little Nemo, smokes cigars in "Little Nemo," which ran sporadically from 1905 to 1927 as does Mutt, the tall woebegone racetrack player (paired with his short friend, Jeff), who puffs on a cigar in a comic strip that ran from 1907 until 1982. In "Bringing Up Father," created by George McManus, Jiggs, a cigar-smoking bricklayer who wins the Irish Sweepstakes, is hounded by his social-climbing wife, Maggie, in a comic strip created in 1913. Daddy Warbucks, Orphan Annie's protector; Dagwood Bumstead's boss, Mr. Dithers; Marryin' Sam, justice of the peace in "Li'l Abner's" Dogpatch; Brenda Starr's editor, Mr. Livwright; Dick Tracy's partner Sam Catchem; and Albert the Alligator, the Okefenokee Swamp sidekick of the opossum in "Pogo" all smoked cigars.

In the 1990s, cigar-smoking cartoon characters have become scarce. Apart from Jiggs and Shoe (the bird), smoking in strips is a rarity. In the top 10 comic strips—"Peanuts," "Garfield," "Calvin and Hobbes," "Blondie," "Hagar the Horrible," "Beetle Baily," "For Better or Worse," "Doonesbury," "Andy Capp," and "The Family Circus"—no smoking characters appear. When cigars do appear, it's usually villains who are doing the puffing. J. Jonah, the nemesis of Spider Man and editor of the *Daily Bugle* chomps on a cigar, and a 300-pound character named Papa Python smokes cigars in "Terry and the Pirates," a revised comic strip.

Cigar Labels

At the turn of the century, when thousands of cigar brands from thousands of small factories flooded the market, cigar makers needed something to set themselves apart from their competitors. Eye appealing labels on the inside lids of cigar boxes attracted customers.

The idea had been used in 1830 by the banking firm of H. Upmann when it began shipping cigars to its directors in London in sealed cedar boxes emblazoned with the bank's emblem. In 1837, Ramon Allones, a Spanish immigrant to Cuba, began printing colorful lithographed labels as a way to distinguish brands. He spawned an industry that has taken stone lithography to new heights of quality.

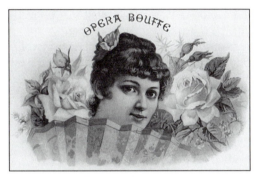

Cigar label with a woman's head.

The labels designed in the twentieth century used new color printing techniques that allowed inexpensive mass production of brilliantly colored images. A broad variety of subject matter was pictured including cowboys and Indians, scenes from operas, celebrity portraits, illustrations of fictional characters like Sherlock Holmes, sports, transportation, animals, beautiful women, and cartoon characters. Wealthy cigar makers spent a great deal of money to create vanity labels featuring themselves, their families, and pets.

Today cigar labels, or *vistas,* have become a collectible art form. When many of the surviving labels were discovered in abandoned cigar factories, box companies, and old lithography firms, they generated little or no excitement in collector circles. By 1979, however, cigar art began to appear in galleries.

On September 7, 1979, the *Wall Street Journal* published a front-page feature story about cigar labels as a growth industry in both the collectible and investment markets. Since then, people in the U.S. and Europe have avidly collected *vistas.* Some rare vintage labels command thousand of dollars.

In Cuba, cigar boxes embellished with lithographs, called *cromos,* have become an art form native to the country. This visual art originated during the nineteenth century when many European artists visited the island. They, together, with local craftsmen, started a revolution in the art of commercial lithography.

The cigar box, made of cedar wood from forests in Honduras, is fitted with the *cromo* by a *filetador.* The *cromos* are glued on the sides and on the lid and also in the interior of the cigar box. The lithograph on the reverse of the cover, called a *vista,* is matched by a *cromo* that hangs from a side of the box, a sort of inner lid. The last leaf must not be printed on high relief, as are all the other *cromos* on the outside of the box and even the *vista* lithograph. If a design had any embossed pattern, when the lid was closed, it would be printed in low relief on the cigar wrapper leaves of the first row of cigars lying in the box. *See also* CIGAR; CIGAR MANUFACTURING, UNITED STATES; CIGAR WRAPPER; CONNECTICUT TOBACCO; LANCASTER COUNTY, PENNSYLVANIA

Cigar Makers' International Union (CIU)

By 1864, with the growth of the factory system and the spread of unionization of the workers, there were enough locals to establish the National Cigarmakers Union (NCU). Czechs, Germans, and Hungarians made up the membership that reached almost 1,000. In 1867, the NCU was renamed the Cigar Makers' International Union (CIU) and it grew to 5,800 members by 1869.

The CIU began to decline partly because of the introduction of the mold that broke down the special skill of the cigar makers, but also because of the growth of the tenement system of manufacturing. In 1871 and

1872, Bohemians emigrated to New York and were employed as unskilled workers in tenement houses. Cigar makers rented the rooms from their employers, furnished their own tools, and put their families to work from early in the morning until late at night, seven days a week.

Because the CIU had membership restrictions and refused to include mold workers, three locals combined and formed a new organization called the United Cigarmakers (UC) that included rollers, bunch breakers, and tenement workers who were excluded from the CIU. The UC drafted a constitution that recognized "the solidarity of the whole working class to work harmoniously against their common enemy—the capitalists." SAMUEL GOMPERS was elected president and Adolph Strasser the financial secretary of the UC. In 1875, the UC joined the CIU as Local 144 at a time when molds, bunching machines, and suction tables threatened the hand-rolled cigar industry.

Weakened by a series of costly strikes in the formative years (1869, 1873, and 1877), the union was reorganized by Gompers and Strasser (both from Local 144), who introduced financial and administrative reforms associated with unions in Great Britain. The rivalry between the Cigar Makers' International Union and the Progressive Cigarmakers (PC) culminated in the formation of the American Federation of Labor (AFL), which absorbed the PC in 1886.

In 1900, continued technological innovations caused fears of job loss and triggered many strikes. Women in the industry gained recognition during the strikes and were encouraged to join the union in 1915.

Between world wars, cigar makers moved from unionized regions such as New York City to other parts of the United States. National membership fell from 40,000 in 1919 to 7,000 in 1940. After the Second World War, the CIU left New York City.

Cigar-Making Machines

The cigar was the last of the tobacco products to become mechanized. In 1917 Rufus Lenoir Patterson produced the intricate mechanism that made the cigar-making machine turn out some 4,000 finished cigars per day.

Machines helped concentrate the cigar trade into fewer hands. In 1910, there were 22,000 cigar factories; in 1929, there were about 6,000. By 1940, the number was reduced to 3,800. Nevertheless, considerable hand industry continues, especially for the exclusive cigar types.

Cigar Manufacturing, United States

The CIGAR first arrived in America in 1762. A British naval officer, Colonel Israel Putnam, returning to his home in Connecticut from a term of service in Cuba, brought back a selection of Havana cigars and large amounts of Cuban tobacco. It was not long before cigar factories were established in Connecticut, New York, and Pennsylvania.

Around the time of the American Revolution, cigar manufacturing took hold in New York City and Philadelphia. At Conestoga, Pennsylvania, long slender cigars were made of the so-called "shoe-string tobacco," a narrow-leafed, coarse variety grown in York and Lancaster Counties as well as in the Connecticut Valley.

In 1810, after a Suffield, Connecticut, cigar manufacturer imported a Cuban cigar roller to teach his skills to American workers, cigar factories became numerous. Since all the work was done by hand, a large number of factories prevailed until machinery was introduced over a century later.

As cigar production grew, a planter in East Windsor, Connecticut, experimented with Maryland seed and grew in 1830 a smooth, broad leaf that made a more attractive wrapper than the "shoestring" leaf. Since the visible wrapper sells the cigar, a demand grew for the Connecticut broadleaf, still grown today, and the shoestring was abandoned.

The practice of using Cuban leaf, whether for wrapper or filler, grew quickly. "Clear Havanas" made of Cuban tobacco were first manufactured in the United States in the 1840s, and cost four to five times more than domestic cigars. During the next decade, "half-Spanish," or 50 percent Cuban leaf,

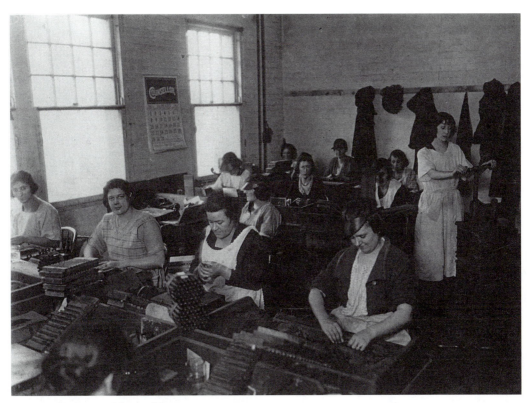

Women rolling cigars. *Library of Congress.*

became true for the industry as a whole. The Havana leaf was used as a filler enclosed by an outer wrapper of smooth New England broadleaf. The amount of Cuban leaf imported for use in U.S. cigar establishments—mostly through New York City—was about equal to the amount grown in all of New England. Despite the use of Cuban leaf, a good proportion of nineteenth-century cigars were still made without it. The CHEROOT, a long and untapered roll of non-blended tobacco was cheap and popular.

Because of the pretension of quality, virtually every New England cigar brand carried a Spanish trademark. Using Spanish words led to odd brand names like La For de Chas. F. Kurtz, made in Millville, New Jersey, and Velocipede Vuelta Abajo Havanas, made in Detroit.

After the Civil War and into the 1870s, when cigar smoking showed an accelerated rate of growth, domestic cigars underwent radical changes. The broadleaf wrapper became a BINDER and a lighter, more bland wrapper was added, first Sumatra-grown, later

Connecticut shade-grown. Havana leaf was used in the FILLER rather than on the outside. Several different types of leaves made blending possible.

Although cigar manufacture developed in New England, it soon spread to virtually every sizeable city in the United States. In 1880, New York City alone had 14,500 workers rolling cigars on a piecework basis in shops, crowded tenement houses, and small enterprises where the shop owner was the main laborer. In all of New England's 503 establishments, the number of workers amounted to 2,300. Big cities had customer demand and a supply of labor. The capital required was small, and new businesses were readily established. Besides urban centers like New York and Philadelphia, cigar manufacturing also took hold in Tampa, Florida, in the 1890s when refugees from Cuba fled there.

By 1880, most states and territories, except for Montana and Idaho, had cigar factories. Most states had plug and pipe tobacco manufacturing as well. In 1880, there were 53,000 cigar makers (as opposed to 33,000 employed in chewing and smoking factories) working for thousands of cigar manufacturers. By the end of the 1800s, there were more than 7,000 cigar factories in the United States, some 500 of them in Florida.

By the early twentieth century, new machines moved the manufacture of cigars out of the tenement houses and into factories. Hand-rolling became a lost art when machine-rolling was perfected in the 1920s. Today, nearly all U.S. cigars are machine-made. But despite the technology, a great amount of hand work still characterizes cigar factories even though most of the actual rolling is mechanized.

The art of cigar manufacture is threefold: blending, rolling, and packing. Since the strength of the delivered smoke varies with the diameter of the roll, thick cigars or *perfectos* require a different combination of heavy, medium, and light leaves than the long, thin *premiers* or *fancy tales*.

About 1900, numerous mergers of cigar manufacturers took place. In 1901 in New Jersey, American, Continental, and Powell, Smith and Company formed the American Cigar Company, the greatest single manufacturer of cigars in the United States, although it never controlled more than one-sixth of the national output. Although cigar manufacturing was distributed all over the nation, Pennsylvania and New York led in quantity. Ohio, Massachusetts, Illinois, New Jersey, Maryland, and California also produced considerable quantities.

In the 1990s, only a few companies sell most of the cigars. Five companies, Swisher International (Bering, King Edward, Swisher Sweets Universal), Havatampa (Havatampa, Phillies), Consolidated Cigar (Antonio y Cleopatra, Backwoods, Dutch Masters, El Producto, La Corona, Muriel, and Roi-Tan), Middleton, and Culbro/General Cigar (Canaria d'Oro, Garcia y Vega, Robert Burns, Macanudo, Partagas,Tijuana Smalls, White Owl, William Penn) control 95 percent of the market in the United States. Except for Havatampa, which only sells machine-made cigars, each of the major companies sells both premium and non-premium brands. In addition to the major companies, some small companies manufacture and import premium cigars.

The market for little cigars is more concentrated, with three companies, Swisher International, Consolidated Cigar, and Tobacco Exporters International controlling 86 percent of the market. Swisher alone has a 42 percent share.

Aside from the use of Spanish words and phrases to indicate or suggest Havana leaf, cigar manufacturers named brands after great men like Senator Henry Clay, famous generals, and notables. *See also* CUBA; GOMPERS, SAMUEL; LANCASTER COUNTY, PENNSYLVANIA

Cigar Regulation

A number of federal and state policies cover tobacco products. In general, cigars are exempted from many of the regulations that apply to other tobacco products, espcially at the federal level.

No law requires health warnings on cigars, except in California and Massachusetts. In 1986, California adopted the Safe Drinking Water and Toxic Substances Enforcement Act, which required warnings on products that contain chemicals that cause cancer or reproductive risks. Cigar manufacturers and retailers agreed to place the following warning on cigars sold in the state: "Warning: This product contains/produces chemicals known to the state of California to cause cancer and birth defects or other reproductive harm." Cigars sold singly generally do not bear the California warning outside the state. In Massachusetts, health warnings appear only on machine-made, not hand-rolled cigars.

The FEDERAL CIGARETTE LABELING AND ADVERTISING ACT OF 1965 required cigarette manufacturers to report annually to Congress the tar and nicotine yield of cigarettes. In 1981, the cigarette makers had to report carbon monoxide as well. But cigar manufacturers are not required by federal law to report tar, nicotine, and carbon monoxide content of their products to the federal government. Texas and Minnesota require nicotine reporting of cigars. The International Committee for Cigar Smoking has stated that, given the range in cigar size and variability of the products, it would be difficult to produce valid tar deliveries, and that ranking cigars by tar content is virtually meaningless and not of value to consumers.

Cigar manufacturers are not required by federal law to disclose added constituents. Texas requires reporting of ingredients added to cigars, and Minnesota requires reporting of constituents in the cigar or cigar smoke that are on the state's hazardous substances list.

In 1973, the Little Cigar Act banned broadcast advertising of "Little Cigars" defined as "any roll of tobacco wrapped in leaf tobacco or any substance containing tobacco as to which one thousand units weigh not more than 3 pounds." The ban did not extend to large cigars and cigarillos, which can still be advertised on electronic media today.

Cigar smoking has been regulated in public places. In 1971, the Civil Aeronautics Board restricted cigarette smoking on airlines to a limited number of seats and at the same time banned cigar and pipe smoking. State and local jurisdictions have regulated cigar smoking as part of ordinances that have restricted cigarette smoking. In general, cigars are more strictly regulated than cigarettes by these ordinances.

At the federal level, the FOOD AND DRUG ADMINISTRATION (FDA) adopted a regulation on August 23, 1996, to prohibit the sale of cigarettes and smokeless tobacco products to persons under 18 years as well as to restrict advertisements and promotions directed towards youth. The FDA rule did not include cigars.

The Federal Alcohol, Drug Abuse and Mental Health Act was amended in 1992 to include a requirement for states to establish 18 years of age as the minimum age for the purchase of tobacco products. If a state did not establish such a requirement, the state would not receive full funding for federal substance abuse block grants. Cigars were not included in the act.

The current federal tax on cigars is broken into two categories. Small cigars are taxed at $1.25 per thousand or approximately one-tenth of a cent per small cigar. The small cigar is defined as having a weight no more than three pounds per 1,000 units, and resembling cigarettes in size and weight. The federal tax on a package of 20 cigarettes is 24¢ while the tax on 20 small cigars is about one-tenth that or 2.25¢ for 20 small cigars.

The federal tax on large cigars, defined as cigars weighing more than 3 pounds per thousand, is 12.75 percent of the wholesale price, but not more than $30 per thousand. At this rate, there is a maximum tax of 3¢ per cigar. Based on this weight classification, cigarillos and manufactured and premium cigars would all be classified as large cigars. The federal tax on a manufactured or premium cigar would be limited to 3¢ a cigar.

As of January 1, 1996, the number of states taxing cigars was 41. Five states have a tax system similar to that of the federal government with multiple rates according to the weight or price of the cigar. Of the 36 states with the single rate, Washington has the highest tax of 74.9 percent of the wholesale price, and North Carolina has the lowest at 2 percent.

All 50 states and the District of Columbia have enacted some form of legislation with respect to the sale of cigars to minors. According to the National Cancer Institute's State Cancer Legislative Database, through November 1997, 29 states and the District of Columbia explicitly prohibited the sale of cigars to minors. The remaining states prohibit the sale of tobacco products to minors, implicitly covering cigars.

Cigar Resurgence

Cigar production peaked around 1907 and then declined throughout the 1920s and into the 1930s. A combination of factors, including anti-cigar images in movies, the "loosies" or single cigarettes, and lower leaf prices, made cigarettes more popular. In 1964, cigars peaked again with 9.1 billion consumed, when many smokers switched to cigars from cigarettes after the first major surgeon general's report on the health risks of smoking appeared. Cigars again fell out of favor from the early 1970s until 1993 when they fell to a low of 2.1 billion, the lowest level since 1950. After 1993, however, a resurgence of interest in cigars worldwide among young men and women led to a rise in sales for premium cigars by about 50 percent.

Cigar smokers in the 1990s are mostly male, white, young (under 40), middle-class, and well educated. Members of minority groups and women are increasingly puffing on cigars as well. Women, who once represented one-tenth of 1 percent of cigar sales now account for up to 5 percent of sales in the United States. Researchers also note that the young are smoking cigars. Almost 27 percent of American teenagers smoked a cigar in 1996, according to a 1997 CENTERS FOR DISEASE CONTROL AND PREVENTION (CDC) study.

The growing popularity of cigars has generated cigar bars in many metropolitan areas of the United States. Trendy restaurants are providing areas for patrons smoking their stogies. There are cigar cruises, cigar magazines like CIGAR AFICIONADO, and catalogs like Dunhill, Thompson & Company, Nat Sherman, and others filled with cigar accessories, including humidors (airtight boxes that keep cigars moist), cutters, lighters, and appointment diaries.

Supermodels, Hollywood stars, and famous athletes also glamorize cigars. Michael Jordan with a cigar in his mouth appeared on the cover of *Sports Illustrated*. Ads for the film *The First Wives Club* pictured Goldie Hawn, Diane Keaton, and Bette Midler with cigars in their mouths. Will Smith smoked cigars in the blockbuster movie *Independence Day*. Wu-Tang Clan's CD "Wu-Tang Forever," which debuted at number one, had a cigar on the cover. An AMERICAN LUNG ASSOCIATION (ALA) survey found that in 133 films, at least 40 percent featured the smoking of cigars or had scenes that "promoted cigars subliminally." *See also* CIGAR AFICIONADO; CIGAR AND HEALTH

Cigar Size and Shape

In English, two words are required to describe cigars—both size (girth of the cigar and its length) and shape. In Spanish, the word *vitola* covers both size and shape. Because manufacturers independently decide which name

goes with which length and girth, the same word may be used by different manufacturers for cigars of different sizes. The basic measurement standard, however, remains the same. Length is listed in inches or centimeters, and girth or diameter, or ring gauge, as it is commonly called, is in 64ths of an inch or millimeters. A classic CORONA size is 6 by 42, which means it is six inches long and 42/64 of an inch thick. Many manufacturers today produce coronas with a 44 ring gauge, not a 42. A double corona is 7 ½ inches by 49 ring gauge. A Churchill measures 7 inches by 47 ring gauge and a robusto is 5 inches by 50 ring gauge. Panetelas measure 7 inches by 38 ring gauge. Lonsdales are 6 ¾ inches by 42 ring gauge.

Today, manufacturers make about 70 different cigar sizes or shapes. They fall into one of two categories: straight or parallel-sided, or *parejos,* and irregular shapes, or *figurados*. The main groups in the straight category are coronas, Churchills, lonsdales, robustos, panetelas, and cigarillos. There are six major irregular shapes: torpedo (a pointed head, bulging in the middle, and a closed foot—the lit end), pyramid (pointed, closed head—the smoked end, widening to an open foot), belicoso (small pyramid-shaped cigar with a rounded head rather than a point), perfecto (two closed rounded ends and bulging in the middle), diademas (a giant cigar 8 inches or longer usually with an open foot), and culebras (three panetelas braided together).

Even with these classic irregular shapes, manufactures vary the basic shape designations greatly so a Churchill from one company doesn't match in size a Churchill from another company.

Cigar Store Indians

Shops selling cigars and other tobacco products identified themselves with distinctive trade symbols, such as wooden American Indians. The use of such figures probably originated in England where, as early as 1617, carved black boys ("Black-more") made their appearance as tobacconist's signs. Not all figures were American Indians. There were

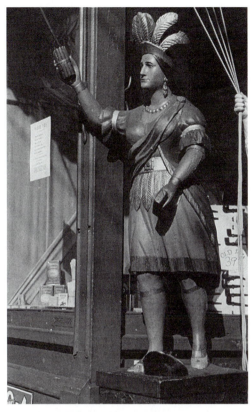

A cigar store Indian. *Library of Congress.*

Scotch Highlanders, Negroes, Canadian trappers, and contemporary females.

A large industry in America turned out these figures, which stood in front of and on counters in tobacco shops—and still do in parts of the United States. With few exceptions, the sculptures were large, armed American Indians. Few of the figures were realistic because carvers rarely used models; some figures were even grotesque or comic. A number had names like "Lo" for "Lo, the Poor Indian," a sentimentalized nineteenth-century embodiment of the vanishing Indian, or insulting names like Big-Chief-Me-Smoke-Em. Some females, named Pocahontas or Maiden, were armed, but many held out a bundle of cigars or tobacco leaves as well as an outstretched, welcoming hand. By the early twentieth century, most wooden cigar store Indians vanished from the streets. Today, they are collector's items.

On October 1, 1986, the United States Postal Service issued "Wood-Carving: Cigar-Store Figure," one of four commemorative folk art stamps depicting wood carved figurines.

Cigar Wrapper

Wrapper leaf for cigars is judged by its texture, elasticity, color, and other factors. Color refers to the shade of the outer wrapper tobacco leaf. Today, there are six major color grades used in Brazil, Cameroon, Cuba, Ecuador, Honduras, Nicaragua, Sumatra, and the United States. They are called claro claro, a light green; claro, a light-tan color, usually grown under shade tents; colorado, brown to reddish-brown, usually shade-grown; natural, light-brown to brown, usually sun-grown; maduro, from the Spanish word for "ripe," a rich, dark-brown color; and oscuro, called negro or black.

Cigarette

Any filler of finely cut tobaccos rolled in paper may be termed a cigarette. Before 1881, all cigarettes were produced by hand by "rollers," and most experienced rollers were foreign born. After 1884, the cigarette industry became highly mechanized.

During most of the seventeenth and eighteenth centuries, the Spanish called the cigarette *papelete* or *cigarillo.* In Brazil, it was called *papelito;* in Italy a paper cigar. The French called it "cigarette." By 1854, the cigarette was known by that name in New York, as observed by Dr. RUSSELL T. TRALL.

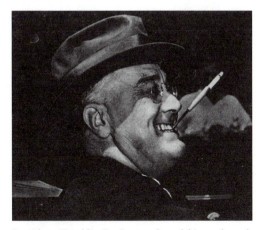

President Franklin D. Roosevelt and his trademark cigarette holder. *Library of Congress.*

Some of the *ladies* of this refined and fashion-forming metropolis are aping the silly ways of some pseudo-accomplished foreigners, in smoking Tobacco through a weaker and more *feminine* article, which has been most delicately denominated cigarette. (Heimann, 1960)

See also FILTERED CIGARETTES

References: Robert K. Heimann, *Tobacco and Americans*, New York: McGraw-Hill Book Company, 1960, p. 204.

Cigarette-Making Machines

As early as 1867, inventors had been working on machinery for making cigarettes. The Paris Exhibition of 1867 featured the Susini invention that claimed to make 3,600 cigarettes per hour. In 1872, Albert Hooks from New York came up with a machine that made cigarettes but they were loosely packed and irregularly shaped. In 1874, the Abadie Company of Paris received a patent for its machine, which failed in test runs. William and Charles Emery introduced their machine with a three-stage process in 1876.

Then in 1881, James Bonsack of Virginia announced his device, which also used a three-stage process and promised to produce 200 cigarettes a minute. Several more machines were developed in the early 1880s, and by the 1890s, at least nine different cigarette makers had been invented. Because the machines made it possible to supply a mass market at reduced costs of production, cigarette prices were kept low. *See also* BONSACK MACHINE

Cigarette Manufacturing History

The modern cigarette came to the United States via SEVILLE, SPAIN, the world's first tobacco-manufacturing center. Early cigarettes were made from scraps of discarded cigar butt, snuff dust, and pipe dottle wrapped in scraps of paper. In Spain and in the Spanish colonies of the seventeenth and eighteenth centuries, the *papelete* (Sevillian name for the smoke) or *cigarillo* took hold throughout most of Europe. The "paper cigar" was considered cheap, a beggar's smoke for people unable to afford cigars.

At some time after 1800, cigarettes moved to Portugal, Italy, and southern Russia. They appeared in France where cigarette smoking was in vogue among revolutionary groups and in Bohemian (artist and writer) circles in most European political centers. In 1843, the French tobacco monopoly, seeking new profits, began manufacturing them. In Russia, the czar's officers copied French cigarettes and made cigarettes from dark and aromatic Turkish and south Russian tobaccos.

British soldiers who encountered cigarettes being smoked by Russians during the Crimean War of 1854–1856, brought them back to London where they gradually caught on. In the 1850s, ROBERT PEACOCK GLOAG and PHILIP MORRIS opened the first British cigarette factories manufacturing cigarettes made from Latakia, smoke-cured Turkish tobacco. About this time, Americans visiting England brought these cigarettes back home with them.

Before the Civil War, the only cigarettes known in the United States were those that came from England and, to a lesser extent, from Cuba. After the war, small-scale manufacturing began in New York where hand rollers from Russian and Poland made the long cigarettes, at first labeled "Turkish" with "Russian" tips. After 1870, a shop operated by the Bedrossian brothers first used a blend of domestic BRIGHT TOBACCO LEAF and Latakia in cigarettes, and soon other New York and RICHMOND, VIRGINIA, manufacturers followed suit formulating new blends. By 1877, there were 121 different brands registered with the government tax authorities.

By 1880, cigarettes were not a national form of tobacco consumption in the way cigars were. There were only a dozen centers with any cigarette production at all. Of these only five (NEW YORK, NEW YORK; Jersey City, New Jersey; Rochester, New York; BALTIMORE, MARYLAND; and Richmond, Virginia) accounted for 75 percent of the 1880 national total. At this stage, the cigarette was a specialty item for big-city markets.

In 1881, cigarettes were produced by hand in a difficult and expensive process. Americans followed the London mode of using European immigrants to roll cigarettes with flat paper rectangles. After rolling the shredded leaf and paper slip into a compact cylinder, the seam was sealed with a touch of flour and water. Even a well-trained cigarette girl could scarcely exceed four per minute at top speed. In 1883, ALLEN AND GINTER, in Richmond, Virginia, had 500 girls working for the company. In 1886, there were 900. One New York visitor commented as follows on the cigarette rollers:

> One of the most surprising features is the intelligent and comely appearance of the girls. This is accounted for by the fact that an applicant for admission into the factory must go through a most thorough examination as to character and habits, and none are admitted who, after careful examination, are discovered wanting in good moral character. (Heimann, 1960)

From 1885 to 1902, the cigarette gained wide popular acceptance. There were 2,100 "cigarettes, cigarros and cheroos" listed in Connorton's Directory, a business directory, along with 9,000 plugs and twists, 3,600 fine cuts, 7,000 smoking tobaccos, and 3,600 snuff brands.

By 1930, however, cigarettes eclipsed all other tobacco products. Mass production of cigarettes, new methods of distribution, the invention of the match, skillful national advertising and marketing, and a change in the tempo of American life resulted in the popularity of cigarettes. *See also* SPAIN.

References: Robert K. Heimann, *Tobacco and Americans*, New York: McGraw-Hill Book Company, 1960, p. 212.

Cigarette Picture Cards, England

By the 1890s, cigarette picture cards began to appear regularly in England, replacing cards with advertisements used to stiffen crush-prone paper packs. The Player brothers issued series of naval and army heroes, castles and abbeys, and "Beauties." In 1899, Ogden started a series of actresses, promi-

nent people, and subjects of general interest. During the 11 years they were printed, 20,000 different sets of cards were issued to smokers. Other companies issued cards picturing music hall artists, authors, wild animals, and political propaganda.

Cigarette cards proliferated through the 1940s but paper and board shortages during the Second World War finally forced their end.

Cigarette Picture Cards, United States

Between 1885 and 1892, dozens of tobacco firms like ALLEN AND GINTER of RICHMOND, VIRGINIA, put small picture cards in cigarette boxes to stiffen the crush-prone paper packs and to attract cigarette buyers to their brands. Every possible subject was pictured, from

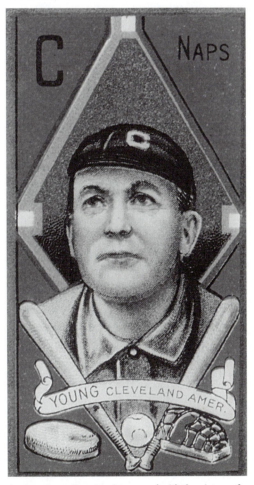

An American cigarette picture card with the picture of a baseball player. *Library of Congress.*

birds, dogs, flags, and flowers to actresses, great American Indian chiefs, presidents, and baseball players. By the mid-1890s, JAMES BUCHANAN DUKE controlled the tobacco business, and the need for cards disappeared along with the tobacco companies gobbled up by Duke's AMERICAN TOBACCO COMPANY. Tobacco companies phased out the cards but brought them back to life after 1910, about the time the U.S. Supreme Court ordered Duke to break up his company. Imported Turkish tobacco products also threatened U.S. tobacco companies, so they reintroduced baseball cards to pep up sales.

Of all the subjects pictured on the cards, baseball cards were most popular and helped to raise cigarette sales. Between 1887 and 1896, several sets of cards were issued. Between 1909 and 1912, more sets were produced, including the 1909 T-206 color lithographed set of 522 cards. A card in this set pictured Honus Wagner, a Pittsburgh National shortstop, now the most desirable and one of the most expensive cards in the sports card hobby world. Only 30 to 50 cards exist (every baseball source quotes a different number). The story is that Honus Wagner opposed cigarette smoking and did not want his face used to endorse cigarettes, especially to children. He insisted the cards be taken out of circulation, but several dozen escaped destruction. These cards have gone on to make history and a fortune for their lucky owners. In 1991, it was reported that Wayne Gretzky, the famous hockey star, bought his Honus Wagner card for $450,000.

Cigarillo

The trade name for a small thin CIGAR, cigarillos range in size from 4 inches to 7 ½ inches. Their ring gauge is below 30. *See also* THE CIGAR AND HEALTH

Cincinnati, Ohio

In June 1994, the city council of Cincinnati voted to remove tobacco advertisements from city bus shelters and buses and to ban all outdoor advertising of tobacco products by June 1996. Cincinnati became the second city, af-

ter BALTIMORE, MARYLAND, to ban tobacco BILL-BOARDS. The ban applied to billboards along highways and in Riverfront Stadium, the home of the Cincinnati Reds and Bengals, in contrast to the Baltimore ban on tobacco ads throughout the city, except in heavily industrialized areas and near stadiums and sports parks.

Cipollone, Rose (1926–1984)

In 1988, a Newark, New Jersey, federal court ruled, for the first time, that a cigarette manufacturer was liable for the death of a smoker and ordered it to pay damages. A New Jersey woman named Rose Cipollone, who had begun smoking at 16 years of age and continued to smoke for 42 years, was diagnosed with lung cancer in 1981. On August 1, 1983, she filed a lawsuit against PHILIP MORRIS COMPANIES INC., Liggett Group Inc., and LORILLARD COMPANY INC., makers of the brands she smoked—VIRGINIA SLIMS, True, and CHESTERFIELD. Seeking unspecified damages, she accused the three companies of failing to provide adequate health warnings and intentionally misleading the public about the dangers of smoking.

On September 21, 1984, in an unprecedented ruling, U.S. District Court Judge H. Lee Sarokin agreed to hear the case, dismissing defense arguments that a federal law requiring health warnings on cigarette packs protected the industry from product liability suits. He said the health warning label, like many government standards, was meant only to fix a minimum level of industry performance, not to provide a shield from liability.

Rose Cipollone died on October 21, 1984, before the case went to trial, but her husband, Antonio, carried on the suit. Explaining why she started smoking, Cipollone said in court papers: "I thought it was cool and lovely and looked nice" ("Turning Points," 1992). After his wife died, Mr. Cipollone amended the complaint to include a wrongful death claim.

On April 7, 1986, the U.S. Court of Appeals for the Third Circuit in Philadelphia ruled that the FEDERAL CIGARETTE LABELING AND ADVERTISING ACT OF 1965, the law requiring warning labels on cigarette packs, protected the tobacco industry from product liability suits, reversing Judge Sarokin's ruling. Cipollone's attorneys appealed to the U.S. Supreme Court. On January 12, 1987, the Supreme Court refused to hear Cipollone's appeal, upholding the circuit court's ruling. Cipollone's case against the cigarette companies continued, but was restricted to events that occurred before January 1, 1966, the date the warning first appeared on cigarette packs.

On February 1, 1988, the case finally went to trial. Cipollone's lawyer, Marc Edell, who had defended asbestos companies in their fight with plaintiffs' lawyers in the 1970s and 1980s, forced the tobacco companies to produce internal memos and research papers on smoking and health. He made the tobacco industry spend an estimated $50 million in legal fees.

On June 13, 1988, the jury in a Newark, New Jersey, federal district court agreed that Rose's cancer had been caused by smoking and that one company, Liggett and Myers, which made the Chesterfields she had smoked primarily, had not warned her of the harmful effects of tobacco prior to 1966—the year government warning labels appeared on cigarette packs. (Philip Morris and Lorillard were let off because Rose smoked their brands after 1966.) The jury did not award Rose's estate any damages because they found the company only 20 percent responsible for her death (New Jersey law requires a finding of 50 percent responsibility), but the jury ordered the company to pay $400,000 in damages to her husband—which was the first time a jury awarded any damages in a tobacco lawsuit.

The cigarette companies asked that the lawsuit be thrown out on the grounds that the federal law that has mandated warnings on cigarette packs since 1966 bars lawsuits based on state law. On January 5, 1990, the circuit court of appeals in Philadelphia set aside the $400,000 judgment. The court ordered that the case be retried, noting the difficulty caused by the "artificial distinction between conduct before and after January 1, 1966" ("Turning Points," 1992). Antonio

Cipollone died five days after the appeals court overturned the $400,000 award.

On December 28, 1990, Thomas Cipollone, a son, filed an appeal to the U.S. Supreme Court (*Cipollone v. Liggett Group Inc.*) and on March 25, 1991, the Court agreed to hear Cipollone's appeal. The Court heard oral arguments on October 8 and 22, 1991, and again on January 14, 1992, when Lawrence Tribe, a Harvard law professor, argued the case for the family in place of Edell. On June 24, 1992, the Court handed down a landmark decision ruling that federal law does not preempt claims by smokers based on the conduct of cigarette manufacturers before 1969, but restricted what claims Cipollone could bring against the companies after 1969, the year Congress, in the Court's opinion, made "substantial changes" to the federal act that mandated warning labels.

Writing for the majority in the 7-to-2 ruling, Justice John Paul Stevens (and Chief Justice William H. Rehnquist, Justices Byron R. White, and Sandra Day O'Connor) wrote that the Federal Cigarette Labeling and Advertising Act, was so narrowly written that it "merely prohibited state and federal rule-making bodies from mandating particular cautionary statements on cigarette labels or in cigarette advertisements" (Sanderson, 1992). But Stevens also wrote that the "broad language" of the amended 1969 law prevented the Cipollones from pursuing two of their claims beyond 1969—that the companies failed to warn the public about the health problems and that they made false claims about the link between smoking and cancer. The justices allowed the family to sue on grounds the cigarette companies breached an "express warranty" that their products did not pose any significant health hazards and that the companies conspired to deprive the public of medical and scientific data on the dangers of smoking.

In a separate opinion, Justice Harry A. Blackmun, writing on behalf of himself and Justices Anthony M. Kennedy and David Souter, argued that all claims should be allowed against cigarette companies. Blackmun wrote that the Court created a crazy quilt by allowing some claims but not others after 1969. In a dissenting opinion, Justice Antonin Scalia argued that the 1969 law protects cigarette companies from any claims under state laws. Justice Clarence Thomas joined Scalia's dissent.

The Court's decision overruled the decisions of five federal courts of appeal, which held that the 1965 Federal Cigarette Labeling and Advertising Act preempted all claims based on the conduct of cigarette manufacturers after the introduction of the warning labels in 1965. The Court made clear that the 1969 act allowed lawsuits that allege the tobacco companies possessed and concealed, or misrepresented, material facts, such as scientific evidence of the dangers of smoking, in channels other than advertising and promotion. These channels could include press releases, toll-free hotlines, and spokespersons on radio and television shows. This meant that failure-to-warn claims can be brought against the industry based on post-1969 as well as pre-1969 conduct.

The Cipollone case was sent back to the U.S. District Court in New Jersey for a retrial, but the loss of Judge Sarokin who was ordered removed as the judge in pending tobacco liability cases because of a perceived bias, the death of Antonio Cipollone, and the lack of enthusiasm in Edell's firm about carrying on an expensive struggle led the Cipollone family to drop the appeal.

References: Bill Sanderson, "Setback for Tobacco Giants," *New York Times*, June 25, 1992, p. A-1.
"Turning Points in Cipollone Case," *The Record*, June 25, 1992, p. A-14.

Civil War. *See* CONFEDERATE GOVERNMENT

Class

Class is one of the major divisions of leaf tobacco based on the distinct characteristics of tobacco caused by differences in varieties, soil, and climate plus the methods of handling, cultivation, and curing. The U.S. government assigns tobaccos of the same type to a common class. Class One includes all flue-cured types; Class Two, fire-cured types; Class Three, air-cured types; Class Four, cigar-filler types; Class Five, cigar binder; Class Six, cigar wrapper; Class Seven, miscellaneous types; and Class Eight, foreign types. *See also* AIR-CURED TOBACCO; BINDER; CIGAR; CIGAR WRAPPER; FILLER; FIRE-CURED TOBACCO; FLUE-CURED TOBACCO; TOBACCO CLASSES

Clemens, Samuel. *See* TWAIN, MARK

Clement, Earle C. (1896–1985)

Former Kentucky congressman and senator and protégé of Senate majority leader Lyndon Johnson in the 1950s, Earle Clement was hired by the six major tobacco companies to be their chief lobbyist and to coordinate a campaign to save the industry from governmental action at a time when stories about health issues of smoking were emerging and beginning to hurt cigarette sales.

Clement advised the manufacturers to play down the health issue, emphasize the importance of cigarettes in the nation's history and economy, remind the media of its financial stake in cigarette advertising, and oppose all regulatory action by the FEDERAL TRADE COMMISSION (FTC) and by state and local governments. But he told the industry to settle for a package warning, if necessary, from Congress rather than risk an FTC-imposed requirement that all advertisements carry a health warning too.

Clove Cigarettes

Clove cigarettes are a mixture of tobaccos and clove spice, rolled into a cigarette. Almost all clove cigarettes are made in Indonesia, where the name for them is *Kreteks*. The smoke of traditional clove cigarettes with brand names like "Djarum" and "Gadang Garum" smells like cloves, not burning tobacco. They are made from dark tobaccos instead of the light or blond tobaccos used in Western-style brands, and have high tar and nicotine yields.

Despite their name, clove cigarettes are primarily made up of tobacco. Because the dark tobaccos produce a harsher smoke, it is believed that cloves are added to make it easier for smokers to inhale the smoke because of the anesthetizing action of eugenol, an active ingredient in cloves. Eugenol has been widely used for years and is regarded as safe by the U.S. FOOD AND DRUG ADMINISTRATION (FDA) when used topically as a dental anesthetic. Clove cigarette users, however, inhale the smoke of burning eugenol. Some scientists believe burning eugenol triggers an acute allergic reaction in some people.

Clove cigarettes constitute an enormous share of the cigarette market in Indonesia. While the government in Jakarta forbade foreign companies from making clove cigarettes, Indonesian clove manufacturers began establishing markets for these cigarettes in Australia, Malaysia, and the United States by the early 1980s.

Coale, John (1946–)

A leading attorney in the Castano class-action lawsuit brought on behalf of 50 million tobacco-addicted smokers, John Coale is a liability lawyer from a wealthy family in BALTIMORE, MARYLAND. A graduate of Baltimore Law School, Coale's career was launched when he got a great deal of publicity collecting clients injured by the releasing of toxic gases in 1984 at the Union Carbide chemical plant in Bhopal, India. He worked with WENDELL GAUTHIER on the case involving the fire in the Dupont Plaza Hotel in San Juan, Puerto Rico. After that, Coale became part of the Castano team of lawyers and represented the Castano group at the June 1997 talks with tobacco executives. At one executive committee meeting, he copied a set of MERRELL WILLIAMS stolen documents and sent them to Congressman Henry Waxman's office. *See also* BROWN AND WILLIAMSON TOBACCO CORPORATION—MERRELL WILLIAMS DOCUMENTS; CASTANO, PETER; *CASTANO V. AMERICAN TOBACCO COMPANY*; TOBACCO SETTLEMENT—JUNE 1997

Coalition on Smoking or Health

In 1982, the AMERICAN CANCER SOCIETY (ACS), AMERICAN LUNG ASSOCIATION (ALA), and AMERICAN HEART ASSOCIATION (AHA) formed the Coalition on Smoking or Health, primarily to coordinate federal legislative activities related to smoking control. Through the coalition, the three voluntary health agencies worked with other organizations. The coalition supported smoking control policies relating to health warning labels, tobacco advertising, airport smoking policies, the tobacco excise tax, and the tobacco price support program. The coalition disbanded in 1996.

Cocke, John Hartwell (1780–1866)

A reformer from Virginia, General John Hartwell Cocke, who cofounded the University of Virginia, adopted anti-slavery, anti-liquor, and anti-tobacco programs. He distributed anti-tobacco tracts to adults and anti-tobacco medals to small boys. A friend of Thomas Jefferson, he stopped raising tobacco leaf and published a sweeping denunciation of the plant entitled *Tobacco, the Bane of Virginia Husbandry.*

Cohausen, Johann

In 1720, a German named Johann Cohausen wrote a satiric commentary about SNUFF:

> I have sometimes wondered to see how lords and lackeys, High Society and the mob, woodchoppers and handy men, broom squires and beadles, take out their snuff-boxes with an air, and dip into them. Box sexes snuff, for the fashion has spread to women: the ladies began it, and are now imitated by the washerwomen. People snuff so often that their noses are more like a dust-heap than a nose; so irrationally that they think the dust an ornament, although, since the world began, all rational men have thought a dirty face unhealthy; so recklessly that they lose the sense of smell and their bodily health.
>
> They snuff without need, at all times, in all places, without rest, as though their fate and fortune, their name and fame, their

life and health, even their eternal salvation depended on it.

Do but notice what grimaces snuff-takers make, how their features are convulsed, how they dip into their snuff-boxes in measured rhythm, cock up their noses, compose their mouths, eyes and all their features to a pompous dignity, and as they perform the solemn rite of snuff-taking, they look as if they scorned the whole world. . . . (Dunhill, 1954)

References: Alfred H. Dunhill, *The Gentle Art of Smoking*, London: Max Reinhardt, 1954, pp. 104–05.

Cohiba Cigar

On October 28, 1492, CHRISTOPHER COLUM-BUS noted in his log that the explorers had met many "Indian" men and women who carried "a little lighted brand made from a kind of plant whose aroma it was their custom to inhale" (Conrad, 1996). The aboriginal Cubans called the plant *cohiba*, a word that has survived 500 years to become the brand name Cohiba, one of the most widely recognized and sought-after cigar brands in the world and a preeminent cigar in Castro's Cuba. It comes in 11 sizes and is one of the 30 brands exported by Cuba.

In Cuba, the Cohiba is a symbol of revolution because the cigar was made for Fidel Castro seven years after the 1959 Cuban revolution brought him to power. It remained his favorite cigar until he gave up smoking for health reasons in the late 1980s.

Eduardo Rivera Irizarri (1941–) is credited with creating the Cohiba, which has an elegant shape that fascinated Castro. Working at the La Corona factory in Havana, Irizarri was a roller of the first rank. Government officials gave Irizarri carte blanche to make Castro's cigars, which soon became a coveted diplomatic gift as well. At first, Castro reserved the Cohibas for his own use and that of associates, but eventually he began handing them out as gifts to heads of state and other foreign visitors.

Because of an economic embargo against Cuba, Cohibas cannot legally be imported into the United States nor, according to Cuban officials, can its trademark and name be registered in the United States.

Despite the Cuban ban, General Cigar Holdings Inc., a New York-based company, began using the Cohiba name in the United States as early as 1978. In 1997, lawyers for Habanos S.A., the Cuban government's cigar exporting and marketing corporation, formally challenged General Cigar's trademark saying its property had been illegally expropriated. Habanos also describes the rival Cohiba as a fraud that neither offers the superior characteristics of its own Cohiba or compares with the quality of any other Cuban brand.

On February 28, 1997, Fidel Castro hosted an event at Havana's Tropicana Club to celebrate the 30th anniversary of the Cohiba and to raise money for Cuban health care. Some 800 people from Europe, Canada, and the United States paid $500 per person to attend. One hundred Americans attended despite warnings from the U.S. government that they could be prosecuted on their return (they were not prosecuted).

Other events associated with the Cohiba anniversary, organized by Habanos S.A., included a trip to the plantations of the Vuelta Abajo, Cuba's premium tobacco-growing region, and a visit for cigar tasting to the newly renovated El Laguito factory, where Cohibas are produced. El Laguito was established in the 1960s as a school to teach women cigar production. Until then, Cuban cigar factories and rolling rooms were almost exclusively male domains. About 180 workers make two million cigars in the El Laguito factory.

A charity auction followed the awards. Humidors, signed by Castro and filled with different sizes of Cohibas, sold for tens of thousands of dollars. After the auction, Castro told the groups that charity cigar auctions of humidors had raised about $1 million for Cuban medical relief. *See also* CIGAR; CUBA; CUBAN TOBACCO HISTORY; VUELTA ABAJO, CUBA

References: Barnaby Conrad III, *The Cigar*, San Francisco: Chronicle Books, 1996, p. 21.

Coleridge, Samuel Taylor (1772–1834)

Samuel Taylor Coleridge, the English poet and critic, wrote about an experience smoking a pipe when he was 18 years old:

> On the assurance that the tobacco was mild, I took half a pipe, filling the lower half of the bowl with salt. I was soon, however, compelled to resign it, in consequence of a giddiness and distressed feeling in my eyes. . . . Soon after, deeming myself recovered, I sallied forth to my engagement. . . . I had scarcely entered the minister's living room, ere I sank back in the sofa in a sort of swoon. . . . My face was like a wall that is white-washing, with cold drops of perspiration running down it from my forehead. . . . I at length awoke from insensibility, my eyes dazzled by the candles which had been lighted in the interim.

College Students and Cigarettes

Tobacco companies have a history of aiming advertising at college students. In 1950, a tobacco industry journal reported that "A massive potential market still exists among women and young adults." At a 1955 press conference, the ad director for PHILIP MORRIS COMPANIES INC. announced "Our ads are now aimed at young people and emphasize gentleness" (Gilbert, 1957).

Philip Morris had targeted college students since the 1930s, but in the late 1950s it established a full-scale campus promotion program. In 1959, Philip Morris paid $50 a month to 165 campus representatives to distribute free cigarettes. Campus reps encouraged fraternities to compete with each other in trying to guess football scores correctly. Scores had to be written on the back of Philip Morris wrappers. Prizes ranged from phonographs and ping-pong tables to trips to Europe. Another contest offered record players in exchange for collected empty cigarette packages. LIGGETT AND MYERS TOBACCO COMPANY awarded cars as prizes in its contests.

For years, the main support of college newspapers and magazines had been cigarette advertising. A 1963 Consumer Union report showed that cigarette ads accounted for an estimated 40 percent of the advertising incomes of 850 college newspapers. The AMERICAN TOBACCO COMPANY campaigned for college sales by giving away samples, advertising LUCKY STRIKES CIGARETTES in college newspapers and football programs and on campus radio stations. The American Tobacco Company aimed its Tareyton brand directly at college students: "Hooray for college students! They're making Dual Filter Tareyton the big smoke on American campuses! Are you part of this movement? If so, thanks. If not, try 'em!"

In 1954, Philip Morris Companies Inc. hired the Gilbert Youth Research Company to survey college students' smoking habits. The survey found that only one out of four college-student smokers started smoking in college. Three out of four college-student smokers chose their brands before entering college. The survey also said general advertising, such as on radio and television and ads in national publications, penetrated the college market and the college mind.

In the fall of 1954, Philip Morris decided that the college market required a "smartly tailored approach." Out of this came the Max Shulman column idea designed to separate Philip Morris from other manufacturers and establish a "climate and receptivity to our sell." In September 1954, humorist Max Shulman started writing "On Campus with Max Shulman." More than one million students and college professors read this column. Philip Morris paid Shulman and for the space in 132 college newspapers. A line at the bottom of the column read: "This column is brought to you by the makers of PHILIP MORRIS, who think you would enjoy their cigarette." The plan worked extremely well and produced "the highest readership and sponsor identity of any advertising" Philip Morris ever placed (Gilbert, 1957).

Cigarette advertisers also pitched cigarettes to college and high school students on plastic-coated book covers that students wrapped around their textbooks. The front cover sported school colors, name, and logos; the back covers carried advertising messages.

In 1953, Lorillard became the first national advertiser to try the back cover. It advertised OLD GOLD CIGARETTES promoting them to students in most of the nation's 1,800 colleges and in more than a third of its high schools.

During the 1960s, college students were exposed to thousands of televised cigarette commercials and increasing numbers of students began to smoke. After the broadcast ban on cigarette advertising in 1971, cigarette smoking among college students fell in the 1970s and early 1980s and remained steady until 1990 when the rate began to increase.

College students and their smoking habits were in the news in the late 1990s. A national survey of about 15,000 students by the Harvard School of Public Health showed that smoking increased substantially in recent years. There were increased rates of cigarette smoking among all students regardless of age, sex, race, type of college, or region of the country. The study found that African American and Asian American students were less likely to smoke than whites. The study appeared in the November 18, 1998, issue of the *Journal of the American Medical Association(JAMA)*.

References: Eugene Gilbert, *Advertising and Marketing to Young People*, Pleasantville, NY: Printers' Ink Books, 1957, p. 184.

Colombia

Tobacco has been important to the Colombian economy for hundreds of years. Tobacco growing became important to the Spanish colonies within 30 years of Columbus's first voyage to the Western hemisphere. Initially, the state was the sole buyer of this product and remained so after independence from Spain in the early nineteenth century. From 1850, when free trade was permitted, until the end of the nineteenth century, tobacco was the principal export. *Tabaco negro* (dark tobacco) was the only variety grown until 1960, when *Tabaco rubio* (light tobacco) production began.

Colombia is the third largest producer of tobacco in Latin America, following Brazil and Cuba. Tobacco agriculture has expanded slightly due to an increase of exports as well as the promotion of tobacco agriculture by the local cigarette manufacturing companies, which provide technical assistance to small growers to increase the yield of tobacco per hectare. In Colombia, the peasant farmer who grows tobacco essentially depends on the cigarette manufacturing industry because the industry sets the prices and loans money to these farmers for each new harvest's expenses.

In 1987, two large cigarette companies were responsible for 92.4 percent of production—Compañía colombiana de Tabaco, S.A., with three factories, and the Productora Tabacalera de Colombia S.A., with one factory. The latter manufactured brands of LIGGETT AND MYERS TOBACCO COMPANY, a multinational tobacco company. The rest of the companies in Colombia are small producers of handmade leaf cigars and *calillas* ("thin" cigars) in the departments of Santander and Valle. In addition, in the tobacco-producing areas such as Sucre and Bolivar departments, cigars and calilas for local consumption are made from tobacco that has been rejected for export purposes.

A substantial illegal trade in foreign cigarettes, especially from the United States, was evident in Colombia in the early 1990s. Through advertising, which is ubiquitous in Colombia, the multinational tobacco companies created a market for U.S.-made cigarette brands in Colombia. This situation was similar to the experience of other Latin American countries that had resisted the entry of multinational tobacco companies into their domestic markets. With intense advertising of illegally sold cigarettes, the domestic industries were subverted and eventually overcome by the multinationals through licensure or direct acquisition.

The cigarette market has changed steadily to the filtered light tobacco, cigarette brands sold by multinational tobacco companies. Because of the increased use of cigarettes, Colombian men and women have experienced increased lung cancer mortality rates directly related to the exposure to cigarettes.

Overall, in Colombia, the largest numbers of smokers are to be found in the low socio-economic stratum, the largest segment of the population. Per capita cigarette consumption in Colombia has been among the highest in countries of the Western hemisphere. *See also* CIGAR; CIGARETTE; GLOBAL TOBACCO USE; LATIN AMERICA

Color of Tobacco Leaves

The color of tobacco leaf is a technical term that involves hue, saturation, and brilliance. In FLUE-CURED TOBACCOS, the most desirable colors are, in order of preference, lemon, orange, red, dark-red, and green.

In Cuba, women called *escogedora* have keen eyes for the color of tobacco leaves that are made into cigars. They can distinguish no less than 68 different tones in the shading of a leaf. *See also* CIGAR; CIGAR WRAPPER

Columbus, Christopher (1451–1506)

In 1492, when Christopher Columbus made his explorations in the Americas, he landed on San Salvador Island where native people offered him food, drink, and handfuls of dried leaves. Columbus noted the following in his journal:

> In the middle of the gulf between the two islands . . . . I found a man alone in a canoe who was going from . . . . Santa Maria to Fernandina. He had food and water and some dry leaves which must be a thing very much appreciated among them, because they had already brought me some of them as a present at San Salvador. (Brooks, 1952)

Later, on another island, Columbus and his men reported seeing people who "drank smoke." In the words of Bartholomio de Las Casas, who edited Columbus' journal,

> They did wrap the tobacco in a certain leaf in the manner of a musket formed of paper . . . having lighted one end of it . . . they sucked, absorbed or received that smoke inside with their breath. (Brooks, 1952)

See also COHIBA CIGAR; CUBA

References: Jerome E. Brooks, *The Mighty Leaf*, Boston: Little, Brown and Company, 1952, p. 11.

Comprehensive Smokeless Tobacco Health Education Act

Passed by the U.S. Congress on February 27, 1986, the Comprehensive Smokeless Tobacco Health Education Act provides for the following:

- Development and implementation of health education programs, materials, and public service announcements to inform the public of the health risks resulting from the use of smokeless tobacco products.
- Public health education technical assistance concerning smokeless tobacco.
- Research on the effects of smokeless tobacco on human health and the collection, analysis, and dissemination of information and studies on smokeless tobacco and health.
- Health warning labels on all smokeless tobacco products and advertisements, except for outdoor billboards, effective February 27, 1987. The labels included the following: WARNING: This Product May Cause Mouth Cancer; WARNING: This Product May Cause Gum Disease and Result in Tooth Loss; WARNING: This Product Is Not A Safe Alternative to Cigarette Smoking.
- Banning of radio and television advertising, effective August 27, 1986.
- Disclosure to the secretary of health and human services of ingredients used in the production of smokeless tobacco as well as the quantity of nicotine in each such product by all manufacturers, packagers, and importers of smokeless tobacco. (U.S. Dept. of Health and Human Services, 1994)

See also HEALTH WARNINGS ON CIGARETTE PACKS AND ADVERTISEMENTS AND SMOKELESS TOBACCO; MARSEE, SEAN

References: U.S. Department of Health and Human Services, *Preventing Tobacco Use Among Young People: A Report of the Surgeon General*, Atlanta: Public Health Service, Centers for Disease Control and Prevention, 1994, p. 258–59, 261.

Comprehensive Smoking Education Act of 1984

After publication of a 1981 FEDERAL TRADE COMMISSION (FTC) report on cigarette advertising, it was clear new warning labels were needed. Most people did not know the specific risks of smoking. Surgeon General C. EVERETT KOOP wanted—but did not get—a warning label on cigarettes that read: "Surgeon General's Warning: Tobacco Contains Nicotine, an Addictive Drug." Although the tobacco companies fought hard against any labels, they agreed to add four warning labels to avoid the addiction warning.

On October 12, 1984, President Ronald Reagan signed the Comprehensive Smoking Education Act. It replaced the previous health warning on cigarette packages and ads with four rotating strongly worded health warnings. They took effect October 12, 1985.

SURGEON GENERAL'S WARNING: Smoking Causes Lung Cancer, Heart Disease, Emphysema, and May Complicate Pregnancy

SURGEON GENERAL'S WARNING: Quitting Smoking Now Greatly Reduces Serious Risks to Your Health

SURGEON GENERAL'S WARNING: Smoking by Pregnant Women May Result in Fetal Injury, Premature Birth, and Low Birth Weight

SURGEON GENERAL'S WARNING: Cigarette Smoke Contains Carbon Monoxide (U.S. Dept. of Health and Human Services, 1994)

The act also required cigarette companies to provide a confidential list of cigarette additives (brand-specific quantities were not required). The bill created a federal OFFICE ON SMOKING AND HEALTH and a new federal interagency council to coordinate and oversee federal and private educational and research efforts concerning health hazards of smoking. The act required the DEPARTMENT OF HEALTH AND HUMAN SERVICES (DHHS) to publish a biennial status report to Congress on smoking and health. *See also* HEALTH WARNINGS ON CIGARETTE PACKS AND ADVERTISEMENTS AND SMOKELESS TOBACCO

References: U.S. Department of Health and Human Services, *Preventing Tobacco Use Among Young People: A Report of the Surgeon General*, p. 258–60. Atlanta: Public Health Service, Centers for Disease Control and Prevention, 1994.

Confederate Government

At first, the Confederate government tried to restrain the growth and manufacture of tobacco. In March 1862, the Confederate Congress passed a joint resolution "recommending the planters of the Confederate States to refrain from the cultivation of cotton and tobacco and devote their energies to raising provisions." Government decrees did not stop tobacco planting or chewing. Finally, An Act to Provide Tobacco for the Army, passed by the Confederate Congress on February 17, 1864, decreed that "one ration of tobacco" be furnished to "every enlisted man in the service of the Confederate States," the first time tobacco rations were supplied at government expense to an American army. (Robert, 1967)

References: Joseph C. Robert, *The Story of Tobacco in America*, Chapel Hill: The University of North Carolina Press, 1949, 1967, p. 120.

Connecticut General Court

The seventeenth-century legal code of Connecticut associated tobacco users with idlers and people who hunted birds for pleasure. In 1647, the Connecticut General Court ordered that no one "under the age of 20 years, nor any other that hath not already accustomed himself to the use thereof" should take tobacco without a physician's certificate that it was "useful for him," plus a license from the court. Tobacco could not be taken in public, or even in the open fields or woods except on journeys of 10 miles or more. A person could smoke at "the ordinary tyme of repast comonly called dynner [sic]," but no more than two could enjoy their after-dinner pipe in the same house at the same time (Heimann, 1960, p. 83).

In New Haven, a fine of sixpence was imposed in 1646 for smoking in public, and in 1655 it was ordered that

> no tobacco shall be taken in the streets, yards or aboute the howses in any plantation or farms in this jurisdiction without dores, neere or aboute the towne, or in the meeting howse, or body of the trayne Souldiors, or any other place where they may doe mischief thereby, under the penalty of 84 pence a pipe or a time, which is to goe to him that informs and prosecuts.(Heimann, 1960, p. 83)

Although the Connecticut magistrates were in theory against tobacco consumption, they recognized its importance as a home industry needing protection. In 1662, the Hartford court held "that whenever Tobacco is landed in this Colony" the master of the vessel or merchant importer should pay the custom master of the port 25 shillings per hogshead. In 1680, the Connecticut governor reported: "We have no need of Virginia trade most people planting so much Tobacco as they spend" (Heimann, 1960, p. 83). After 1700, the New England tobacco crop, concentrated in the Connecticut River valley around the original river towns of Windsor, Hartford, and Wethersfield increased beyond home consumption needs. By 1704, tobacco was exported from Wethersfield to the West Indies. *See also* CONNECTICUT TOBACCO; CONNECTICUT TOBACCO FARMING

References: Robert K. Heimann, *Tobacco and Americans*, New York: McGraw-Hill Book Company, 1960, p. 83–84.

Connecticut Havana. *See* HAVANA SEED

Connecticut Tobacco

When New Englanders withdrew from competing in CIGAR manufacturing, they turned their attention to filling the demand for CIGAR

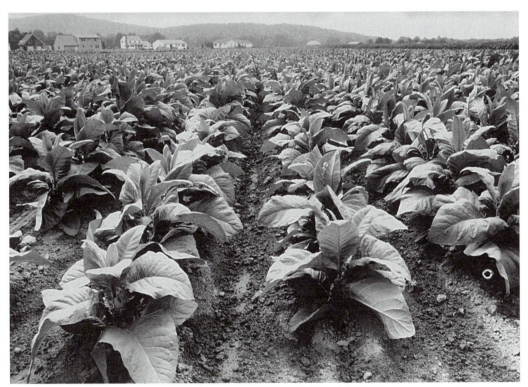

Rows of Connecticut tobacco. ©*Doris Friedman.*

WRAPPER and BINDER leaves. A combination of good soil, adequate rainfall, and abundant sunshine made the Connecticut Valley one of the world's premium tobacco-growing regions. The tobaccos were grown mostly in Connecticut, part of Massachusetts, a small portion of Vermont, and New Hampshire on lands bordering the Connecticut River. They include Connecticut shade-grown used for cigar wrappers, Connecticut broadleaf, and Havana seed used for cigar binders.

The excellent quality of Connecticut tobacco was recognized by the 1850s. As one farm manual published at the time explained,

> The tobacco grown in Connecticut is used for making cigars, but chiefly for the outside, or wrappers for cigars made of imported tobacco. For this purpose only the best leaves are used, and it is in order to obtain these best leaves (the prime wrappers) that the tobacco is cultivated. ("Wrapped Up," 1992)

Shade-grown tobacco, a highly specialized product, is the most expensive tobacco grown in the United States. Filtered sunlight gives the wrapper a light color and a milder taste than sun-grown tobacco. A full-grown Connecticut wrapper leaf plant can grow as high as 10 feet, its giant leaves nearly a half-yard across and twice as long. The leaves are delicate in the field and break easily. *See also* CONNECTICUT GENERAL COURT; CONNECTICUT TOBACCO FARMING

References: "Wrapped Up: Some of the World's Best Cigars Use Connecticut Tobacco Wrapper Leaves," *Cigar Aficionado*, (online) Library Archives, Winter 1992, p. 5.

Connecticut Tobacco Farming

When the first settlers came to the Connecticut Valley in 1635, the native population had already been growing tobacco. The use of CONNECTICUT TOBACCO as a CIGAR WRAPPER leaf began in the 1820s; by 1830, several farmers were experimenting with different seeds. By 1870, more than eight million pounds of tobacco were produced by local farmers. At the time, there were 235 factories making hand-rolled cigars with imported FILLER to-

bacco and Connecticut wrapper leaf. Around 1900, growing wrapper leaf in shaded fields was introduced in the Connecticut Valley. Four years later, Connecticut shade-grown won awards in international competitions. By 1924, 15,000 acres of tobacco were being cultivated under shade in the valley. *See also* CIGAR; CONNECTICUT GENERAL COURT

Connolly, Gregory (1949–)

An expert on spitting-tobacco products, Dr. Gregory Connolly has directed the Massachusetts Department of Public Health's efforts to curb smoking since 1986. A dentist, he also directs the Massachusetts Tobacco Control Program (MTCP), created after voters approved "Question 1" in November 1992. Question 1 established a health Protection Fund with a 25¢ increase in the state's excise tax on CIGARETTES and SMOKELESS TOBACCO.

As director of the MTCP, Dr. Connolly has developed a program that is designed to prevent young people from starting to use tobacco and to reduce their access to tobacco, to persuade and help adults to stop smoking, and to protect nonsmokers from adverse health effects by reducing their exposure to environmental tobacco smoke. The MTCP has more than 300 local programs throughout the state.

Dr. Connolly began his career in public health in the late 1970s as a dentist with the Veterans Administration Hospital in Brockton, Massachusetts. He has been with the state Department of Public Health since 1980 and directs the Office on Non-Smoking and Health.

Dr. Connolly is nationally recognized for his work on smokeless tobacco and was instrumental in the passage of the federal COMPREHENSIVE SMOKELESS TOBACCO HEALTH EDUCATION ACT OF 1986. Besides testifying numerous times before Congress, he has traveled throughout the country educating major league baseball players on the dangers of smokeless tobacco and conducted research on smokeless tobacco use among professional baseball players. He has written over 50 scientific articles for prestigious medical journals such as the *New England Journal of Medicine* and the *Journal of the American Medical Association (JAMA)*.

Connor, Jean (1946–1995)

After Jean Connor, a bank office supervisor and mother of three, contracted lung cancer in 1995 and died, her family filed a wrongful death lawsuit against R.J. REYNOLDS TOBACCO COMPANY. For 22 years, Connor smoked Salem and Winston cigarettes, both manufactured by R.J. Reynolds. Before she died, Connor hired NORWOOD "WOODY" WILNER to represent her, and RON L. MOTLEY teamed up with Wilner. After her death, Connor's claim was continued by her three adult children and her sister.

After a month-long trial in Jacksonville, Florida, the jury found R.J. Reynolds not responsible for the lung cancer death of Connor. The jurors had been instructed by the judge to absolve Reynolds if they found the risks of smoking were "commonly known." Not only did Ms. Connors have access to "common knowledge of smoking risks," in a videotape deposition made before her death, she herself said that she understood the health risks of smoking. She smoked three packs a day of Winston and Salem cigarette brands for 20 years. On camera, she admitted that she had managed to stop, in 1993, after her doctor insisted on it before she had minor surgery. Connor's cancer was discovered shortly after the surgery and she never returned to smoking. *See also* CARTER, GRADY; CIPOLLONE, ROSE; MADDOX, ROLAND; ROGERS, RICHARD

Consolidated Omnibus Budget Reconciliation Act (COBRA) of 1985

Because the tobacco price support program was in jeopardy and needed to be reformed, Title I of the Consolidated Omnibus Budget Reconciliation Act (COBRA) of 1985, Public Law 99-272-April 7, 1986, was enacted to solve problems with the program. The act consisted of agricultural program savings and tobacco program improvements. Congress found that the maintenance of a viable tobacco price support and production adjustment program was in the interests of tobacco producers, purchasers of tobacco, persons employed directly or indirectly by the tobacco industry, and the localities and states whose economies and tax bases are dependent on the tobacco industry.

The purpose of COBRA was to encourage cooperation among tobacco producers, tobacco purchasers, and the secretary of agriculture in reducing price support levels, assessment costs, the size of inventories of producer associations, and the exposure of taxpayers to large budget outlays. By amending the AGRICULTURAL ADJUSTMENT ACT OF 1938 and the Agricultural Act of 1949, COBRA adjusted the method by which price support levels and production quotas were calculated to reflect actual market conditions. It facilitated the purchase and sale of FLUE-CURED and BURLEY TOBACCO in the inventories of producer associations and provided that purchasers and producers of domestic tobacco share equally in the cost of maintaining the tobacco price support program at no net cost to the taxpayers. Finally, the law expedited reform of the system of grading tobacco so that grades assigned to tobacco more accurately reflect the quality of such tobacco.

Because the levels of price support for tobacco resulted in market prices for tobacco that were not competitive on the world market, extremely large quantities of domestic tobacco were put under loan and placed in the inventories of producer-owned cooperative marketing associations that administer the tobacco price support program. The increased inventories led to a significant increase in the assessments producers had to pay to maintain the tobacco price support program on a "no net cost" basis. Because increasingly large assessments created a severe hardship on the producers and posed a threat to the orderly marketing of future crops of tobacco, inventories of producer associations had to be significantly reduced and disposed of, under the supervision of the agriculture secretary, so the tobacco price support program would not collapse. Finally, Congress found that restoring stability to the tobacco price support program through a sharing of the cost of that program by purchasers and producers of tobacco was necessary to prevent undue burdens on interstate and foreign commerce in tobacco. *See also* Tobacco Classes

Corona

Corona is a term applied to a large CIGAR that is cut off squarely at the tuck end and is round and tight. Originally, corona was a size marking for a popular clear Havana cigar in the United States. At one time a Corona was a brand name of a Havana made in Havana, Cuba. The name originally came from the plant and meant the leaves taken from the corona or crown, the top leaves of the *Nicotiana* plant. Later, a manufacturer appropriated the name. For almost 100 years, the corona size has been the most popular. *See also* Cigar Size and Shape

Council for Tobacco Research (CTR)—USA

A nonprofit organization funded primarily by five tobacco companies that contribute in proportion to their revenues, the Council for Tobacco Research (CTR)—USA gave grants to independent researchers who were assured scientific freedom and encouraged to publish their results. A scientific advisory board made up of prominent researchers reviewed grant applications for CTR. Although CTR calls itself "the sponsoring agency of a program of research into questions of tobacco use and health," it has funded grants that sometimes have little connection to the health effects of smoking. Between its inception in 1954 and 1994, CTR gave 1,038 researchers more than $243 million. In 1994, CTR awarded $19.5 million in grants.

Tobacco industry critics argued that, regardless of the eminent scientific advisory board members, CTR funded research that questioned whether tobacco causes disease. In 1994, CTR president James Glenn, a urologist and former dean of the Emory University and Mount Sinai medical schools, testified at Henry Waxman's congressional hearing that it was his personal view that while there are risk factors associated with tobacco use, "[n]o one has been able to demonstrate that smoking, per se, causes any diseases." By funding research through CTR, he said, "we believe that we are providing the best opportunity for understanding the processes and mechanisms of disease, specifically those that are statistically associated with smoking." Arguing that CTR had been unfairly attacked, he said, "I think it is by inference that we are supporting smoking, which is certainly the furthest thing from the truth" (Cohen, 1996, p. 492). During the same testimony, Dr. Glenn named six eminent medical institutions CTR had funded and noted that three of their grantees had subsequently won Nobel Prizes.

A number of institutions and scientific researchers wrestled with the idea of accepting CTR funding. In July 1995, the *Journal of the American Medical Association (JAMA)* published five papers criticizing the tobacco industry's support of scientific research and in an editorial wrote: "Medical schools and research institutions, as well as individual researchers, should refuse any funding from the tobacco industry and its subsidiaries to avoid giving them an appearance of credibility" (Cohen, 1996, p. 488). In December 1995, two journals published by the American Lung Association (ALA) announced they would no longer accept papers if the work was funded by tobacco money. In January 1996, editors of the *British Medical Journal* branded the policy "misguided," and said it was "a threat to medical science, to journalism, and ultimately to a free society" (Cohen, 1996, p. 492).

Some institutions debated the issue of rejecting or accepting tobacco industry monies and accepted the funding. But other academic institutions forbade their researchers from accepting CTR money or funding from its cousin, the Smokeless Tobacco Research Council. In 1994, Boston's Massachusetts General Hospital (part of Harvard Medical School); Roswell Park Cancer Institute, in Buffalo, New York; and Wadsworth

Center for Labs and Research in Albany, New York, barred tobacco industry support.

In early 1996, *Science* magazine interviewed dozens of researchers on both sides of the debate as to whether scientific researchers should take money from the tobacco industry. Defenders like Sydney Brenner, renowned molecular biologist at Scripps Memorial Hospital in LaJolla, California, argued that he viewed his tobacco funding as a gift. Michael Van Dyke, a biochemist at M.D. Anderson Cancer Institute in Houston, Texas, whose researchers voted unanimously in 1995 to turn down tobacco money, said he was thankful for CTR funding and would have applied again. Molecular biologist Lynne Maquat of Roswell Park Cancer Institute said "I was grateful to have received the funds, and it allowed us to take on a project I otherwise would not have been able to do—and it was very productive."

The CTR was dissolved in 1998 as a result of the settlement of the MINNESOTA MEDICAID CASE.

References: Jon Cohen, "Tobacco Money Lights Up a Debate," *Science*, vol. 272, April 26, 1996, pp. 488, 490, 492.

Counterblaste to Tobacco

An anti-tobacco tract written by James I of England in 1604 and published anonymously, the *Counterblaste to Tobacco* argued that the smoking habit resulted in laziness. James I also questioned the medicinal value of the plant. *See also* JAMES I

Crawford, Victor (d. 1996)

An ex-tobacco lobbyist who turned tobacco-control advocate, Victor Crawford worked as a lobbyist for the TOBACCO INSTITUTE from 1985 until his throat cancer was diagnosed in 1991. According to Crawford, an attorney and former Maryland legislator, he made at least $20,000 during the six years he helped the tobacco industry fight public health efforts to restrict smoking. After 1991, Crawford began speaking out against smoking to undo the harm he said he believed he caused as a lobbyist.

Crawford, a Democrat, was elected to the Maryland House of Delegates in 1966 and appointed to the state senate in 1969 to fill a term. He retired from the senate in 1983. A legendary figure at Maryland's state house, Crawford, as a lobbyist for the tobacco industry, buttonholed old friends in the legislature to try to persuade them to drop anti-smoking measures. After he was diagnosed with cancer, Crawford switched gears. In declining health, he spoke out not only about the dangers of smoking but also about the evils of marketing campaigns designed, he said, to hook teenagers on CIGARETTES.

Featured on the CBS news program *60 MINUTES*, Crawford spoke on President Bill Clinton's weekly radio address of August 12, 1995.

Crimean War (1853–1856)

During the Crimean War, the Russians fought an alliance of Turkish, English, French, Austrian, and Italian soldiers. British and French soldiers began smoking the dark-leaf CIGARETTES wrapped with special papers so popular with their Turkish allies as well as their Russian rivals. After the Western European soldiers returned home, they took their cigarette habit with them. When they tried to purchase Turkish and Russian cigarettes, it prompted several tobacco merchants to manufacture them and cash in on the developing fad. *See also* GLOAG, ROBERT

Crow Tobacco Society

The Crow Tobacco Society was a sacred society believed to have been organized after a mystical star-being who appeared on earth and transformed itself into the holy tobacco plant. The society is considered beneficial to the welfare of all the Crow people. Its membership includes both men and women. Initiates are ritually adopted into the society after receiving instructions from their sponsors, completing the required preparations, and assembling payment fees. Then they have the right to sow the seed of *Nicotiana multivalvis,* the holy or medicine tobacco associated with the society. The species is distinct from that grown for ordinary use; it is ritually planted on an annual basis in May, cared for, and harvested by members of the society who observe certain rules between planting and harvesting.

Many subdivisions, or chapters, of the society developed over time, generally as the result of visions. Each chapter possesses unique features, including sacred songs, symbols, and ceremonies.

Cuba

Tobacco has played an important role in the Cuban economy and culture. Today Cuba is the second largest producer and exporter of tobacco in LATIN AMERICA after BRAZIL. Tobacco is one of the country's traditional crops. During CHRISTOPHER COLUMBUS's first voyage, tobacco was seen growing in the eastern part of the island, near Gibara. Tobacco production continues to be an important factor in the Cuban economy, but it has fluctuated over the years with variations caused by adverse climate conditions, pests, and diseases. BLUE MOLD was a problem in 1980.

Tobacco manufacturing is concentrated in rural tobacco-growing areas, and is largely a manual process. Most of the production is for domestic consumption, especially in the case of the CIGARETTE, as opposed to other tobacco products such as cigars, which accounted in 1990 for 15.4 percent of the tobacco consumed in Cuba.

From the earliest times, Cuba has been renowned for growing fine cigar leaf, and superior cigars are synonymous with Cuba. At the top of the scale is the Cuban-made tobacco rolled from leaf grown in the renowned VUELTA ABAJA region where a time-honored pattern of growth, cure, and manufacture by hand ensures the quality. Four other key tobacco-growing districts are Semi-Vuelta, Oriente, Remedios, and Partidos.

The tobacco harvest in Cuba usually begins in January and might last until the end of April. It takes about 80 to 90 days for a tobacco plant to develop from a seed to a full-grown plant ready for picking. Tobacco seeds are grown in special beds and transplanted to fields at a certain height. With constant hoeing, irrigating, and fertilizing, the plants become full grown. Sixteen to 17 leaves of a tobacco plant are picked by hand, tied together in pairs, and hung on long poles in wooden barns. About 100 leaves dry on each pole, a process that takes from 40 to 45 days.

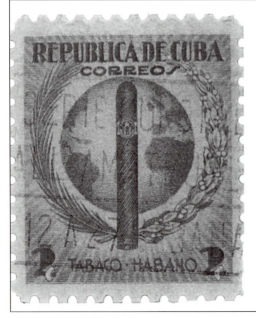 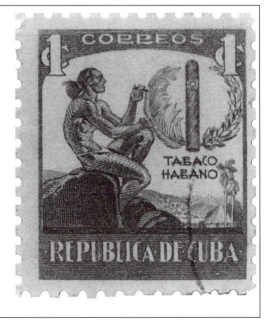

Two stamps depicting cigar manufacturing issued by the Republic of Cuba.

Afterwards, leaves are removed from the poles and placed in piles of 50 leaves in a nearby warehouse. The small piles arranged into larger stacks ferment to remove impurities for about 35 to 40 days. Afterwards, the leaves are stored in warehouses for up to two years in large bales wrapped in burlap. The aging process mellows the tobacco's harsh components.

The Cubans have three names for the tobacco according to where the leaf is on the plant: the *ligero* at the top, *seco* in the middle, and *volado* at the bottom.

Tobacco is stemmed and sorted according to color, size, and texture, and then placed in piles and fermented at high temperatures a second time for about 45 to 60 days, depending on the classification of the tobacco. After the second fermentation, bundled tobacco is aged for up to three years before being sent to one of hundreds of factories on the island. Then the leaves are ready for manufacture. The key factories, mostly in Havana, are Romeo y Julieta, La Corona, H. Upmann, Partagas, and El Laguito. Each factory usually specializes in particular brands and shapes.

Once tobacco is delivered from the warehouses to the factories, the leaves are further classified by color, texture, and size. Then the tobacco goes to the blending rooms. Each cigar brand and shape has its own blend and recipe. Cigar rollers, who have studied a minimum of nine months in schools run by the factories, make an average of 92 cigars a day. Skilled workers, or *torcedores,* who need five to six years to develop, can roll between 100 and 150 cigars a day, depending on the size. It takes 20 years for a cigar roller to become a master *torcedor.* Today, many fine *torcedors* in Cuba are women. After the revolution, they were permitted to be rollers. In 1962, a cigar-rolling school for women was opened in the El Laguito factory.

Cuba has seven grades of cigar rollers. The first three grades perform other functions such as sorting and stemming. Grades four through seven make increasingly more difficult and specialist shaped cigars.

While the rollers blend and shape their cigars, they listen to the *lector de tabaueria* or reader seated up high or in front of them. The man reads aloud from a book while hundreds of men roll cigars in Havana cigar factories. The tradition dates back to the mid-nineteenth century. The reader, paid by the rollers, reads from the daily newspaper and from the works of national heroes such as José Marti, Che Guevara, or Fidel Castro as well as from novels by William Shakespeare and Ernest Hemingway.

Tobacco is Cuba's fourth biggest export behind sugar, nickel, and citrus fruit. The key markets for finished cigars are Spain, France, the United Kingdom, Switzerland, Belgium, Germany, and Asian countries. In 1961, Cuban cigars imports were banned from the United States.

Three branches of the Cuban government oversee the cigar industry. The Ministry of Agriculture manages the growing, the Ministry of Industry controls the production of cigars, and the organization of Cubatabaco under the auspices of the Ministry of Foreign Trade directs the marketing and sales of Cuban cigars. At one time, Cuba sold hundreds of cigar brands, but the number has declined to about 36. *See also* CIGAR; COHIBA CIGAR; CUBAN TOBACCO HISTORY; HAVANA

Cuban Tobacco History

Since 1676, when the first cigar factories appeared in SEVILLE, SPAIN, Cuba, a Spanish colony, shipped tobacco leaf to Spain to be made into cigars. When it was clear that cigars made from Cuban leaf survived the trans-Atlantic voyage much better than the leaf itself, *fabricas,* cigar factories, were born in Cuba. They sprang up from eighteenth-century tobacco plantations, each offering its own brand or brands of cigars.

In 1810, the first names to be registered in Havana's trademark office were the forerunners of the renowned industry. Preserved in the Cuban National Archives is the permit issued for the establishment of one factory and shop that reads: "Francisco Cabanas, born in Havana, single, has opened a shop in Jesus del Monte Avenue, which previously operated at 112 Jesus Maria Street." A factory with 16 workers in 1810, by 1833

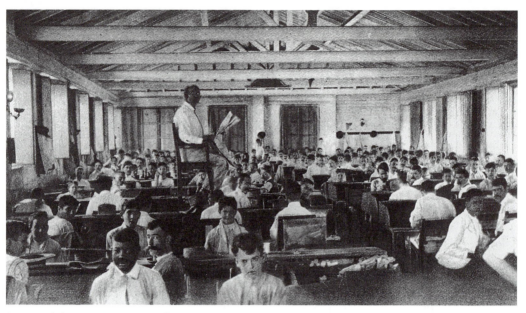

A postcard showing a Havana cigar factory with a reader seated up high.

Cabanas's cigars were selling in a shop in London, England. Between 1830 and 1850, the great brands were founded, many of which survive today: Por Larranaga, 1834; Ramon Allones, 1837; Punch, 1840; H. Upmann, 1844; and LaCorona and Partagas, 1845. In 1850, CIGAR BANDS were introduced on cigars as a way of distinguishing prestigious brands. By 1855, virtually all Cuban cigar makers banded their exports, registered their bands with the government, and advised consumers to insist on buying banded cigars.

After King Fernando VII signed a royal decree in 1817 allowing free trade for the island of Cuba, ships headed for Cuba and distributed Cuban cigars all over the world. The rush for cigars by power brokers, heads of state, kings, presidents, and dictators established the reputation of the Cuban cigar as a symbol of wealth, power, and prestige.

When Fidel Castro came to power on January 2, 1959, Cuban cigar companies, many of which were financed by American firms, were placed under a state monopoly. After Castro nationalized the industry, the decorated cigar bands and cigar boxes disappeared. From at least 960 brands of Cuban cigars that flourished before Castro's takeover, only one new label emerged—the

Siboney, available in four sizes and of uneven quality.

In 1961, the United States imposed a trade embargo on Cuba, in response to Castro's expropriation of more than $1 billion in American businesses. Cuban tobacco could not be imported into the United States. President John F. Kennedy, who signed the embargo order, stockpiled up to 1,000 Havanas before it went into effect so he could have his own personal supply. Some manufacturers still bought Cuban tobacco by going through other countries, but they saw the prices steadily rise from $150 a bale to over $1,000. To offset the price increases and supply problems, importers and distributors replanted operations in Jamaica and the Dominican Republic.

After the world refused to buy Cuba's nationalized cigars, Castro, after consulting with ZINO DAVIDOFF, the most prominent cigar dealer in the world, reintroduced many of the great brands from Cuba's cigar tradition. Eventually, 330 types and sizes were made available. Gradually, after the excellent 1964 tobacco harvest, the Cuban cigar industry regained its quality and reputation. By 1970, the HAVANA had reacquired its status as the best cigar in the world. The Davidoff organization continued its relationship with Cuba until 1989 when it pulled out of Cuba and established itself with better terms and control in the Dominican Republic.

In 1975, the World Court ruled that exiled cigar workers had the right to use their former brand names. Many cigar families, including the the Menendezes of Montecristo and the Cifuentes of Partagas, had left their homelands determined to resume production using their old names. Since many of these families developed their own tobacco and cigar bands, there are now two versions, Cuban and non-Cuban, of prestigious brands such as Partagas, Montecristo, Upmann, Hoyo de Monterrey, and Romeo y Julieta.

During the 1990s, shortages of raw materials, such as fertilizers and packaging, have hampered Cuba's efforts to revitalize its cigar industry. The state company, Cuba tobacco, refinanced and restructured by Spain as Habanos S.A., is doing better.

The majority of cigar factories are located in Havana, including six that were founded in the first half of the nineteenth century. Renamed for communist heroes (in parentheses), they are still called by their original names: H. Upmann (Jose Marti); Partagas (Francisco Perez German); Romeo y Julieta (Briones Montoto); La Corona (Fernando Roig); El Laguito and El Rey del Mundo (Heroes del Moncado). *See also* CIGAR; CUBA

Cured Tobacco

Tobacco leaf is not suitable for smoking when it is harvested; it quickly becomes moldy unless it is cured. There are four main methods of curing:

1. **Flue-cured tobacco** involves the most widely used method, in which tobacco leaves are dried from heat radiating from pipes or flues connected with a furnace. The principal type used in North America and the United Kingdom, flue-cured tobacco forms almost the whole content of cigarettes and a large part of the ingredients of pipe tobaccos;

the leaves turn a bright golden color.
2. **Air-cured tobacco** is made by suspending tobacco leaves on lathes in barns for about five weeks, exposed to a flow of air. The leaves turn a light reddish-brown.
3. **Sun-cured tobacco** requires that leaves be placed in racks in sunshine for set daily periods over four weeks, depending on the weather. The leaves look similar to air-cured ones.
4. **Fire-cured tobacco** leaf is hung in barns, and cured by wood fires lit in trenches. The leaves turn a dark-brown because the smoke comes in direct contact with them.

See also AIR-CURED TOBACCO; FIRE-CURED TOBACCO; FLUE-CURED TOBACCO

Currency in Colonial North America

Because of an unfavorable balance of trade in colonial North America, a shortage of the supply of gold and silver coins resulted. That shortage plus the termination of wampum as currency resulted in the circulation of various commodity currencies. Several colonies that produced crops of tobacco adopted it as legal tender even though leaves were of uneven quality and perishable, not readily divisible, and not as portable as coin.

In the Chesapeake region, tobacco was, in the colonial era, the accepted medium of exchange. Fees, debts, and taxes were paid in cured leaf. In Virginia, Maryland, and other southern colonies, the services of the clergy were paid for in tobacco. In the early eighteenth century, Virginia clergymen received 16,000 pounds of tobacco annually as a salary. When prospective wives arrived at Jamestown in 1619, bachelors and widowers purchased their brides with 120 pounds of Virginia leaf. When the crop became overproduced and adulterated, its status as currency was nullified in 1633.

In the Carolinas, New Jersey, and Pennsylvania, tobacco was one of many media of exchange, circulating alongside items like wheat, corn, pork, and beef. In New York, tobacco coexisted with beaver as a medium of exchange.

In addition to being used for purchasing goods, tobacco currency was also used to pay fines and taxes. For example, owners that allowed Negro slaves to keep horses were fined 500 pounds of tobacco.

The "One Penny Tax of 1673" specified that all tobacco exported from Virginia or Maryland to another colony be taxed one penny per pound. The income from this tax was used to enable the youth of Maryland to attend the College of William and Mary in Virginia. When it was established, the college received as part of its total grant, the right to received income from the tax, arguably the first example of tobacco being used for education.

Currency in Post-World War II Europe

In Germany and other parts of Europe after WORLD WAR II, a currency system based on American CIGARETTES, Luckies, Camels, and Chesterfields in particular, existed from 1945 to 1949. The cigarettes possessed the basic qualifications for a currency: uniform, easily recognizable, universally accepted, fairly durable, divisible, difficult to counterfeit, and easy to carry.

In 1946, the army set up official barter exchanges where soldiers and civilians brought goods for which they received "barter units." The Germans brought valuables to the market where military personnel evaluated them. A silver tea service might be "priced" at 400 units. American soldiers traded toothbrushes, pens, and other products.

At the Berlin Barter Center a carton of cigarettes was valued at first for 20 barter units. After it rose to 95, the chief of staff in Berlin ordered the value drastically cut to 55 barter units. Twenty-three cartons of cigarettes bought a Leica, a famous well-made German camera. Cigarettes also bought works of art and antiques at bargain prices. *See also* CAMEL CIGARETTES; CHESTERFIELD CIGARETTES; LUCKY STRIKE CIGARETTES

D

Dark-Fired Tobacco

Dark-fired tobacco is a synonym for FIRE-CURED TOBACCO, and is another name for DARK VIRGINIA TOBACCO. Dark-fired tobaccos are used in making SNUFF, plug, or twist. *See also* CURED TOBACCO

Dark Tobacco District Planters' Protective Association

The Dark Tobacco District Planters' Protection Association consisted of farmers who opposed tobacco monopolists of the early twentieth century. *See also* NIGHT RIDERS

Dark Virginia Tobacco

Dark Virginia tobacco is a common name for one of the FIRE-CURED TOBACCOS raised principally in the Piedmont and mountain sections of Virginia.

Davidoff, Zino (1906–1994)

The founder of a renowned cigar company that named its Cuban cigars after French wines, Zino Davidoff, was born in Russia to a family that fled the pogroms in a covered wagon in 1912. Zino's father, Henry, a tobacco merchant in Kiev, settled his family in Geneva, Switzerland, where he operated a shop. In his father's shop, Davidoff learned to blend the Turkish-style CIGARETTES that were the favorite of Vladimir Lenin and other Russian exiles in Switzerland. When he was 18, his father sent him to visit tobacco plantations in ARGENTINA, BRAZIL, and CUBA to gain experience in CIGAR making. For two years he worked at a *finca* (tobacco farm) where he developed an appreciation for HAVANA cigars.

In 1929, Davidoff returned to Geneva and opened his shop. An idea came to him to name cigars after French Bordeaux wines. In 1969, when the Davidoff brand was established, the French wine names were retained. Zino associated cigars with the world's greatest wines in the belief that cigars held a place in the epicurean lifestyle.

In 1970, Davidoff sold his shop and brand to Oettinger Imex A.G., a Swiss importer headed by his friend Ernst Schneider. With Davidoff's help, Schneider increased the brand's worldwide presence and expanded into other luxury products such as fragrance and cognac. Davidoff helped his friend launch the Zino brand of Honduran cigars in 1987 and developed the blend for the Dominican Davidoff when Oettinger moved its production there in 1990.

Zino Davidoff wrote a book published in 1967 and entitled *The Connoisseur's Book of the Cigar,* now an out-of-print collector's item. Of the cigar, he wrote: "I owe it everything: my pleasures and my anguish, the joys of my work as well as the pleasant leisure hours it affords." *See also* CUBAN TOBACCO HISTORY

Davis, Ronald M. (1957–)

Dr. Ronald M. Davis has been a renowned figure in tobacco control. Trained in medicine at the University of Chicago, he was elected at 24 to the AMERICAN MEDICAL ASSOCIATION (AMA) House of Delegates. He began speaking out on policy issues like smoking, about which he felt the AMA was out of date. In 1984, he became the first resident physician with full voting authority to serve on the AMA's ruling 16-member board of trustees, where he spoke up about the need for the AMA to be in front on the smoking issue. As a result, in 1985, the AMA sent a spokesman to testify before Congress in favor of making the higher federal cigarette tax permanent.

Dr. Davis also endorsed an extension of the ban on broadcast advertising of CIGARETTES to include all forms of advertising of the product as well as on all forms of promotion, including cultural and sports events that carried the name of cigarette brands.

When U.S. Representative MIKE SYNAR of Oklahoma introduced a House bill to impose the sweeping ban, Davis was sent to testify in its favor in 1986.

After his residency, Dr. Davis joined the preventive medicine training program at the Public Health Service's CENTERS FOR DISEASE CONTROL AND PREVENTION (CDC) and was sent to the DOMINICAN REPUBLIC to oversee government immunization efforts. There, he observed the saturation of cigarette advertising, including street signs that bore the MARLBORO design, colors, and logo.

In 1987, Davis became director of the OFFICE ON SMOKING AND HEALTH where he became a forceful anti-smoking advocate. After four years, he left the job. His budget never allowed him to carry out studies into the possible dangers of tobacco additives that the industry was using according to lists provided to his office under the 1984 cigarette labeling law. He became chief medical officer, the ranking public health official for the Michigan Department of Public Health. Now director of the Center for Health Promotion and Disease Prevention, Henry Ford Health System, Dr. Davis also edits TOBACCO CON-TROL, an international journal published in London, England. *See also* ADVERTISING AND CIGARETTES AND SMOKELESS TOBACCO

Day One

On February 28 and March 7, 1994, ABC's news magazine television program *Day One* reported that cigarette companies controlled the content of nicotine in cigarettes as a way of increasing the pleasure of inhaling and as a way of possibly addicting smokers. The report, titled "Smokescreen," directly accused the tobacco industry of "artificially spiking" cigarettes with nicotine to keep smokers hooked. It charged that tobacco companies used a secret process that included adding a "nicotine rich" tobacco extract from outside suppliers. Fifteen months in the making, the report, which focused on R.J. REYNOLDS TOBACCO COMPANY but in essence accused all major cigarette makers, was later mentioned on ABC's *World News Tonight*, *World News This Morning*, *Nightline*, and *20/20*. The report later won the 1994 George Polk Award in the category of network television reporting.

The industry immediately denied the allegations, saying it never added any nicotine that wasn't in the original leaf. In March 1994, PHILIP MORRIS USA, the largest of the U.S. companies, brought a $10 billion libel suit against ABC News arguing that it made false, defamatory, and reckless statements about how Philip Morris makes cigarettes. Filed in RICHMOND, VIRGINIA, the lawsuit, the biggest libel claim on record, said that Philip Morris suffered "massive harm" as a result of statements made on *Day One*. R.J. Reynolds filed a similar lawsuit in February 1995.

In what one newspaper called "an extraordinary act of contrition," ABC News publicly apologized twice, on August 21 and August 24, 1995, for asserting in a news program that two giant tobacco companies added extra nicotine to their cigarettes. The apologies were read during halftime on "Monday Night Football" and during *Day One*. The statement said, in part: "We now agree that we should not have reported that Philip Morris and R.J. Reynolds add significant amounts of nicotine from outside sources. We apologize to our audience, Philip Morris and Reynolds" (Lander, 1995)

Under the terms of the settlement, ABC reportedly paid at least $15 million dollars in legal fees incurred by Philip Morris and R.J. Reynolds, making it one of the costliest settlements of a libel case.

The case against ABC turned on a single word: "spike." In its report on how Philip Morris made cigarettes, ABC argued the company "spiked" cigarettes by adding nicotine in the manufacturing process. Philip Morris said ABC misconstrued the process. In almost all its cigarettes, Philip Morris said it uses reconstituted tobacco with a lower nicotine content than pure tobacco. The lower nicotine results because Philip Morris removes the nicotine when it manufactures the filler. After the filler is rolled into the cigarette, the company adds back the nicotine to heighten its flavor. As a result, Philp Morris contends it is "recombining" ingredients, not spiking the cigarettes.

The out-of-court settlement drew harsh criticism from opponents of cigarette smoking as well as from John Martin, the correspondent for the *Day One* segment and his producer, Walt Bogdanich, both of whom opposed the agreement and reportedly declined to sign it. The two journalists hired separate lawyers and refused public comment. They both received new contracts. ABC lawyers concluded that secret cigarette industry documents obtained from Philip Morris in the course of pretrial fact finding did not support the broadcast's statement about spiking cigarettes with nicotine and ABC corporate management signaled it wanted a settlement. The settlement stunned people in the news media who expected ABC to defend itself. According to Jonathan Alter, "Much of ABC News was devastated by the deal" (Alter, 1995). *See also* David Kessler

References: Jonathan Alter, "The Cave in on Tobacco Road," *Newsweek*, September 4, 1995, p. 29.

Mark Lander, "ABC News Settles Suits on Tobacco," *New York Times*, August 22, 1995, pp. A1, D6.

Daynard, Richard (1943–)

A professor of law at Northeastern University School of Law, Richard Daynard is president of the Tobacco Control Resource Center and chairman of the Tobacco Products Liability Project, an advocacy group and clearinghouse that supports litigation against tobacco companies as a public health strategy. He is editor-in-chief of the *Tobacco Products Litigation Reporter*. Daynard is widely regarded as one of the most influential attorneys in the third wave of tobacco litigation—the explosion of lawsuits from 1994 until the present characterized by a focus on the behavior of cigarette executives.

He has conducted broad-ranging research in tobacco control policy from 1975 to the late 1990s, authored dozens of publications, and lectured on tobacco control policy to lawyers, doctors, and public health professionals in 10 countries. He comments frequently to national and international media. *See also* Tobacco Litigation: First, Second, and Third Waves

Death in the West

In 1976, filmmaker Peter Taylor went to the western plains of the United States and interviewed six real-life American cowboys for his 27-minute documentary film titled *Death in the West*. Taylor contrasted the macho image of the Marlboro Man, a rugged cowboy featured in Marlboro cigarette ads, with the lives of six cowboys, all heavy smokers at one time and all suffering from lung cancer or emphysema. The filmmaker mixed in statements from doctors who blamed heavy smoking for the cowboys' diseases. Taylor also interspersed Marlboro cigarettes commercials and interviews with two executives of the Philip Morris Companies Inc. (makers of Marlboros) who refused to concede the health hazards of smoking. Here are several excerpts from the documentary:

- Bob Julian (a Wyoming cowboy stoking a campfire) stated, "I started smoking when I was a kid following these bronco busters. I thought that to be a man you had to have a cigarette in your mouth. It took me years to discover that all I got out of it was lung cancer. I'm going to die a young man." (He died a few months after the interview at 51.) "In my opinion, Mr. Julian has lung cancer directly as a result of his smoking," said the doctor.

- John Holmes (a New Mexico cattle-man with emphysema shown riding the range with an oxygen tank draped over his horse, tubes running into his nose) said, "I just have to stop and gasp for breath and it feels like someone has their fingers down in my chest cutting all the air passages off." "Cigarette smoking, I'm sure, is the cause of John Holmes' pulmonary emphysema," said his doctor.

Shortly after *Death in the West* was shown on British television, the American Cancer Society's and CBS-TV's news magazine *60 Minutes* expressed interest in American broadcast rights to the film. Philip Morris went to High Court in London to prevent Thames Television from selling the film or showing it again. Thames and Philip Morris secretly settled out of court. All copies of the film except one (locked in Thames's vault) were handed over to Philip Morris.

On December 1, 1981, Dr. STANTON GLANTZ, an associate professor at the University of California at San Francisco, received a copy of *Death in the West*. Five months later, in May 1982, *Death in the West* was shown again on television in San Francisco. By the time the film was shown in the United States, five of the six cowboys were dead.

In December 1983, Pyramid Film and Video of Santa Monica, California, a major supplier of educational films in the United States, made copies of *Death in the West* available. A five-lesson curriculum for fifth through tenth graders was developed from the film by researchers at the University of California at Berkeley and the AMERICANS FOR NONSMOKERS RIGHTS (ANR). *See also* AMERICAN CANCER SOCIETY (ACS)

References: "Death in the West," British Broadcasting Company, 1976; 32 minutes, color. Distributed by Pyramid Film and Video.

DeNoble, Victor and Mele, Paul

On April 28, 1994, two PHILIP MORRIS USA researchers, Victor DeNoble and Paul Mele, appeared before the Subcommittee on Health and the Environment of the House Committee on Energy and Commerce to testify about their research at Philip Morris from 1980 to 1984.

Both men worked for Philip Morris at the company's research labs in RICHMOND, VIRGINIA. They described how they used experimental techniques developed by the National Institute on Drug Abuse (NIDA) to determine the addiction potential of NICOTINE in rats. DeNoble's and Mele's experiments involved primarily nicotine self-administration studies in rats. They found that rats would self-administer nicotine—one of the hallmark characteristics of an addictive drug. The rats also developed the condition known as "tolerance" to the drug. As time went on, they needed more nicotine to achieve the same effect. Although the implications of the study were enormous for Philip Morris, DeNoble pointed out that a single observation in rats was not enough to project the results to humans with any scientific certainty.

DeNoble and Mele's work held great interest for top Philip Morris executives. According to their testimony, in mid-1983 they were flown to New York to brief senior management on their work. Then in November 1983, the president of Philip Morris, Shep Pollack, flew to Richmond to observe rats injecting nicotine in one of DeNoble and Mele's self-administration experiments. At that time, DeNoble informed Pollack that the procedures he observed were "exactly the same tests" NIDA uses to "determine whether a drug has a potential for abuse" (Kessler, et al., 1996).

Despite Philip Morris's interest in their work, DeNoble and Mele were abruptly terminated in April 1984, due to concerns that their findings could be used against the company in product liability lawsuits. DeNoble was told to shut down his experiments, kill the rats, and clear out his office. Subsequently, Philip Morris threatened the two researchers, who had signed confidentiality agreements covering the work they had done for the company, with litigation if they disclosed their research activities in journals or at public forums.

DeNoble and Mele found other jobs but wanted to publish their work. At the end of 1985, they took the risk and resubmitted their paper to *Psychopharmacology*. They also delivered a paper on rat tolerance to nicotine to the Federation of American Societies for Experimental Biology. Philip Morris sent the researchers a warning letter. After hearing about DeNoble and Mele's troubles with Philip Morris, the FOOD AND DRUG ADMINISTRATION (FDA) asked them to help the agency with its inquiries into the tobacco industry. Denoble and Mele's paper was received by Congressman Henry Waxman's Health and Environmental Subcommittee. Waxman released the paper from his office in March 1994, forcing Philip Morris to release the men from the confidentiality agreement. The release of DeNoble and Mele's research showing at least one tobacco company had knowledge of nicotine's potential for addiction gave the Food and Drug Administration one of its first insights into the internal knowledge and actions of a tobacco company.

References: David Kessler et al, "The Food and Drug Administration's Regulation of Tobacco Products," *The New England Journal of Medicine*, vol. 335, no. 13, September 26, 1996, p. 989.

Department of Health and Human Services (DHHS)

A cabinet-level department in the United States government, the Department of Health and Human Services (DHHS) resulted from the reorganization of the Department of Health, Education, and Welfare (HEW). In 1979, when the Department of Education Organization Act was signed into law, providing for a separate Department of Education, HEW became DHHS on May 4, 1980.

Agencies in the DHHS that concern themselves with tobacco-related diseases, control, and prevention are the OFFICE ON SMOKING AND HEALTH; the CENTERS FOR DISEASE CONTROL AND PREVENTION (CDC); the FOOD AND DRUG ADMINISTRATION (FDA); the NATIONAL CANCER INSTITUTE (NCI), the largest of 17 biomedical research institutes and centers at the National Institutes of Health located in Bethesda, Maryland; and the National Institute on Drug Abuse, also part of the National Institutes of Health.

Diaz del Castillo, Bernal (c. 1492– c. 1581)

Bernal Diaz del Castillo, a Spanish soldier and historian, observed the following after-dinner custom of Montezuma, Aztec ruler of Mexico at the time of Spanish conquest:

> They also set upon the table three painted and gilded tubes containing liquidambar mixed with a certain plant they call *tobaco*; and when he finished eating, after they had sung and danced for him, and the table was cleared, he took the smoke of one of those tubes, and little by little with it he fell asleep. (Heimann, 1960)

References: Robert K. Heimann, *Tobacco and Americans*, New York: McGraw-Hill Book Company, 1960, p. 20.

Dickens, Charles (1812–1870)

English novelist Charles Dickens was not as avid a smoker as his friend WILLIAM MAKEPEACE THACKERAY, but he did indulge in tobacco. Dickens has a cigar named after him. According to *Tobacco Talk,* in 1897 "The London tobacco manufacturers elected to pay Charles Dickens a Cuban compliment. A neat little cigar costing only a penny, was devised and christened the 'Pickwick,' which still retains its popularity" (Infante, 1985, p. 259).

One tobacco habit Dickens deplored was the careless spitting he encountered in the United States. In his *American Notes* published in October 1842, Dickens commented on the presence everywhere of spittoons, or spit-boxes, for people who chewed tobacco.

In the court of law the judge has his spittoon, the crier, his, the warden his, and the prisoner his; while the jury-men and spectators are provided for as so many men who, in the course of nature, must desire to spit incessantly. In the hospitals, the students of medicine are requested by notices upon the wall to eject their tobacco-juice into the boxes provided for that purpose and not to discolour the stairs. In public buildings visitors are implored through the same agency to squirt the essence of their quids, or "plugs," as I have heard them called by gentlemen learned in this kind of sweet-meat, into the national spittoons, and not about the bases of the marble columns. In some parts this custom is inseparably mixed up with every meal and morning call, and with all the transactions of social life. (Infante, 1985, p. 258)

References: G. Cabera Infante, *Holy Smoke.* London: Faber and Faber, 1985, pp. 258, 259.

DiFranza, Joseph (1954–)

A family physician in Fitchburg, Massachusetts, as well as a member of the Department of Family and Community Medicine at the University of Massachusetts Medical School in Worcester, Joseph DiFranza has done research on the promotion of CIGARETTES to children. In 1991, Dr. DiFranza and six other authors published a landmark study about how children respond to OLD JOE CAMEL, the cartoon character used to advertise CAMEL CIGARETTES. Titled, "RJR Nabisco's Cartoon Camel Promotes Camel Cigarettes to Children," it was one of three studies published in the December 1991 issue of the *Journal of the American Medical Association* (*JAMA*).

R.J. REYNOLDS TOBACCO COMPANY, maker of Camel cigarettes, served subpoenas on DiFranza and on JOHN P. PIERCE of the University of California, San Diego, and PAUL FISCHER of the Medical College of Georgia, lead authors of the other two papers published in the same *JAMA* issue. The subpoenas arose from a lawsuit filed in December 1991 in San Francisco Superior Court by attorney Janet Mangini. She charged Reynolds with violating California's Unfair Business Practices Act by distributing T-shirts, mugs, and other items without including the surgeon general's warning that appears on cigarette advertising. Cited in the suit were the papers by DiFranza, Fischer, and Pierce published in *JAMA*.

The tobacco company requested the researchers' materials, notes, and correspondence, along with the name of children interviewed in the studies. After DiFranza received a court order to obey the subpoena, he turned over his files, minus the children's names, to Reynolds. After the judge exempted DiFranza from identifying his subjects, Reynolds withdrew its request for the names, but argued that it needed the papers to check up on whether the studies were biased or possibly fraudulent.

Reynolds turned over the research documents to a reporter from the company's hometown newspaper, the *Winston-Salem Journal,* after the tobacco company concluded DiFranza's work was slanted by an anti-tobacco bias. RJR wanted "to set the record straight" by letting a reporter read them. In her article, "Study on Old Joe Ads May Be Flawed," *Journal* business reporter Stella Eisele reported that Dr. DiFranza had a bias against the cigarette company. She quotes him as acknowledging that a potential bias was introduced into the study by the order in which he asked questions. In response to the reporter's accusation that he omitted data that didn't support his conclusions, Dr. DiFranza said Reynolds and Eisele misinterpreted his notes and hand-drawn graphs.

Dr. DiFranza authored two more studies in 1992. In one study published in the August 1992 *Journal of Family Practice*, he concluded that a tobacco industry campaign called "Tobacco: Helping Youth Say No" portraying smoking as an adult activity actually encourages children to smoke by making it appear to be a forbidden fruit. He said that scientific studies have shown that an approach that encourages children to make mature decisions about smoking actually makes them more likely to smoke.

In his second study published in the September 1992 *American Journal of Public Health,* the doctor said that a TOBACCO

INSTITUTE'S 1989 campaign called "It's the Law" did not discourage stores from selling cigarettes to children. The "It's the Law" campaign involves the distribution to stores of literature and signs pointing out that the sale of tobacco to children is illegal. DiFranza found that 86 percent of stores participating in the program sold cigarettes illegally to children. Four years later, in another piece published in the February 1986 *American Journal of Public Health,* DiFranza found merchants participating in the "It's the Law" program were just as likely to make illegal sales as those merchants who were not participating in the program.

Diversification

In the late 1950s, cigarette companies began diversifying. Tobacco companies, once confined solely to making one or two brands of cigarettes, branched out and bought businesses of all kinds. Recognizing that health campaigns were stepping up, that new generations were learning about the dangers of smoking, and that a single-product business was vulnerable to unforeseen challenges, the big cigarette suppliers in the United States and Great Britain began to ease themselves out of complete dependence on tobacco in general and CIGARETTES in particular.

Other motives have also been attributed to tobacco industry diversification. One explanation holds that tobacco companies are afraid of product liability suits and hope diversifying protects as many assets as possible. According to Professor Robert H. Miles, author of *Coffin Nails and Corporate Strategies,* tobacco companies were looking for legitimacy when they bought consumer products and insurance companies.

After diversifying, tobacco companies dropped the word "tobacco" from their main corporate files and stepped up the acquisitions of companies outside their industry or engaged in mergers. To reflect its diversification, the R.J. REYNOLDS TOBACCO COMPANY became R.J. Reynolds Industries and then RJR NABISCO HOLDINGS CORPORATION in 1987. In 1969, the AMERICAN TOBACCO COMPANY be-

came American Brands. In England, Imperial Tobacco eventually incorporated as Imperial Group. In 1974, BROWN AND WILLIAMSON TOBACCO CORPORATION became Brown and Williamson Industries. Philip Morris and Lorillard never had the word tobacco in their names.

Philip Morris led the way in diversifying. In 1957, it acquired Milprint, a manufacturer of packaging, some of which could be used for cigarettes, and in 1958 Polymer Industries, a chemical company. In the 1960s and 1970s, Philip Morris acquired consumer goods, including American Safety Razor, Burma-Vita, Clark Gum, and Miller Brewing Company. Later, Philip Morris diversified into land development.

In 1956, R.J. Reynolds amended its corporate charter to permit investment in nontobacco enterprises. In 1963, it turned to convenience foods and beverages, recognizing the growth potential in this industry. The company purchased Pacific Hawaiian Products, Vermont Maid syrup, My-T-Fine desserts, and other food and consumer products. It also diversified into petroleum and packaging and in 1969 brought into the corporation Sea-Land Service, the world's largest containerized freight operation that speeds cargoes of every kind across continents and oceans.

American Tobacco diversified in 1966, when it purchased Sunshine Biscuits and James Beam Distilling Company and later acquired Swingline, a manufacturer of office equipment; Acme Visible Records; Master Lock; and Andrew Jergen, a cosmetics company. By 1970, half of American Tobacco's sales and profits were derived from non-tobacco products and services. To signal its independence from cigarettes, the company changed its name to American Brands Inc.

Liggett and Myers followed American into the liquor business by purchasing control of Paddington, the importer of J and B Scotch, Bombay Gin, and other brands, and Star Industries, a liquor distributor. It controlled Allen Products, the canner of Alpo dog food and a leader in that industry. In 1976, LIGGETT AND MYERS TOBACCO COMPANY changed its name to Liggett Group to signal its new composition.

Lorillard purchased Usen Canning, the second largest firm in the cat food business, then Golden Nuggets Sweets, a candy manufacturer. Unable to make a go with candy and pet foods and unable to expand its cigarette business, Lorillard was acquired by Loews Corporation in 1969.

The anti-smoking movement feared diversification would hamper their efforts to destroy the tobacco companies of the 1960s. Tobacco companies began to take over corporations that advertised heavily in newspapers, and magazines. Tobacco control advocates feared tobacco advertising clout would encourage publications to ignore or de-emphasize the dangers of smoking. *See also* LORILLARD COMPANY INC.; PHILIP MORRIS COMPANIES INC.

Doctors Ought to Care (DOC)

Doctors Ought to Care (DOC), a national nonprofit organization of health professionals founded in 1977 and located in Houston, Texas, is renowned for its national advertising campaign to counteract the promotion of what it calls lethal lifestyles, especially tobacco advertising. DOC was founded to try to bring to the public's attention, in innovative and offbeat ways, the major preventable causes of poor health and high medical costs and to increase activism within the medical profession.

DOC counters these problems with advertising campaigns. It was the first organization to buy advertising space to counter seductive imagery found on buses, subways, and billboards. DOC pays for counter ads that spoof real tobacco ads and has sponsored a Dead Man Chew Softball Tournament, an Emphysema Slims Celebrity Tennis Tournament, and a Smoke-Free Jazz Fest.

In 1993, when DOC decided to undermine the Marlboro Adventure Team's United States debut, it repainted a Volkswagen van, calling it a Barfmobile. It printed thousands of Barfboro Barf Bags—in red and white, Marlboro package colors—and created the Barfboro Barfing Team. In 1994, the Barfing Team coordinated dozens of community activities designed to get young people to laugh at the Marlboro Adventure team. It sells a Barfboro line of items, including lunch bags, posters, T-shirts, stickers, pins, and posters titled "Virginia Slime" and "New Corpse" as well as a "Throw Tobacco Out of Sports" cardboard boomerang. DOC's *Journal of Medical Activism* covers its activities.

DOC was the creation of Dr. ALAN BLUM, a family practitioner, who got the idea for the organization while he was speaking to cigarette-puffing teens at a drug rehabilitation clinic. By the end of his talk, in which he made fun of ads in the teen magazines, he noticed that everyone had put out their cigarettes. *See also* MARLBORO CIGARETTES

Dogs and Cigarette Testing. *See* AUERBACH, OSCAR

Doll, Richard and Hill, A. Bradford

In September 1950, four months after the ERNST L. WYNDER and EVARTS GRAHAM study appeared ("Tobacco Smoking as a Possible Etiological Factor in Bronchiogenic Carcinoma"), the *British Medical Journal* carried the first preliminary report on the same subject of smoking and lung cancer by Drs. Richard Doll and A. Bradford Hill. Doll, a scholar-biostatistician on Britain's Medical Research Council, and Hill, his colleague, examined the smoking rates of 1,732 cancer patients at 20 London hospitals and compared them with 743 non-cancer patients. In "Smoking and Carcinoma of the Lung," their 1950 article, they concluded lung cancer occurred at a higher percentage in smokers. While Doll and Hill obtained data similar to those of Wynder and Graham, the British study incriminated smoking more than the American study finding that heavy smokers were 50 times as likely as nonsmokers to contract lung cancer.

After the final Doll-Hill report on London hospital patients was published, the *British Medical Journal* wrote in late 1952 that it was "incumbent on tobacco manufacturers" to undertake intensive research on the chemical ingredients of smoke to try to isolate carcionogenic agents "so that smoking will become a less dangerous occupation than it appears to be now" (Kluger, 1996).

Doll and Hill also gathered information on smoking behavior from nearly 40,000 physicians in Great Britain aged 35 years and older who returned questionnaires. The researchers kept track of the doctors for four and a half years, obtaining death certificates whenever deaths occurred. In a 1954 article entitled "The Mortality of Doctors in Relation to Their Smoking Habits" published in the *British Medical Journal* (June 26 issue), they concluded that "Mild smokers are 7 times as likely to die of lung cancer as nonsmokers, moderate smokers are 12 times as likely to die of lung cancer as nonsmokers, immoderate smokers are 24 times as likely to die of lung cancer than nonsmokers" (Whelan, 1984). *See also* AUERBACH, OSCAR; FILTERED CIGARETTES

References: Kluger, *Ashes to Ashes*, New York: Alfred A. Knopf, 1996, p. 148.

Elizabeth M. Whelan, *A Smoking Gun: How the Tobacco Industry Gets Away with Murder*, Phildelphia: George F. Stickley Co., 1984, p. 85.

Dominican Republic

Tobacco is a major agricultural product in the Dominican Republic. Most tobacco agriculture is in the north part of the island.

In the early 1990s, E. León Jiménez, a subsidiary of the PHILIP MORRIS COMPANY INC. controlled 70.7 percent of the market while the state-owned company, Compañia Anónima Tabacalera, which became a subsidiary of R.J. REYNOLDS TOBACCO COMPANY, controlled 29.3 percent. There are other manufacturing companies, but they are mainly involved in CIGAR production.

The multinational tobacco companies, especially Philip Morris, succeeded in shifting both consumer tastes and national revenue from dark tobacco produced by a national monopoly to Virginia (blond) tobacco manufactured primarily under the cachet of the world's most widely marketed consumer product, MARLBORO CIGARETTES. Heavily promoted throughout the country,

Marlboros have been the most popular brand in the Dominican Republic.

In the 1990s, the Dominican Republic became one of the world's largest producers of hand-made premium cigars. Yaque Valley, the prime tobacco growing region in the country, is one of two of the world's greatest locations for growing premium cigar tobacco. (VUELTA ABAJO, CUBA, is the other premier location). Cigar tobacco farming is centered around the tobacco villages of Villa Gonzalez, Jacagua, Navarette, La Canela, Palmar, and Las Cienagas in the Yaque Valley. Because each village has its own climate and soil type, the character of the tobacco differs depending on the village where it is grown.

Three key tobacco types are grown in the Dominican Republic for premium cigars. Piloto, with its intense flavor, is the best, with its seed originating in Cuba's Vuelta Abajo. San Vincente, a hybrid of piloto that also developed in the Vuelta Abajo, is slightly less powerful than piloto. The third type, Olor, is neutral in flavor. Cigar producers use varied amounts of all three in their blends.

Most cigars produced in the dozens of Dominican factories are a blend of tobaccos from nations other than CUBA, including Nicaragua, Honduras, Ecuador, BRAZIL, Indonesia, Mexico, Cameroon, and the United States. For the most part, Dominican tobacco is used for FILLER, although some cigar makers use it for BINDER as well. *See also* LATIN AMERICA

Drake, Sir Francis (c. 1540–1925)

In 1573, Sir Francis Drake brought quantities of tobacco leaves and seeds as well as West Indian clay pipes from the West Indies to England. In 1586, he brought back pipes and tobacco from Virginia as well as from the West Indies. The imports led to the PIPE becoming a national institution of England.

Duke, James Buchanan (1856–1925)

James Buchanan "Buck" Duke revolutionized the tobacco industry by building a corporate structure. His modern approach to the tobacco business through the use of large-scale capital, modern machinery, aggressive sales-manship, and monopolistic organization made him famous. Buchanan, who was named in honor of Democratic President James Buchanan, was the third child of Artelia and Washington Duke, a North Carolina tobacco farmer. Armed with a six-month business education in bookkeeping and accounting, Buchanan began a formal partnership in 1878 with his father. The company was called W. Duke Sons and Company.

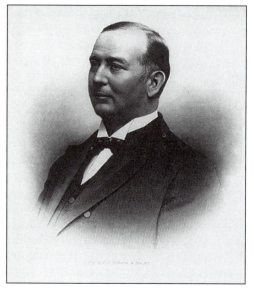

James Buchanan Duke was president of the American Tobacco Company. *North Carolina Division of Archives and History.*

Unable to compete with the manufacturers of BULL DURHAM SMOKING TOBACCO, James Duke decided in the 1880s to go into the business of CIGARETTES, a product popular in England and growing in demand in New York circles. A key factor in his decision to manufacture cigarettes was a bill in Congress to reduce the federal cigarette tax from $1.75 per 1,000 to 50¢.

After Duke set up a team of hand rollers in Durham, he investigated the BONSACK MACHINE, invented by James Bonsack of Virginia, that made cigarettes on a continuous rod principle—an endless tube of wrapped tobacco that was cut by a circular saw to produce 200 cigarettes a minute. He figured that smokers would end up preferring "tailor mades" or manufactured cigarettes to the roll-your-own type. In 1883, Duke ordered two for his Durham, North Carolina, factory and began replacing hand rollers with machines. After the machines proved to be both productive and profitable, Duke, in 1885, made a contract with Bonsack to use the machines on a royalty basis, which made Duke's firm the first company to produce machine-made cigarettes on a large scale. The Bonsack Company also agreed in a secret codicil to rebates if it leased its machines to other manufacturers.

Duke realized that cigarettes appealed to urban dwellers and knew the marketing of the output of the Bonsack machine required global selling and distribution organizations. In 1884, Duke established a branch in New York City, set up a factory, and developed national and international purchasing, distributing, and marketing techniques and networks. Duke, who once said that if manufacturers advertised extensively enough, they could make smokers out of all Americans, attracted customers with promotions like cash coupons, payments to individuals who handed in the most empty packs, and numbered sets of CIGARETTE PICTURE CARDS that were illustrated with actors and sports figures.

By 1889, W. Duke Sons and Company was the largest cigarette producer in the United States. Because this was the era of great combinations, especially in such areas as oil and sugar, Duke proposed that the leading cigarette firms combine. Although ALLEN AND GINTER held out for a while, 33-year old Duke formally merged most of his competition—Allen and Ginter of RICHMOND, VIRGINIA; William Kimball and Company of Rochester; Kinney Tobacco Company of New York City; and Goodwin and Company of New York City—into the AMERICAN TOBACCO COMPANY with himself as president. The company, also known as the Tobacco trust, was valued at $25 million; it incorporated in New Jersey on January 31, 1890. Over the next 14 years, Duke spent enormous amounts of money to enlarge his company, crush his competition, and control prices. He bought at least 250 other tobacco companies, some of which he closed, and paid other competitors large sums of money to promise not to compete for 20 years or to go out of the tobacco business permanently.

As opposition to cigarettes increased at the turn of the century, Duke diversified and expanded his trust into other lines of tobacco. By 1900, Duke and his organization produced more than 90 percent of American cigarettes, 80 percent of SNUFF, 62 percent of plug, and 60 percent of pipe tobacco. Duke never dominated in the field of CIGAR manufacturing because it remained largely in the hands of small, independent producers. Duke's trust also absorbed businesses involved in the production of licorice paste (used in making chewing tobacco), tin foil, cotton bags, and wooden boxes. American Tobacco expanded into overseas markets, especially JAPAN and CHINA.

Finally, in July 1907, President Theodore Roosevelt's attorney general went after Duke's American Tobacco Company for violating the Anti-Trust Act of 1890 which outlawed monopolies. Named as defendants were Duke and 28 other individuals as well as 65 American corporations and 2 English corporations. On May 29, 1911, the U.S. Supreme Court handed down its decision holding Duke and his trust guilty of violating the anti-trust law in securing control of four-fifths of the total non-cigar manufactured tobacco industry. The Court ordered the dissolution of the trust.

After Duke's trust was dissolved, he found "nothing attractive" in managing any of the smaller companies, so he became interested in the money-making potential of hydro-electric power. In 1912, he formed the Southern Power Company, later renamed the Duke Power Company. He also plunged into the textile and aluminum industries. Duke gave sizeable amounts of money to Trinity College (now Duke University in Durham, North Carolina), less than an hour's walk from the old Duke homestead. His contributions to Trinity reached the millions when, in 1924, Duke created the Duke Endowment, originally valued at some $40 million. He made plans to transform Trinity into Duke University after the trustees accepted a huge bequest and his philanthropy extended to aiding other colleges, hospitals, and churches.

Duke, who died of bronco-pneumonia on October 10, 1925, detested cigarettes; he never smoked them. He chewed tobacco as a young man and took up cigars later in his life. The statue that commemorates his life at Duke University in Durham, North Carolina, depicts him with a cigar in his hand. *See also* IMPERIAL TOBACCO COMPANY OF GREAT BRITAIN AND IRELAND

Duke, Washington (1820–1905)

Washington Duke, an Orange County, North Carolina, farmer who planted his first tobacco crop around 1859, decided to quit farming and manufacture tobacco instead. After the Civil War, along with his children, Duke began a factory on his homestead near Durham Station. During the Civil War, although the family homestead had been looted of livestock, a small crop of cured bright tobacco remained in a log barn, a hoard that laid the foundation for a corporate empire. Duke and his sons produced chewing plug; they packed it into muslin bags, each with a hand-lettered yellow tag attached bearing the words *Pro Bono Publico,* meaning "for the public good."

Duke and his youngest son, James, also known as "Buck," peddled these products in eastern North Carolina, bringing back supplies and coin. Within a few years, the Dukes' business grew to include two more tobacco processing factories located at the family homestead. In 1866, the factory produced 15,000 pounds; in 1872, 125,000.

In 1874, Duke moved his operation to Durham. Duke and his three sons (James, Ben, and Brodie) formed a successful business team and incorporated in 1878 as W. Duke and Sons. In 1880, Duke retired and his son, JAMES BUCHANAN DUKE, became president of the company. Unable to compete with the manufacturers of BULL DURHAM SMOKING TOBACCO, James Duke decided in the 1880s to go into the CIGARETTE business.

Under James Duke's leadership, W. Duke and Sons became part of the AMERICAN TOBACCO COMPANY. Embarrassed by preachers, doctors, and women crusading against the evils of smoking and targeting the Duke family in particular, Washington Duke wished his son had never put his family into the American Tobacco Company. He reportedly told a friend: "You know, there are three things I just can't seem to understand: ee-lec-tricity, the Holy Ghost, and my son, Buck" (Tate, 1995). As a child, Washington Duke converted to Methodism. Between 1895 and 1900, Washington Duke gave more than $300,000 to Trinity College (now Duke University), which was administered by the Methodist Episcopal Church South.

References: C. Cassandra Tate, "The American Anti-Cigarette Movement, 1880–1930." (Ph.D. dissertation) Seattle: University of Washington, 1995. (UMI Number 9609793.)

E

Eastern and Central Europe

Tobacco is one of the greatest public health hazards in Eastern and Central Europe (World Health Organization, 1997). In many countries in this area, smoking rates among men are especially high, and in a number of countries these rates are greater than 50 percent. Among women, smoking prevalence is greater than 20 percent and in some cases as high as 30 percent. In the majority of countries in Eastern and Central Europe, cigarette use is increasing among young people.

In 1995, the WORLD HEALTH ORGANIZATION (WHO) estimated that tobacco caused about 700,000 deaths in that region, about 25 percent of the world total. Seventy to 75 percent of these deaths were in people of middle age (35-69 years). WHO estimated that in 1995, 41 percent of all deaths among middle-aged men were caused by tobacco. WHO projects that in 2020, Eastern and Central Europe will have the highest adult male risk of death largely due to the impact of tobacco. It also predicts that while tobacco-related diseases have already reached an unprecedented high level in Eastern European men, further increases among women are expected between 2020 and 2040.

Countries in Eastern Europe have received considerable attention from transnational tobacco companies, not only in terms of advertising and promotion, but in terms of considerable investment in their tobacco manufacturing sectors. The move to free markets led to the acquisition of the former East Germany tobacco industry by the multinational corporations in 1989 and a purchase in 1992 of majority interest in the Czechoslovakian and Hungarian tobacco industry. In 1996, Philip Morris purchased a 32 percent interest in the Polish government's biggest tobacco factory. British-American Tobacco (BAT) manufactures Sobieski cigarettes in a plant it also bought from the Polish government.

In the Eastern European market, tobacco companies have launched marketing and public relations campaigns aimed at getting consumers to identify with brand names. The campaigns began in the 1990s after communism collapsed and Eastern Europe's tobacco sector opened to privatization. According to Euromonitor, a market research company in London, between 1992 and 1996 overall consumption in the region grew 6 percent to 689 billion cigarettes.

After London-based BAT bought the Hungarian market leader Sopiane, the cigarette brand grew to command a market share of 39 percent. Besides changing the packaging and adding a cellophane wrapper and a seal, BAT added light, extra-light, ultra-light, and menthol varieties.

In Hungary, hospitals, schools, student scholarship programs, police and fire departments, orphanages, senior citizens, athletes, and cultural institutions have received tobacco monies from BAT and Philip Morris. BAT officials said its giving programs not only are legitimate public relations efforts, but a way of shouldering a welfare burden. In 1997, BAT spent $17.1 million on community projects globally, mostly in Eastern Europe and the former Soviet Union, places that need money for welfare projects.

Although some countries in Eastern and Central Europe have established comprehensive tobacco control policies, international public health officials worry that community sponsorships by tobacco companies, while legal, will sway government officials and public opinion to oppose anti-smoking measures. *See also* BAT INDUSTRIES PLC; GLOBAL TOBACCO USE; PHILIP MORRIS INTERNATIONAL INC.

References: World Health Organization, "The Tobacco Epidemic Rages on in Eastern and Central Europe," Fact Sheets, May 1997.

Eclipse

In 1994, R.J. REYNOLDS TOBACCO COMPANY announced that it had developed a cigarette that eliminated most smoke and ash by heating instead of burning the tobacco. According to the tobacco company, the CIGARETTE, called Eclipse, eliminated SECONDHAND SMOKE up to 90 percent, had no lingering odor and none of the staining associated with other cigarettes. Although Eclipse looks like a regular cigarette and has tobacco in it, only a highly purified piece of carbon in the tip is lit. Warm air is drawn over the tobacco, which is mixed with glycerine, and the glycerine vapor carries nicotine and tobacco flavor through a filter to the smoker. Reynolds did not call Eclipse, the result of seven years of research, a safer cigarette because the cigarette still generates substantial amounts of carbon monoxide and NICOTINE. Because Eclipse burns a small amount of tobacco in its tip, it has tar levels ranging between a light and an ultra-light cigarette.

Reynolds, which marketed Eclipse in Chattanooga, Tennessee, said more than 12,000 smokers in 20 states tried Eclipse, but nearly all the research was directed at developing the marketing program. At a meeting of public health officials, Reynolds released studies showing dramatic reductions in the hazardous components of Eclipse's smoke. Scientists cautioned, however, that much of the data was based on animal studies or smoking machines that, like the FEDERAL TRADE COMMISSION (FTC) method, has been discredited for failing to mimic human smoking behavior.

RJR Tobacco urged critics of tobacco companies to accept Eclipse because millions of smokers deserved an option with reduced risk. Tobacco control groups contended that Eclipse was not a cigarette but a drug delivery device that must undergo the rigorous testing procedures of the FOOD AND DRUG ADMINISTRATION (FDA) before being sold over the counter. Some well-known researchers like Neil Benowitz, a leading nicotine expert at the University of California at San Francisco, thought Eclipse should come under FDA supervision. In November 1998, the Roswell Park Cancer Institute investigators published a report that said Eclipse cigarettes were contaminated with glass fibers and other fragments and particles, that when inhaled or ingested, may pose an additional health risk to users. *See also* ARIEL, PREMIER

Edison, Thomas Alva (1847–1931)

American inventor Thomas A. Edison condemned CIGARETTES. He wrote that cigarette paper, when burned, released "acrolein," which if inhaled could destroy brain cells. In a letter to Henry Ford, he wrote: "I employ no person who smokes cigarettes" (Tennent, 1971). But Edison smoked cigars and also chewed on strong plug.

References: Richard B. Tennent, *The American Cigarette Industries*, New York: Archon Books, 1971, pp. 134–35.

Engle v. R.J. Reynolds Tobacco Company et al. (1999)

The nation's first class-action lawsuit by sick smokers to go to trial was decided on July 7, 1999, when a Florida jury ruled against the tobacco industry. It found cigarette makers addicted and defrauded smokers. The case was named after the lead plaintiff, Dr. Howard Engle, a retired pediatrician in Miami Beach, Florida, who began smoking during his first year of medical school. Dr. Engle alleged that smoking caused his asthma. On October 31, 1994, a Florida state court judge in Miami granted the plaintiff's motion for class certification. The class certified in *Engle* consisted of the following:

> All Florida citizens and residents, and their survivors, who have suffered, presently suffer or who have died from diseases and medical conditions caused by their addiction to cigarettes that contain nicotine. The class shall specifically exclude officers, directors, and agents of the defendants. ("First Class Certifications," 1994)

The landmark trial opened on October 14, 1998, in Dade County Circuit Court, seeking damages from five major tobacco companies (PHILIP MORRIS COMPANIES INC., R.J. REYNOLDS TOBACCO COMPANY, BROWN AND WILLIAMSON TOBACCO CORPORATION, LORILLARD COMPANY INC., and Liggett Group) on behalf of all Florida residents injured by smoking and the survivors of such residents. The smokers are represented by the husband-and-wife team of Stanley and Susan Rosenblatt, the attorneys who filed the 1991 *BROIN V. PHILIP MORRIS COMPANIES INC.* class action on behalf of a class of approximately 60,000 flight attendants. The Rosenblatts have estimated that there are anywhere from 40,000 to one million claimants.

The eight-count complaint asserts that the tobacco industry knew that NICOTINE was addictive, claimed that it was not, and made every effort to suppress scientific and medical evidence of nicotine's addictiveness. The plaintiffs' claims focused on the tobacco companies' allegedly intentional manipulation of the levels of nicotine in their tobacco products to make them addictive, while concealing information about the addictive nature of nicotine. In the next phases of the trial, jurors will review the cases of smokers and decide whether to award damages. *See also* CASTANO V. AMERICAN TOBACCO COMPANY; LIGGETT AND MYERS TOBACCO COMPANY; To-

BACCO LITIGATION: FIRST, SECOND, AND THIRD WAVES

References: "First Class Certifications in the Third Wave of Tobacco Litigation Herald the Beginning of the End for the Tobacco Industry," *Tobacco on Trial*, October, 1994.

Environmental Protection Agency (EPA) 1993 Report

In August 1993, the Environmental Protection Agency (EPA) released its report entitled "Respiratory Health Effects of Passive Smoking: Lung Cancer and Other Disorders." Because the mission of the EPA requires it to protect human health and to safeguard the natural environment, air, water, and land, upon which life depends, the agency researched the effects of ENVIRONMENTAL TOBACCO SMOKE (ETS) on human beings.

The report said that in adults, environmental tobacco smoke is a human lung carcinogen, responsible for approximately 3,000 lung cancer deaths annually in U.S. nonsmokers. ETS has subtle but significant effects on the respiratory health of nonsmokers, including reduced lung function, increased coughing, phlegm production, and chest discomfort.

The report said that in children, ETS exposure is causally associated with an increased risk of lower respiratory tract infections such as bronchitis and pneumonia. The report estimated that 150,000 to 300,000 cases annually in infants and young children up to 18 months of age are attributable to ETS. Exposure to ETS is causally associated with increased prevalence of fluid in the middle ear, symptoms of upper respiratory tract irritation, and a small but significant reduction in lung function. ETS is causally associated with additional episodes and increased severity of symptoms in children with asthma; the report estimates that 200,000 to one million asthmatic children have their condition worsened by exposure to ETS. Exposure to ETS is a risk factor for new cases of asthma in children who have not previously displayed symptoms.

The EPA report formally classified environmental tobacco smoke as a Group A carcinogen like benzene and asbestos. *See also* ENVIRONMENTAL PROTECTION AGENCY (EPA) AND 1998 U.S. DISTRICT COURT RULING

Environmental Protection Agency (EPA) and 1998 U.S. District Court Ruling

In July 1998 in Greensboro, North Carolina, U.S. District Judge WILLIAM L. OSTEEN declared that the 1993 Environmental Protection Agency (EPA) study, "Respiratory Health Effects of Passive Smoking: Lung Cancer and Other Disorders," overstated the link between ENVIRONMENTAL TOBACCO SMOKE (ETS) and cancer. In the report, the EPA declared ETS to be a Group A carcinogen, the most definitive link that the regulator can make between a chemical and cancer.

The EPA findings, which said ETS smoke killed at least 3,000 nonsmokers a year, spurred regulations and ordinances around the country curbing smoking in public buildings, workplaces, restaurants, and domestic airplane flights. The report did not begin the movement to protect nonsmokers from SECONDHAND SMOKE. It did, however, escalate efforts to restrict smoking in public places. After 1993, the number of clean air ordinances in cities and states across the nation jumped.

The 1998 ruling came in a case filed by the tobacco industry against the EPA. In his 92-page decision, Judge Osteen said that the agency reached its conclusion before doing its research, disregarded information and made findings on selective information, did not disseminate significant epidemiological information, deviated from its "Risk Assessment Guidelines," failed to disclose important opposing findings, left significant questions unanswered, and excluded the tobacco industry during the process. He also said the EPA aggressively used the report's findings "to establish a de facto regulatory scheme intended to restrict plaintiff's products and to influence public opinion" (Herbert, 1998).

The court's ruling supports the long held belief of tobacco companies that ETS smoke has not been scientifically proven to cause disease in nonsmokers and that science does not justify smoking bans by state and local governments. Industry lawyers also said Judge Osteen's decision was a major setback for nonsmokers seeking to win damages from CIGARETTE smokers. The EPA's finding that "environmentally transmitted smoke" ranks among the deadliest carcinogens has been used as evidence in secondhand smoke court cases. The EPA stated it was standing by its conclusions. *See also* ENVIRONMENTAL PROTECTION AGENCY (EPA) 1993 REPORT

References: H. Josef Herbert, "EPA Stands by Its Warning," *Record*, July 20, 1998, p. 6.

Environmental Tobacco Smoke (ETS)

Air pollution resulting from SIDESTREAM SMOKE that comes off the burning tip of a cigarette and MAINSTREAM SMOKE that smokers draw into their lungs is called environmental tobacco smoke (ETS) or SECONDHAND SMOKE. People who breathe this smoke are known as passive smokers or involuntary smokers.

ETS has been determined by almost a dozen major governmental bodies and dozens of scientific, medical, and public health organizations both in the United States and abroad to cause lung cancer and other diseases in nonsmokers. In the 1970s, researchers showed that children exposed to ETS have higher rates of respiratory diseases. In 1981, a Japanese study by TAKESHI HIRAYAMA published in the *British Medical Journal*, and widely reported in the press, showed that nonsmoking women married to smokers have a higher risk of dying from lung cancer than nonsmoking women married to nonsmokers.

Reports by respected groups like the National Cancer Institute, National Institute for Occupational Safety and Health, National Research Council of the National Academy of Sciences, the U.S. Occupational Safety and Health Administration, and the U.S. surgeon general confirmed the evidence that ETS endangers children and causes lung cancer in adults. The report of the Scientific Committee on Tobacco and Health in Great Britain, the National Health and Medical Research Council in Australia, and the World Health

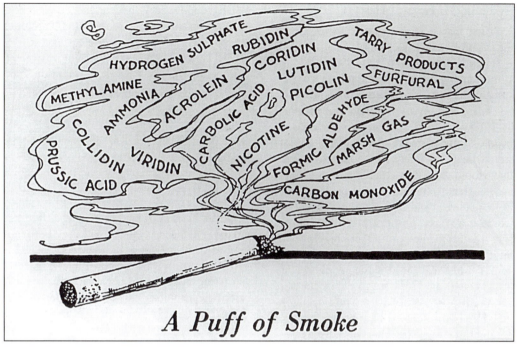

HYDROGEN SULPHATE
RUBIDIN
CORIDIN
TARRY PRODUCTS
METHYLAMINE
AMMONIA
ACROLEIN
LUTIDIN
FURFURAL
CARBOLIC ACID
PICOLIN
FORMIC ALDEHYDE
NICOTINE
MARSH GAS
COLLIDIN
VIRIDIN
PRUSSIC ACID
CARBON MONOXIDE

A Puff of Smoke

This 1922 image depicts the chemicals found in a puff of tobacco smoke.

Organization (WHO) also found exposure to ETS causes lung cancer.

An ENVIRONMENTAL PROTECTION AGENCY (EPA) 1993 REPORT listed ETS as a Class A (known human) carcinogen and a major source of respiratory problems in children. Subsequent studies have shown that exposure to ETS also increases the risk of heart disease.

In the October 18, 1997, *British Medical Journal,* an editorial summary of the research into the effects of tobacco smoke on non-smokers concluded that

Public health action to eliminate exposure to environmental smoke is long overdue . . . . A total ban on smoking is preferred on three grounds: it provides maximum protection of nonsmokers, it avoids exposing smokers to extremely high levels of environmental tobacco smoke in designated smoking areas, and it avoids the costs of constructing separately ventilated smoking areas. Health advocates should pursue all strategies that would help accomplish that goal, including education, legislation, regulation, and litigation. ("Passive Smoking," 1997)

Nonsmokers also have won many lawsuits against employees and others for exposure to ETS. The courts have repeatedly held there is no right to smoke. In at least 15 states where the issue has been raised, courts have held that parents who subject their children to tobacco smoke can lose custody, and in a few cases they have. In a 1991 case (*Mitchell v. Mitchell III*) heard in the Tennessee Court of Appeals, Robert C. Mitchell III gained custody of his son. The boy's mother and grandmother smoked around him aggravating his asthmatic condition.

Persons who are especially sensitive to smoke are protected under the AMERICANS WITH DISABILITIES ACT (ADA). At least one court has held that they can sue to ban all smoking in a retail area. Nonsmoking employees may also file a formal complaint under the Occupational Safety and Health Act, even though the Occupational Safety and Health Administration has yet to issue a formal rule limiting smoking. *See also* ENVIRONMENTAL PROTECTION AGENCY (EPA) AND 1998 U.S. DISTRICT COURT RULING

References: "Passive Smoking: History Repeats Itself," *British Medical Journal,* October 18, 1997: 961–62.

Eysenck, Hans J. (1916–)

A British psychologist who is an expert on the creation and extinction of habits, Hans J. Eysenck is one of the founders of the "constitutional hypothesis" that smokers were essentially born, not made. In his book, *Smoking, Health, and Personality,* published in 1965, Eysenck laid out his theory that people of an extraverted type of personality would be more likely to smoke CIGARETTES than would more introverted people. Further, he theorized that extraverted people would be more prone to suffer from lung cancer than would introverts. Eysenck concluded therefore that lung cancer and smoking were related, not because smoking causes lung cancer, but because the same people predisposed genetically to develop lung cancer were also predisposed genetically to take up smoking. His book deals with the relationships among three variables: smoking; disease, especially lung cancer and coronary thrombosis; and personality.

Eysenck stated that while smoking clearly was not likely to promote anyone's health and suspicion was strong that cigarette smoking may indeed be a killer, the evidence was inconclusive, circumstantial rather than direct, and did not demonstrate the case against smoking beyond any reasonable doubt. He cautioned against using the statistical correlation between smoking and lung cancer because numerical values have been subject to so many errors and inaccuracies. He argued that the populations studied were clearly not representative and that the refusal rate among those asked to take part in investigations was too large. He also argued that the ascertainment of smoking habits was subject to errors of memory and of estimation. Worst of all, he argued that the smokers and nonsmokers were self-selected, thus allowing alternative hypotheses to that of a direct causal relation between smoking and lung cancer to be put forward to explain the statistical correlations.

Eysenck's book gave evidence that persons of an extraverted temperament are both more likely to smoke cigarettes and to develop cancer than persons of an introverted temperament. As a result, he hypothesized that, "while this evidence is not based on sufficient numbers of cases to establish the point definitively," persons constitutionally predisposed to start smoking are also constitutionally predisposed to develop cancer (Eysenck, 1965).

The book concludes that two main hypotheses exist on the market, both explaining the facts, both having certain difficulties in the evidence to contend with, and both failing to provide that definitive proof that scientists require. He stated that "Cigarette smoking is neither a necessary nor a sufficient cause of lung cancer; the evidence suggests but does not prove that it is an important contributory cause." Eysenck wrote that because the evidence suggested that atmospheric pollution was probably an even more important factor, it was unwise to concentrate all available research efforts and legislative measures on smoking. He suggested that research be directed at the search for "direct, causal physiological and neurological variables, rather than for circumstantial evidence supporting purely statistical calculations" (Eysenck, 1965).

The tobacco industry in Great Britain and the United States responded favorably to Eysenck's hypothesis and funded his research. He worked at London University's Institute of Psychiatry, where, according to the Merrell Williams documents, he received more than £70,000 from Special Account Number 4 and nearly £900,000 in research grants between 1977 and 1989. *See also* BROWN AND WILLIAMSON TOBACCO CORPORATION—MERRELL WILLIAMS DOCUMENTS

References: Hans J. Eysenck, *Smoking, Health and Personality*, New York: Basic Books, 1965, p. 152.

F

Fairness Doctrine of the Federal Communications Commission (FCC)

In 1967, the Federal Communication Commission ruled that all radio and television stations broadcasting CIGARETTE commercials donate "significant" free air time for anti-smoking messages.

In 1966, John Banzhaf III, a young lawyer, filed a complaint with the FCC asking it to apply the "fairness doctrine" to cigarette commercials on television and radio. The FCC "fairness doctrine" is basic to this country's system of commercial broadcasting. To receive a broadcasting channel, a radio or television station must be licensed, and this license is periodically reviewed. One of the requirements for receiving a license is that the broadcaster agree to operate in the public interest, and one of the criteria is whether he or she gives a fair cross-section of opinion in the coverage of public affairs and matters of public controversy.

The FCC unanimously rejected petitions of the tobacco industry and the broadcasters to rescind its fairness doctrine order. FCC Commissioner Lee Loevinger declared "suggesting cigarette smoking to young people, in the light of present-day knowledge, is something very close to wickedness" (Soper, ·p. 1). In its September 15, 1967, ruling, the FCC said:

> We believe that the licensee's statutory obligation to operate in the public interest includes the duty to make a fair presentation of opposing viewpoints on the controversial issue of public importance posed by cigarette advertising (i.e., the desirability of smoking), that this duty extends to cigarette advertising which encourages the public to use a product that is habit forming and, as found by the Congress and Governmental reports, may in normal use be hazardous to health, and that the licensee's compliance with this duty may be examined at license renewal time.

The fairness doctrine did not require a station to give as many minutes to anti-smoking information as it gave to cigarette ads. But it did have a responsibility during each broadcasting week to give a significant presentation to the other side. Nor did the FCC ruling require that a station necessarily use spot messages to inform the public of the hazards of smoking. Many kinds of programming—news shows, panel discussions, special features—were capable of telling the story. But spot messages were the method that most stations used. *See also* ANTI-SMOKING MESSAGES, 1967–1970; BROADCAST BAN ON CIGARETTE ADVERTISING

References: Francis A. Soper, "John Banzhaf and the Giants." *Listen, Journal of Better Living*, vol. 21, no. 7, n.d.

Farone, William

As director of applied research with Philip Morris's research complex in RICHMOND,

VIRGINIA, from 1976 to 1984, William Farone gave a sworn statement to the FOOD AND DRUG ADMINISTRATION (FDA) on how the tobacco company focused on lowering levels of tar while still giving smokers adequate levels of NICOTINE. He authored a paper entitled "The Manipulation and Control of Nicotine and Tar in the Design and Manufacture of Cigarettes." Farone, who also explained how the industry added ammonia compounds to deliver more nicotine to smokers, succeeded in developing a filter that removed virtually all of the carbon monoxide from CIGARETTE smoke. Although the filter was patented, it never left the research lab. Frustrated by the way Philip Morris handled the research that would have made cigarettes safer Farone cooperated with the FDA inquiry into the tobacco industry.

Farone, who graduated from Clarkson University in upstate New York, has long been inventive in developing new technology for products, working for Lever Brothers and PVO International before going to work for Philip Morris in 1976. *See also* FILTERED CIGARETTES; PHILIP MORRIS COMPANIES INC.

Federal Cigarette Labeling and Advertising Act of 1965

The Federal Cigarette Labeling and Advertising Act of 1965 was the first federal statute to enact labeling requirements for tobacco products. The text of the act began by declaring it was the intention of Congress to establish a federal program to inform the public of the possible health hazards of smoking. The act required a package warning label—"Caution: Cigarette Smoking May be Hazardous to Your Health" (other health warnings were prohibited). The act required no labels on CIGARETTE advertisements (in fact, it implemented a three-year prohibition of any such labels). The act required the FEDERAL TRADE COMMISSION (FTC) to report to Congress annually on the effectiveness of cigarette labeling, advertising, and promotion. The law also required the Department of Health, Education and Welfare to report annually to Congress on the health consequences of smoking.

Congress appropriated $2 million shortly after the act was passed to establish the NATIONAL CLEARINGHOUSE FOR SMOKING AND HEALTH in the PUBLIC HEALTH SERVICE; the clearinghouse's function was to carry out educational campaigns and collect data on smoking and health research. *See also* HEALTH WARNINGS ON CIGARETTE PACKS AND ADVERTISEMENTS AND SMOKELESS TOBACCO

Federal Regulation of Tobacco Production

Producers and consumers of tobacco in the United States have been subject to a variety of different regulations since 1613, when JOHN ROLFE cultivated tobacco in colonial Virginia. Notwithstanding the attitude of King JAMES I, who despised tobacco, England encouraged—and regulated—the growth of the tobacco industry. The Crown granted monopolies to court favorites to import tobacco from the colonies. In 1622, James I granted the import monopoly to the Virginia and Bermuda companies and prohibited the domestic cultivation of tobacco.

The competition of colonies in the marketplace led to legislation regulating importing and exporting of tobacco. In 1679, Virginia prohibited the importation of Carolinian tobacco and did not permit North Carolina to export its tobacco from Virginia ports. In 1658, Virginia and Maryland, vying for customers, enacted laws prescribing the dimensions of the hogshead in which tobacco was packaged. The two colonies gradually enlarged the statutory size of the hogshead until, under edict from the English privy council, Maryland was ordered to pass a gauge act establishing the size of the hogshead in the same dimensions as those fixed in Virginia.

It was not long before colonial planters were faced with a serious problem of overproduction, which caused a decline in prices as well as in quality of the leaf. Legislation was passed to restrict production. In 1619, the first tobacco inspection law was passed by the Virginia House of Burgesses, ordering the lowest grade of tobacco to be destroyed and prohibiting "second growth" tobacco and the marketing of trash leaves. In 1621, each cultivator was required to limit his growth to 1,000 plants of nine leaves each. After the act failed to restrict production, a 1629 act permitted each planter to grow 3,000 plants with an additional allowance of 1,000 for non-laboring "women and each child." Carolina, Maryland, and Virginia even reached a decision to prohibit the planting of tobacco from February 1667 to February 1668. After the Virginia assembly failed to pass a similar act, some planters burned their own crops and the plants of their neighbors. The surfeit of tobacco led to a warehouse system to enforce tobacco inspection to "prevent the sending to market such trash as is unfit for any other use but Manure" (*Maryland and Tobacco,* 1971).

The initial hogshead inspection system gave way to the sale of loose-leaf tobacco by auction. In 1849, the Virginia Code recognized these methods in lieu of the sale of HOGSHEADS and by 1865, the tobacco auction had completely replaced the earlier marketing techniques in Virginia. Decades later, Maryland followed suit. In 1939, the loose-leaf auction warehouse system was introduced to replace the hogshead system.

In the 1930s, the federal government enacted several bills to aid growers. In 1935, it passed the Tobacco Inspection Act, which directed the secretary of agriculture to establish quality standards and to designate auction markets. In 1936, the Tobacco Control Act was passed giving congressional approval to state compacts that regulate the production of tobacco and subsidize the expenses of the state commissions involved. The AGRICULTURAL ADJUSTMENT ACT OF 1938 also regulated quantity. In addition, the secretary of agriculture is authorized to set national marketing quotas with regard to each kind of tobacco produced, to apportion the quotas among the states, and to allot the portions among the farms. Penalties are imposed for overproduction. Thus, two elements of initial colonial regulation were preserved— the encouragement of quality and the discouragement of quantity.

References: *Maryland and Tobacco,* Washington, D.C.: Tobacco Institute, 1971, p. 23.

Federal Trade Commission (FTC)

Established by Congress in 1914 to compensate for the perceived weakness of the 1890 Sherman Antitrust Act for combatting the abuses of monopolies, the Federal Trade Commission (FTC) was originally designed to give advice and guidance to businesses and protect businesspeople from unfair methods of competition. It had the authority to demand reports from corporations, investigate and publish reports about corporate activities, and issue "cease-and-desist" orders to stop unfair business practices.

By the late 1920s, when CIGARETTES were mass produced, widely distributed, and skillfully advertised and marketed on a national scale, the FTC began monitoring the business practices of tobacco companies. In1929, FTC commissioners summoned AMERICAN TOBACCO COMPANY lawyers to its offices and advised them to discontinue the company's implicit claim that LUCKY STRIKE CIGARETTES were weight-reducing devices.

In 1938, Congress passed the Wheeler-Lea Act, which widened the commission's powers. It gave the FTC authority to regulate "unfair or deceptive acts or practices in commerce" (Taylor, 1984). The agency had the authority to subpoena documents, lay down fair-practice guidelines, and seek civil penalties in the federal courts of up to $10,000 per day per violation. Congress, however, denied the commission power to enjoin the suspect practice throughout the proceedings against wrongdoers. A typical action took four years.

From 1938 to 1997, the FTC acted against false and misleading advertising claims of tobacco companies 51 times. In August 1942, for example, the FTC told tobacco manufacturers to stop making false and misleading claims: Pall Mall cigarettes did not protect throats from irritation; LUCKY STRIKE CIGARETTES were not toasted, as that term was commonly understood by the public, nor did they contain less NICOTINE than other brands; CAMELS did not aid digestion; and Kools did not give extra protection against colds. In 1950, when the FTC investigated OLD GOLD CIGARETTES' claim that the brand contained less nicotine than other brands, it was discovered that the difference was only two-fifths of 1 percent, a margin that was found to be physiologically without significance. The FTC ordered the manufacturer to stop making its claim. In 1955, the FTC barred from ads all phony testimonials and any medical approval of cigarette smoking.

Although the FTC tried to halt the tobacco industry's explicit health and other kinds of claims, it never did so aggressively or on its own initiative. It moved against a tobacco company when an aggrieved customer or competitor brought cases to it. In the late 1950s, U.S. representative John A. Blatnik (D-MN) showed, when investigating deceptive filter-cigarette advertising, that the FTC had not done its job at all.

In 1957, Blatnik, chairman of the Legal and Monetary Subcommittee of the Government Operations Committee, conducted hearings to define the responsibility of the FTC regarding advertising claims for cigarettes. The Blatnik subcommittee concluded that

> The Federal Trade Commission has failed in its statutory duty to "prevent deceptive acts or practices" in filter-cigarette advertising. The activities of the Commission to prevent this deception were weak and tardy. As a result, the connection between filter-tip cigarettes and "protection" has become deeply embedded in the public mind. (Wagner, 1971)

After trying to work out a standard testing procedure for tar and nicotine content, the FTC decided no reliable test existed. Weary of deciding the legal merits of individual tobacco company claims, the FTC decided to knock the tar and nicotine claims out of cigarette advertising altogether. On December 17, 1959, it sent a letter to manufacturers stating "We wish to advise that all representations of low or reduced tar or nicotine, whether by filtration or otherwise, will be construed as health claims . . . . Our purpose is to eliminate from cigarette advertis-

ing representations which in any way imply health benefit" (Wagner, 1971).

It was not until the early 1960s, however, that major regulatory moves against tobacco use began in earnest. Shortly after the release of the U.S. SURGEON GENERAL'S REPORT OF 1964, which declared cigarette smoking a major hazard, the FTC proposed a strong health warning regarding the risk of death from disease caused by tobacco use. Congress agreed a warning was needed, but in 1965 passed the FEDERAL CIGARETTE LABELING AND ADVERTISING ACT, a law with a weaker warning than the kind the FTC wanted. As of January 1, 1966, cigarette packs had to carry a nine-word warning: "Caution: Cigarette smoking may be hazardous to your health." The law temporarily prohibited the FTC and states from requiring health warnings in cigarette advertising.

The law also required that, beginning in 1967, the FTC report annually to Congress about the effectiveness of the warning label and the practices of cigarette advertising and promotions, with "recommendations for legislation that are deemed appropriate."

After passage of the act, the FTC developed a machine system for measuring tar and nicotine yield of cigarettes and provided, in the annual report to Congress, the yields of tar and nicotine of the most popular brands. The system was modified in 1981 to include carbon monoxide. Cigarette manufacturers disclose tar and nicotine yield of their brands in advertisements.

In its first report to Congress, the FTC recommended extending the health warning to cigarette advertising and strengthening the wording. The subsequent PUBLIC HEALTH CIGARETTE SMOKING ACT OF 1969 strengthened the package warning label to read: "The Surgeon General Has Determined That Cigarette Smoking Is Hazardous to Your Health." Again, the FTC was temporarily restricted from issuing regulations that would require a health warning in cigarette advertising.

After the second congressional moratorium expired in late 1971, the FTC announced its intention to file complaints against cigarette companies for failure to warn in their advertising that smoking is dangerous to health. Negotiations among the companies and the FTC resulted on March 30, 1972, in consent orders requiring that all cigarette advertising in newspapers and magazines or on BILLBOARDS "clearly and conspicuously" display the same warning required by Congress for cigarette packages.

In 1981, the FTC sent a staff report to Congress that concluded that the warning appearing on cigarette packages and in advertisements had become overexposed and "worn out" and thus was no longer effective. The report pointed out that the existing warning was too abstract and recommended changing the shape of the warning, increasing the size of the warning, and replacing the existing single warning with a rotational system of warnings. The 1981 FTC staff report eventually helped pass the COMPREHENSIVE SMOKING EDUCATION ACT OF 1984. Although Congress increased the size, number, and specificity of the warnings, they were not as restrictive as the FTC recommended. *See also* FEDERAL TRADE COMMISSION AND TAR AND NICOTINE LEVELS

References: Peter Taylor, *The Smoke Ring: Tobacco Money, and Multinational Politics*, New York: Pantheon Books, 1984, p. 168.

Susan Wagner, *Cigarette Country, Tobacco in American History and Politics*, New York: Praeger Publishers, 1971, p. 89.

Federal Trade Commission (FTC) Act

In September 1914, at President Woodrow Wilson's recommendation, Congress passed the Federal Trade Commission Act. Originally designed to give advice and guidance to businesses and protect businesspeople from unfair methods of competition, the act set up the FEDERAL TRADE COMMISSION (FTC), a bipartisan agency with five commissioners nominated by the president and confirmed by the Senate, each serving a seven-year term. The president chooses one commissioner to act as chair. Today, the FTC has law enforcement powers and polices businesses and protects consumers from deceptive business practices.

Federal Trade Commission (FTC) and Joe Camel Advertising

In 1991 and 1992, Surgeon General Antonia Novello, the American Medical Association, and several health groups requested that the FEDERAL TRADE COMMISSION (FTC) take action against the R.J. REYNOLDS TOBACCO COMPANY cartoon character OLD JOE CAMEL and order Reynolds to stop using it in its cigarette advertising, promotion, and marketing. They argued that Camel cigarette sales to children spiked after the introduction of Joe Camel in 1988, increasing more dramatically than sales to adults.

In 1993, the FTC staff recommended that the agency seek an outright ban on the Joe Camel advertising campaign. In 1994, after reviewing tens of thousands of pages of Reynolds documents, the agency found no grounds for action and voted not to pursue the complaint that the company's advertising was aimed at children. In 1996, however, the agency reopened its investigation of Reynolds advertising practices after receiving a bipartisan petition from 67 members of the House of Representatives and one from seven senators arguing that the Joe Camel campaign was in part responsible for an alarming increase in smoking among teenagers.

On May 28, 1997, the FTC filed an unfair advertising complaint against R.J. Reynolds alleging that its Joe Camel advertising campaign was illegally aimed at minors and tried to entice youngsters to smoke CAMEL CIGARETTES. This was the first time the FTC accused the tobacco industry of aiming its products at minors. The commission voted three to two, largely on the strength of new evidence that was not available in 1994 when the FTC decided not to act. The FOOD AND DRUG ADMINISTRATION (FDA) supplied the FTC with many of the documents it acquired through its own investigation of tobacco companies.

In the complaint filed with an administrative judge within the FTC, the agency said the campaign violated federal law that prohibits marketing of cigarettes to children. The campaign, the complaint said, was so successful that Camel's market share among kids exceeded its share among adults. Before the Joe Camel campaign began in 1987, Camel's share of the youth smoking market was less than 3 percent. In two years, its share jumped to almost 9 percent and by 1993 the brand was used by 13.2 percent of minors.

R.J. Reynolds denounced the FTC complaint. In a written statement, the tobacco company denied that it focused on underage smokers and said that it had a First Amendment right to advertise its products in an appealing way. On July 10, 1997, without any mention of the FTC, Reynolds announced it would phase out the cartoon camel character in domestic advertising and replace it with a stylized version of Camel's original camel trademark that has appeared on Camel cigarette packs since the brand's introduction as the first nationally advertised cigarette in 1913. The company insisted that dropping the cartoon camel was a marketing decision. Joe Camel and his camel buddies disappeared from BILLBOARDS, print advertisements, display signs, and door store stickers, although they will continue to appear in advertising overseas.

In November 1998, opening arguments began in a trial over Joe Camel's future use. The FTC wanted an administrative judge to bar the tobacco company from ever again using Old Joe or his fellow cartoon camels in advertisements. The FTC also wanted the company to pay for an anti-smoking campaign targeted to teens. The case was dismissed after the Tobacco Settlement of November 1998 banned cartoon characters in tobacco advertising. *See also* FISCHER, PAUL; TOBACCO SETTLEMENT—NOVEMBER 1998

Federal Trade Commission (FTC) and Tar and Nicotine Levels

Following the publication of the first Surgeon General's Report on Smoking and Health in 1964, the FEDERAL TRADE COMMISSION (FTC) began to provide lists of its estimates of the amount of tar and NICOTINE delivered by various brands of CIGARETTES. In the late 1960s,

after the outgrowth of a "tar derby" among cigarette manufacturers touting their lower-tar products on the basis of different test methods, smokers became confused. To head off government regulation, the industry volunteered in 1970 to disclose the results of FTC testing in ads. The industry took over the job of testing in 1987, under the FTC's oversight, using a smoking machine that smokes cigarettes almost to the butt and then filters out the tar and nicotine for measurement. The system was not designed to predict actual tar and nicotine intake among humans, only to provide a relative measure between brands. Under a 1971 consent agreement with the FTC, cigarette makers agreed to disclose tar and nicotine yield of their brands in cigarette ads.

Although tar and nicotine levels have dropped over the last few decades, sound evidence indicates that FTC-published estimates have little to do with either the content of tobacco or the way people smoke cigarettes. Rather, the FTC method of estimating tar and nicotine levels has been based on the amount of smoke obtained by cigarette-smoking machines. FILTERED CIGARETTES have a band of microscopic air vents that are designed to dilute the intake of tar and nicotine. Researchers have found that many smokers who have switched to lower-tar brands for a safer smoke compensate by taking more frequent puffs, inhale more deeply, plug up the filter's air vents with their fingers or lips, or smoke more cigarettes a day. Smokers who are not aware that holes exist may plug them unwittingly.

In late 1998, the FTC decided to revamp the way tobacco companies measure tar and nicotine yields and then disclose these numbers in ads. The new system will show a range of yields per brand instead of a single number. The new system will require every ad to include a disclaimer that the amount of tar and nicotine smokers get from a cigarette depends on how deeply they breathe in the smoke. *See also* HEALTH WARNINGS ON CIGARETTE PACKS AND ADVERTISEMENTS AND SMOKELESS TOBACCO; PERTSCHUK, MICHAEL; SURGEON GENERAL'S REPORT OF 1964

Fight Ordinances and Restrictions to Control and Eliminate Smoking (FORCES)

FORCES is a Political Action Committee (PAC), with membership funded by private individuals; it is based in San Francisco, California. It is pro-choice on the smoking issue, and it lobbies on behalf of smokers in the legal arena. FORCES believes the media has suppressed vital information about the tobacco issue, allowing only one side to have a voice. It believes the media issues, without verification, false or distorted information provided by anti-smoking forces.

Filler

In the cigar industry, this term is used specifically to indicate the core or inner part of the CIGAR that is encased in the BINDER and CIGAR WRAPPER. "Long fillers" are made of leaves that have been folded together and that run the entire length of the cigar. "Short fillers" are composed of scrap and small broken leaves.

In the CIGARETTE industry, the term is used to indicate tobacco that has gone through the cutting machine.

Filtered Cigarettes

Filters are any porous substance, such as paper, cotton, cork, or silicate jelly, attached to the end of a CIGAR or CIGARETTE to absorb moisture, tars, NICOTINE or other impurities. A filter can also be a separate holder in which a cigar or cigarette is inserted.

For some years, processes for filters using crepe-paper filler, sometimes with a cellulose wadding, had been available from a Hungarian inventor, Boris Aivaz. The crepe-paper filter-tipped cigarettes sold well in Switzerland and South Africa. British manufacturers, however, did not like the papery taste of the products and felt cigarette holders were the answers for smokers who wanted a filter.

In the 1950s, numerous scientific studies informed the public that cigarette smoking was linked to lung cancer and other serious diseases. The May 1950 issue of the *Journal of the American Medical Association (JAMA)* reported how medical researchers found cigarette smoking to be an important factor in bronchiogenic cancer. The December 1952 issue of *Reader's Digest* ran the story "Cancer by the Carload." During 1953 and 1954, the stories increased. Researchers at New York's Memorial Center for Cancer and Allied Diseases announced that they produced cancer in mice with tar condensed from cigarette smoke. *Consumer Reports* published a report on the tar and nicotine content of cigarette smoke and health hazards of smoking. In 1954, doctors at the AMERICAN CANCER SOCIETY (ACS) reported conclusions of a large study that found men with a regular history of smoking cigarettes had a considerably higher death rate than men who never smoked or who smoked only cigars or pipes.

Cigarette sales slumped, so cigarette manufacturers responded to the growing public concern by promoting filter tips. The filter-tipped brands of the 1950s evolved from old nineteenth-century devices such as cork mouthpieces, as well as from a late 1930s device found attached to VICEROYS—a cardboard tube filled with cotton tufts and folded wads of paper. Tobacco companies brought back filters to reassure smokers it was all right to keep on smoking despite the health scare.

In 1952, the first filter-tipped cigarette that was highly promoted was Lorillard's KENT CIGARETTES. They had a "micronite" filter tip developed by Lorillard in atomic energy plants. After Kent filter tips appeared on the market, other cigarette manufacturers developed competing filters. In the filter war that followed, all brands claimed the best combination of good taste with low tar and nicotine. L and M appeared in 1953 with a "Pure White Miracle Tip of Alpha-Cellulose." Winston appeared in 1954 and became the leading filter brand by 1956. MARLBORO filtered was introduced in 1954, and so was Herbert Tareyton with a "new Selective Filter" containing charcoal. In 1954, Viceroy changed its hollow tube to a cellulose acetate filter, the material that quickly became the "normal" filter throughout the industry. Salem, the first filter-tipped menthol cigarette, was introduced in 1956. Newport, another filter-tipped menthol brand, appeared in 1957.

Tobacco companies outdid one another in making claims for their filter-tip brands. In fierce and expensive advertising campaigns in the late 1950s, each company tried to differentiate its brand from competing brands. Expenditures in selected media jumped from over $55 million in 1952 to approximately $150 million in 1959. These advertising campaigns led to the first attempts by the FEDERAL TRADE COMMISSION (FTC) to regulate the industry.

Filter-tip brands were supposed to reduce the amount of tar and nicotine content in smoke that gets inhaled directly into the lungs. In March 1957, Consumers Union tested 33 brands of cigarettes for the content of nicotine and tar in their smoke. After test results showed little difference between filtered and unfiltered smoke, the Federal Trade Commission (FTC) and cigarette companies made a voluntary agreement barring from all ads any mention of filters and tar and nicotine levels.

The so-called "tar derby" ended in 1960. Earl W. Kintner, then FTC chairman, stated that in "the absence of a satisfactory uniform testing method and proof of advantage to the smoker, there will be no more tar and nicotine claims in advertising." Kintner called the tar and nicotine blackout "a landmark example of industry-government cooperation in solving a pressing problem" (Kluger, 1996).

In 1950, filter-tipped cigarettes accounted for only 0.6 percent of cigarette sales. Six years later, filter-tips had zoomed to almost 50 percent of sales. In 1975, filters accounted for 87 percent of sales. Most people switched to filter tips because they wanted "health protection." *See also* HOROWITZ, MILTON

References: Richard Kluger, *Ashes to Ashes*, New York: Alfred A. Knopf, 1996, p. 190.

Fire-Cured Tobacco

Tobacco cured by means of an open fire is grown in western Kentucky and Tennessee and in central Virginia in heavy loam soils, which contain a high percentage of clay or silt. The principal characteristics of fire-cured tobacco are leaves with dark color, high NICOTINE content, heavy body, and a smoky aroma from being cured by the smoke of an open fire. The greater portion of this type of tobacco is used domestically for making smoking and CHEWING TOBACCO as well as SNUFF and plug wrapper. The U.S. Department of Agriculture grades fire-cured tobacco Class Two. *See also* AIR-CURED TOBACCO; DARK-FIRED TOBACCO; FLUE-CURED TOBACCO; TOBACCO CLASSES

Fischer, Paul (1953–)

Paul Fischer is a family doctor practicing in Augusta, Georgia; editor of a medical journal on family medicine; and a teacher at the Medical College of Georgia (MCG). In 1989, Dr. Fischer conducted an experiment involving children and cigarette advertising. He created a game with cards of advertising symbols like McDonald's golden arches, Apple Computer's apple, and Camel's Joe Camel and a game board with well-known products like a hamburger, a computer, and a lit CIGARETTE. Dr. Fischer tested the game on his own children and then on 229 children, ages three to six, at local day care centers. Parents signed a written permission form.

The children were asked to place each card with an advertising symbol on the product the symbol advertised. One-third of the three-year-olds and 91 percent of six-year-olds put Joe Camel's face on the picture of cigarettes. Less than 61 percent of the six-year-olds identified the MARLBORO MAN.

Dr. Fischer sent the results to the *Journal of the American Medical Association (JAMA)*, which published his findings, along with two other related studies on CAMEL CIGARETTES and children, in the December 1991 issue. His findings, which upset the public health community, drew "an avalanche of newspaper and TV coverage" and resonated with the FOOD AND DRUG ADMINISTRATION (FDA), which was looking for new ways to regulate cigarettes and curb youth smoking. A coalition of the AMERICAN CANCER SOCIETY (ACS), AMERICAN HEART ASSOCIATION (AHA), and AMERICAN LUNG ASSOCIATION (ALA) petitioned the FED-

ERAL TRADE COMMISSION (FTC) to ban all Joe Camel advertising, calling it "one of the most egregious examples in recent history of tobacco advertising that targets children."

R.J. REYNOLDS TOBACCO COMPANY challenged Fischer's study, demanding all of his notes, and the names and telephone numbers of the children he interviewed and their parents. The tobacco company maintained it needed the researcher's notes to defend itself in a California lawsuit. R.J. Reynolds eventually got possession of the doctor's notes. Two years after the study was published, Dr. Fischer resigned from the MCG and established a private practice. He also became a paid expert witness in anti-tobacco litigation. He was a witness in the Florida and Mississippi lawsuits against the tobacco industry concerning Medicaid costs. *See also* FEDERAL TRADE COMMISSION (FTC) AND JOE CAMEL ADVERTISING; FLORIDA MEDICAID CASE; MISSISSIPPI MEDICAID CASE; OLD JOE CAMEL

Florida Medicaid Case

On August 25, 1997, Florida settled its tobacco lawsuit against the tobacco industry, the second state to do so after Mississippi. The companies agreed to pay $11.3 billion over 25 years, which includes $200 million to underwrite an educational program aimed at reducing teen smoking. In September 1998, Governor Lawton Chiles announced a deal to increase by $1.7 billion the amount of money Florida would get in its settlement with the tobacco industry. (The increase came under a provision in the settlement guaranteeing that Florida could renegotiate to match better deals reached by other states.) The companies will continue paying the state for 25 years. Each company's payment will be based on its market share.

The industry also agreed to eliminate cigarette advertising BILLBOARDS within 1,000 feet of a public or private school, finance anti-smoking campaigns aimed at reducing youth smoking, and stop advertising in sporting arenas and on mass transit (trains, buses, and taxis, and at airports). But the industry reserved the right to put signs outside stores and at special sporting or other events. The industry also agreed to support legislative initiatives in Florida to ban the sales of cigarettes in vending machines accessible to youth but such sales remained permissible in premises like bars that are frequented only by adults. They also agreed to support a new state law that would strengthen penalties against shop owners found to be selling cigarettes to people under 18 years of age. The Florida agreement also called for a court review of about 400 industry documents that were sealed in Florida's lawsuit.

In some ways, Florida was considered to have one of the strongest cases because its legislature passed a law stripping the industry's traditional legal defense that smokers know the health risk of smoking and choose to smoke anyway. The law allowed the state to aggregate damage claims and use mathematical models to arrive at a number.

As jury selection proceeded in the state court in West Palm Beach, damaging corporate documents were revealed under rulings by state judges. Further, in pretrial depositions in August 1997, the chairmen of RJR NABISCO HOLDINGS CORPORATION (the company that owns R.J. REYNOLDS TOBACCO COMPANY) and PHILIP MORRIS COMPANIES INC. testified about the risks of smoking. Asked by RONALD MOTLEY, a lawyer representing the state, whether he believed that smoking caused disease, RJR's STEVEN F. GOLDSTONE said: "I have always believed that smoking plays a part in causing lung cancer. What the role is, I don't know, but I do believe it." GEOFFREY BIBLE, Philip Morris CEO, answered that cigarettes "might have" killed 100,000 Americans (Meier, 1997).

The settlement of the Florida case, which was filed in 1995, was marred by a dispute over the fees for some of the private lawyers hired by the state to take the tobacco lawsuit to trial. The state's contract with the lawyers gave them a 25 percent contingency fee if they won. The settlement with the tobacco companies called for "reasonable attorney fees" to be determined by a panel of independent arbitrators. *See also* MINNESOTA MEDICAID CASE; MISSISSIPPI MEDICAID CASE; TEXAS MEDICAID CASE

References: Barry Meier, "Chief of R.J. Reynolds Says Smoking Has Role in Cancer," *New York Times*, August 23, 1997, p. 7.

Flue-Cured Tobacco

Tobacco cured in barns from heat radiating from pipes or flues is grown in Virginia, northern and eastern North Carolina, eastern South Carolina, southeastern Georgia, and northern Florida. Also called BRIGHT TO-BACCO, the flue-cured tobacco leaf is used principally in making cigarettes, but it is also found in smoking and chewing tobaccos and is exported as well. The bright yellow color of the leaf is due to the character of the soil in which it is grown and the method of curing. Typical soils include light sands, coarse sandy loams, sandy loams, and fine sandy loams with yellow or red sandy subsoils. The U.S. Department of Agriculture grades flue-cured tobacco Class One. *See also* AIR-CURED TOBACCO; FIRE-CURED TOBACCO; TOBACCO CLASSES

Food and Drug Act of 1906

In 1906, Congress passed the Pure Food and Drug Act, the first food and drug law intended to ensure the safety of products sold as food or drugs. The law set up the FOOD AND DRUG ADMINISTRATION (FDA) and gave the agency the power to regulate any drug that appeared in the *United States Pharmacopoeia (USP)*, a national list of substances that affect the functioning of the human body in any way.

Before 1906, tobacco was listed in the *USP* because it was widely used as a medicine, especially during the colonial period, because of the properties of NICOTINE. "Nicotine therapy" was used as an analgesic, an expectorant, a laxative, and a salve. During the nineteenth century, the medical uses of tobacco declined, but it remained in the *USP* until 1905.

In 1906, tobacco was dropped from the eighth edition, the same year the Food and Drug Act became law, so it was no longer considered a drug and was no longer subject to FDA jurisdiction. Legend has it that legislators from states where tobacco was grown got tobacco removed from the national drug list to avoid FDA regulation in return for their support of the 1906 act. No deal, however, is mentioned in the *Congressional Record* or the papers of Dr. Harvey Washington Wiley, a physician/pharmacist who headed the precursor to the FDA.

Food and Drug Administration (FDA)

The United States Food and Drug Administration (FDA) is an agency of the federal government within the U.S. DEPARTMENT OF HEALTH AND HUMAN SERVICES (DHHS). It was founded in 1906 to ensure compliance with the FOOD AND DRUG ACT OF 1906 and the Meat Inspection Act of 1906—laws enacted to prohibit interstate commerce in misbranded and adulterated foods, drinks, and drugs—and to enforce sanitation in meat-packing plants.

In 1998, the FDA had more than 9,000 employees in 157 cities, including 2,000 chemists and microbiologists in 40 laboratories. Annually, 1,100 investigators and inspectors visited 15,000 facilities as part of their oversight of the 95,000 U.S. businesses that the FDA regulates. The FDA regulates the purity of consumer products such as food, cosmetics, medication, medical devices, and radiation-emitting products, as well as feed and drugs for pets and farm animals.

The FDA has not been a well-regarded agency. For years it has been criticized by congressional committees, public interest groups, and executives of industries it tries to regulate. A 1990 advisory committee, appointed by secretary of Health and Human Services Louis W. Sullivan, reported that the FDA operated on a threadbare budget, with a shortage of inspectors and laboratories in abysmal condition, and without a clear-cut mission. Under the leadership of the FDA's new commissioner, Dr. DAVID KESSLER, who brought a new sense of purpose to the agency when he took the position in November 1990, the FDA began restoring its credibility. Kessler's activism encouraged staffers to take on issues that had been ignored during the Reagan administration.

In April 1991, Jeffrey Nesbit, an FDA spokesperson, told Dr. Kessler that if the FDA was a public health agency, it ought to protect public health by taking on tobacco, a politically explosive issue. Nesbit showed the committee many years' worth of petitions containing hundreds of thousands of signatures calling for the agency to regulate tobacco products as drugs.

Kessler hesitated at first, in part because the FDA did not have enough scientific evidence to support a claim that cigarettes were drug delivery devices that disperse nicotine and should be regulated by the agency. Kessler, however, assigned several dozen FDA scientists, lawyers, and other staffers to collect data. Dr. Kessler was aware that the COALITION ON SMOKING OR HEALTH, a Washington group of health lobbyists, had been pressing the government to regulate cigarettes since the late 1980s and had recently petitioned the FDA to regulate low-tar cigarettes.

Kessler was also intrigued by a Philip Morris brand of cigarettes called Next, a "denicotined" cigarette developed in 1989. The company had extracted virtually all of Next's nicotine. The commissioner reasoned that if nicotine could be taken out of one brand, why was it not taken out of all brands? Kessler's team shifted its focus to the question of whether manufacturers deliberately set nicotine levels and began assembling evidence.

In the autumn of 1993, ABC News informed the FDA of its in-depth, year-long investigation of the tobacco industry's manipulation of nicotine levels in cigarettes and introduced FDA officials to key confidential sources. In January 1994, an informer named Deep Cough, who was sent to the FDA, described the steps taken by tobacco companies to control the precise levels of nicotine in cigarettes. This information gave the agency the foundation it needed to open its own investigation into nicotine manipulation and to begin building its case for regulating nicotine as a drug and cigarettes as drug delivery devices.

In the spring of 1994, the FDA observed a trend that suggested that the tobacco industry manipulated and controlled the levels of nicotine in cigarettes. Tobacco companies are required to report the levels of nicotine and tar in their products to the FEDERAL TRADE COMMISSION (FTC). When FDA investigators analyzed these reports, they found that the amount of nicotine delivered had been increasing since 1982, with the greatest increases in lowest tar cigarettes. Tar levels, however, showed no increases, contradicting the industry's claim that "nicotine follows the tar level." It seemed unlikely that nicotine could increase independently of the delivery of tar unless the manufacturers had done so deliberately. FDA scientists also learned that certain cigarettes advertised as having the lowest tar content actually contained the blends of tobacco richest in nicotine.

In the spring and summer of 1994, Kessler and his team learned more about the actions of tobacco companies. In April 1994, two former Philip Morris scientists, VICTOR DENOBLE and PAUL MELE, testified before Congress about the company's efforts in the 1980s to find an analogue of nicotine that would "mimic nicotine's effect on the brain" without affecting the cardiovascular system. In May, more evidence about nicotine's addictiveness emerged when the *New York Times* published an article describing confidential documents obtained from BROWN AND WILLIAMSON TOBACCO CORPORATION that showed that in the 1960s company officials acknowledged that "smoking is a habit of addiction," and said "we are, then, in the business of selling nicotine, an addictive drug." Besides learning that the company had conducted dozens of studies of the drug-like properties of nicotine, FDA investigators also learned from an anonymous phone tip that Brown and Williamson had created a new variety of tobacco, code named Y-1, with twice the normal level of nicotine.

In addition to a series of meetings in May 1994 with JEFFREY WIGAND, a former Brown and Williamson research scientist and the tobacco industry's highest-ranking whistle blower, another piece of evidence surfaced. It was a section of one tobacco company's handbook on leaf blending and product development that showed that tobacco companies used chemical additives to affect the delivery of nicotine. The FDA investigation also revealed that manufacturers conducted and funded research into the pharmacokinetics of nicotine and methods of delivery.

By the end of 1994, the FDA had collected enough information to begin work drafting a proposed rule that would give the agency the authority to regulate nicotine as a drug and cigarettes as drug delivery devices. After months of preparing the legal paper, the agency submitted for review a two-part proposal to the White House. The agency threw the matter to the president rather than use its own authority because of the delicate nature of the issue.

The first part of the paper was a long technical document asserting that the FDA has the authority to control tobacco under the FOOD, DRUG, AND COSMETIC ACT OF 1938, an assertion that, according to the FDA, did not require White House or congressional approval. (This assertion was challenged; see FOOD AND DRUG ADMINISTRATION (FDA) REGULATIONS: FEDERAL DISTRICT COURT RULING.) The second part included proposals for regulating tobacco that focused only on combating smoking by children and teens. The FDA confined itself to modest proposals on the politically surer ground of limiting young people's access to tobacco rather than on broader controls. Polls showed that even in pro-tobacco states, voters would support some kind of tobacco regulation aimed at protecting children.

On August 10, 1995, President Bill Clinton announced at a news conference that the FDA's scientific and legal evidence and analysis supported a finding, subject to public comment, that nicotine in cigarettes and SMOKELESS TOBACCO products is a drug and addictive and that these products are drug delivery devices. Clinton became the first president in U.S. history to assert authority over the tobacco companies when he ordered FDA regulation governing the sale of cigarettes. But the Clinton administration determined that there should be regulations only with respect to minors, not adults. In the news conference, the president said, "We do not . . . seek to address activities that sell, that seek to sell, cigarettes only to adults. We are stepping in to protect those who need our help, our vulnerable young people" ("Excerpts from Clinton News Conference," 1995).

The authority asserted by the FDA to regulate tobacco products was challenged immediately by the tobacco companies in federal district court charging that the administration overstepped its authority and was heading down the path towards prohibition of all tobacco products. Although Judge William L. Osteen, Sr., ruled on April 25, 1997, that the FDA had jurisdiction under the Food, Drug, and Cosmetic Act of 1938 to regulate nicotine-containing cigarettes and smokeless tobacco, his decision was overturned by the U.S. Court of Appeals for the Fourth Circuit on August 14, 1998. The Clinton administration appealed the Court of Appeals decision. On April 26, 1999, the Supreme Court announced it would decide whether the Food and Drug Administration has authority to regulate tobacco products as drugs and cigarettes as "drug delivering devices." The case, *Food and Drug Administration v. Brown and Williamson Tobacco Corp.*, is scheduled to be argued in November 1999. *See also* BROWN AND WILLIAMSON TOBACCO CORPORATION—MERRELL WILLIAMS DOCUMENTS; *DAY ONE*; FOOD AND DRUG ADMINISTRATION (FDA) 1995 PROPOSAL FOR REGULATING TOBACCO; FOOD AND DRUG ADMINISTRATION (FDA) 1997 TOBACCO REGULATIONS; FOOD AND DRUG ADMINISTRATION (FDA) REGULATIONS: U.S. COURT OF APPEALS FOR THE FOURTH CIRCUIT RULING; KESSLER, DAVID; Y-1 TOBACCO

References: "Excerpts from Clinton News Conference on His Tobacco Order," *New York Times*, August 11, 1995, p. A18.

Food and Drug Administration (FDA) 1995 Proposal for Regulating Tobacco

The proposed rule was set out in a 324-page section in the *Federal Register*. The proposals would prohibit sales to those under 18 years of age and require photo ID for proof of age. The rules would ban sales through vending machines and mail order, ban the sale of individual cigarettes or packs of 20 or fewer cigarettes, and prohibit free samples. They would forbid brand-name tobacco sponsorship of sporting or entertainment events, permitting only corporate name sponsorship, and prohibit the sale or giving away of promotional items (T-shirts, gym bags, cigarette lighters, caps) with brand names or logos to children. BILLBOARD ads less than 1,000 feet from schools and playgrounds would be banned, but black-and-white, text advertising for all other outdoor ads and ads at the point of sale in stores would be permitted. Tobacco advertising would be limited to black-and-white text only in publications like *Sports Illustrated* with more than 15 percent readership under 18 or more than two million young readers. Finally, tobacco companies would have to create a multimillion-dollar fund for anti-smoking campaigns directed at young people.

The regulations covered CIGARETTES and SMOKELESS TOBACCO, but not pipe tobacco or cigars. Unlike the evidence relating to cigarettes and smokeless tobacco, the FOOD AND DRUG ADMINISTRATION (FDA) had insufficient evidence to move ahead with regulations regarding cigars and pipes at the time the agency proposed the rules.

Under the federal regulatory process, the FDA was required to take public comment for 90 days, but the agency extended the period until January 1, 1996. More than 700,000 comments on its finding of jurisdiction and on its proposed regulations were sent to FDA headquarters, more comments than had been received about any other federal rule in history. The cigarette and smokeless tobacco industries alone sent 2,500 pages of text and nearly 50,000 pages of exhibits.

On August 23, 1996, President Bill Clinton authorized the final FDA rule to regulate tobacco products (cigarettes and smokeless tobacco). The rule, the most far-reaching measure ever instituted to reduce tobacco use by young people, differed in some ways from those rules the FDA initially proposed. It allowed more leeway for sales of tobacco products clearly aimed at adult purchasers and dropped language that called for a $150 million annual fund maintained by the tobacco industry to conduct a national education campaign. In response to business complaints, the president changed one of the FDA proposals to ban all vending machine sales of cigarettes to locations where children have access and he rejected another proposal to prohibit tobacco sales through the mail. The final rule permitted color imagery in ads only in adults-only areas such as bars and nightclubs, provided the image cannot be seen from the outside and cannot be removed easily. The provisions were scheduled to take effect one year later to allow the industry time to comply. *See also* FOOD AND DRUG ADMINISTRATION (FDA) 1997 TOBACCO REGULATIONS; FOOD AND DRUG ADMINISTRATION (FDA) REGULATIONS: FEDERAL DISTRICT COURT RULING; FOOD AND DRUG ADMINISTRATION (FDA) REGULATIONS: U.S. COURT OF APPEALS FOR THE FOURTH CIRCUIT RULING; KESSLER, DAVID

Food and Drug Administration (FDA) 1997 Tobacco Regulations

On February 28, 1997, under new regulations issued by the U.S. FOOD AND DRUG ADMINISTRATION (FDA), retailers (drug, convenience stores, food stores, gasoline stations, restaurants) were prohibited from selling cigarettes, loose cigarette tobacco, and smokeless tobacco to anyone under age 18. To verify that anyone buying tobacco products is at least 18 years old or older, retailers must check identification of everyone under 27 showing the buyer's picture and date of birth. Retailers must sell cigarettes or smokeless tobacco only in a direct, face-to-face exchange, without the help of any electronic or mechanical device. Retailers must not break open any tobacco package or sell any number or quantity of cigarettes or smokeless tobacco that is less than the smallest package (20 cigarettes) distributed by the manufacturer for individual consumer use.

To ensure that the federal rule would be followed, the FDA contracted with the states to carry out unannounced compliance checks during which adolescents, accompanied by state or local officials commissioned by the FDA, tried to purchase cigarettes and smokeless tobacco from retailers. The first compliance checks began during the summer of 1997. Under the FOOD, DRUG, AND COSMETIC ACT OF 1938, retailers selling tobacco products to minors are held responsible for violating regulations. Enforcement procedures involve correspondence notifying the retailer of a violation or a penalty proceeding and civil money penalties that escalate from $250 to $10,000 for violations observed and documented during compliance checks conducted by or for the FDA. Retailers who refuse to sell tobacco products to minors will also receive letters stating that they were found to be in compliance. Finally, state or local authorities may also impose their own sanctions for retailers who fail to comply with state and local laws. In March 2000, the Supreme Court ruled that the FDA did not have the authority to regulate tobacco. The court's ruling invalidated the FDA identification rule.

Food and Drug Administration (FDA) Regulations: Federal District Court Ruling

After President Bill Clinton's 1995 news conference, cigarette and smokeless tobacco manufacturers, contending that the FEDERAL DRUG ADMINISTRATION (FDA) lacked the authority to regulate cigarettes and smokeless tobacco, filed a lawsuit to block the proposals in a Federal District Court in Greensboro, North Carolina, the heart of tobacco country. WILLIAM L. OSTEEN, SR., was appointed to examine the case. Trade associations representing advertising agencies and convenience stores, distributors, and others also filed a lawsuit in the same North Carolina court, claiming that FDA chief DAVID KESSLER's advertising ban would violate the

"commercial free speech" interpretation of the First Amendment.

On April 25, 1997, Judge Osteen ruled that the FDA had jurisdiction under the FOOD, DRUG AND COSMETIC ACT OF 1938 to regulate nicotine-containing cigarettes and smokeless tobacco. The court held that tobacco products fit within the act's definitions of "drug" and "device," and that the FDA can regulate cigarettes and smokeless tobacco products as drug delivery devices. The court upheld all restrictions involving youth access and labeling, including the two provisions that went into effect on February 28, 1997: (1) the prohibition on sales of cigarettes and smokeless tobacco products to children and adolescents under 18 years of age, and (2) the requirement that retailers check photo identification of customers who are under 27. The court also upheld access and labeling restrictions scheduled to go into effect August 28, 1997, including a prohibition on self-service displays and the placement of vending machines where children have access to them. Distribution of free samples was banned, as was the sale of so-called kiddie packs of less than 20 cigarettes and the sale of individual cigarettes.

In his ruling, Judge Osteen said Congress never expressly excluded the agency from controlling nicotine in cigarettes. Osteen found that nicotine alters the bodily function just as other drugs do. Further, he said cigarettes deliver nicotine so they are drug delivery devices. Therefore the FDA was empowered to regulate tobacco products under its charter even though the tobacco companies did not advertise their products as drug delivery devices.

Although Judge Osteen rejected the industry's arguments opposing FDA jurisdiction, he ruled that the agency could not impose controls on tobacco advertising and the promotion of tobacco products. His ruling was based on the scope of the Food, Drug, and Cosmetic Act of 1938, which does not provide the FDA with the authority to regulate the advertising and promotion of tobacco products. Because Judge Osteen based his ruling on statutory grounds, he declined to consider the First Amendment challenge to those parts of the rule. Both sides appealed

Judge Osteen's decision. *See also* FOOD AND DRUG ADMINISTRATION (FDA) REGULATIONS: U.S. COURT OF APPEALS FOR THE FOURTH CIRCUIT RULING

Food and Drug Administration (FDA) Regulations: U.S. Court of Appeals for the Fourth Circuit Ruling

On August 14, 1998, the U.S. Court of Appeals for the Fourth Circuit in RICHMOND, VIRGINIA, overturned the decision of the U.S. District Court for the Middle District of North Carolina and ruled that the FOOD AND DRUG ADMINISTRATION (FDA) had no authority to regulate cigarettes and smokeless tobacco and that the agency needed explicit authority from Congress to regulate tobacco products. In a 58-page opinion, the panel's majority wrote that there is "strong evidence that Congress has reserved for itself the regulation of tobacco products rather than delegating that regulation to the F.D.A." (Meier, 1998). The FDA, therefore, needed explicit authority from Congress to regulate tobacco products. The majority opinion, written by Circuit Judge H. Emory Widener, Jr., noted that from 1914 until its attempt to regulate tobacco in 1996, the FDA had consistently said tobacco products were outside its authority. In the 60 years following the passage of the act in 1938, the FDA repeatedly informed Congress that cigarettes marketed without therapeutic claims do not fit within the scope of the act. The court, however, did not reject the FDA's conclusion that these products fall within the Food, Drug and Cosmetic Act's definitions of "drugs" and "devices." Instead, the majority opinion concluded, based on several sources of evidence, there was a lack of regulatory tools in the act appropriate for the regulation of tobacco products.

Because the majority found that the agency lacked jurisdiction, it invalidated the FDA's August 1996 regulations that restricted the sale and distribution of tobacco products to children and adolescents. The restrictions in effect since February 1997 remained in effect pending the court's review of the government's request for a rehearing. *See also* FOOD AND DRUG ADMINISTRATION (FDA) REGULATIONS: FEDERAL DISTRICT COURT RULING; FOOD, DRUG AND COSMETIC ACT OF 1968; OSTEEN, WILLIAM L.

References: Barry Meier, "Court Rules F.D.A. lacks Authority to Limit Tobacco." *New York Times*, August 15, 1998, p. 1.

Food, Drug and Cosmetic Act of 1938

According to the Food, Drug and Cosmetic Act of 1938, an article (other than food) is a drug or a device subject to regulation by the FOOD AND DRUG ADMINISTRATION (FDA) if its manufacturer intends that it affects the structure or function of the body when used. Under this law, which was amended to include oversight of "medical devices" such as syringes, the FDA has oversight over any substance for which the manufacturer has claimed a health benefit. In the 1950s, the FDA challenged the claims made for some cigarettes. Advertising leaflets for Fairfax claimed it prevented "the common cold, influenza, pneumonia . . . scarlet fever, whooping cough, measles, meningitis, tuberculosis . . . [and] parrot fever." The FDA's complaint was upheld because the material contained a therapeutic claim.

Food for Peace Program

From 1954 through the early 1980s, tobacco was included in the Department of Agriculture's Food for Peace Program. Under this tax-supported program, the U.S. Department of Agriculture purchased and shipped millions of dollars worth of surplus domestic tobacco, along with much-needed food, to hungry nations of the world. Between 1971 and 1974, the average annual value was over $650 million and represented 1 percent of total exports. In 1979, $2.15 billion worth of tobacco products and leaf was exported.

Republican Senator Jesse Helms of North Carolina justified the existence of tobacco in a food aid program by noting that, in addition to supplying an outlet for surplus tobacco leaf, "historically these sales have developed new markets for American tobacco" (Taylor,

1984). The practice of sending tobacco was abandoned in response to criticism from international health officials. *See also* GLOBAL TOBACCO USE

References: Peter Taylor, *The Smoke Ring: Tobacco, Money, & Multinational Politics*, New York: Pantheon Books, 1984, p. 262.

Foote, Emerson (1906–1992)

A founder of Foote, Cone and Belding and former board chairman of McCann-Erickson, a New York ad agency, Emerson Foote handled the LUCKY STRIKE CIGARETTES account. Foote, a "reformed' smoker, joined the health forces not, he explained, because he disliked smoking, "I am not against tobacco. I am against cancer, heart disease, and emphysema" (Wagner, 1971). Though he wrote many of the slogans that helped popularize smoking, he felt no progress could be made until cigarette advertising was curbed. He favored health warnings in advertising. In the summer of 1965, Foote became the first chairman of the NATIONAL INTERAGENCY COUNCIL ON SMOKING AND HEALTH.

Foote became one of the few advertising authorities to speak against tobacco promotion. In a 1980 statement he made to the Toronto Transit Commission (which voted unanimously to reject future tobacco advertising, Foote said that, from his experience, he was not convinced that competition among cigarette brands was the most important purpose of advertising). He felt that creating a positive climate of social acceptability for smoking, which encourages new smokers to join the market, was more important to the industry. The implied message is "if it is alright to advertise, the product can't be that bad." The converse of this, of which the industry is aware, is that if it is not acceptable to advertise, then there must be something wrong with the product.

He also said that in recent years, the cigarette industry had been maintaining that cigarette advertising had nothing to do with total sales.

I am always amused by the suggestion that advertising, a function that has been shown to increase consumption of virtually every other product, somehow miraculously fails to work for tobacco products. The argument is only advanced to undermine efforts to restrict tobacco promotion. (Foote, 1981)

References: Emerson Foote, "Advertising and Tobacco, " *JAMA*, vol. 245, no. 16, April 24, 1981, p. 1668.

Susan Wagner, *Cigarette Country: Tobacco in American History and Politics*, New York: Praegar Publishers, 1971, p. 154.

Ford, Henry (1863–1947)

Henry Ford was convinced cigarettes caused criminality, and swore that no cigarette smoker would work for the Ford Motor Company. Ford watched the personal habits of his employees through the company's "Sociological Department," which spied on workers by making surprise visits to their homes. He discouraged, but did not prohibit the use of other forms of tobacco. After World War I, he abandoned his efforts to keep cigarette smokers off his payroll. It was no longer practical given the popularity of the habit.

Henry Ford wrote about his views in a self-published book, *The Case Against the Little White Slaver*, published in four volumes between 1914 and 1916. The book consists of statements from employers about the undesirability of cigarette smokers as employees and testimonials from athletes and other celebrities about the virtues of tobacco-free living.

France

Tobacco was introduced into France around 1650 by the explorer ANDRÉ THEVET, and, more prominently, by JEAN NICOT. As ambassador to the Portuguese court in the sixteenth century, Nicot became familiar with the plant and sent it as a gift to Catherine de Médicis, queen mother of France. Nicot and the court were the primary influences in France in the spread of knowledge about tobacco and its reputation for healing almost every complaint. It was in honor of Nicot that, in 1570, the plant was dubbed *Nicotiana* and the active ingredient was later called NICOTINE.

The history of tobacco in seventeenth- and eighteenth-century France is distinguished by the spread of snuffing, the decline of opposition to tobacco, the rise of dependence on it for revenues, and the spread of monopolies. During the reign of Louis XIII (1610–1643), smoking spread among the lower classes. The court, nobility, and clergy increasingly turned to SNUFF. Although the king gave no encouragement, the habit grew.

Cardinal Richelieu, the chief minister of France, personally objected to smoking, and thought by imposing a duty on imported tobacco, the growing habit might be checked by making it expensive. But he also thought tobacco might be an inexhaustible spring of wealth. He believed that taxation would be better and more profitable than direct prohibition.

In the reign of Louis XIV (1643–1715), the tobacco habit was widespread and continued despite the king's personal dislike. The king's physician, Fagon, voiced dissent, attacking tobacco fiercely for shortening life. Most writers of the age celebrated tobacco for its pleasures. Molière in *Don Juan* (1665) called tobacco "the passion of all proper people"; Corneille in *Le festin de Piere* (1677) wrote that "tobacco is divine"; and the Marquis de Prade praised tobacco in *Histoire de tabac* (1677) (Austin, 1978).

Louis XIV and Colbert, his finance minister, issued an edict in September 1674 introducing the tobacco monopoly that reserved for the king the privilege of manufacturing and selling tobacco, which the king farmed out to contractors. The French system of tax and trade monopolies imitated the tobacco monopolies of the Italian and Austrian states. Tobacco policy was typical of government mercantilism aimed at making the country self-sufficient, in part by increasing the wealth from which taxes were drawn. The French government relied on methods for increasing taxable wealth, and it realized quickly that tobacco was an especially profitable source of revenue.

Although Louis XIV never attacked tobacco, he disliked it so much that tobacco was never used in his presence. Once tobacco spread in France, the king was powerless against its use. But once he discovered the profitable returns that could be gained from the trade, he willingly protected it.

During the French Revolution, there was hostility towards the tobacco monopoly, and the barriers to tobacco trading were swept away. But in 1810, Napoleon needed huge sums of money for his continental wars, and he reestablished the monopoly by imperial decree, declaring that tobacco could bear taxation better than other articles. Direct control of the tobacco industry became the system in France and its favorable monetary return attracted the attention of other governments. The French system became the model for other major European countries.

It was in France that snuff-taking first became fashionable. Its appeal to the aristocracy and clergy played an important role in the spread of tobacco throughout Europe by 1700. SNUFF remained in vogue in France and England until the French Revolution. After that, its use declined. A large-scale industry developed in France to produce snuff and exquisite snuff boxes. *See also* SNUFF EQUIPMENT; SNUFF MILLS

References: Examples from Gregory A. Austin, *Perspectives on the History of Psychoactive Substance Use*, Rockville, MD: National Institute on Drug Abuse, 1978, p. 14.

Frédéric, François Alexandre (1747–1827)

French philanthropist François Alexandre Frédéric, the Duc de la Rochefoucauld-Liancourt, authored one of the oldest known tributes to the CIGAR. Sent by the French revolutionary government to the United States in 1794, he wrote about cigars on his sea voyage.

> The cigar is a great resource. It is necessary to have traveled for a long time on a ship to understand that at least the cigar offers you the pleasure of smoking. It raises your spirits. Are you troubled by something? The cigar dissolves it. Are you subject to aches and pains (or bad temper)? The cigar will change your disposition. Are you harassed by unpleasant thoughts?

Smoking a cigar puts one in a frame of mind to dispense with these. Do you ever feel a little faint from hunger? A cigar satisfies the yearning. If you are obsessed by sad thoughts, a cigar will take your mind off of them. Finally don't you sometimes have some pleasant remembrance or consoling thought? A cigar will reinforce this. Sometimes they die out, and happy are those who do not need to relight too quickly. I hardly need to say anything more about the cigar, to which I dedicate this little eulogy for past services rendered. (Conrad, 1996)

References: Barnaby Conrad III, *The Cigar*, San Francisco: Chronicle Books, 1996, p. 24.

Freud, Sigmund (1856–1939)

An Austrian neurologist and the founder of psychoanalysis, Sigmund Freud was rarely without a CIGAR and usually smoked 15 to 20 per day. He began smoking at the age of 24, emulating his father, Jacob, who smoked until he was 81 years old. For almost 50 years, Freud maintained a highly ritualized daily schedule that included a visit to the neighborhood tobacconist. For much of his life, Freud kept a diary in which he recorded these visits to the store and the cigars he purchased. Freud's options were limited because the Austrian government had strict control over the tobacco industry.

According to *The Diary of Sigmund Freud 1929–1939: A Record of the Final Decade,* translated by Michael Molnar, Freud usually smoked a cigar called a *trabucco,* which was a small, mild cigar produced by the Austrian monopoly. However, he favored Don Pedros and Reina Cubanas, which he acquired on trips to the Bavarian town of Berchtesgaden and Dutch Liliputanos. Freud received boxes of cigars as gifts from patients, an unorthodox practice, and from friends who kept him supplied with his favorite brands.

Freud, for whom not smoking was unthinkable, smoked from the time he awoke to the time he went to bed. As patients lay on his couch, he sat behind them, hidden from view in his armchair, smoking and taking notes. Freud was so fond of smoking that when men around him did not smoke, he became irritated. Nearly all of Freud's inner circle, therefore, were cigar smokers.

Inconsolable if he could not smoke, Freud ignored warnings from his physician friend, Wilhelm Fliess, who wanted him to give up cigars. Even after he developed a cancerous growth in his mouth in 1923 at age 67, he waited for years before showing it to anyone for fear smoking would be suspected as the cause. When his physician advised him to give up cigars, he resisted. During one seven-week period of abstinence, he wrote Dr. Fliess a letter telling him that life was unbearable and that he experienced cardiac symptoms and depression. Abstinence also left Freud incapable of working. Once he resumed smoking, he was able to work. Even when he was terminally ill with cancer, Freud smoked until the end of his life. Before he died, on his brother Alexander's 72nd birthday, he bequeathed him his stock of fine cigars, and wrote: "I would like you to take over the good cigars which have been accumulating with me over the years, as you can still indulge in such pleasures, I no longer can" (Elkin, 1994).

References: Evan J. Elkin, "More than Cigar: Sigmund Freud, the Father of Psychoanalysis, Revered His Cigars and Defended His Right to Smoke Above All Else." *Cigar Aficionado: The Library Archives*, Winter 1994, p. 9 (online).

G

Garfinkel, Lawrence

In 1981, Lawrence Garfinkel of the AMERI-CAN CANCER SOCIETY (ACS) published the findings of a major epidemiological study on the role of secondhand cigarette smoke in causing lung cancer. Appearing in the *Journal of the National Cancer Institute,* the study's results contradicted those of Dr. TAKESHI HIRAYAMA, which had appeared six months earlier.

Garfinkel detected no increase in lung cancer deaths in 375,000 nonsmoking women and 148,000 nonsmoking men over the 17½-year study period. He found no significant differences in lung cancer rates between women whose husbands smoked and those whose husbands did not smoke. *See also* SECONDHAND SMOKE

Garner, Donald

A law professor at the University of Southern Illinois, Donald Garner, who has studied the tobacco industry's legal history, came up with the idea of suing tobacco companies for reimbursement of Medicaid expenses. In an article entitled "Cigarettes and Welfare Reform," published in the spring 1977 issue of the *Emery Law Journal,* Professor Garner noted the increasing economic waste caused by CIGARETTE smoking, especially when it came to health costs. He suggested that the states get the appropriate cigarette manufacturer to pay the direct medical cost "of look-ing after patients with smoking diseases." He acknowledged that there might be a problem proving that the illnesses were caused by smoking, but felt that issue could be overcome using a method similar to that used to assess the eligibility of coal miners for black lung disease benefits.

Gaston, Lucy Page (1860–1924)

Anti-cigarette crusader Lucy Page Gaston was born in Delaware, Ohio, and grew up in a family of nonsmokers and total abstainers. Immersed in the temperance movement, she led raids on saloons and gambling halls while a student at Illinois State Normal School in the early 1880s. During the late 1880s, she taught school in small towns in Illinois and, disturbed by boys sneaking behind the building to smoke cigarettes, developed an interest in cigarettes as a social issue. Along with her mother, Gaston worked for the Women's Christian Temperance Union (WCTU) and wrote for various WCTU publications. By 1892, Gaston had aroused the WCTU, the Young Men's Christian Association (YMCA), and other groups to the dangers of smoking. In 1895, she began speaking before legislative bodies, asking them to ban the manufacture and sale of cigarettes. Influenced at least in part by Gaston's efforts, 11 states passed anti-cigarette laws by 1913.

In the early 1890s, as a leading worker of the WCTU, she wrote and lectured about the physical and moral dangers of smoking, which Gaston saw as a launching pad to moral decay. By the late 1890s, Gaston focused almost exclusively on the issue of cigarettes, a target largely ignored by the reform community, and rarely spoke out against CIGARS, PIPES, or SNUFF. She believed the state had the authority and an obligation to intervene because cigarettes were making inroads among youth and, in her opinion, youthful smoking led to alcohol abuse, delinquency, disease, and vice.

In 1899, with financing from a group of Chicago businessmen who regarded cigarettes as impediments to efficiency, she founded the Anti-Cigarette League of America whose objective was to enact legislation "to combat and discourage by all legitimate means, the use of and traffic of cigaretts [sic]" (Tate, 1995). It sent recruiters like Gaston around the country to give speeches; pass out pamphlets and gentian root, which was supposed to have tonic qualities when chewed; and solicit donations from church, temperance, and business groups. In 1901, Gaston organized the National Anti-Cigarette League and made complete prohibition of cigarettes its goal. For a while, Gaston seemed on the brink of bringing down James Buchanan Duke's AMERICAN TOBACCO COMPANY, and he was at a loss as how to deal with the forceful, humorless woman and her scores of anti-cigarette converts.

Combining flamboyant tactics, unflagging zeal, an evangelical spirit, and uncompromising attitude, this self-described "extremist of extremists," who signed letters to supporters "Yours for the extermination of the cigarette," was determined to stop everyone from smoking—even the president of the United States. On December 20, 1920, she sent a letter to President-elect Warren G. Harding, a cigarette smoker with what she called a "cigarette face," asking him to quit: "The United States has had no smoking President since McKinley. Roosevelt and Taft and Wilson all have clean records. Is not this a question of grave importance?" (Whelan, 1984). President Harding wrote Gaston back congratulating her for her zeal, but he ignored her appeal. (He stopped smoking in public, how-

ever.) President Harding died at 59 years of age of "stroke of apoplexy," a condition some doctors today believe was caused by smoking.

Eventually, owing to her intemperate tone and financial mismanagement, Gaston was forced in 1920 to resign as superintendent of the Anti-Cigarette League; but she remained dedicated to her cause. She announced her availability for the Republican presidential nomination, entered the South Dakota primary, and received a few votes, but dropped out of the race. In 1921, Gaston organized a new National Anti-Cigarette League, but conceded defeat as far as the nation's male population and cigarettes were concerned. Her new motto was "save the Girl," and her goal was "The Abolition of the Cigarette in America by 1925."

Until she was struck by a streetcar while on her way home from an anti-cigarette rally in Chicago, Gaston zipped through the streets of Chicago snatching cigarettes out of the mouths of boys and girls and made them sign Clean Life Pledges. She died on August 20, 1924, ironically of throat cancer, a disease associated with smoking. In the middle of her funeral service, four children rose, pointed to her coffin, and said together: "Miss Gaston, we thank you for what you have done for us" (Tate, 1995). Then they repeated the Clean Life Pledge. In 1901, when she started the National Anti-Cigarette League, 4.4 billion cigarettes were consumed. When she died, more than 73 billion cigarettes were sold. *See also* ANTI-TOBACCO MOVEMENTS, UNITED STATES; Duke, JAMES BUCHANAN

References: C. Cassandra Tate, "The American Anti-Cigarette Movement, 1880–1930," Ph.D. dissertation, Seattle: University of Washington, 1995, p. 115. (UMI Number 9609793).

Elizabeth M. Whelan, *A Smoking Gun: How the Tobacco Industry Gets Away with Murder*, Philadelphia: George F. Stickley Co., 1984, p. 51.

Gauthier, Wendell Haynes (1943–)

In 1994, New Orleans attorney Wendell Haynes Gauthier devised a new legal theory for suing tobacco companies that became the basis for the first and largest national class-action suit against cigarette makers. Although the suit was ultimately dismissed, Gauthier's idea was to create a class of more than 50 million smokers nationwide who would sue the tobacco companies for the costs of medical monitoring to pay for checkups of addicted smokers and smoking cessation programs, compensation for being addicted, as well as punitive damages. He contended that smokers were not forewarned that smoking was habit forming and nothing on cigarette packs spelled out that cigarettes were addictive.

Wendell Gauthier was a close friend of PETER CASTANO, a New Orleans lawyer who died at the age of 43 in 1993 from lung cancer caused by smoking. A nonsmoker who was familiar with the work of renowned thoracic surgeon Dr. ALTON OCHSNER of New Orleans, Gauthier, at the request of Castano's widow, filed a lawsuit on her husband's behalf. He did so after learning about a February 25, 1994, letter from Dr. DAVID KESSLER to the COALITION ON SMOKING OR HEALTH and after viewing ABC's news program DAY ONE on February 28, 1994.

Gauthier saw a new way to sue the tobacco companies based on the theory that addiction, not failure to warn of the health dangers of smoking, was a new legal issue. He recruited 65 of the top U.S. trial lawyers, many of them friends of Castano, to sue on behalf of addicted smokers and to defray the cost of filing a class-action suit. On March 29, 1994, Gauthier's coalition filed CASTANO V. AMERICAN TOBACCO COMPANY in the U.S. District Court in New Orleans. Although the lawsuit carried Castano's name, it was in actuality the world's largest class action on behalf of all nicotine-addicted smokers, potentially tens of millions of Americans. The tobacco companies predicted correctly that the suit would fail. See also ENGLE V. R.J. REYNOLDS TOBACCO COMPANY ET AL.

Gilboy v. American Tobacco Company

An example of a cigarette case litigated during the second wave of tobacco litigation (1983–1992) was the case of Gilboy v. American Tobacco Company. It was argued under the theory of strict liability. The plaintiff, Robert C. Gilboy (1928–), alleged he developed brain and lung cancer from smoking cigarettes manufactured by the defendant, AMERICAN TOBACCO COMPANY.

Gilboy began smoking cigarettes at 12 or 13 years of age. After a seizure on March 31, 1986, he was diagnosed as having cancer of the lung and brain. Gilboy filed suit in 1987. The trial court granted a judgment in favor of the tobacco company, principally on the theory that Gilboy voluntarily encountered the risks associated with cigarette smoking, and dismissed the suit.

In 1990, the Court of Appeals for the First Circuit examined whether strict liability should be applied to tobacco litigation. In rendering its decision, the court affirmed the judgment that cigarettes are not unreasonably dangerous. The court refused to find unreasonableness, holding that cigarette smoking is a voluntary act and the presence of warning labels on cigarette packs alerts the consumer to any potential dangers. The court reasoned that to allow a recovery based on strict liability would open other products to litigation. The court used alcohol as an example. Under the plaintiff's theory, drinkers who suffer from alcohol-related diseases would be able to seek compensation from liquor manufacturers under strict liability. This theory could result in the abandonment of individual responsibility, and products adequately labeled with warnings would provide no protection to manufacturers. See also TOBACCO LITIGATION: FIRST, SECOND, AND THIRD WAVES

Ginter, Lewis (1824–1897)

One of the pioneers in the field of cigarette manufacturing during the late 1870s and early 1880s, Lewis Ginter, a native of New York, established himself as a CIGARETTE manufacturer in RICHMOND, VIRGINIA. He was a good salesman and packaged his product well. Ginter was also acknowledged as a master of cigarette advertising who had a worldwide reputation for stuffing packages with puzzles, maps, and pictures of boats, flags, actors, and actresses in numbered sets. *See also* ALLEN AND GINTER; CIGARETTE PICTURE CARDS, UNITED STATES

Glantz, Stanton (1946–)

Anti-tobacco activist Stanton Glantz has been involved in the battle for nonsmokers' rights. A professor of medicine and member of the Institute for Health Policy Studies at the University of California, San Francisco, he earned a doctorate at Stanford University in engineering and economics, studying the heart muscle and pump mechanisms.

In his research on the heart, he looked at drugs that affect the pump rate, including NICOTINE. When he learned about how the tobacco companies concealed their research and what they knew about nicotine's effects on the heart, he decided to devote his life to exposing them. He has lectured and gone to conferences all over the world. Dr. Glantz, an editor of the *Journal of the American College of Cardiology,* one of the world's leading heart journals, has served as a consultant to the National Institutes of Health, Environmental Protection Agency, Occupational Safety and Health Administration, National Science Foundation, and numerous scientific publications. Besides authoring six books, he has written over 90 scientific papers, including the first major review that identified involuntary smoking as a cause of heart disease, and was one of the founders of AMERICANS FOR NONSMOKERS RIGHTS (ANR).

In 1982, Professor Glantz received a package containing a copy of the film *DEATH IN THE WEST,* which had been suppressed by Philip Morris. He was instrumental in getting the film aired on television and he also developed a curriculum used by an estimated one million students. He also helped write and produce the films *Secondhand Smoke,* which concerns the health effects of involuntary smoking, and *On the Air,* which describes how to create a smoke-free workplace.

In 1983, Glantz helped defend the San Francisco Workplace Ordinance against a tobacco industry attempt to repeal it by referendum. The victory represented the tobacco industry's first electoral defeat and is now viewed as a major turning point in the battle for nonsmokers' rights.

On May 12, 1994, Dr. Glantz received a Federal Express box containing 4,000 pages of Brown and Williamson's company documents stolen by paralegal Merrell Williams. The anonymous sender's name was "Mr. Butts," the cartoon character in "Doonesbury." After examining the documents, many of which were about NICOTINE addiction, Glantz put the papers in the university library until Brown and Williamson discovered them. The tobacco company tried to block publication of the documents by the university, but the California Supreme Court rejected the company's request to stop the university library from making the documents available to the public. The library put the papers on the World Wide Web as well as on CD-ROM.

After the documents were made available to the public, the industry's congressional lobbyists tried and failed to persuade Congress to cancel the National Cancer Institute funding of Glantz's tobacco control studies. One of the reports tracked the effects of tobacco money on state legislators' voting patterns. Another examined the industry's role in grassroots smokers' rights campaigns.

A citizens' group, Californians for Scientific Integrity, filed a lawsuit against the University of California at San Francisco charging that Glantz skewed data in a 1994 study of the effect of smoking bans in restaurants and used state funds illegally to promote tobacco control. Glantz's study concluded there was no economic impact. The group, which obtained a court order to "lock up" Glantz's computer and prevent him from destroying data, demanded that the *American Journal of Public Health,* the journal where the 1994 study was published, reexamine it. After the journal did so and concluded the article was sound, the journal's editor wrote in the October 1997 issue that "plainly, the aim is to destroy Glantz's career." *See also* BROWN AND WILLIAMS TOBACCO CORPORATION; BROWN AND WILLIAMSON TOBACCO CORPORATION—MERRELL WILLIAMS DOCUMENTS; SECONDHAND SMOKE

Gloag, Robert Peacock (1825–1891)

As paymaster to the Turkish allied forces in the CRIMEAN WAR, Scotsman Robert Gloag watched British troops smoke hand-made Russian and Turkish smoking tubes. He imported a small quantity of Latakia, granulated the small leaves, and poked them into preformed paper tubes in the French manner. He gave these Turkish cigarettes brand names like Xanthe and Kohinoor. Gloag is credited with opening the first full-fledged British CIGARETTE factory in 1856. He first employed foreigners skilled in hand manufacture and later well-trained women to make cigarettes for Gloag and Company.

By the 1860s, cigarette smoking, or the "Crimea fad," as one newspaper called it, had declined and Gloag turned his attention to marketing CIGARS.

In an 1890 interview in the trade journal *Tobacco*, Gloag described the cigarettes that led to his historic decision to open a factory.

> The tobacco used was Latakia dust and the paper yellow tissue...the mouthpiece was of cane. The mode of manufacture was first to make the canes, into which the tobacco had been pressed. In order to keep the dust tobacco from escaping, the ends were turned in. The size of the cigarettes was that which is now known as an Oxford, and they were put up in bundles of ten, to be retailed at 6d.

See also TURKEY

Global Tobacco Control Measures

Of major concern to public health officials is the fact that the burden of smoking related diseases will be shifted during the 1990s and the next decades from developed nations to newly developed ones. According to the WORLD HEALTH ORGANIZATION (WHO), in the early 1990s tobacco products were estimated to have caused around 3 million deaths a year throughout the world, a figure WHO predicts will increase to 10 million annual deaths during the 2020s, with 7 million of these deaths occurring in developing countries. According to WHO, progress made in curbing deaths from malnutrition and infectious disease in less-developed countries will be lost to deaths caused by smoking.

Cigarettes smoked in less-developed countries usually have a higher-tar content than do the same brands purchased in the United States. Tar is believed to be one of the more carcinogenic components of cigarettes. Since health education may be almost nonexistent in some regions, smoking higher-tar cigarettes may set the stage for an epidemic of smoking-related diseases.

To curb disease and death caused by tobacco products, about 25 countries have enacted laws in the 1990s to prohibit the sale of cigarettes to minors, with the age of prohibition ranging from 16 to 21 years of age. In some cases, other related measures have been enacted, including bans or restrictions on cigarette sales from vending machines, prohibitions on sales of tobacco products and smoking in schools, as well as the sale of single cigarettes and the offering of free samples of cigarettes.

In the early 1990s, about 80 countries required health warnings to appear on packages of tobacco products. However, in most of these countries, the warnings are small, inconspicuous, and provide little information about the serious health consequences of tobacco use. By the mid-1990s, however, a number of countries adopted more stringent warning systems, involving direct statements of health hazards, multiple messages, and large and prominent displays. Such warnings are required in a number of countries including Australia, Canada, Iceland, Norway, Singapore, South Africa, and Thailand.

A number of countries have successfully passed laws to ban all or nearly all forms of tobacco advertising. As of 1990, 27 countries reportedly had total or near-total bans on advertising. Since then, however, the number has declined. Tobacco advertising bans that had been in place became inoperative in Canada and the independent states of Central and Eastern Europe.

In 1998, the European Parliament, the legislative body of the 15-nation European Union (EU), agreed to phase out tobacco advertising and sponsorships in the EU. The move will abolish almost all tobacco advertising in the 15 countries by 2006. Most advertising will be illegal by 2004, and cigarette makers will have until October 2006 to stop sponsoring major sports and cultural events.

A number of countries have successfully used a portion of tobacco taxation revenue to offset the cost of operating their comprehensive tobacco control programs. In several Australian states, tobacco taxes are used to finance Health Promotion Foundations. A similar foundation in New Zealand is funded from general revenues. In Finland, almost half of tobacco taxation is allocated for tobacco control activities. In Nepal, Portugal, Romania, and Switzerland, a portion of tobacco tax revenue is used to finance specific health or social programs. *See also* CHINA, TOBACCO, AND HEALTH; APPENDIX 4: TOBACCO TAXATION IN COUNTRIES OF THE EUROPEAN UNION

Global Tobacco Use

By the end of the twentieth century, cigarettes were the predominant form of tobacco consumption around the world. Between 65 and 85 percent of global tobacco consumption is in the form of cigarettes including *bidis* (tobacco wrapped in a temburni leaf widely consumed on the Indian subcontinent) and *kreteks* (clove-flavored cigarettes especially popular in Indonesia). An additional 15 percent to 35 percent of tobacco is consumed in the form of all other tobacco products.

According to estimates made by the WORLD HEALTH ORGANIZATION (WHO), there are around 1,100 million smokers in the world, about one-third of the global population aged 15 years and over.

In the 1990s, tobacco use declined in many countries of North America and Western Europe, but increased in many developing countries. In CHINA, the world's most populous country with about 300 million smokers, the growth in estimated per capita consumption of cigarettes has been rapid, increasing by 260 percent from the early 1970s to the early 1990s. For China, WHO estimated consumption of 1,900 cigarettes per adult per year. India, the world's second most populous country, ranks second globally for total cigarette consumption when *bidis* are taken into account.

WHO found a dramatic shift in the groups of countries with the highest rates of per adult tobacco consumption from the early 1970s to the early 1990s. In the early 1970s, Australia, Canada, Switzerland, and the United Kingdom had the highest consumption while in the early 1990s, Greece, Hungary, JAPAN, Poland, and the Republic of KOREA had the highest.

A 1996 WHO report revealed that globally, approximately 47 percent of men and 12 percent of women smoked. Smoking among women was most prevalent in the countries of EASTERN AND CENTRAL EUROPE, countries with established market economies, and Latin American and Caribbean countries. In all other regions, fewer than 10 percent of women smoked. About one-third of regular smokers in developed countries were women, compared with only about one in eight in the developing world. In many countries, the median age of smoking initiation was under the age of 15.

Tobacco Production and Trade

Most of the global tobacco manufacturing industry is controlled by a small number of state monopolies and multinational corporations. The largest is the state monopoly in China, which in 1993 represented 31 percent of the global market. In 1993, the seven largest multinational tobacco corporations accounted for nearly 40 percent of global cigarette sales.

While tobacco is grown in over 100 countries, the 25 leading producers accounted for over 90 percent of global tobacco production. China, the world's dominant producer of unmanufactured tobacco, produced as much as the next seven largest producers combined. Worldwide, in 1994, four countries, China, the United States, Japan, and Germany, accounted for over half of the global production of cigarettes.

Countries that are major importers of cigarettes include France, Germany, Hong Kong, Japan, the Netherlands, the Russian Federation, and Singapore. The United States is the world's leading exporter of manufactured cigarettes.

For a number of years, the United States was the world's leading exporter of unmanufactured tobacco, but by 1994 it was surpassed by Brazil, the world's largest tobacco-leaf exporter, and Zimbabwe. These two countries became the leading sources of internationally traded unmanufactured tobacco by the mid-1990s. By the late 1990s, Brazil, Italy, Turkey, the United States, and Zimbabwe accounted for half of all global exports of unmanufactured tobacco.

Economics of Tobacco

Although tobacco is grown in more than 100 countries, tobacco leaf and manufactured tobacco exports account for more than 8 percent of export earnings in just two countries, Malawi and Zimbabwe. Tobacco represents a much smaller proportion of export earnings in all other countries.

All countries that have devoted more than 1 percent of their total import expenses to purchasing tobacco are either developing countries or countries of Central and Eastern Europe. In the latter, tobacco import expenditures are relatively large. *See also* ASIA AND U.S. TRADE POLICY; CIGARETTE; CIGAR; LATIN AMERICA

References: The statistics used in this entry come from World Health Organization, "The Tobacco Epidemic: A Global Public Health Emergency," (Factsheets) May 1996.

Godfrey, Arthur (1903–1983)

In 1972, Arthur Godfrey, a retired radio personality who smoked for 35 years, had lung cancer surgery. When he was told cigarettes had damaged him, he replied: "It couldn't be that—I got a $1.5 million contract with Chesterfield." He changed his tune after surgery and branded smoking "a stupid habit." *See also* CHESTERFIELD CIGARETTES

Goldstone, Steven

Steven Goldstone, since 1995 the chairman and chief executive officer of RJR NABISCO HOLDINGS CORPORATION, had been an attorney with the Wall Street firm Davis Polk and Wardell. In 1995 he became president and CEO of RJR Nabisco Inc., whose cigarette

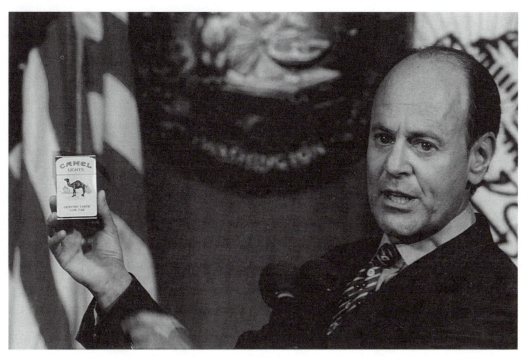

RJR Nabisco CEO Steven Goldstone holds a pack of Camel cigarettes during a luncheon address at the National Press Club in Washington in April 1998. *AP/Wide World Photos.*

unit, R.J. REYNOLDS TOBACCO COMPANY, is the second largest tobacco company in the United States.

Well-skilled at complex negotiations, Goldstone was assigned the job of rescuing his company from tobacco litigation. RJR Nabisco Inc. was in considerable debt from a leveraged buyout of the company a decade before.

Goldstone, who felt it was best to fight state lawsuits all at once, led his fellow chief executive officers of tobacco companies into historic negotiations with the state attorneys general in the $368.5 billion proposed tobacco settlement of June 1997. In the months that followed the signing of the settlement, the White House, Congress, and the public health community all believed the settlement was too small. When Senator John McCain, an Arizona Republican, introduced a bill that would nearly double the tax on a cigarette pack proposed in the settlement with the states, Goldstone pulled out of the agreement. *See also* TOBACCO SETTLEMENT—JUNE 1997

Gompers, Samuel (1850–1924)

An immigrant from London, England, who founded the American Federation of Labor, Samuel Gompers was given the choice at 10 years of age whether to work in the shoemaking trade or become an apprentice in CIGAR making. He chose the latter because "there was a society among the cigar makers but none among the shoemakers" (Gompers, 1925). He was legally indentured to David Schwab, a cigar maker.

One of the practices in the shop angered Gompers every time he remembered the scene. Unlike American cigar shops, English cigar makers were not entitled to a number of cigars to smoke. Every night, the foreman lined up the work force at the door and frisked each person to make sure no cigars were being carried away.

Gompers and his family sailed for the United States in June 1863 and settled in New York City where he worked as a cigar maker.

He and his father took out a card in the Cigarmakers' Local Union Number 15 after they arrived in New York. At the factory where he rolled cigars, he loved the camaraderie among the workers and took pride in his workmanship, becoming highly skilled at rolling tobacco leaves.

In his autobiography published in 1925, *Seventy Years of Life and Labor: An Autobiography,* he described working conditions in a cigar shop around 1872, the year he became a citizen.

Any kind of an old loft served a cigar shop. If there were enough windows, we had sufficient light for our work; if not, it was apparently no concern of the management. There was an entirely different conception of sanitation both in the shop and in the home of those days from now. The toilet facilities were a water closet and a sink for washing purposes, usually located by the closet. In most cigar shops our towels were the bagging that came around the bales of Havana and other high grades of tobacco. Cigar shops were always dusty from the

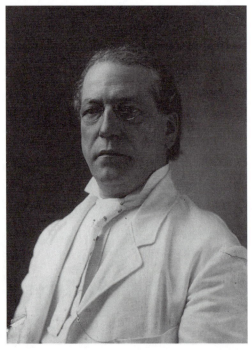

Labor leader Samuel Gompers began as an expert cigar roller. *Library of Congress.*

tobacco stems and powdered leaves. Benches and work tables were not designed to enable the workmen to adjust bodies and arms comfortably to work surface. Each workman supplied his own cutting board of lignum vitae and knife blade.

The tobacco leaf was prepared by strippers who drew the leaves from the heavy stem and put them in pads of about fifty. The leaves had to be handled carefully to prevent tearing. The craftsmanship of the cigar maker was shown in his ability to utilize wrappers to the best advantage to shave off the unusable to a hairbreadth, to roll so as to cover holes in the leaf and to use both hands so as to make a perfectly shaped and rolled product. These things a good cigar maker learned to do more or less mechanically, which left us free to think, talk, listen, or sing. I loved the freedom of that work, for I had earned the mind-freedom that accompanied skill as a craftsmen. I was eager to learn from discussion and reading or to pour out my feeling in song. Often we chose someone to read to us who was a particularly good reader, and in payment the rest of us gave him sufficient of our cigars so he was not the loser. The reading was always followed by discussion, so we learned to know each other pretty thoroughly. We learned who could take a joke in good spirit, who could marshal his thought in an orderly way, who could distinguish clever sophistry from sound reasoning. The fellowship that grew between congenial shopmates was something that lasted a lifetime.

Gompers, who was bothered by cigar workers doing piecework in crowded tenement quarters and working long hours for little pay, headed a drive for better working conditions in the cigar-rolling trade. Gompers managed to interest New York state assemblyman Theodore Roosevelt in remedial legislation. Roosevelt introduced laws to eliminate sweated tenement labor.

In 1873, Gompers organized the United Cigarmakers, which joined the CIGAR MAKERS' INTERNATIONAL UNION (CIU) as Local 144 in 1875, and he was a member until his death nearly 50 years later. He also became an organizer for the CIU in December 1875.

In 1877, Gompers was first elected by Local 144 as its delegate to the Cigar Makers' International Union convention. (He represented his local in every convention but one from that year until he died.) Gompers's rise to national leadership was based on his policy of setting the union on a strong foundation. In the process of moving Local 144 into the international union, he won acceptance for unskilled workers in the trade.

He headed the union's constitutional committee during the 1880s, introducing several measures that revitalized the union. In the 1880s, conflicts between the Cigar Makers' International Union and the Progressive Cigarmakers resulted in the formation of the American Federation of Labor (AFL). Elected president of the AFL in 1886, Gompers endorsed the mayoral candidacy of Henry George, launched by a coalition of unions in 1886, and was adviser to the Social Reform Club, which promoted workers' compensation, union labels, and collective bargaining. He testified at state assembly hearings on production in tenements and conditions in sweatshops and urged legislators to enact stricter factory codes.

In 1886, Gompers was also elected first vice president of the international union. His father, Solomon Gompers, proud of his son's position in the union, often referred to him, not as the president of the AFL, but as the vice president of the CIU.

In later years, Gompers spoke at rallies organized by garment workers and helped to settle disputes involving teamsters (1910), furriers (1912), and transit workers (1916).

References: Samuel Gompers, *Seventy Years of Life and Labor: An Autobiography*, New York: E. P. Dutton & Company, Inc., 1925, p. 18.

Gottlieb, Mark (1963–)

A staff attorney at the Tobacco Control Resource Center (TCRC), Mark Gottlieb is the legal editor of *Tobacco on Trial* and *Tobacco Products Litigation Reporter* and Webmaster for the TCRC < (http://tobacco.neu.edu). > Gottlieb has authored or coauthored several journal and magazine articles in addition to regular contributions to the two publications he edits. His recent research has focused on using the AMERICANS WITH DISABILITIES ACT (ADA) to require workplaces and public places to adopt smoke-free policies to provide access to people with severe medical conditions affected by SECONDHAND SMOKE. *See also* DAYNARD, RICHARD; KELDER, GRAHAM; SWEDA, EDWARD L.; TOBACCO LITIGATION: FIRST, SECOND, AND THIRD WAVES

Grading of Tobacco

The U.S. Department of Agriculture grades tobacco by dividing it into seven classes based on methods of curing as well as types of leaf groups. Classes one, two, and three are the non-cigar leaf classes that include CIGARETTE, smoking, and chewing tobaccos and SNUFF. Class one includes FLUE-CURED TOBACCO, class two FIRE-CURED TOBACCO, and class three, AIR-CURED TOBACCO. Classes four, five, and six cover the cigar-leaf groups. Class four includes the cigar-filler type; class five, the cigar binder; and class six, the cigar-wrapper type. Class seven includes "miscellaneous types." *See also* BINDER; CIGAR WRAPPER; FILLER; TOBACCO CLASSES

Graham, Evarts A. (1883–1957)

Dr. Evarts A. Graham was the head of the chest service at Barnes Hospital in St. Louis, Missouri, and one of the first surgeons to successfully remove an entire cancerous lung. In 1949, the AMERICAN CANCER SOCIETY (ACS) commissioned the first of many studies by awarding a grant to Graham and one of his medical students, ERNST L. WYNDER of the Washington University School of Medicine in St. Louis.

Dr. Graham, a heavy smoker, was dubious about the hypothesis that the increased incidence of lung cancer was related to cigarette smoking. Other faculty members also thought Wynder's in-depth interviews with lung cancer patients at Bellevue Hospital in New York City a waste of time. Graham, who saw no harm in doing a study, became supportive once the results began to accumulate.

In 1950, Drs. Wynder and Graham published an influential study showing that smokers had a greater risk of lung cancer than did nonsmokers. In 1953, they published an article about their research with mice that had cigarette tar painted on their backs.

Grant, Ulysses S. (1822–1885)

Tobacco appeared in the detailed obituary of Ulysses S. Grant, the 18th president of the United States from 1869–1877. Published in the July 24,1885, issue of the *New York Times,* the obituary stated that

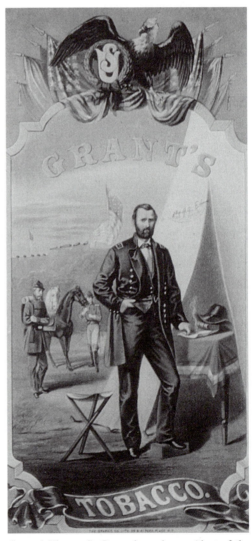

General Ulysses S. Grant, later the president of the United States, was a lifelong cigar smoker. *Library of Congress.*

On June 2, 1884, while eating lunch at Long Branch, the General, as he tasted some fruit, felt a lump in the roof of his mouth and found that swallowing was painful. The lump grew more troublesome day by day. The General was an inveterate smoker, and his cigar on the battlefield has become as much a matter of history as the story itself. To give up a life-long habit . . . was no easy task and the physicians, recognizing this fact, confined their advice to requesting him to limit his indulgence in tobacco. (*New York Times*, 1885)

References: *New York Times*, July 24, 1885, p. 1.

Great American Smokeout

An annual quit-smoking-for-a-day event is conducted by the AMERICAN CANCER SOCIETY (ACS). In 1974, LYNN SMITH, publisher of the Monticello, Minnesota, *Times,* suggested that the townspeople try to quit smoking for 24 hours. Three hundred out of a total population of 1,800 tried, and three months later 10 percent of them succeeded in staying tobacco free. In November 1974, the event (referred to as "D-Day" in Minnesota) spread statewide. Surgeon General Julius Richmond heard about the Minnesota smokeout and suggested making it national.

In 1977, the ACS launched its first Great American Smokeout, an annual event held on the third Thursday in November to foster community-based activities that encourage cigarette smokers to stop smoking for at least 24 hours in the hope of giving up tobacco forever. According to the ACS, more Americans try to kick the habit on the smokeout day than at any other time of the year. Of those who are able to quit for a day, a number give up smoking for good. During the Great American Smokeout, millions of people have reported quitting or reducing the number of cigarettes smoked that day. Activities have included distributing materials to interested schools, hospitals, businesses, and other organizations that discourage tobacco use; encouraging retail businesses not to sell tobacco products and restaurants and other businesses to be smoke free for the day; and providing media coverage of prominent lo-

cal citizens who have pledged to stop smoking for the day. *See also* GREENFIELD, IOWA; SMITH, LYNN; WORLD NO-TOBACCO DAY

Greeley, Horace (1811–1872)

Horace Greeley, publisher of the *New York Tribune* and one of the most active reformers in the United States in the nineteenth century, popularized the description of the cigar as "a fire at one end and a fool at the other" (Kluger, 1996).

References: Richard Kluger, *Ashes to Ashes*, New York: Alfred A. Knopf, 1996, p. 16.

Green, John Ruffin (d. 1869)

About 1860, John Ruffin Green of Durham Station, North Carolina, built up a business manufacturing a good quality of smoking tobacco that was disrupted by the Civil War. In his tobacco factory, Green made his product from the new BRIGHT TOBACCO LEAF. He shredded it, rather than pressing the leaf into twist or plug, foreseeing the trend towards smoking and away from chewing. Green's factory stock of his "Best Flavored Spanish Smoking Tobacco" was consumed by soldiers of both the Union and the Confederacy.

After the war, soldiers throughout the nation sent letters to Durham Station all desirous of getting more of the "Best Flavored Spanish." To protect himself against the numerous imitations that immediately appeared, he adopted a picture of a Durham bull as his trademark. Not only was he impressed with his neighbor's bull, he liked the bull's head on jars of Colman's Mustard, manufactured in Durham, England. He also adopted a brand name and chose for a label the name of his town, shortened to Durham. The official name of the granulated straight bright tobacco in a sack was "Genuine Durham Smoking Tobacco," but it has always been known as "Bull Durham." For the next 50 years, it was the first truly national tobacco brand.

Green's advertising campaign for BULL DURHAM SMOKING TOBACCO helped to create a wide demand for the product. He advertised on BILLBOARDS and posters, in newspapers, comic books, and on premium clocks. Green's campaign was significant in creating a national and international brand, an abrupt departure from the hundreds of brands that preceded it that depended on local renown and word-of-mouth recommendation for sales growth.

Before his death, he took into partnership WILLIAM T. BLACKWELL, a merchant and tobacco peddler.

Green, Samuel

In 1836, Samuel Green blasted tobacco in the *New England Almanack and Farmer's Friend.*

> Smoking—That tobacco may kill insects on shrubs and that one stench may overpower another is possible enough; but that thousands and tens of thousands die of diseases of the lungs generally brought on by tobacco smoking, is a fact as well known in the whole history of disease. How is it possible to be otherwise? Tobacco is a poison. A man will die of an infusion of tobacco as of a shot through the head. Can inhaling this powerful narcotic be good for men? Its operation is to produce a sensation of giddiness and drowsiness—is it good to be within the next step of perpetual drunkenness? It inflames the mouth and requires a perpetual flow of saliva, a fluid known to be among the most important to the whole economy of digestion; it irritates the eyes, corrupts the breath and causes thirst. No doubt the human frame may become so far accustomed to this drain, that the smoker may go on from year to year making himself a nuisance to society, yet there can be no doubt whatever, that the custom is as deleterious in general as it is filthy. (Whelan, 1984)

References: Elizabeth M. Whelan, *A Smoking Gun: How the Tobacco Industry Gets Away with Murder*, Philadelphia: George F. Stickley Co., 1984, p. 37.

Green Tobacco Sickness

Green Tobacco Sickness is an illness resulting from skin exposure to dissolved NICOTINE from wet tobacco leaves. It is characterized by nausea, vomiting, weakness, and dizziness and sometimes fluctuations in blood pressure or heart rate. This illness affects tobacco harvesters whose hands, forearms, thighs, and backs receive the most dermal exposure to wet tobacco. When rain is uncharacteristically heavy, it potentially increases a worker's exposure to wet tobacco. Dew from tobacco leaves also saturates workers' clothing within minutes of beginning field work. Water-resistant protective clothing and rubber gloves reduce the amount of nicotine absorbed by workers in contact with green tobacco.

Green v. American Tobacco Company

An example of a cigarette case litigated during the first wave of tobacco litigation (1954–1973) was *Green v. American Tobacco Company.* The case was argued according to the theory of breach of implied warranty. In December 1957, Edwin Green (1909–1958) filed a $1.5 million lawsuit in a Florida state court against AMERICAN TOBACCO COMPANY, manufacturer of LUCKY STRIKE CIGARETTES, charging that the company's cigarettes caused his illness. Green's lawyer argued that American Tobacco Company, in selling its product to the public, had warranted by implication its fitness and merchantability and should be held liable for any damages incurred by breach of that warranty.

A smoker since the age of 16, Miami, Florida, contractor Edwin Green smoked Lucky Strikes in the 1920s and smoked up to three packs a day until 1956 when his lung cancer was diagnosed. Green died two months after filing the suit and his administrator was substituted as plaintiff; his widow also filed suit under the Florida Wrongful Death Statute.

When the case first went to the Florida jury in a federal appeals court in 1961, the jurors concluded that smoking Lucky Strikes caused Mr. Green's lung cancer but they did not award any money damages to Green's wife and son. The jury reasoned that the tobacco company could not have known that smoking Lucky Strikes would cause cancer. The verdict was reversed by the court and a new trial ordered when the Florida Supreme

Court ruled, in a different case, that a company was responsible under the doctrine of "implied warranty" for its product's purity.

During the second trial, the judge instructed the jury to consider first whether cigarettes are reasonably fit for human consumption, and if not, how much in damages should be assessed against the company. The judge also charged the jury to decide whether cigarettes endangered a substantial number of persons who smoked them. Faced with the complicated task of deciding whether cigarettes were dangerous to the general public, the jury came back for the defendants.

The U.S. Court of Appeals for the Fifth Circuit reversed the decision and remanded for a new trial. Final disposition of the case came in 1970, 13 years after the case was filed in 1957, when the Supreme Court de-nied review. *See also* Tobacco Litigation: First, Second, and Third Waves

Greenfield, Iowa

In 1969, the town of Greenfield, Iowa, went "cold turkey." Some 376 smokers threw their cartons of cigarettes into a bonfire and signed no-smoking pledges. The town helped promote *Cold Turkey,* a movie being filmed in the town at the time. In the movie, a millionaire promises the fictional town of Eagle Rock, Iowa, $25 million if all the residents stop smoking. In real life, United Artists promised $6,000 if Greenfield smokers signed a pledge to quit puffing for 30 days. At the end of the month, merchants reported that cigarette sales in Greenfield were off 30 percent, and 134 townsfolk claimed to have gone the full 30 days without smoking.

H

Hammond, Edward Cuyler (1912–1986)

Two researchers for the AMERICAN CANCER SOCIETY (ACS), Drs. Edward Cuyler Hammond and DANIEL HORN, with the help of 22,000 trained volunteers, in January 1952 enrolled 187,784 men between the ages of 50 and 69 in a massive study dealing with their smoking and nonsmoking habits. The researchers thought that three years would be required before significant differences between smokers and nonsmokers would be detectable. But after 22 months, in October 1953, they took a preliminary look. After the doctors looked at the death rates of smokers and nonsmokers, they became alarmed because it was obvious that the overall death rate of smokers was one and a half times that of nonsmokers. Dr. Horn, who smoked one pack a day, and Dr. Hammond, who smoked four packs a day, switched to PIPES.

Of 11,870 men in the study group who had died, 7,316 were smokers and 4,652 were nonsmokers. The doctors concluded that the deaths of 2,665 smokers had to be considered "excess" deaths over the nonsmoking group.

In absolute numbers, heart disease claimed the most deaths among the smokers. Death from lung cancer was 10 times as frequent in smokers as in nonsmokers. The chances of the heavy smoker dying of lung cancer were found to be 64 times that of the nonsmoker. Ex-smokers had significantly lower death rates than those who continued to smoke regularly. The longer the ex-smoker abstained, the more his death rate resembled that of a nonsmoker. On June 21, 1954, the American Cancer Society reported on the Hammond-Horn study at a meeting of the AMERICAN MEDICAL ASSOCIATION (AMA).

Hanes, Pleasant Henderson (1845–1925)

A North Carolinian, Pleasant Henderson Hanes organized a tobacco firm in Winston, North Carolina—P.H. Hanes and Company. By the late 1880s, the firm was one of Winston's largest, employing more than 300 people and annually producing almost a million pounds of flat tobacco (i.e., tightly compressed plugs of tobacco). Hanes and his brothers sold out to R.J. REYNOLDS TOBACCO COMPANY in 1900.

Hariot, Thomas (1560–1621)

Surveyor-historian Thomas Hariot, a survivor of the first unsuccessful English settlement at Roanoke Island, North Carolina, wrote about tobacco in his "Briefe and True Report of the New Found Land of Virginia" (1588).

> There is an herb called uppowoc, which sows itself. In the West Indies it has several names, according to the different place

where it grows and is used, but the Spaniards generally call it tobacco. Its leaves are dried, made into powder, and then smoked by being sucked through clay pipes into the stomach and head. The fumes purge superfluous phlegm and gross humors from the body, but if there are any obstructions it breaks them up. By this means the natives keep in excellent health, without many of the grievous diseases which often afflict us in England . . . .

While we were there we used to suck in the smoke as they did, and now that we are back in England we still do. We have found many rare and wonderful proofs of the uppowoc's virtues, which would themselves require a volume to relate. There is sufficient evidence in the fact that it is used by so many men and women of great calling, as well as by some learned physicians. (Heimann, 1960)

References: Robert K. Heimann, *Tobacco and Americans*, New York: McGraw-Hill Book Company, 1960, p. 35.

Havana

The term, referring to tobacco raised in Cuba, comes from Havana, the capital of Cuba; when the export of leaf began, it was the island's only port. Havana also refers to cigars grown in Cuba. Superior cigars are synonymous with Havana. The term "Genuine Havanas" refers to cigars made entirely of the highest-quality Cuban tobacco leaf and hand manufactured in Cuba.

At the top of the scale is the Cuban-made tobacco rolled in Havana from leaf grown in the renowned VUELTA ABAJA region where a time-honored pattern of growth, cure, and manufacture by hand ensures the quality. Such cigars bear the Guarantee Seal of the Cuban government, a green band 2 3/16 inches wide.

In the United States, domestic U.S. "Havana" leaves grow in the Connecticut Valley— known as Connecticut Havana or HAVANA SEED—and in New York State. *See also* CIGAR; CIGAR MANUFACTURING; COHIBA CIGAR; CONNECTICUT TOBACCO; CONNECTICUT TOBACCO FARMING; CUBA; CUBAN TOBACCO HISTORY

Havana Seed

Havana seed is one of the principal types of cigar tobaccos raised in the United States, especially in Connecticut. It is more commonly known as Connecticut Havana but is also called Havana Seed. *See also* CONNECTICUT TOBACCO; CONNECTICUT TOBACCO FARMING; HAVANA

Hawkins, Sir John (1532–1595)

In 1564, Sir John Hawkins, an English naval commander, landed at the French colony of Fort Caroline (Florida), and is believed to have brought the first tobacco back to England with him in 1565. In Florida, he observed PIPE smoking among the native people.

The Floridians when they travel have a kind of herb dried, which with a cane, and an earthen cup at the end, with fire, and the dried herbs put together, do suck through the cane the smoke thereof, which smoke satisfieth their hunger, and therewith they live four or five days without meat or drink. (Heimann, 1960)

References: Robert K. Heimann, *Tobacco and Americans*, New York: McGraw-Hill Book Company, 1960, p. 17.

Health Warnings on Cigarette Packs and Advertisements and Smokeless Tobacco

Shortly after the surgeon general's landmark 1964 report was released, the FEDERAL TRADE COMMISSION (FTC) proposed three administrative rules that would have required health warnings on all CIGARETTE packs and advertisements, and would have imposed certain restrictions on cigarette advertising. In part, the FTC proposed that every cigarette advertisement and every pack, box, carton, and other container in which cigarettes were sold to the public carry one of the following messages:

- CAUTION—CIGARETTE SMOKING IS A HEALTH HAZARD: The Surgeon General's Advisory Committee on Smoking and Health has found that cigarette smoking contributes substantially to mortality from certain specific diseases and to the overall death rate.

- CAUTION: Cigarette smoking is dangerous to health. It may cause death from cancer and other diseases.

In preparing its final ruling, published in June 1964 after a six-month comment period, the FTC found that cigarette advertisements were false and deceptive because they failed to disclose known health hazards. The ruling therefore required all cigarette advertising and every container in which cigarettes were sold to consumers to disclose prominently that cigarette smoking is dangerous and may cause death from cancer and other diseases. However, the final rule left the specific wording of the warning to the discretion of the tobacco manufacturers.

In 1965, Congress preempted the FTC and passed a law with a less stringent warning than the FTC regulations they replaced. As of January 1, 1966, the FEDERAL CIGARETTE LABELING AND ADVERTISING ACT OF 1965, the first federal statute to enact labeling requirements for tobacco products, required nine words on all cigarette packages: "CAUTION: Cigarette Smoking May Be Hazardous to Your Health."

This statutory warning was weaker than the earlier proposed FTC warning in that it did not specifically mention the risk of death from cancer and other diseases. Further, whereas the FTC would have required warning disclosures on product advertisements, the Federal Cigarette Labeling and Advertising Act of 1965 temporarily (through June 1969) prohibited any governmental body (including federal regulatory agencies such as the FTC) or individual state from requiring a health warning on cigarette advertising. The laws also prohibited any other health warning on cigarette packs.

The act required the FTC to transmit an annual report to Congress describing the effectiveness of cigarette labeling, discussing current cigarette advertising and promotional practices, and making recommendations for

legislation. In its first report to Congress in 1967, the FTC recommended extending the health warning to cigarette advertisements and strengthening the wording as follows "WARNING: Cigarette Smoking Is Hazardous to Health and May Cause Death from Cancer and Other Diseases."

In mid-1969, just before the expiration of the congressionally imposed temporary restrictions on its actions, the FTC proposed a rule that would have required all cigarette advertising "to disclose, clearly and prominently that cigarette smoking is dangerous to health and may cause death from cancer, coronary heart disease, chronic bronchitis, pulmonary emphysema, and other diseases."

The subsequent law passed by Congress in 1969, the PUBLIC HEALTH CIGARETTE SMOKING ACT OF 1969, banned cigarette advertising on television and radio after January 1, 1971, and strengthened the cigarette package warning label to read, effective November 1970, as follows: "WARNING: The Surgeon General Has Determined That Cigarette Smoking Is Dangerous to Your Health." This law did not affect SMOKELESS TOBACCO products.

Nevertheless, the labeling provisions of this law, like the 1965 law before it, were substantially less stringent than the FTC regulations they preempted. Furthermore, the statutory language of the act continued to omit specific references to the risks and consequences of smoking and extended the preemption on requiring any additional health warnings for cigarette packages. The FTC was again temporarily restricted (through June 1971) from issuing regulations that would require a health warning in cigarette advertising.

After the second congressional moratorium expired in late 1971, the FTC announced its intention to file complaints against cigarette companies for failure to warn in their advertising that smoking is dangerous to health. Negotiations among the companies and the FTC resulted on March 30, 1972, in consent orders requiring that all cigarette advertising "clearly and conspicuously" display the same warning required by

Congress for cigarette packages. That consent order specified the type size of the warning in newspaper, magazine, and other periodical advertisements of various dimensions; for BILLBOARD advertisements, the size of the lettering was specified in inches.

In 1981, the FTC sent a staff report to Congress that concluded that the warning appearing on cigarette packages and in ads had become overexposed and "worn out" and was thus no longer effective. The report noted that a single warning did not communicate sufficient information on the specific risks of smoking and recommended replacing the single warning with a rotational system of warnings.

During the early 1980s, although the tobacco companies fought hard against any labels, they agreed to add four warning labels to cigarette packs and ads to avoid an addiction warning. On October 12, 1984, President Ronald Reagan signed the COMPREHENSIVE SMOKING EDUCATION ACT OF 1984. It replaced the previous health warning on cigarette packages and ads with four rotating, strongly worded health warnings, which took effect October 12, 1985.

- SURGEON GENERAL'S WARNING: Smoking Causes Lung Cancer, Heart Disease, Emphysema, and May Complicate Pregnancy.
- SURGEON GENERAL'S WARNING: Quitting Smoking Now Greatly Reduces Serious Risks to Your Health.
- SURGEON GENERAL'S WARNING: Smoking by Pregnant Women May Result in Fetal Injury, Premature Birth, and Low Birth Weight.
- SURGEON GENERAL'S WARNING: Cigarette Smoke Contains Carbon Monoxide.

The warning statement had to be conspicuous and clear, printed in two lines of type and enclosed within a black-bordered rectangle. The congressional warnings were substantively more passive in their wording than those suggested by the FTC.

In 1986, Congress extended requirements for warning labels to smokeless tobacco prod-

ucts by passing the COMPREHENSIVE SMOKELESS TOBACCO HEALTH EDUCATION ACT OF 1986. The act required tobacco manufacturers to display and regularly rotate the following three warnings on all smokeless tobacco packages and on all smokeless tobacco advertising, except billboards:

- WARNING: This product may cause mouth cancer.
- WARNING: This product may cause gum disease and tooth loss.
- WARNING: This product is not a safe alternative to cigarettes.

The act stipulates that the warnings displayed in ads appear in the circle-and-arrow format. The act prohibits federal agencies as well as state or local jurisdictions from requiring any other health warnings on smokeless tobacco packages and ads. However, states are not preempted from enacting additional advertising restrictions.

An unintended consequence of the federally mandated warning disclosures concerns product liability. The display of a federally mandated warning eventually shielded tobacco manufacturers from product liability and insulated them from lawsuits. *See also* TOBACCO LITIGATION: FIRST, SECOND, AND THIRD WAVES

References: Surgeon General's Report, *Preventing Tobacco Use Among Young People*. 1994, p. 257.

Helling v. McKinney (1993)

On June 18, 1993, in *Helling v. McKinney*, the U.S. Supreme Court held that forcing a prisoner to breathe the tobacco smoke from his cell mate's smoking may constitute cruel and unusual punishment under the Eighth Amendment. The Court said the prisoner need not show that the smoke has created or is creating a current health problem, but rather can rely on evidence based on "possible future effects of" the smoke. The Court also rejected arguments that such evidence did not exist.

McKinney, an inmate in the Nevada State Prison in Carson City, Nevada, filed suit in the U.S. District Court against prison officials claiming that his involuntary exposure to ENVIRONMENTAL TOBACCO SMOKE (ETS) from his cell mate's and other inmates' cigarettes posed an unreasonable risk to his health, thus subjecting him to cruel and unusual punishment in violation of the Eighth Amendment. In his complaint, McKinney said he was assigned to a cell with another inmate who smoked five packs of cigarettes a day. The complaint also stated that cigarettes were sold to inmates without properly informing them of the health hazards a nonsmoking inmate would encounter while sharing a room with them. McKinney complained about certain health problems caused by his exposure to CIGARETTE smoke.

The parties consented to a jury trial before a magistrate who concluded that McKinney had no constitutional right to be free from cigarette smoke. The magistrate found that McKinney could state a claim for deliberate indifference to serious medical needs by the prison, if he could prove the underlying facts, but held that the prisoner had failed to present evidence showing medical problems that were traceable to cigarette smoke. The magistrate granted judgment for the prison officials.

The Court of Appeals affirmed the magistrate's verdict that McKinney did not have a constitutional right to a smoke-free prison environment. On the issue of deliberate indifference, the Court of Appeals held that the prison officials were immune from liability for damages, since there was at the time no clearly established law imposing liability for exposing prisoners to ETS. The court found that McKinney had stated a valid cause of action under the Eighth Amendment by alleging that he had been involuntarily exposed to ETS levels that could endanger his health. The court also concluded that society's attitude had evolved to the point that involuntary exposure to unreasonably dangerous levels of ETS violated current standards of decency. And the court held that the magistrate erred by not permitting McKinney to prove his ETS exposure was sufficient to constitute an unreasonable danger to his future

health. The prison officials sought review in the Supreme Court.

Justice Byron White delivered the opinion of the Court in which Chief Justice William Rehnquist and Justices Blackmun, Stevens, O'Connor, Kennedy, and Souter joined. Justice Clarence Thomas filed a dissenting opinion in which Justice Antonin Scalia joined.

Henley, Patricia (1947–)

Patricia Henley, a smoker who sued PHILIP MORRIS USA after being diagnosed with inoperable cancer, won $51.5 million from a state jury in San Francisco, California on February 10, 1999. Hers was the largest judgment ever awarded in a smoking-related lawsuit. The verdicts were for $1.5 million in compensatory damages (for Henley's medical costs and pain and suffering) and $50 million in punitive damages. Henley, an amateur country-western singer from Los Angeles, smoked as many as three packs of MARLBORO CIGARETTES a day since she was 15. She quit smoking after being diagnosed with lung cancer in January 1998, shortly after the state law granting tobacco companies immunity from lawsuits expired. She sued Philip Morris, maker of Marlboros, the brand she primarily smoked, claiming there were no health warnings on cigarettes when she began smoking and that major tobacco companies failed to warn smokers that addiction might mean they would not be able to give up the habit. Her lawsuit included charges of negligence, strict liability, and fraud.

Henley's attorney, MADELYN CHABER, a former New York City elementary schoolteacher, provided the jury with more than 1,000 Philip Morris documents pulled from the company's files and made public in 1998 during a separate suit brought by the state of Minnesota. The documents detailed Philip Morris's efforts to conduct biological research in Europe to keep from disclosing the results in the United States. The documents also quoted internal discussions of industry executives about the addictiveness and cancer risks of smoking. Chaber also relied on several experts, including Neal Benowitz, a University of California, San Francisco, toxicologist who worked on the 1988 Surgeon General's Report on smoking and who testified about the addictive nature of tobacco. Philip Morris officials said they would appeal the California verdict.

Henley's case was the first to reach trial since the repeal of a 1987 California tort reform law that banned product liability lawsuits by cigarette smokers on the basis that the risks of smoking were well known. Dozens of cases pending at the time were dismissed. In 1997, California joined other states in suing the tobacco industry and the state legislature responded to criticism of the ban by repealing it.

Juries have awarded smokers damages in health claims against tobacco companies only three other times—and all of them were overturned on appeal. *See also* CARTER, GRADY; CIPOLLONE, ROSE; MADDOX, ROLAND; MINNESOTA MEDICAID CASE

Hennepin, Louis (1640–c. 1701)

A French Roman Catholic friar and explorer, Louis Hennepin accompanied French explorer Robert La Salle on a journey to the Mississippi by way of the Great Lakes. Father Hennepin wrote the following description of the pipe of peace in 1678:

> We sent three men to buy provisions in the village, with the Calumet or Pipe of Peace which those of the Island (in Lake Huron) had given us. And because the Calumet of Peace is the most sacred thing among the savages, I shall here describe the same. It is a large Tobacco Pipe of a red, black, or white Marble. The head is finely polished. The Quill, which is commonly two foot and a half long, is made of a pretty strong Reed or Cane, adorned with Feathers of all colors, and interlaced with locks of women's hair. Every Nation adorns it as they think fit, and according to the Birds they have in their Country. Such a Pipe is a safe conduct among all the Allies of the Nation who has given it. And in all Embassies the Calumet is carried as a symbol of Peace. The savages being generally persuaded that some great misfortune would befall them

if they should violate the public Faith of the Calumet. They fill this pipe with the best Tobacco thy have, and then present it to those with whom they have concluded any great affair, and then smoke out the same after them. (Dunhill, 1969)

See also PIPE; PIPE SMOKING AND NATIVE AMERICANS

References: Alfred Dunhill, *The Pipe Book*, New York: Macmillan Company, 1924, 1969, p. 57

Henningfield, Jack E.

An expert on the pharmacology of NICOTINE, Jack E. Henningfield is chief of the clinical pharmacology branch of the Addiction Research Center at the National Institute on Drug Abuse. He is also as associate professor of behavioral biology in the Department of Psychiatry and Behavioral Sciences at Johns Hopkins University in Baltimore, Maryland.

Dr. Henningfield was a scientific editor of the 1988 Surgeon General's Report on nicotine addiction, and a scientific consultant on the surgeon general's report on SMOKELESS TOBACCO in 1986.

Herz, Henri (1806–1888)

Henri Herz, born in Vienna, toured the United States in 1846. Twenty years later, Herz, a concert pianist and composer, wrote a witty description of his adventures in the United States. Entitled *Mes Voyages en Amérique* (1886), the work tells, in the following excerpt, about Herz's experience smoking cigars in the streets of Boston, Massachusetts:

> In the barroom I saw a score of Americans smoking away in a very original and comic position, which has furnished the material for so many joyous criticisms. They were seated with their legs elevated above their heads and exposed a view of the soles of their boots to the passers-by outside. These soles were so evenly aligned, they might have been suspended for inspection.
>
> For that matter, everything in Boston is well aligned, buildings as well as streets, most of which are bordered with trees in a

manner charming to the vision, and useful in purifying the air. Walking about, I lit a cigar. I had not proceeded ten feet when a constable stopped me, shocked:

"Sir, smoking is forbidden."

"You are joking, constable."

"Not at all. Smoking in the streets is forbidden. If you cannot contain yourself, go home to smoke."

"But yesterday I saw twenty people smoking with their legs in the air. Is that the only position in which smoking is permitted?"

"You may smoke in any position you like, but only in your own home. The law forbids any smoking in the streets, and your infraction is all the more shocking and blameworthy on Sunday, the day consecrated to the glory of God."

I could not help but consider this taboo, in the land of all the liberties, tyrannical. But I had to obey. (Handlin, 1949)

References: Oscar Handlin, ed. "Obbligato by Herz," *This Was America*, New York: Harper & Row Publishers, 1949, pp. 186–87.

Hill, A. Bradford. *See* DOLL, RICHARD AND HILL, A. BRADFORD

Hill, George Washington (1885–1946)

One of the most aggressive executives in American business history, George Washington Hill succeeded his father, Percival S. Hill, as president of the AMERICAN TOBACCO COMPANY in 1925. He was a genius in advertising and sales psychology and arguably the most dynamic figure in the tobacco business.

Just out of Williams College in 1904, Hill worked in a leaf market in Wilson, North Carolina, and managed the Wells-Whitehead Tobacco Company, making Carolina bright cigarettes. In 1907, he managed Butler-Butler Inc., a company manufacturing various tobacco products. After he made up his mind that cigarettes were the future of the tobacco business, he persuaded his father to let him concentrate on that product. He focused on PALL MALL CIGARETTES, a Turkish item and the firm's leading brand. He turned it into a money maker with dealer displays, advertising on magazine back covers, and the first of his many slogans: "a shilling in London, a quarter here."

Young Hill used gimmicks to attract smokers. He stuck coupons into Sovereign cigarettes that could be redeemed for ½¢ in cash. In Mecca cigarette packages, he inserted postcards (without stamps) that he said were "eminently suited for the U.S. mail." For a while, he stashed "flag blankets" in Hassan smokes and then switched to coupons that could be redeemed for "useful presents of unusual value." Presents included shaving sticks, talcum powder, razors, shears, knives, clocks, and cigarette cases.

Promoted to head the cigarette division, Hill turned his attention away from promotional work and concentrated on packaging and distribution to reduce his company's loss on damaged stocks of cigarettes. He worked out the most complete salesmen-routing system American business had yet seen, so that cigarettes reached customers in the same condition they left the factory. Hill bought a fleet of autos and sent salesmen to remote areas to deliver cigarette stock to dealers. He wrapped cartons in glassine paper, dated cartons and cases, and inspected cigarette stocks to make sure they were still fresh.

About 1916, the American Tobacco Company launched LUCKY STRIKE CIGARETTES, formerly a PIPE tobacco, to compete with CAMEL CIGARETTES, introduced by R.J. REYNOLDS TOBACCO COMPANY in 1913. According to the company's history, Hill was thrilled with the aroma of the smoke, likening it to morning toast. The brand's first slogan was, "It's toasted," and advertising copy said: "The Burley tobacco is toasted; makes the taste delicious. You know how toasting improves the flavor of bread. And it's the same with tobacco exactly."

In 1928, Hill and advertising man ALBERT LASKER launched a new Lucky Strike advertising campaign "Reach for a Lucky Instead of a Sweet," one of the most successful and profitable themes in the history of advertising. The idea behind the advertising theme was to suggest to women that cigarette smoking would help them slim down. Ads showed fit and trim young women with shadows of double chins and fat bodies in the background. One story goes that the ad evolved from a chance moment when Hill saw two women, one slender and smoking a cigarette, the other stout and eating a big piece of candy. He noticed the contrast and figured the stout one ought to be smoking instead of munching on sugar. Candy companies were furious. A chain of New York candy stores inserted this paragraph in its advertisement: "Do not let anyone tell you that a cigarette can take the place of a piece of candy. The cigarette will inflame your tonsils, poison with nicotine every organ of your body, and dry up your blood—nails in your coffin." In one ad, the National Confectioners' Association reminded people: "Don't neglect your candy ration!" Hill shot back with a booklet on dietetics. One statement in it said

> Sugar is undermining the nation's health. By this I mean cane sugar, beet sugar, and, to a much less degree, maple sugar. The average American consumes daily a quarter pound of cane sugar . . . . Sugar is very bad for children . . . . It not only destroys a child's appetite, but takes the place of essential food elements in the diet . . . . Pastries and puddings are in general detrimental to health. (Wagner, 1971)

The FEDERAL TRADE COMMISSION (FTC) ended the war of words when it told tobacco companies not to sell cigarettes as weight-reducing devices. Women had already bought the message, however. They grabbed up the cigarette, which promised weight reduction without the bother of hard work.

By 1929, Hill thought it was time for women to smoke in public places, so he brought in EDWARD L. BERNAYS, a public relations expert, and asked him: "How can we get women to smoke on the street? They're smoking indoors. But, damn it, if they spend half the time outdoors and we can get 'em to smoke outdoors, we'll damn near double our female market. Do something. Act!" (Tyler, 1998). Once Bernays learned that women not only associated cigarettes with men but

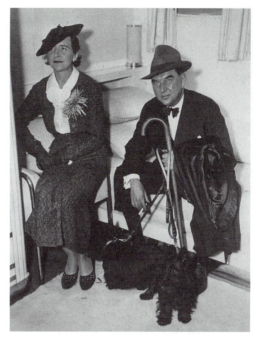

George Washington Hill, president of the American Tobacco Company, returns from Europe in 1934 with his wife and his two dogs, Lucky and Strike. *AP/Wide World Photos.*

viewed cigarettes as torches of freedom, he held a parade of women lighting cigarettes. Not only did the parade make front-page news all over the nation, the idea of women smoking in public became more acceptable.

The Lucky Strike campaigns increased profits for the American Tobacco Company from $21 million in 1925 to $46 million in 1931. Years later, another president of the American Tobacco Company wrote that the Lucky Strikes campaign created more women smokers than any other single promotional effort. Between 1930 and 1950, Lucky Strikes alternated with Camels as the number-one selling brand in the United States.

Hill chose the radio as a medium for his advertising messages. He created the Lucky Strike Dance Orchestra that debuted on 39 radio stations in September 1928. To test the power of radio advertising, he stopped advertising in other media. Two months after Lucky Strike commercials were first heard on the radio, sales skyrocketed by 47 percent. Hill sponsored many radio programs including "Hit Parade," "Information

Please," and the programs of the Metropolitan Opera, Jack Benny, Eddy Duchin, and columnist Dorothy Thompson.

Before Hill, who always had a Lucky in his mouth, died of heart disease in 1946, he left behind memorable trademarks. Hill hired tobacco auctioneers to sound their incomprehensible nasal chants climaxed by "So-o-o-old American!" Another was the slogan "Lucky Strike Green Has Gone to War," which emerged during WORLD WAR II. American Tobacco claimed green dyes used in the paper for Lucky packages were scarce and crucial to military production, and therefore had to be discontinued. In 1942, Hill dreamed up "L.S.M.F.T." or "Lucky Strike Means Fine Tobacco." *See also* CIGARETTE; HILL, PERCIVAL SMITH

References: Larry Tye, *The Father of Spin: Edward L. Bernays and the Birth of Public Relations*, New York: Crown Publishers, Inc., 1998, p. 28.

Susan Wagner, *Cigarette Country*, New York: Praeger Publishers, 1971, pp. 59–60.

Hill, John

A well-known eighteenth-century London physician, botanist, columnist, and playwright, John Hill suggested a relationship existed between SNUFF and "swellings and excrescences." Dr. Hill, a 1750 medical graduate of the Scottish University of St. Andrew, wrote a tract entitled *Cautions against the Immoderate Use of Snuff* (1761). In it, he described six cases related to the excessive use of snuff. One case involved a woman "of sober and virtuous life" who snuffed a vast quantity of tobacco and developed a terrible ulcer in her nose.

> She had been long accustomed to Snuff, and took it in very great quantity. After the use of about a quarter of a pound of Snuff, which she perceived to be particularly acrid; she felt a strange soreness in the upper part of her left nostril; running, as she expressed it, toward the gristle of the nose; she left off that particular parcel of Snuff, but continued to take the usual kind as much as ever. No swelling was perceived; but, after a little time came on a discharge of a very offensive matter; not in great

quantity, but of an intolerable smell, and the more so to her, as she was naturally a person of great delicacy. The discharge increased, and it soon became necessary for her to leave off Snuff. A surgeon was employed, but to very little purpose; the symptoms continued; the ulcer increased, and, from time to time, pieces of the bone came away. Death, from another disease, put an end to that misery, which all the art of physick and surgery seemed very little able to relieve. (Whelan, 1984)

Although Dr. Hill did not label cases of "polypusses" as cancers, he made the following observation:

> Whether or not polypusses, which attend Snuff-takers, are absolutely caused by that custom; or whether the principles of the disorder were there before, and Snuff only irritated the parts, and hastened the mischief, I shall not pretend to determine: but even supposing the latter only to be the case, the damage is certainly more than the indulgence is worth: for who is able to say, that the Snuff is not the absolute cause, or that he has not the seeds of such a disorder which Snuff will bring into action. With respect to the cancer of the nose, they are as dreadful and as fatal as any others . . . . It is evident therefore that no man should venture Snuff, who is not sure that he is not so far liable to a cancer: and no man can be sure of that. (Whelan, 1984)

References: Elizabeth Whelan, *A Smoking Gun: How the Tobacco Industry Gets Away with Murder*, Philadelphia: George F. Stickley Co., 1984, p. 35.

Hill, Percival Smith (1862–1925)

Percival Smith Hill, a Harvard-educated manager of William T. Blackwell's Durham Tobacco Company in Philadelphia, was selected by JAMES BUCHANAN DUKE to run the AMERICAN TOBACCO COMPANY (ATC) after its dissolution. Duke made him vice president in charge of sales.

Hill, who became known as James Buchanan Duke's detail man, performed well as a general overseer of operations, but he had few innovative ideas. In *Sold American!* a company-sponsored history published in

1954, it was written of Hill: " For the first ten years of Percy Hill's presidency, both the sales and manufacturing departments were on a kind of shakedown cruise" ("*Sold American,*" 1954). At his death, his son, GEORGE WASHINGTON HILL, one of the vice presidents of the company, took over. *See also* BLACKWELL, WILLIAM T.

References: *"Sold American!" The First Fifty Years.* American Tobacco Company, 1954, p. 51.

Hirayama, Takeshi

In 1981, Takeshi Hirayama published a major study ("Non-smoking Wives of Heavy Smokers Have a Higher Risk of Lung Cancer: A Study from Japan") in the *British Medical Journal.* A 14-year epidemiological study conducted at the National Cancer Center Research Institute in Tokyo, Japan, Dr. Hirayama's study concluded that wives of Japanese men who smoked were up to twice as likely to die of lung cancer as were wives of nonsmokers. Hirayama asserted his results "appear to explain the long-standing riddle of why many women develop lung cancer although they themselves are nonsmokers" (Whelan, 1984).

Some prominent scientists criticized Hirayama's study for improper experimental design and analysis. Some problems cast doubts on the results of the study. The age-adjusted lung cancer mortality rates for the entire study population and all of its subcategories were higher than those in Japan as a whole. Even nonsmoking women with nonsmoking husbands had higher lung cancer death rates than did smokers, passive smokers, and nonsmokers in the rest of Japan, indicating another factor may have been responsible for the lung cancer studied by Hirayama. Another problem was that the majority of the lung cancer that occurred in his study population was a type not generally associated with CIGARETTE smoking. Finally, the magnitude of the effect of passive smoking on the women in Hirayama's study led many epidemiologists to question the plausibility of his results.

The TOBACCO INSTITUTE responded to the study, which received international attention, by hiring Nathan Mantel, a well-known epidemiologist, to critique the study and then cited his criticisms in a widely reported press release. The institute also reprinted several critical news articles as full-page advertisements in newspapers and magazines. The *British Medical Journal* responded to the attacks on Hirayama's study by opening correspondence on his work so that the scientist could respond publicly to the criticisms.

The tobacco industry and Tobacco Institute have maintained the public position that Hirayama's study was flawed and that the health dangers of passive smoking have not been proven. The tobacco industry also publicizes the study as an example of shoddy and insubstantial evidence used to indict tobacco. The scientific community, however, regards Hirayama's work as a landmark study on the health effects of ENVIRONMENT TOBACCO SMOKE (ETS). Hirayama's findings have been confirmed by several other studies showing a link between passive smoking and lung cancer. *See also* GARFINKEL, LAWRENCE

References: Elizabeth M. Whelan, *A Smoking Gun: How the Tobacco Industry Gets Away with Murder*, Philadelphia: George F. Stickley Co., 1984, p. 194.

Hogshead

A hogshead is a large cask or container in which tobacco is stored in warehouses after curing, and in which tobacco ages for at least a year to give it its mellowness. In the late colonial period, hogsheads averaged nearly a 1,000 pounds, a bit more in the early national period, and about 1,200 soon after the War of 1812.

By necessity, the hogsheads had to be rolled by hand to the nearest tobacco wharf, sometimes a considerable distance, over rough trails, called "rolling roads" or "tobacco roads." One or two horses were hitched to the hogshead by means of shafts attached to spikes driven in the hogshead. The hogshead was rolled along on its own staves. Even a mile over such a road resulted in bruised, dirtied tobacco and 10 or 20 miles could ruin a season's work. From wharves, the hogsheads were swung by block and tackle onto ships or taken by barge to ships built to stow hogsheads seven deep.

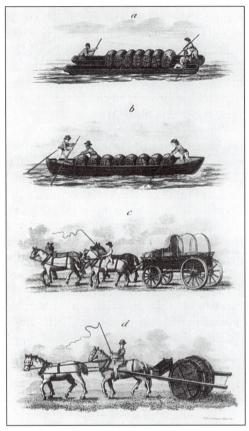

Various modes of conveying hogsheads of tobacco. *Arents Collection, The New York Public Library, Astor, Lenox and Tilden Foundations.*

Besides being carried on wagons, hogsheads were carried on the nation's inland waterways by canoes, flat-bottomed boats, heavy canal cargo boats, and steamboats to the time of the Civil War. Eventually, tobacco was taken to market by steam locomotives. Although certain forms of tobacco are still sold in hogsheads, most tobaccos are now auctioned off in leaf form.

Holmes, Sherlock

Sherlock Holmes, a fictional character created by British physician and novelist Arthur Conan Doyle (1859–1930), is one of the most famous pipe smokers in English literature. Holmes smoked several different pipes, but never a meerschaum. In the morning, Holmes cooked for himself a mixture of all the plugs and dottles left from smokes of the day before and smoked it all before breakfast.

Holmes, who smoked a calabash pipe, could tell the past of a man from the pipe he smoked. In *A Study in Scarlet*, Holmes said:

> "Come along doctor," he said; "we shall go and look him up. I'll tell you one thing which may help you in the case," he continued, turning to the two detectives. "There has been murder done, and the murderer was a man. He was more than six feet high, was in the prime of life, had small feet for his height, worse coarse, square-toed boots, and smoked a Trichinopoly cigar . . . ."
> Lestrade and Gregson glanced at each other with an incredulous smile. (Infante, 1985)

Holmes, an expert who wrote a monograph on the ashes of cigars titled "Upon the Distinction Between the Ashes of the Various Tobaccos," boasted that he could distinguish, at a glance, the ashes of any brand of CIGAR known to man. In *The Boscome Valley Mystery*, he deduced, at a glance, that the killer smoked Indian cigars. *See also* PIPE; PIPE, CALABASH; PIPE, MEERSCHAUM

References: G. Cabrera Infante, *Holy Smoke*, London: Faber and Faber, 1985, p. 273.

Horn, Daniel (1916–1992)

A Harvard University-trained behavioral psychologist, Daniel Horn, was coinvestigator with AMERICAN CANCER SOCIETY (ACS) epidemiologist EDWARD CUYLER HAMMOND of a massive ACS-sponsored study about the effects of smoking on health from 1952 to 1954. Next Dr. Horn studied 22,000 high school students in Portland, Oregon, in his quest to understand why the smoking habit took hold. He published his findings in 1958, reporting that three out of four smokers had begun smoking before they finished secondary school. One-third of all the Portland high school students smoked—38 percent of the boys and 20 percent of the girls. Dr. Horn found that family role models were the most influential factor in young people starting to smoke. The second most important factor was that smoking was "a compensatory form of behavior" that reflected "failure to achieve peer group status or satisfactions" whether academically, socially, or extracurricularly. The third main reason young people smoked, according to Horn, was rebellion against authority or discipline.

In 1965, Dr. Horn became the first director of the NATIONAL CLEARINGHOUSE ON SMOKING AND HEALTH, a small unit added to the U.S. Public Health Service that had a data-gathering function. During the nine years Dr. Horn directed it, the clearinghouse never employed more than 30 people or had an annual budget much above $2 million. After ordering field surveys, he was able to draw from the data insights into the nature of smoking. In 1970, for example, he discussed the alarming rise of teen smoking by noting that the phenomenon, marked in houses where one or both parents were no longer present, was a manifestation of the disintegrating structure of the American family.

In 1974, after the clearinghouse became part of the Centers for Disease Control and moved to Atlanta, Georgia, Horn left Washington, D.C., and went to work for the WORLD HEALTH ORGANIZATION (WHO).

Horn, who had a deep understanding of the smoking problem, developed a 12-page pamphlet entitled "The Smoker's Self-Help Kit," available from the Government Printing Office for 10¢. In the pamphlet was a series of tests that showed would-be quitters, on the one hand, how their tobacco habit seemed to help them manage their emotions, and, on the other hand, how tobacco made their hair, clothes, and breath reek. Horn proposed that people quit "cold turkey."

In May 1964, Dr. Horn gave an address at the National Conference on Smoking and Youth. He shared with the nation's teenage delegates his thoughts on why adults and teens smoke.

Why do people smoke? You do not get much help by asking people this question, whether teenagers or adults. There is probably no other question you can ask of the general public and get such contradictory answers! I have had people tell me that they smoke to be different. Others say that they smoke to be like everyone else. Some smoke to keep thin, others say that they smoke to gain weight. Some smoke to look older, others smoke to look younger. Some smoke to look more sophisticated and glamorous, others smoke to look more rugged and earthy. Some smoke to look more masculine, some smoke to look more feminine. (Horn, 1964).

See also CENTERS FOR DISEASE CONTROL AND PREVENTION

References: Daniel Horn, "Confidentially, It's Worse!" *Smoke Signals*, vol. 10, no. 8, August, 1964, p. 2.

Horowitz, Milton (1926–1996)

In September 1995, a state court jury in San Francisco, California, awarded university professor, clinical psychologist, and former smoker, Milton Horowitz $2 million for the mesothelioma (a fatal form of lung cancer caused by "blue" asbestos) resulting from the use of asbestos in the micronite filters of the KENT CIGARETTES he smoked in the 1950s. On August 12, 1997, the California Court of Appeals issued a unanimous opinion upholding the jury verdict against LORILLARD COMPANY INC., manufacturer of KENT CIGARETTES, and codefendant Hollingsworth and Vose Co., a supplier of asbestos-laden cigarette filters. The opinion represented the first time a jury verdict against a tobacco company survived appeal. The former smoker's lawsuit circumvented a California law that banned lawsuits against manufacturers for tobacco-related illnesses. The jury awarded Mr. Horowitz $1.3 million in compensatory damages and $700,000 in punitive damages, meant to punish misconduct. Dr. Horowitz was represented by MADELYN CHABER.

Mr. Horowitz alleged that Lorillard and Hollingsworth and Vose exposed him to asbestos in the filters of Kent cigarettes, which he smoked from 1952 to 1963. Lorillard was held liable for $1.21 million and Hollingsworth and Vose was liable for the rest of the award. Lorillard appealed, arguing it should not have to pay for the wrongdoing of its predecessor, P. Lorillard. The Supreme Court rejected the appeal. The California Court of Appeals concluded that "substantial evidence supports the punitive damage award against Lorillard." It said the evidence is "sufficient to show that in the 1950s P. Lorillard knew or should have known that smoking asbestos-containing filter cigarettes could result in irreversible and fatal asbestos-related illness" (Tobacco Products Liability Project Press Release, 1997). *See also* CARTER, GRADY; CIPOLLONE, ROSE; MADDOX, ROLAND

References: Tobacco Products Liability Project Press Release, August 13, 1997, p. 1.

Horton, Nathan (1936–1987)

In 1986, Nathan Horton, a 50-year-old black carpenter from Mississippi who smoked two packs a day, brought a lawsuit against the AMERICAN TOBACCO COMPANY (ATC), maker of PALL MALL CIGARETTES, the brand he smoked for more than 30 years. He blamed the tobacco company for his inoperable lung cancer. DON BARRETT, a lawyer who graduated from the University of Mississippi Law School class of 1969, represented Horton on a contingency fee.

Since Mississippi is one of 10 states with a tort statute of "pure" comparative fault (a plaintiff can win damages if a jury decides the maker of the product bears even a fraction of the blame for the injury), Barrett felt the Horton case looked good enough to confront the tobacco industry. Horton's suit also claimed that the tobacco company had knowingly sold cigarettes contaminated with pesticides. After Horton died in January 1987, his wife Ella took up the case on his behalf. American Tobacco hired five Mississippi law firms to defend the case.

The trial in Lexington, Mississippi, began January 5, 1988, and the jury retired January 28 with instructions from the judge that the tobacco company could not be held responsible in comparative fault unless the jury agreed it had been selling cigarettes it knew to contain harmful contaminants. The judge also told the jury (11 blacks and 1 white) that they would have to find the company had a reckless disregard for public health in failing to test their cigarettes properly if they wanted to award punitive damages. The lawsuit ended in a mistrial.

The retrial took place in Oxford, Mississippi, because the judge ruled there had been so much publicity and conflict between the two sides that a new Lexington jury would be prejudiced. After listening to 11 days of evidence, the jury decided that cigarette smoking caused Nathan Horton's lung cancer but refused to award damages, saying both the company and Horton were at fault.

Hubbell, Charles B.

In 1893, Charles B. Hubbell, president of the New York Board of Education, began a crusade against cigarettes in public schools because he felt the cigarette habit was "more devastating to the health and morals of young men than any habit or vice that can be named" (Taylor et al., 1991). He decided to form an anti-cigarette smoking league in every boys' school in New York City. Eventually, 25,000 New York schoolboys joined leagues established in almost all of the 63 male grammar schools. *See also* ANTI-CIGARETTE LEAGUE (ACL), NEW YORK CITY

References: C. Barr Taylor, Joel D. Killen, and the Editors of Consumer Reports Books, *The Facts About Smoking*, Yonkers, NY: Consumer Reports Books, 1991, p. 7.

Humidor

A humidor is a place for storing cigars where the percentage of moisture is regulated. It also is a small box or case fitted for the same purpose, or a glass or wooden container with a lid and moistening device for keeping pipe tobacco. *See also* CIGAR; PIPE

I

Imperial Tobacco Company of Great Britain and Ireland

Imperial Tobacco Company of Great Britain and Ireland was a union of tobacco manufacturing companies created in 1901 to defend their markets, fight the monopolistic AMERICAN TOBACCO COMPANY (ATC), and "hold the British trade for British people." Originally founded by 13 firms, Imperial tried from the outset to avoid the worst features of the American structure. Imperial proposed that wholesale and retail dealers sign a Bonus Agreement. To qualify for a bonus, a distributor had to sign a written agreement with a clause precluding the trader from stocking the goods of the American Tobacco Company founded by JAMES BUCHANAN DUKE.

Duke retaliated with a price-cutting war. The trade war went on for a year until 1902 when Imperial's directors reached a détente with American Tobacco Company. The historic agreement, which divided the world between the two great combines, created an Anglo-American tobacco alliance and formidable profit-making machine and provided for the transfer of the export and overseas trade of both Imperial and American Tobacco to a new company to be formed in the United Kingdom, the BRITISH-AMERICAN TOBACCO COMPANY LTD. or BAT Co. or simply BAT. The Americans owned two-thirds of the stock and the British one-third. As a result of the agreement, American Tobacco withdrew from the United Kingdom market and Imperial agreed not to enter the United States market.

American Tobacco acquired the right to nominate three directors to the Imperial board. The companies assigned brand rights to each other for home sales. James Buchanan Duke joined the Imperial board in October 1902, an appointment he held for nine and a half years. He was also elected the first chairman of British-American Tobacco.

After Duke's monopoly was broken up by the U.S. Supreme Court in 1911, he was forced to sell his majority shareholding in BAT and cancel the trans-Atlantic agreement. BAT was then free to conduct business all over the world. *See also* BAT INDUSTRIES PLC

Impotence and Smoking

In the United States, researchers have found that smoking increases impotence by at least 50 percent even among healthy young men aged 31 to 49, a problem that apparently increases with age according to a seminal study published in a 1995 issue of the *American Journal of Epidemiology*. The study said that the problem is even worse in older men, and that 70 percent of the patients attending impotence clinics were smokers. An earlier report in the *New England Journal of Medicine* said that the probability of impotence in men who both smoked and were being treated for heart disease was 56 percent, compared with only 21 percent of men who didn't smoke.

Scientists have studied the links between smoking and sexual problems for years. Urologists, too, have warned male patients to avoid cigarettes. Smoking clogs blood vessels in the penis just as it clogs those in the heart and brain. NICOTINE also constricts blood vessels, and may interfere with the nervous system and production of sperm. In addition, smoking decreases general physical fitness and vitality to the point that smokers tend to be physiologically eight years older than their chronological age.

Doctors at the Impotency and Fertility Medical Centre in Jerusalem, Israel, have found that men readily abstain from smoking in hopes of boosting their sexual performance. A Centre study showed that 80 percent gave up smoking in the interest of improving sexual performance.

In November 1998 in Thailand, where 90 percent of all smokers are male, one of a series of rotating warnings on cigarette packs read: "Cigarette smoking causes sexual impotence." *See also* SMITH, LYNN R.

Indian Health Service (IHS)

In 1983, Dr. Rice C. Leach, service unit director of the Phoenix Indian Medical Center, launched an educational campaign to establish the "smoke-free hospital" as a standard for all hospitals. He obtained the support of the local Indian Health Board to implement the standard at the center. At first, some employees strongly opposed, and with the potential for union grievances, the plan was indefinitely postponed.

Dr. Leach and Dr. Leland L. Fairbanks, acting director of the Indian Health Service (IHS) Clinical Support Center and champion of a smoke-free environment, discussed their experiences with Dr. Charles North, service unit director of the Public Health Service Indian Hospital on the Hopi Reservation at Keams Canyon, Arizona. Dr. North organized an effort to implement a smoke-free policy that included employee involvement and support from the community and tribal leadership. The smoke-free standard was adopted in December 1983.

In May 1984, Dr. C. EVERETT KOOP, surgeon general of the U.S. Public Health Service (USPHS), issued a challenge to the nation to develop a "smoke-free society" by the year 2000. As the nation's leading public health officer, he was eager to use any opportunity to promote his new initiative. He publicly acknowledged the Keams Canyon effort only one month later at the USPHS Professional Association meeting in Scottsdale, Arizona. The hospital was presented a special citation from the Stanford Heart Disease Prevention Program and a second citation from the American Academy of Family Physicians.

In February 1985, Dr. Koop met with IHS Director Dr. Everett R. Rhoades to endorse and discuss system-wide implementation of a smoke-free standard. Dr. Rhoades appointed an IHS Smoke-Free Task Force that reaffirmed the "Smoke-Free IHS" as realistic and developed a national plan.

In April 1995, Don Davis, director of the IHS Portland Area, instructed all Portland Area offices and facilities that had not already done so to become smoke-free within 30 days. Thus, Portland became the first smoke-free IHS area. Shortly afterwards, in July 1995, the Albuquerque Area announced it had achieved the smoke-free standard at all facilities.

In November 1985, the AMERICAN CANCER SOCIETY (ACS) presented a special citation to the IHS "For its pioneering efforts to bring about the achievement of a totally smoke-free environment in all IHS clinics, hospitals, and administrative offices nationwide" (The Provider, 1997).

On December 12, 1985, in a letter to the editor of the *New England Journal of Medicine,* Dr. Rhoades publicly declared the commitment to ban all indoor smoking in IHS facilities.

On September 16, 1986, union employees in Tahlequah, Oklahoma, challenged the right of the IHS to deny their "right" to smoke in the Indian Hospital. Dr. Rhoades testified before the Federal Labor Relations Authority in Muskogee that the authority to establish smoke-free environments was essential to the

IHS mission of raising the health status of American Indians and Alaska Natives to the highest possible level. The judge agreed, setting a precedent allowing officials to prohibit smoking in federal buildings.

On August 13, 1987, Dr. William H. Foege, executive director of the Carter Center at Emory University and past director of the Centers for Disease Control, proclaimed IHS smoke-free environments a major Public Health Service accomplishment. *See also* CENTERS FOR DISEASE CONTROL AND PREVENTION (CDC); PUBLIC HEALTH SERVICE (PHS)

References: *The Provider*, November 1997, p. 98.

INFACT

INFACT, headquartered in Boston, Massachusetts, is a national grassroots organization whose purpose is to stop life-threatening abuses by transnational corporations such as PHILIP MORRIS COMPANIES INC. and R.J. REYNOLDS TOBACCO COMPANY and to increase their accountability to people around the world. Since 1977, INFACT has been educating the public about dangerous abuses of power by giant corporations and organizing millions of people to take action to change corporate behavior.

In 1993, INFACT organized centers around two major programs. Through the Tobacco Industry Campaign, consumers and health advocates are challenging Philip Morris and RJR NABISCO HOLDINGS CORPORATION to stop addicting new young customers around the world and to stop manipulating public policy in the interest of tobacco profits. The second program, the Tobacco Industry Boycott, fosters shareholder pressure to free Philip Morris's Kraft and RJR's Nabisco food brands from their deadly association with tobacco.

The Human Toll of Tobacco Project, a collection of photos and stories in the memory of loved ones lost to tobacco, is a powerful tool used by INFACT for community-based organizing and educational outreach.

Insurance Coverage and Smoking

Differential insurance premiums exist for smokers and nonsmokers. In 1984, the NATIONAL ASSOCIATION OF INSURANCE COMMISSIONERS called for higher health insurance premiums for smokers. Since then, insurance companies have charged tobacco users more than their nonsmoking coworkers for health insurance.

For people who don't smoke, insurance rates may be lowered in the following categories:

1. **Automobile Insurance:** Some insurance companies offer nonsmokers a reduction from regular rates because they have fewer accidents.
2. **Homeowners Insurance:** Some companies offer discounts to owners who do not smoke because the risk of fires from smoking and matches is decreased.
3. **Disability-income Insurance:** Some insurers offer nonsmokers discounts while laid up.
4. **Life Insurance:** Some of the nation's life insurers either provide discounts from regular rates or market special, preferred-risk life insurance plans for people who don't smoke.

See also NATIONAL ASSOCIATION OF INSURANCE COMMISSIONERS (NAIC)

International Network of Women against Tobacco (INWAT)

The International Network of Women against Tobacco, headquartered in Metuchen, New Jersey, was founded in 1990 by female tobacco control leaders to address the complex issues of tobacco use among women and young girls. INWAT provides contacts, primarily women, to individuals and organizations working in tobacco control. It collects and distributes information regarding global women and tobacco issues, shares strategies to counter tobacco advertising and promotion, and supports the development of women-centered tobacco use prevention and cessation programs. INWAT assists in the organization and planning of conferences on tobacco control and collaborates on the development of publications regarding women and tobacco issues.

International Tobacco Use. *See* GLOBAL TOBACCO USE

International Union against Cancer (UICC)

The International Union against Cancer, an international non-governmental organization devoted exclusively to all aspects of the worldwide fight against cancer, was founded in 1933. Today the UICC has 250 member organizations in 80 countries, all working to control or eliminate cancer.

The UICC's Tobacco and Cancer program was first established in 1976 with the objectives of promoting an agreed international policy on tobacco control and providing expertise to advise on the analysis of local problems and the development of national programs. Through international and national conferences, workshops, symposia, and consultative visits, the UICC provides assistance to member organizations in all matters relating to the tobacco problem. The Tobacco and Cancer program is operated by an international team of expert volunteer project chairpersons and consultants.

The UICC believes that measures to deal with the tobacco problem should include the following:

- a ban on all advertising and promotion of tobacco products (including sponsorship and other forms of indirect advertising)
- effective government health warnings on all tobacco products
- a low TAR and NICOTINE policy
- tax and pricing policies
- alternative economic policies

- policies to protect young people from tobacco promotion and sales and prevent the onset of tobacco use
- policies to protect the rights of non-smokers and establish in law the right to smoke-free common environments, including workplaces
- policies to prohibit new methods of nicotine delivery and block future marketing strategies of the tobacco industry
- policies to ensure the wide availability of help for tobacco users who wish to stop

The UICC helped to organize International No Smoking Day, first held in November 1992 in 10 countries in EASTERN AND CENTRAL EUROPE. *See also* GLOBAL TOBACCO USE

Interreligious Coalition on Smoking or Health

Composed of organizations from all faith traditions, the Interreligious Coalition on Smoking or Health, headquartered in Washington, D.C., is committed to educating religious communities and the wider public on policy initiatives to control tobacco. The focus is on federal and state policies in both the executive and legislative branches of government.

The coalition, along with the AMERICAN CANCER SOCIETY (ACS) and NATIONAL CENTER FOR TOBACCO-FREE KIDS, helped organize the first national conference on religion and tobacco control held on January 21, 1998. Representatives of over 30 religious groups, with tens of millions of members, met at the White House with the president's Domestic Policy Council staff. Coalition cochairs reminded conferees that the churches had historically led the fights against slavery and gender and racial discrimination and urged them to regard saving the lives of half-a-million people a year from smoking as an urgent moral imperative. *See also* SEVENTH DAY ADVENTIST CHURCH

Iowa

In 1896, the state of Iowa passed the second anti-cigarette law in the nation. The Iowa statute, which was repealed in 1921, stated in part:

> No one, by himself, clerk, servant, employee or agent, shall, for himself or any person else, directly or indirectly, or upon any pretense, or by any device, manufacture, sell, exchange, barter, dispense, give in the consideration of the purchase of any property, of any services, or in evasion hereof, or keep for sale, any cigarettes or cigarette paper or cigarette wrappers, or any paper made or prepared for the purpose of making cigarettes, or for the purpose of being filled with tobacco for smoking; or own or keep, or be in any way concerned, engaged or employed in owning or keeping, any such cigarettes or cigarette paper or wrappers, with intent to violate any provision of this section, or authorize or permit the same to be done Iowa Code Ann. §5006 (West 1897). (Widerman, 1992)

Iowa also led the way when, in 1921, it became the first state to impose an excise tax on cigarettes. *See also* ANTI-TOBACCO MOVEMENTS, UNITED STATES; STATE REGULATION OF TOBACCO; TAXATION IN THE UNITED STATES

References: Rivka Widerman, "Tobacco is a Dirty Weed. Have We Ever Liked It? A Look at Nineteenth Century Anti-Cigarette Legislation" *Loyola Law Review*, vol. 38, no. 2, 1992, p. 400.

Iroquois Tobacco Invocation

Addressed to the "Creator," this speech, contents of which are determined by the occasion, is performed twice a year during the Midwinter Ceremony and during the summer. A chant accompanies the tobacco offering. Tobacco is esteemed by the Iroquois as one of the blessings bestowed on them by the Creator and is viewed as a helper to aid people in communicating with the Creator. It is burned, usually in a stove or fireplace, as well as smoked, as an offering to carry messages to the Creator and other spirits. The offering is a way of pledging a sincere mind and heart. The tobacco used in the ceremonies is grown and cured by the Iroquois for sacred purposes. *See also* NATIVE AMERICANS; PIPE SMOKING AND NATIVE AMERICANS

Italy

The fashion of smoking was first adopted by court circles in Italy in the sixteenth century and was little known among the masses. Prominent clerics also spread its use because they regarded tobacco as a medical plant. In 1560, Prospero Santa Croce, papal nuncio, brought back with him from his mission to the Portuguese court tobacco seeds that were planted in the Vatican gardens. Tobacco became known as *herba Santa Croce.* By 1585, tobacco was found in abundant quantities in Rome, thanks to Cardinal Santa Croce, although it was not yet widely smoked.

By the mid-seventeenth century, smoking had increased so dramatically among the clergy in Italy and Spain that clerics indulged in it even in church and during Mass. The Diocese of Seville in Spain appealed to Pope Urban VIII to stop the practice. The pope issued the bull (papal edict) *Ad futuram rei memoriam* to punish offenders by immediate excommunication. A special clause, however, exempted certain high personages and rendered the bull ineffective. Clerical use continued and Urban's successor, Pope Innocent X, issued another bull forbidding tobacco use in St. Peter's Basilica, under penalty of excommunication. Again, the pope's bull provided for special exemptions and had little effect. Other clergy also denounced the tobacco habit strongly, arguing smoking in church was a deadly sin and tobacco the work of the devil. A bitter controversy in the church led to an official pronouncement that while using tobacco was not a sin, it should not be done. In 1655, Pope Alexander VII issued yet another edict forbidding the import and cultivation of tobacco.

By 1700, there was little opposition to tobacco use. By that time, a majority was smoking in Italy. The lower classes used clay pipes; the upper classes china pipes. SNUFF taking was fashionable among the court, nobility, and clergy. On January 10, 1725, Pope

Benedict XIII, a smoker and snuff taker, repealed Pope Innocent's bull and permitted the use of snuff in St. Peter's.

While the popes were trying to forbid tobacco use, the republic of Venice succeeded in profiting from the habit. In 1626, it taxed tobacco, and in 1651 began to limit its cultivation and sale, while granting certain private parties the privilege of growing tobacco.

In 1659, the first tobacco *appalto* was founded, a contract giving a private person exclusive right to import, manufacture, or trade in tobacco in return for a payment. This contract became a model monopoly imitated in most European states. In the course of time, the rising revenues from tobacco taxes and monopolies led Italy and other governments to lift the ban on tobacco. *See also* PIPE

J

James I (1566–1625)

James I, king of England and Scotland, was a fanatical hater of tobacco and made the plant a royal monopoly to control its growth, discourage its use, and profit from the revenue it generated. He prohibited the sowing of tobacco seed in his kingdoms, but such decrees were not effective in curbing the smoking habit. One of the first acts by James to stifle smoking, which continued through smuggling, was to raise the duty on imported tobacco leaf from 2 pence per pound to 6 shillings and 8 pence.

In 1604, the king published anonymously (his authorship was not revealed until 1616) a long pamphlet entitled *A Counterblaste to Tobacco* attacking the habit of smoking with fury and some fact. In the pamphlet, James discovered in his kingdoms "a generall sluggishnesse, which makes us wallow in all sorts of idle delights." Users of tobacco, the king said, would become "feeble, his spirits dull, and in the end, as dwosie lazie bellygod, he shall evanish in a Lethargie." The use of the "precious stink" was a sin. The document also attacked Sir WALTER RALEIGH for making fashionable in England "so vile and stinking a custom." In London alone at the time there were some 7,000 establishments selling tobacco. The *Counterblaste* concluded as follows:

> Have you not reason then to be ashamed, and to forbear this filthy novelty so basely grounded, so foolishly received and so grossly mistaken in the right to use thereof? In your abuse thereof sinning against God, harming yourselves both in persons and goods, and taking also thereby the marks and notes of vanity upon you: by the custom thereof making yourselves to be wondered at by all foreign civil Nations, and by all strangers that come among you, to be scorned and condemned. A custom loathsome to the eye, hateful to the nose, harmful to the brain, dangerous to the lungs, and in the black stinking fume thereof, nearest resembling the horrible Stygian smoke of the pit that is bottomless.

In 1605, the king arranged the first public debate at Oxford University on the evils of tobacco. To prove his point, he displayed black brains and black viscera allegedly obtained from bodies of smokers. To discourage tobacco sales and use, James increased the tax 40-fold, but when use and smuggling increased, he reduced the tax in 1608 to one shilling per pound of tobacco and sold the monopoly right to collect it. In 1613, he barred anyone from dealing in tobacco without a Letter Patent (a holder was required to turn over half their profits to the royal treasury). In 1615, tobacco imports had risen so greatly that James revoked his 1608 monopoly grant and reassigned it at a higher price. Since smuggling continued unabated, James decreed in 1620 that all tobacco sold should bear a government stamp.

When the Virginia Company resisted the royal orders for a stamp on tobacco, James lowered the duty to one shilling a pound, half the impost on the rival Spanish tobacco. To help the colonial planters, he also tried to limit the growing of tobacco in England, saying that the growing of food for the colonies would be jeopardized. In 1621, the House of Commons passed an act providing for a system of preferential tariffs for tobacco to help foster the colonial enterprise. In 1624, the king declared a Royal Tobacco Monopoly to protect his colonial suppliers, and decreed that only Virginia tobacco be imported. He refused legal imports of any tobacco from other sources and English tobacco growers used force to resist the king's embargo.

James I died in 1625. Although his reign began with an assault on tobacco, it ended with thousands of pounds of Virginia leaf passing with his approval through London customs.

References: James I, *Counterblaste to Tobacco*, 1604.

Jamestown, Virginia Colony

In 1610, Englishman JOHN ROLFE settled in Jamestown in Virginia (the first permanent English settlement in North America), a colony near financial collapse. After obtaining the seeds of *NICOTIANA TABACUM* from the Spanish West Indies and planting them in the sandy soil of Virginia, the Spanish tobacco thrived.

The dramatic success of Jamestown's tobacco crop, which made the colony economically viable, is credited not only to Rolfe's importation of the Spanish strain, but to his finding better ways of growing and curing it. Some scholars feel he was guided in the techniques by Pocahontas, daughter of American Indian chief Powhatan; Rolfe married Pocahontas in April 1614. That year, the first shipment of Virginia tobacco was sold in London.

Despite James I's disapproval of Jamestown's dependence on a crop he despised, he could not ignore the enormous import duties Rolfe's Virginia tobacco brought to the royal treasury. Londoners and others around the world who liked its taste demanded it. Since all sales had to be made through London, where hefty excise taxes were levied, the English treasury grew with every transaction. In 1615, Jamestown exported 2,300 pounds of tobacco; three years later, 20,000 pounds; and in 1620, 40,000 pounds.

By 1619, the Virginia staple exceeded the popular large-leaf Spanish tobacco product on the London market. The Spanish monopoly had been broken. Jamestown exported 10 tons of tobacco to Europe. In 1620, Virginia exports doubled the 1619 quantity. By 1639, the colony exported 750 tons of tobacco, making it the main source of revenue for Virginia and the chief export.

Tobacco dominated the lives of the Jamestown colonists. It grew in the streets, in houses, and anywhere a plant could be

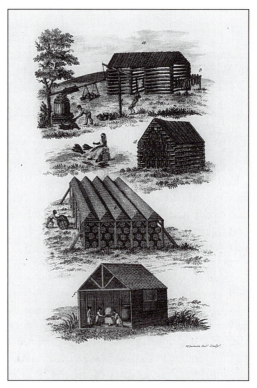

Tobacco culture became the economic salvation of the Jamestown Colony. These scenes depict the growing and preparing of tobacco on a Virginia plantation c. 1800. *Arents Collection, The New York Public Library, Astor, Lenox and Tilden Foundations.*

squeezed in. People were so deeply involved with tobacco that at one time in the early days of the colony, Rolfe expressed concern over the lack of attention given to growing food. Laws were written to control the tobacco fever. One act limited colonists to growing 1,000 plants. In 1629, it was changed to 3,000. In a 1617 report, Captain John Smith wrote that he "found but five or six houses, the Church down, the 16 palisades broken, the bridge in pieces, the well of fresh water spoiled . . . [because] the colony was dispersed all about, planting tobacco" (Brooks, 1952).

By 1619, tobacco was being used as currency. The first cargo of African slaves was deposited in Virginia by the Dutch, who were paid with tobacco. The Africans were bought as indentured servants from the Dutch who were low on food. Two years later, transportation charges for brides from England came to 120 pounds "best leaf" tobacco per wife. The salaries of clergy were also paid in tobacco.

Although Virginia tobacco did not equal Spanish in quality, the English king gave it customs preference. Under the Navigation Acts of 1651 and 1660, tobacco grown in the tidewater could only be shipped in English vessels to northern European countries: England, Holland, Germany, Scandinavia, and France.

To the colony of Virginia, tobacco was equivalent to gold. It brought the colony from wretched failure to heady success. In 1847, S.J.W. Tabor, a historian, described it as follows:

> [T]he herb [tobacco] was almost the potable gold of the alchemists. It was their solace and their coin. It ministered to their bodily gratifications, furnished them employment, paid their taxes, discarded their debts, and might be said to serve them spiritually and temporally . . . . In the ports of Virginia alone, at Christmas 1648 the great staple had brought 31 ships from various quarters for trade: seven from New England, ten from London, two from Bristol, and twelve from Holland. (Tabor, 1847)

See also JAMES I

References: Jerome E. Brooks, *The Mighty Leaf: Tobacco Through the Centuries*, Boston: Little, Brown and Company, 1952, p. 54.

S. J. W. Tabor, M.D. "Historical Sketch of Tobacco from 1640 to 1662." *The Boston Medical and Surgical Journal*, vol. 37, no. 17, 1847, p. 471.

Japan

Japan was probably the first nation in Asia to adopt the habit of smoking tobacco both for recreation and for medicinal purposes. In 1542, a group of Portuguese sailors, kidnapped by Chinese pirates and driven by a sudden storm into a Japanese port, brought tobacco with them. A commerce between the Portuguese and Japanese began. Portuguese seamen taught the inhabitants of Kiushiu, an independent island, to smoke.

The smoking habit spread quickly and in 1596, the emperor himself ordered tobacco seeds planted in the Royal Gardens of the capital city of Kyoto. In 1605, cultivation of tobacco began in Japan when it was planted around Nagasaki. In 1607, a Nagasaki doctor named Saka wrote: "Of late a new thing is come into fashion called tobacco, it consists of large leaves which are cut up and of which one drinks the smoke" (Dunhill, 1969). Smoking spread to all classes of society and smoking clubs flourished in the capital city. At first tobacco was smoked rolled up in a piece of paper, later in pipes of bamboo, then of copper and other metals.

In 1603, the young regent Hideyori issued an edict prohibiting tobacco, but to little effect. Two further edicts were issued making cultivation a penal offense. One of the chief motives of anti-tobacco laws was the fear that cultivation would interfere with the production of rice and corn. In 1612, a proclamation forbid trade in tobacco. Smoking, sale, and cultivation of tobacco were also prohibited. Hideyori's shogun decreed that the property of any man detected selling tobacco would be handed over to his accuser. Anyone arrested for "trafficking" on horseback would lose both the tobacco and the horse. Despite the attempts at repression, smoking became so general that even officers at the royal court indulged in the habit. Three years later, another edict warned those in the army that their property would be confiscated if they were caught smoking. A year later, in 1616, penalties were increased to include both prison and fines. Nevertheless, tobacco use spread rapidly, even among the upper classes who were responsible for the prohibition.

During the early seventeenth century, authorities viewed tobacco with suspicion because it was a foreign habit. They also disapproved of the excesses of smoking enthusiasts who belonged to smoking clubs. Fires were also blamed on smokers. Royal orders issued against planters of tobacco and smokers failed to control the use or stop the spread of tobacco. After the laws were abandoned, cultivation of the plant was allowed in 1625 except in rice fields and vegetable gardens.

Smoking was so widespread in polite society that tobacco accompanied the ceremonial tea offered to guests. By 1650, tobacco use spread to include respectable women and SNUFF was introduced by Jesuit missionaries and Portuguese traders. In 1651, tobacco smoking was recognized as legal. The Japanese medical profession on the whole appeared to be in favor of smoking in moderation while others praised its soothing and pleasing recreational qualities. Still others feared tobacco as a fire and health hazard.

References: Alfred Dunhill, *The Pipe Book*, New York: Macmillan Company, 1924, 1969, pp. 88–89.

Japan Tobacco Inc.

Japan Tobacco Inc., with its primary business of production, sale, and export of tobacco products, has also been actively engaged in the area of pharmaceuticals, food, agribusiness, and engineering and real estate since the company was privatized in 1985. The president of the company is Masaru Mizuno, and it is headquartered in Tokyo.

Japan Tobacco has offered a total of 92 cigarette brands since February 1998. The total reaches 114 if cigars (10), pipe tobac-

cos (11), and cut tobacco (91) are included. Among them are the popular Mild Seven, which is the world's second biggest-selling CIGARETTE, and Cabin. *See also* ASIA AND U.S. TRADE POLICY; CIGAR; JAPAN

Joe Camel. *See* OLD JOE CAMEL

Jones, Okla, II (1946–1996)

The son of a cotton sharecropper, Okla Jones II was a federal judge on the New Orleans District Court, Louisiana. He certified *CASTANO V. AMERICAN TOBACCO COMPANY*, the first national class-action lawsuit against the tobacco industry seeking damages on behalf of millions of smokers. Jones began his career as a civil rights and public interest attorney and then turned to private practice, which included personal injury cases and culminated in his becoming New Orlean's first African-American city attorney. In 1990, he was elected a state judge.

Judge Jones was sworn onto the federal bench six days before he heard arguments on whether to allow the tobacco class action to go forward. He certified *Castano* for trial on February 17, 1995. The ruling formally granted class-action status to the 1994 lawsuit by three smokers and Peter Castano's widow and gave plaintiffs a broad boundary line for their class. The tobacco companies appealed Judge Jones's decision to the U.S. Court of Appeals for the Fifth Circuit, which agreed to review the case. As the lawyers prepared their appeal arguments, Judge Jones died suddenly from leukemia in January 1996. *See also* CASTANO, PETER; TOBACCO LITIGATION: FIRST, SECOND, AND THIRD WAVES

Jordan, David Starr (1851–1931)

The first president of Stanford University, David Starr Jordan believed that NICOTINE in cigarettes served as a "nerve irritant" that disrupted the nervous system and left the smoker vulnerable to other vices. Jordan also objected to the effects of smoke on nonsmokers because it irritated their eyes, nostrils, and lungs. Shortly after Stanford University opened in 1891, students adopted a no-smoking policy that pleased Jordan.

For more than 20 years, Jordan was involved with several anti-cigarette groups and donated cash and his time to them, serving as an officer of the Anti-Cigarette League from 1904 to 1925. He allowed his epigrams, including "Cigarette-smoking boys are like wormy apples: they drop long before the harvest time," to be used in posters and cards circulated by anti-cigarette activists. The Anti-Cigarette League was permitted to use "The boy who smokes cigarettes need not be anxious about his future. He has none." *See also* ANTI-TOBACCO MOVEMENTS, UNITED STATES; KELLOGG, JOHN HARVEY

K

Karbiwnyk, Joann (1938–)

In November 1997, a jury in a state circuit court in Jacksonville, Florida, ruled in favor of the R.J. REYNOLDS TOBACCO COMPANY and declined to order the cigarette maker to pay damages to Joann Karbiwnyk, a smoker for 30 years who developed lung cancer in 1995. Karbiwnyk, who quit smoking in 1984 when she took up running, was represented by NORWOOD "WOODY" WILNER, the Jacksonville lawyer who filed several hundred tobacco lawsuits.

The Duval County Circuit Court judge permitted the jury to see BROWN AND WILLIAMSON TOBACCO CORPORATION internal documents stolen from the company's law firm by former paralegal, MERRELL WILLIAMS, as well as an editorial in the *Journal of the American Medical Association (JAMA)* saying "the U.S. public has been duped by the tobacco industry. No right thinking individual can ignore the evidence" (Geyelin, 1997). Jurors remained unsympathetic to Karbiwnyk, especially because she quit smoking the first time she tried. The majority of the jurors also believed the health risks of smoking were known well enough when she started smoking. *See also* BROWN AND WILLIAMSON TOBACCO CORPORATION—MERRILL WILLIAMS DOCUMENTS; CONNOR, JEAN; ROGERS, RICHARD

References: Milo Geyelin, "Reynolds Wins Ex-Smoker's Cancer Suit," *Wall Street Journal*, November 3, 1997, p. 12, Section B.

Kelder, Graham (1957–)

An attorney at the TOBACCO CONTROL RESOURCE CENTER and Tobacco Products Liability Project, Graham Kelder has authored numerous journal articles on tobacco control and has been a media resource on tobacco issues. He specializes in local tobacco control and policy, and has spearheaded review boards to help ensure that local tobacco regulation is legally sound and can withstand tobacco industry challenges. *See also* DAYNARD, RICHARD; TOBACCO LITIGATION: FIRST, SECOND, AND THIRD WAVES

Kellogg, John Harvey (1852–1943)

The founder of a breakfast cereal dynasty, Dr. John Harvey Kellogg was a forceful critic of smoking. The medical director of the Battle Creek, Michigan, Sanitarium in 1876, he regarded tobacco as a threat to health. He believed that the CIGARETTE was dangerous because its smoke was inhaled and could damage internal organs. Although he thought smoking was harmful to both sexes, he said that women were at greater risk because of reproduction. Labeling tobacco a heart poison, he did not allow its use in any form at the sanitarium. Neither as head of the sanitarium nor as director of the Michigan Board of Health would he hire anyone who snuffed, chewed, or smoked a PIPE, CIGAR, or cigarette.

Kellogg wrote a book, published pamphlets, produced a film and a lantern slide

Tobacco is a Heart Poison

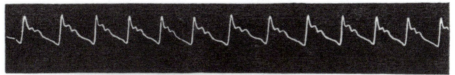

NORMAL PULSE—EACH VERTICAL LINE REPRESENTS A HEART BEAT

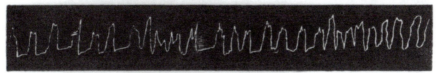

IRREGULAR PULSE OF TOBACCO HEART

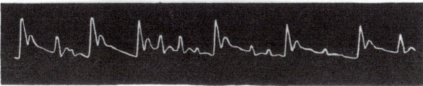

A SMOKER'S PULSE

"Tobacco is a heart poison"—a depiction of the irregular pulse of a smoker's heart illustrates Kellogg's belief.

show, and lectured on the theme "How Tobacco Kills."

In an article condemning the distribution of cigarettes to soldiers in WORLD WAR I, he wrote the following:

> The cigarette is known to be an enemy of scholarship, of culture, of morals, of health and vigor, and yet it is tolerated, even encouraged. The millions of cigarettes now being fired at our soldiers will every one hit its mark and do its mischief. More American soldiers will be damaged by the cigarette than by German bullets. (Tate, 1995)

See also JORDAN, DAVID STARR; WORLD WAR I

References: C. Cassandra Tate, "The American Anti-Cigarette Movement, 1880–1930," Ph.D. Dissertation, Seattle: University of Washington, 1995, p. 218. (UMI Number 9609793.)

Kent Cigarettes

In 1952, in response to numerous scientific studies linking cigarette smoking and life-threatening diseases, LORILLARD COMPANY INC. introduced the micronite filter for Kent cigarettes. The brand was named after Lorillard executive Herbert A. Kent and given a heavy promotional campaign. In full-page advertisements, Lorillard said Kent filters, a blend of paper, cotton acetate, and crocidolite, a form of asbestos, took out "more nicotine and tars than any other leading cigarette" (Kluger, 1996).

Smokers found it difficult to draw in smoke because of the filters and when they succeeded Kent cigarettes tasted flavorless. "People complained that puffing on a Kent was like smoking through a mattress" (Kluger, 1996). The filters were loosened up to allow more flavor through, making them easier to smoke. NICOTINE and tar levels went up, so in 1957, without publicity, Kent abandoned its original micronite filter. *See also* FILTERED CIGARETTES

References: Richard Kluger, *Ashes to Ashes*, New York: Alfred A. Knopf, 1996, p. 186.

Kessler, David (1951–)

Appointed in November 1990 as commissioner of the FOOD AND DRUG ADMINISTRATION (FDA) by President George Bush, David Kessler waged a crusade against the tobacco industry until his departure in late 1996. A pediatrician with a medical degree from Harvard Medical School and a law degree from the University of Chicago and management training at New York University School of Business, Dr. Kessler worked as a consultant on health issues for the Senate Committee on Labor and Human Resources chaired by Republican Senator Orrin Hatch of Utah. A registered Republican himself, Kessler was basically apolitical. When nominated to head the FDA, *Time* called him "almost certainly the most capable person ever put in charge of the Food and Drug Administration" (Campbell, 1994).

As a medical doctor, Dr. Kessler was concerned about public health issues related to smoking. When Kessler first looked into the possibility of regulating the tobacco industry in 1991, FDA agency veterans told him it was a "fool's mission." Although he turned his attention to attacking deceptive food labels, curtailing silicone implants, and speeding up the review of new drugs, he kept thinking about the idea of regulating cigarettes. Prodded by Jeff Nesbitt, an FDA spokesman who had tried to get the FDA to regulate tobacco, Kessler and his team became interested in the way tobacco companies controlled the level of NICOTINE in cigarettes.

On February 25, 1994, Kessler, in a sudden change of FDA policy, charged in a letter to the Coalition on Smoking and Health's chairman Scott Ballin that the FDA had received "mounting evidence" that the tobacco companies controlled nicotine levels in cigarettes to satisfy the smoker's addiction. He suggested that these conclusions, if established in an administrative or judicial proceeding, would justify regulating cigarettes as a drug and ultimately banning tobacco products "containing nicotine at levels that cause or sustain addiction."

The change was partly an outgrowth of a secret investigation made by the agency as well as the result of an inquiry by the staff of the ABC news program *DAY ONE*. Kessler's charge came three days before *Day One's* February 28 telecast on the tobacco industry's manipulation of nicotine levels in their products to addict smokers. On March 25, Kessler testified at a congressional hearing chaired by Henry Waxman, a Democrat from California, that cigarette manufacturers have long known of tobacco's addictive qualities and manipulated nicotine levels to keep smokers hooked. He spoke about several tobacco company patents that mentioned ways of "adding nicotine" or "maintaining or increasing nicotine content." The proof, he said, was in volumes of tobacco company papers that showed the tobacco industry conducted or funded studies in both animals and humans. Kessler admitted that none of the evidence meant the patents had been used.

Dr. Kessler, who knew it was politically undesirable to propose a ban on tobacco, devised with his staff a new way to look at nicotine. On March 9, 1995, in a speech at Columbia University School of Law, Kessler redefined smoking as "a pediatric disease." He said it was easy to think of smoking as an adult problem because it is adults who die from tobacco-related diseases. Seeing adults light up in a restaurant or a bar was something like entering a theater in the third act, after the plot has been set in motion. He pointed out that

> [A] person who hasn't started smoking by age nineteen is unlikely to ever become a smoker. Nicotine addiction begins when most tobacco users are teen-agers, so let's call this what it really is: a pediatric disease. (Hilts, 1995)

Kessler shifted the debate away from the concept of smoking as an "adult choice," forcing the tobacco industry to agree with him that children should not smoke.

Besides Kessler's drive for cigarette regulation, he wanted a comprehensive program to prevent young people from becoming addicted to nicotine and he felt it was the responsibility of the U.S. government to deliver that program.

In November 1996, Kessler left the Food and Drug Administration. He became dean of the Yale University School of Medicine in New Haven, Connecticut.

In July 1997, at the request of a bipartisan group of congressmen led by Henry Waxman, Kessler and former surgeon general C. EVERETT KOOP formed an advisory committee on tobacco policy and public health to study the proposed $368.5 billion tobacco settlement of June 1997 between state attorneys general, plaintiffs' lawyers, health advocates, and tobacco executives and their lawyers. *See also* TOBACCO SETTLEMENT—JUNE 1997; WAXMAN HEARINGS

References: Andrew Campbell, "Doctor, Lawyer, Agency Chief," *University of Chicago Magazine*, December 1994, p. 22.

Philip J. Hilts, "FDA Head Calls Smoking a Pediatric Disease," *New York Times*, March 9, 1995, p. A 22.

Key West, Florida

At the turn of the century, Key West, Florida, was the nation's number-one producer of clear HAVANA cigars. Between 1868 and 1900, thousands of Cuban cigar workers relocated to Key West, only 90 miles from Havana, Cuba, where they were able to escape Spanish rule and continue to produce the best cigars. In 1885, cigar factories numbered 86. By 1890, the number of factories grew to almost 130. By that time, it was the beginning of the end of Key West's prominence as a cigar-making location. Businessmen induced Key West cigar manufacturers to relocate to Tampa, Florida. Vincente Martinez Ybor was one of the first major cigar makers to relocate, and others soon followed. By 1900, only 44 factories remained in Key West. Increased labor unrest and hurricane damage combined in 1909, 1910, and 1919 to all but stamp out the industry in Key West. *See also* CIGAR; YBOR CITY, FLORIDA

Kieft, Wilhelmus (c. 1600–1647)

During the term of Wilhelmus Kieft as governor of New Netherlands in the first half of the seventeenth century, he raised a great fury among the Dutch colonists when he issued an edict prohibiting the smoking of tobacco. A story in Washington Irving's satirical *History of New York* (1809) deals with the extremes to which colonists went to protect their freedom to smoke.

> Wilhelmus Kieft . . . . issued an edict, prohibiting the smoking of tobacco throughout the New Netherlands. . . . Had he lived in the present age and attempted to check the unbounded license of the press, he could not have struck more sorely upon the sensibilities of the million. The pipe, in fact, was the great organ of reflection and deliberation of the New Netherlander. It was his constant companion and solace: was he gay, he smoked; was he sad, he smoked; his pipe was never out of his mouth; it was a part of his physiognomy; without it his best friends would not know him. Take away his pipe? You might as well take away his nose!
>
> The immediate effect of the edict of William the Testy was a popular commotion. A vast multitude, armed with pipes and tobacco-boxes, and an immense supply of ammunition, sat themselves down before the governor's house, and fell to smoking with tremendous violence. The testy William issued forth like a wrathful spider, demanding the reason of this lawless fumigation. The sturdy rioters replied by lolling back in their seats, and puffing away with redoubled fury, raising such a murky cloud that the governor was fain to take refuge in the interior of his castle.
>
> A long negotiation ensured through the medium of Antony the Trumpeter. The governor was at first wrathful and unyielding, but was gradually smoked into terms. He concluded by permitting the smoking of tobacco, but he abolished the fair long pipes used in the days of Wouter van Twiller, denoting ease, tranquility, and sobriety of deportment; these he condemned as incompatible with the dispatch of business, in place whereof he substituted little captious short pipes, two

inches in length, which, he observed, could be stuck in one corer of the mouth, or twisted in the hatband, and would never be in the way. Thus ended this alarming insurrection, which was long known by the name of The Pipe-Plot, and which, it has been somewhat quaintly observed, did end, like most plots and seditions, in mere smoke. (Ehwa, 1994)

References: Carl Ehwa, Jr. *The Book of Pipes & Tobacco*, New York: Random House, 1994, pp. 53–56.

Kinney, F.S.

In 1868, tobacconist F.S. Kinney opened a small shop in lower Manhattan, hired some foreign-born rollers, and packaged his Russian and Turkish cigarettes in paper packs to lower prices. In 1869, Kinney experimented with a cigarette made wholly from Bright tobacco, calling it Caporal. He added sugar and licorice to the tobacco to produce a more flavorful cigarette, and renamed it Sweet Caporal. It became New York City's leading brand and made Kinney, for a period, the nation's leading cigarette manufacturer. By 1870, Sweet Caporals made their way to Boston and Philadelphia via visitors who heard about them. Kinney hired jobbers to sell his smokes along the eastern seaboard.

In 1889, Kinney, then the third largest factory in the tobacco industry behind Duke and ALLEN AND GINTER, was one of the first to accept JAMES BUCHANAN DUKE's offer to merge with his new AMERICAN TOBACCO COMPANY (ATC). *See also* BRIGHT TOBACCO

Kinnikinnick

"Kinnikinnick" is an Algonquian term for a blend of tobacco with other products, usually the inner bark of dogwood, sumac leaves, some pungent herbs, and oil to provide a milder smoke than produced by NICOTIANA RUSTICA.

Koop, C. Everett (1916–)

Appointed by President Ronald Reagan, C. Everett Koop, a family doctor, became U.S. surgeon general in 1981; he resigned shortly before his term of office officially expired in November 1989. During the years he served as surgeon general, Koop presided over some of the most pressing health issues of the late twentieth century. Before Koop left office, he became a leader in the nation on smoking and AIDS.

While Surgeon General Koop was in office, seven reports on the health hazards of smoking were released. In February 1982, the surgeon general's report dealt with cancer, and it was one of the strongest anti-smoking reports the U.S. PUBLIC HEALTH SERVICE had written. Newspaper headlines around the country scared people with the news: "Cigarette Smoking Contributes to Bladder, Kidney, Pancreatic Cancer," "Report Finds Smoking Top Cancer-Death Cause," "Cigarettes Blamed for 30 Percent of All Cancer Deaths." At the press conference where Koop released the report, he said for the first time what he repeated countless times afterwards: "Cigarette smoking is the chief preventable cause of death in our society." He also said that 85 percent of lung cancer deaths would not have happened if the victims had never smoked. The report called for more study of SECONDHAND SMOKE, because it "may pose a carcinogenic risk to the nonsmoker" (Koop, 1991). The report, press conference, and Koop's picture received front-page coverage from most major newspapers.

The next three years brought three more hard-hitting reports. The public recognized smoking's connection with cancer, but it was not widely known that smoking caused more deaths from heart disease than from cancer. Koop's 1983 Surgeon General's Report dealt with the connection between cigarette smoking and heart disease. The 1984 report dealt with the connection between cigarette smoking and chronic bronchitis and emphysema. In 1985, Koop's report pointed out that for American workers, cigarette smoking represents a greater cause of death and disability than their workplace environment. Koop's 1986 report delivered proof that secondhand smoke endangered smokers. The same year Koop targeted SMOKELESS TOBACCO—chewing (or spit tobacco) and SNUFF. He appointed an advisory committee that found "The oral use of smokeless tobacco represents a significant health risk. It is not a safe substitute for smoking cigarettes. It can cause cancer . . . and can lead to nicotine addiction" (Advisory Committee, 1986).

After Koop's advisory committee published the smokeless tobacco report, he turned his attention to NICOTINE addiction, the heart of the smoking and smokeless tobacco issue. In 1988, the surgeon general's report branded nicotine a highly addictive substance, like heroin and cocaine, that makes the smoker physically crave tobacco. Koop wanted—but didn't get—cigarettes to carry a warning label that read: "Surgeon General's Warning: Tobacco Contains Nicotine, an Addictive Drug." Although the tobacco companies fought hard against any labels, they agreed to add four health warning labels to cigarette packs and ads to avoid the addiction warning.

In July 1997, at the request of a bipartisan group of congressmen led by Henry Waxman, Surgeon General Koop and former FOOD AND DRUG ADMINISTRATION (FDA) commissioner DAVID KESSLER formed an advisory committee on tobacco policy and public health to study the proposed $368.5 billion tobacco settlement between state attorneys general, plaintiffs' lawyers, health advocates, and tobacco executives and their lawyers.

In 1991, the former surgeon general published his memoirs, *Koop: The Memoirs of America's Family Doctor.* An entire chapter is devoted to tobacco, the first health problem he addressed as surgeon general. He told how every time he gave a public lecture about smoking, he got people's attention by opening with the statement: "A thousand people will stop smoking today. Their funerals will be held sometime during the next three or four days" (Koop, 1991). *See also* HEALTH WARNINGS ON CIGARETTE PACKS AND ADVERTISEMENTS AND SMOKELESS TOBACCO; SURGEON GENERAL'S REPORTS, 1964–1998; STEINFELD, JESSE; TERRY, LUTHER; WAXMAN HEARINGS

References: Advisory Committee to the Surgeon General, *The Health Consequences of Using Smokeless Tobacco*, Bethesda, MD: U.S. Depart-

ment of Health and Human Services, 1986, p. vii.

C. Everett Koop, *Koop: The Memoirs of America's Family Doctor*, New York: Random House, 1991, pp. 166–67.

Korea

Introduced into Korea by the Japanese around 1610, the tobacco plant was called "nambanpoy" after the "namban," or Southern Barbarians, a term the Japanese used for Europeans who introduced tobacco to them. About 50 years later, Henri Hemel, a French traveler who spent time in Korea, remarked on the popularity of tobacco: "They take so much at present that there are very few of either sex but what smoke, and the very children practice it at four or five years of age" (Dunhill, 1969). *See also* GLOBAL TOBACCO USE

References: Alfred Dunhill, *The Pipe Book*, New York: Macmillan Company, 1924, 1969, p. 89.

Kornegay, Horace (1924–)

A congressman from North Carolina, Horace Kornegay left Congress to become chairman of the TOBACCO INSTITUTE. In 1964, Kornegay, a member of the House Interstate and Foreign Commerce Committee, brought a potted tobacco plant to hearings on the issue of labeling cigarette packs with health warnings. He said: "This tobacco plant stands as a defendant in this trial" (Whelan, 1984).

References: Elizabeth M. Whelan, *A Smoking Gun: How the Tobacco Industry Gets Away with Murder*, Philadelphia: George F. Stickley Co., 1984, p. 106.

Kyte v. Store 24 Inc. (1991)

In 1987, 17-year-old Theresa Kyte and her father sued PHILIP MORRIS USA and Store 24 of Waltham, Massachusetts, because the teen was ill and nicotine-dependent. Theresa blamed the cigarette maker and the store for conspiring to sell cigarettes to minors like herself. Theresa had been buying her cigarettes, made by Philip Morris, from Store 24 since she was 14 years old despite a state law prohibiting cigarette sales to people under 18.

Theresa's lawsuit also said that Philip Morris had conspired to increase its profits and "hook" a new generation of smokers. The tobacco company tried to get the case dismissed, but failed.

In 1991, in the landmark case of *Kyte v. Store 24 Inc.,* the Massachusetts Supreme Judicial Court decided the cigarette maker had no control over the stores that sell its products. However, a judge did rule that retailers are liable for any NICOTINE addiction that customers suffer from CIGARETTES. As part of the settlement, Store 24 promised to closely monitor its sales and demand positive identification from young tobacco purchasers to prevent young people under 18 from buying cigarettes. *See also* CHILDREN AND TEENS, UNITED STATES

L

La Rochefoucauld-Liancourt, Duc François Alexandre Frederic, De. *See* FRÉDÉRIC, FRANÇOIS ALEXANDRE

Lancaster County, Pennsylvania

Lancaster County, Pennsylvania, has a rich tradition of tobacco farming and CIGAR production. Both the early Mennonite and Amish settlers in the county took to tobacco farm-

ing. The term "stogie" originated in Lancaster, home of the Conestoga wagon that carried families in the 1800s. Wagon masters smoked long cigars made from coarser leaves that gave off a strong aroma. They became known as "stogies."

Until the 1970s, Pennsylvania tobacco was a top FILLER of choice for many of the country's premier cigar companies. The Amish in Lancaster County, the second larg-

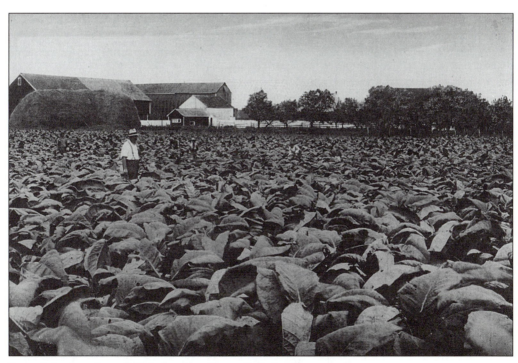

Postcard showing tobacco fields in Lancaster County, Pennsylvania.

est Amish community in the United States, were the primary growers, but tobacco farming among the Amish is declining. Tobacco acreage in Lancaster has dropped from a high of 25,000 in the late 1950s to fewer than 9,000 acres. The Amish have turned to dairy farming instead. Despite less acreage, tobacco remains Lancaster County's largest cash crop.

About 1,000 Amish and Mennonite farmers farm tobacco. They plant some tobacco designated by the U.S. Department of Agriculture as "Pennsylvania 41," a heavy-bodied, dark-colored leaf sold mostly for cigar filler and CHEWING TOBACCO. About 20 years ago Amish farmers started growing Maryland 609 tobacco, now more than half the county's tobacco crop.

The Amish use horse-drawn carts, not tractors and automated planters, to plant the tobacco in the ground in early summer and haul the plants to the tobacco shed for curing. In 1839, the first year a census was available on tobacco in Pennsylvania, records show Lancaster County produced 48,860 pounds of tobacco. The 1995 crop was approximately 17 million pounds. *See also* CONNECTICUT TOBACCO

Lancet

In the December 10, 1825, issue of the *Lancet,* a prestigious medical journal, a description was given of British soldiers returning from Wellington's Napoleonic campaigns in the Iberian Peninsula (1808–1814). They are credited with introducing cigarette smoking to England.

> In Spain and Portugal, a thin paper manufactured from straw, and without size, is used for making segars, by rolling up some tobacco in paper, until the whole is about the size of a pencil and the length of a finger.
> The tobacco itself cannot get into the stomach or lungs, as in the case of snuff-taking, nor can the raw juice of the tobacco do it, as in the case of quid-chewing; but the mouth, nasal passage and (I think) the lungs, gullet and stomach must be powerfully coated with smoke and whatever that contains.
> Turks are perpetually smoking; Spaniards and Portuguese use tobacco profusely; and since the army returned from the peninsula, the habit has become fashionable; the increased number of tobacco shops must be evident to every observor. (Ravenholt, 1990)

In the years 1856–1857, the *Lancet* featured a series entitled "The Great Tobacco Question." Over 50 physicians presented their viewpoints, both pro and con. To prove the evils of tobacco, the physicians presented clinical cases from America and England. One physician, Dr. Hodgkin, associated tobacco with an increase in crime. He also claimed that the use of tobacco, by drying the stomach, caused a craving for alcohol, thus leading the smoker into the dangerous and immoral cult of Bacchus. Indeed, Dr. Hodgkin thought the word tobacco was derived from "to Baccho!" Dr. Solly associated tobacco with nervous paralysis and a loss of intellectual capacity. Dr. Schneider claimed that "So frequently is vision impaired by the constant use of tobacco that spectacles may be said to be part and parcel of a German, as a hat is to an Englishman . . . . Americans wear themselves out by the use of tobacco" (Whelan, 1984).

At the end of the series, the *Lancet* gave tobacco a passing grade:

> The use of tobacco is widely spread, more widely spread than any one custom, form of worship, or religious belief, and that therefore it must have some good or at least pleasurable effects; that, if its evil effects were so dreadful as stated the human race would have ceased to exist. (Whelan, 1984)

In the March 14, 1857, issue of the *Lancet*, a commentary appeared that condemned tobacco for all the health problems it causes.

> Tobacco is said to act on the mind by producing inactivity thereof; inability to think; drowsiness; irritability . . . . On the respiratory organs, it acts by causing consumption, haemoptysis [coughing up blood] and inflammatory condition of the mucous membrane of the larynx, trachea and bronchae, ulceration of the larynx, short

irritable cough, hurried breathing. The circulating organs are affected by irritable circulation. (Whelan, 1984)

References: R.T. Ravenholt, *Tobacco's Global Death March, Population and Development Review*, vol. 16, no. 2 (June 1990), pp. 218–19.

Elizabeth M. Whelan, *A Smoking Gun: How the Tobacco Industry Gets Away with Murder*, Philadelphia: George F. Stuckley Co., 1984, p. 38.

Lartigue, Frank (1890–1955)

An example of a case tried during the first wave of tobacco litigation (1954–1973) was the 1963 case of *Lartigue v. R.J. Reynolds Tobacco Company*. It was argued under the theory of breach of implied warranty and negligence.

Frank Lartigue smoked at least two packs of cigarettes per day for over 40 years, from 1913 until his death. He developed cancer of the larynx, and less than three months after successful surgery he developed lung cancer. Frank's lung cancer caused his death on July 13, 1955, at the age of 65. His wife, Victoria, filed a $779,500 suit for wrongful death against R.J. REYNOLDS TOBACCO COMPANY and LIGGETT AND MYERS TOBACCO COMPANY charging that her husband's use of their tobacco products caused his death. She claimed the tobacco companies were negligent in not warning the public that use of their CIGARETTE products would cause cancer.

Two days after the case first came to trial, federal judge Herbert W. Christenberry ordered a mistrial in March 1958. It was revealed that one of Mrs. Lartigue's two lawyers had hired an investigator to gather information about the smoking habits of prospective jurors.

More than two years later, in September 1960, when the Lartigue case went to trial again, Mrs. Lartigue asked for $150,000 in damages. H. Alva Brumfield, a former Louisiana state senator, argued that the two tobacco companies killed Frank Lartigue "not by running over him with one of their trucks, but causing his death just as effectively by the use of products manufactured and sold by them." He said Liggett and Myers and Reynolds

had a responsibility, a duty, to make their products wholesome, to make their product in such a manner that it wouldn't kill people or cause them harm . . . that there was a breach and a violation of that chargeable responsibility, not only was it so unwholesome that it made Mr. Lartigue ill, it gave him the cancer of the throat . . . that these products, Camel cigarettes, Picayune cigarettes and King Bee tobacco have cancer producing substances in them. As he smoked he inhaled cancer producing substances . . . condensate known as tar. [The two companies] never gave any warning of any kind . . . that these products were unwholesome. (Wagner, 1971)

The deposition of one Lartigue expert witness, Dr. ERNST L. WYNDER, was read before the court. His experiments with mice in the 1950s showed that mice who had cigarette "tar" painted on their backs were more likely to develop malignant tumors than control mice that were not painted with tobacco tar. Dr. ALTON OCHSNER, renowned thoracic surgeon who arguably treated more cancer patients than any doctor alive and who had done extensive epidemiological research on the smoking-cancer link also testified at the trial.

R.J. Reynolds attorney Theodore Kiendl, who described Lartigue as an unhealthy man who had had many diseases in his early life and who smoked to an "absurd excess," told the jury there was no basis for monetary recovery. He said evidence produced by the tobacco companies showed that nonsmokers get lung cancer and that the overwhelming number of smokers do not get lung cancer. The defense counsel said the tobacco companies had nothing to do with starting Lartigue on his smoking habit and that the plaintiff tried to "capitalize on the death of her husband" and wasn't entitled to a single dollar.

Dr. Thomas H. Burford, professor of surgery at Washington University in St. Louis, Missouri, who trained under Dr. EVARTS GRAHAM, testified for the defense. He said he and other members of the scientific community remained unconvinced that cigarette smoking was a major cause of lung cancer. When asked by the defense attorney whether he could say with certainty that Mr. Lartigue's lung cancer was caused by cigarette smoking, he testified: "No, I cannot." He went on to testify as follows:

> My opinion is that cigarette-smoking does not cause cancer of the lung. I base this opinion upon my clinical experience and upon my observations. Dr. Evarts Graham and I, I presume, have as large a collective experience in cancer of the lung as any two surgeons in the world, and in that collective experience, we saw only two, I mean four, cancers of the structure called the trachea.
> Now, the trachea . . . has the same type of epithelial lining that the major windpipes do. This structure gets the blast of cigarette smoke coming and going, and yet, as I have said, on our large experience we only saw four cases of cancer of the trachea. (Wagner, 1971)

The 17-day trial produced 20 volumes of testimony and many medical exhibits. The jury had chemical, epidemiological, and animal studies; pathology reports; clinical observations; and testimony of renowned doctors. The trial court instructed the jury that for the tobacco company to be found negligent, it must have had some knowledge as to the inherent danger or defective condition of its cigarette. The plaintiff had the burden of proving that the manufacturer knew or should have known of the defective condition before the cancer developed. The court instructed the jury that medical knowledge obtained after the development of the plaintiff's cancer was not to be used as a measure to determine if the manufacturer should have known of product defects. Because the jury found the plaintiff did not prove that the manufacturer had knowledge of the defect of its product at the time the plaintiff developed cancer, an action for negligence could not be maintained. The jury deliberated for one hour and 40 minutes and returned with a verdict for the tobacco companies. *See also* TOBACCO LITIGATION: FIRST, SECOND, AND THIRD WAVES

References: Susan Wagner, *Cigarette Country: Tobacco in American History and Politics*, New York: Praeger Publishers, 1971, p. 111.

Lasker, Albert Davis (1880–1952)

Albert Davis Lasker was president of Lord and Thomas advertising agency in Chicago, the most powerful and famous firm in the advertising field. In 1923, Lasker began creating campaigns for American Tobacco Company's LUCKY STRIKE CIGARETTES. At first, Lasker gathered testimonials from actresses, opera singers, and sports personalities. Then, in campaigns that showed that cigarettes could be a substitute for candy, Lasker helped to make Luckies the leading cigarette in the 1920s. He also popularized open smoking for middle-class women.

In 1942, Lasker retired at the age of 62. He liquidated Lord and Thomas and sold the assets to three associates, EMERSON FOOTE, Fairfax Cone, and Don Belding who formed Foote, Cone, and Belding. Foote, named president, serviced the Lucky Strike account. *See also* AMERICAN TOBACCO COMPANY

Latin America

Tobacco is grown is a number of countries in Latin America. The number of hectares devoted to tobacco cultivation ranges from 25,000 hectares in countries such as COLOMBIA and Peru to more than 50,000 hectares in large producing countries such as ARGENTINA, BRAZIL, and CUBA. Only a few countries of Latin America have economies that are largely dependent on tobacco production. Brazil is the largest tobacco producer in Latin America, and the third largest producer of tobacco in the world, with over 700,000 hectares under cultivation.

After rapid growth in per capita tobacco consumption in Latin America during the 1960s and 1970s, a severe economic downturn in the 1980s led to a decline in tobacco consumption, which for many countries continued into the 1990s. In the late 1990s, smoking prevalence in Latin America was reported to be 37 percent for men and 20 percent for women. Studies conducted in a number of Latin American countries indicated that three-fourths of smokers started smoking between the ages of 14 and 17.

Smoking was more prevalent in urban areas, where in some cities 50 percent of youths smoked. Rural populations, especially indigenous populations, recorded relatively low smoking rates. Smoking was reported to be increasing substantially among women and more common among groups with higher income than among those with the least education and economic capability. In general, smokers in Latin America and the Caribbean smoked fewer cigarettes per day than smokers in the United States and CANADA. But because of unreported sales, illegal trade in cigarettes, and substantial duty-free sales, cigarette consumption data has been underestimated.

Multinational tobacco companies dominate the tobacco industry in most countries of Latin America. Recent socio-demographic changes have facilitated the expansion of markets for manufactured cigarettes. Before people smoked manufactured cigarettes made with blond tobacco (i.e., Virginia blend, bright tobacco, light tobacco, *tabaco rubio*), people consumed dark tobacco (i.e., black tobacco, *tabaco negro*). In most countries, particularly in South America, dark-tobacco consumption has decreased and blond tobacco has increased. Cigarettes containing blond tobacco has dominated most markets in Latin America.

The marketing and advertising of manufactured cigarettes made with blond tobacco proliferated in the 1970s and 1980s. By the early 1990s, multinational tobacco companies saturated Latin countries with tobacco product advertising and promotions. They sponsored cultural and sports events to promote product identification.

In Latin America, public awareness of the health risks of tobacco use as well as the motivation to quit was generally low. Although many countries in Latin America have enacted laws to limit smoking in public places, advertising of tobacco products, and access to tobacco by young persons, there is not enough compliance with the laws. In some cases, cigarette tax revenues were used to fund research on or interventions against smoking. In some Latin American countries,

non-governmental organizations, such as medical associations, anti-cancer associations, and churches provided leadership in policy, school-based education, and public information on tobacco-related issues.

The health consequences of smoking in Latin America and the Caribbean may not be as striking because there is not enough data to demonstrate the effects of smoking on the population's health. In 1998, studies estimated that 150,000 people die per year from tobacco-related illnesses in Latin America; by 2020, projections showed that 400,000 people would die every year. *See also* DOMINICAN REPUBLIC; PANAMA

Latrobe, Benjamin Henry (1764–1829)

English architect and civil engineer Benjamin Henry Latrobe came to the United States in 1796. He was a leading exponent of Greek Revival and, in rebuilding the Capitol after the War of 1812, he used a tobacco motif in designing the capitals for the 16 columns in the small rotunda of the north wing.

Lawsuits. *See* TOBACCO LITIGATION: FIRST, SECOND, AND THIRD WAVES

Le Moyne, Jacques (d. 1588)

Part of the French expedition to North America in 1564 headed by René de Laudonnière, Jacques Le Moyne was the earliest artist to visit the continental United States. He accompanied Laudonnière to Florida, Georgia, and the Carolinas. Le Moyne not only made dozens of watercolors of the natives, he described their life as well. One of several paintings that illustrated smoking was captioned as follows:

> They also have a plant which the Brazilians call *petun* and the Spanish *tapaco*. After carefully drying its leaves, they put them in the bowl of a pipe. They light the pipe, and, holding the other end in their mouths, they inhale the smoke so deeply that it comes out through their mouths and noses . . . . (Heimann, 1960)

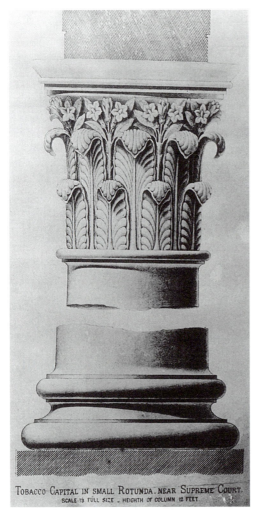

TOBACCO CAPITAL IN SMALL ROTUNDA. NEAR SUPREME COURT.
SCALE ⅓ FULL SIZE – HEIGHTH OF COLUMN 12 FEET.

Tobacco capital designed by Benjamin Latrobe for columns in the small rotunda of the U.S. Capitol, which was rebuilt after its destruction during the War of 1812. *Library of Congress.*

Le Moyne's watercolors were published by the Flemish engraver Theodore de Bry.

References: Robert K. Heimann, *Tobacco and Americans*, New York: McGraw-Hill Book Company Inc., 1960, p. 17.

LeBow, Bennett (1938–)

In 1996, financier Bennett LeBow, chairman of the BROOKE GROUP LTD. INC., of which Liggett Group is a unit, broke rank with other large tobacco companies and became the first tobacco company CEO to settle a lawsuit out of court with class-action lawyers and five states. Known for going after high-risk deals,

LeBow, a one-time computer scientist and scuba diver, has bought companies in distress, rebuilt them, and tried to sell them for a profit. Since the early 1960s, he had purchased companies that made jewelry, computers, microfilm, and planes. In 1986, LeBow bought LIGGETT AND MYERS TOBACCO COMPANY for $137 million, became the company's CEO, and changed its name to the Liggett Group. In 1990, Liggett merged with Brooke Group Ltd., also controlled by LeBow at the time.

LeBow hoped a settlement between Liggett and plaintiffs' lawyers in a group of CIGARETTE liability lawsuits would help him win the fight to control RJR and make Liggett look more desirable for sale. Marc Kasowitz, a New Yorker and LeBow's personal lawyer, believed that if LeBow were the first to settle the state cases, he could extinguish or at least significantly limit the company's financial exposure. Despite his reputation for complicated and clever financial dealings, LeBow tried but failed to engineer a merger of Liggett with a bigger player. He tried to take over RJR NABISCO HOLDINGS CORPORATION, the nation's second largest cigarette maker, so he could then have RJR buy Liggett from him. RJR's shareholders rejected LeBow's attempt to take control.

At the end of 1995, Kasowitz met DON BARRETT, one of the attorneys representing Mississippi in its tobacco litigation, while the two were on opposing sides in a class action unrelated to tobacco. With LeBow's approval, Kasowitz approached Barrett, and informal talks between the two began and led to secret meetings between the two sides in Houston, Miami, and New York City. In March 1996, LeBow settled with five states (Florida, Louisiana, Massachusetts, Mississippi, and West Virginia). Liggett neither admitted nor denied liability for tobacco-related illnesses, but LeBow agreed to pay the five states $1 million immediately, $440,000 a year over the next nine years, and 2 1/2 percent of annual pretax income over the next 25 years. He also agreed to many of the FOOD AND DRUG ADMINISTRATION's (FDA) proposals to curb youth sales of cigarettes including a ban on promotional T-shirts and other clothing, elimination of BILLBOARDS within 1,000 feet of schools, black-and-white-only ads in magazines, an end to free distribution of cigarettes at rock concerts and other youth events, plus a ban on cartoon characters. In exchange, Liggett would be freed from lawsuits filed to recover state Medicaid money spent treating sick smokers.

On March 20, 1997, one year and a week after the Liggett Group settled with the five states, LeBow signed a new and broader settlement with an additional 17 states (Arizona, Connecticut, Hawaii, Illinois, Iowa, Kansas, Maryland, Michigan, Minnesota, New Jersey, New York, Ohio, Oklahoma, Texas, Utah, Washington, and Wisconsin; California was added later) that expanded the 1996 agreement.

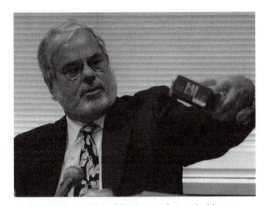

Bennett LeBow, CEO of the Ligget Group, holds a carton of his company's L&M cigarettes as he testifies before a Massachusetts Department of Public Health panel in Boston in June 1997. *AP/Wide World Photos.*

In exchange for immunity from the state Medicaid claims and from all current and future class actions and individual lawsuits, LeBow became the first tobacco CEO to declare NICOTINE is addictive and smoking causes cancer. This was also the first time a tobacco company took responsibility for tobacco-related diseases. He admitted that some tobacco marketing had been directed at teenagers as customers. He agreed to cooperate in suits against other companies. Liggett also agreed to add a warning to its cigarettes (Eve, L and M, Chesterfield, and Pyramid) that "smoking is addictive." The company agreed to pay 25 percent of its pretax profits to the

states annually over the next 25 years, and an additional $25 million if it merged with another tobacco company. In return, Liggett was removed as a defendant in 22 state Medicaid cases and in class-action lawsuits that had been or would be filed.

LeBow agreed to turn over thousands of pages of Liggett's documents considered privileged, including notes taken by Liggett lawyers at joint defense meetings with other tobacco company lawyers in the so-called Committee of Counsel. The documents, which could help anti-tobacco forces in their litigation against the rest of the tobacco industry, chronicled Liggett's research and marketing plans and confidential discussions involving the four biggest tobacco companies: PHILIP MORRIS COMPANIES, INC., R.J. REYNOLDS TOBACCO COMPANY, BROWN AND WILLIAMSON TOBACCO CORPORATION, and LORILLARD COMPANY INC. The four companies obtained a restraining order from a North Carolina state judge barring Liggett from turning over the documents. The companies claimed the proceedings of the Committee of Counsel were covered by the lawyer-client privilege. For a while, the documents were sealed.

Within a month of LeBow signing the second deal on March 20, 1997, the CEOs of Philip Morris and R.J. Reynolds began negotiations with anti-tobacco forces.

Despite tobacco producers branding him a traitor, LeBow testifed on behalf of plaintiffs in smoking-related lawsuits. He appeared as a witness for the state of Minnesota suing tobacco manufacturers for money spent treating smoking-related illnesses. At the trial, he testified that he broke rank with the tobacco industry because he didn't want to have to go to court and lie about smoking. He said he began admitting that cigarettes cause cancer and nicotine is additive because it was time someone told the truth. LeBow also said he settled in part for financial reasons, to keep his struggling company afloat. Liggett cigarette sales fell 50 percent since it added a warning label that nicotine is addictive.

LeBow released information on cigarette ingredients and additives. He also agreed to cooperate with the Justice Department's long-running criminal investigation of the tobacco industry, without a promise of immunity. LeBow agreed to provide information about industry knowledge of the health consequences of smoking cigarettes and the addictive nature of nicotine, the targeting of children and adolescents as customers, and the manipulation of nicotine levels in tobacco products. He also promised to disclose the involvement by lawyers in drafting misleading or false statements to regulators or Congress and research undertaken by the COUNCIL FOR TOBACCO RESEARCH.

In the tobacco settlement of November 1998, the attorneys general of 46 states accepted a $206-billion plan to settle state lawsuits filed against cigarette makers to recover Medicaid money spent treating diseases related to smoking. LeBow and Liggett and Myers, although not directly involved in the negotiations, agreed to join the November 1998 settlement. As a result, the company was released from earlier agreements. Liggett and Myers would not have to contribute financially to the settlement unless its sales rose 25 percent above current levels. *See also* CHESTERFIELD CIGARETTES; TOBACCO SETTLEMENT—NOVEMBER 1998

Lewis, Michael T. (1944–)

Michael T. Lewis was one of the first to have the idea to sue tobacco companies to recover monies the state spent in Medicaid bills treating poor patients for cigarette-related illnesses. He wanted to move the focus away from the personal choice of smokers. His initiative eventually led to a settlement of the MISSISSIPPI MEDICAID CASE against tobacco companies.

Lewis was a small-town lawyer who ran a personal-injury law practice with his wife Pauline in Clarksdale, Mississippi. Initially, he wanted to recoup state monies that paid for the care of his bookkeeper's mother, Jackie Thompson, who after a lifetime of smoking died from lung cancer. He called fellow University of Law School classmate MICHAEL MOORE, attorney general of Mississippi, to tell him about his idea to sue to-

bacco companies to recover state money spent in Medicaid bills for cigarette-related illness. Lewis's idea was similar to a plan of Moore's law school friend RICHARD F. SCRUGGS, an asbestos litigator who saw the potential for collecting billions of dollars in Medicaid bills incurred by countless smokers.

In June 1993, Lewis and Scruggs joined forces to help finance and litigate the state's Medicaid case. Mr. Lewis, who quietly started it all, got a cut of the lawyer's fees in the $3.4 billion settlement of the Mississippi Medicaid lawsuit.

Liggett and Myers Tobacco Company

Established in 1822 by Christopher Fouls, the Liggett and Myers Tobacco Company is the fifth largest tobacco company in the United States. It was the first cigarette maker to sign a settlement agreement with several states in 1996, the first company to acknowledge a link between smoking and cancer, and the first company to concede that tobacco products are addictive.

Liggett and Myers first manufactured SNUFF in Belleville, Illinois. In 1847, Fouls's grandson, John Edmund Liggett entered the business and when his brother William joined the firm, it was called J.E. Liggett and Brother. In 1873, George S. Myers bought William Liggett's share in the company, and the name Liggett and Myers appeared for the first time.

The company's leading brand of plug tobacco was Star. A row of small tin stars was placed across the plug so that each cut had a star attached to it. This caught the public's eye and the plug was called "tin star tobacco." By 1885, Liggett and Myers was the largest producer of plug tobacco in the world until it was absorbed into the AMERICAN TOBACCO COMPANY (ATC), a tobacco trust.

When the trust was broken up in 1911, Liggett and Myers emerged with 12 manufacturing branches and some 625 brand names, the top sellers being Star, a smoking tobacco called Duke's Mixture, and Piedmont and Fatima cigarettes. In 1912, the company introduced CHESTERFIELD CIGARETTES, one of the brands Liggett and Myers was given when the tobacco trust was dissolved. The company has also made Lark, L and M, Eve, Pyramid, and a variety of generic cigarettes.

In 1986, Liggett and Myers changed its name to Liggett Group to signal its new composition. Tobacco companies in the United States and Great Britain, recognizing that a single-product business was vulnerable to unforeseen challenges, branched out and bought up businesses of all kinds, ending their complete dependence on tobacco in general and cigarettes in particular.

In 1986, BENNETT LEBOW bought Liggett and Myers for $137 million and became the company's CEO. Two years later, using revenues from cigarettes, he paid off a substantial portion of the debt he accumulated when he bought Liggett. In 1990, Liggett merged with Brooke Group Ltd., also controlled by LeBow at the time. As the industry's smallest tobacco company with just about 2 percent of the U. S. market and pretax profits of $11 million, Liggett was barely staying alive.

In March 1996, the Liggett Group Inc., the smallest of the nation's five major tobacco companies, became the first tobacco company to settle cigarette lawsuits out of court with five states. A year later, LeBow, agreed to a broader settlement with 22 states and to turn state's evidence. As a result of the settlement, all of Liggett and Myers tobacco product lines included an additional warning statement beyond the traditional surgeon general's warning. The labels on Liggett brands declare: "Warning: Smoking Is Addictive."

In the tobacco settlement in November 1998, Liggett and Myers, although not directly involved in the negotiations, agreed to join the plan. In agreeing to the November 1998 settlement, the company was released from earlier agreements. Liggett and Myers would not have to contribute financially to the settlement unless its sales rose 25 percent above current levels.

At the end of November 1998, PHILIP MORRIS COMPANIES INC. struck a deal to buy Lark, L and M, and Chesterfield brands from the Liggett Group for $300 million. Philip Morris has owned the international rights to the three brands for about two decades.

The packs Philip Morris sells outside the United States are not required to have the addiction warning label. *See also* TOBACCO SETTLEMENT—NOVEMBER 1998

Liggett Group. *See* LEBOW, BENNETT; LIGGETT AND MYERS TOBACCO COMPANY

Lighters

During WORLD WAR I, when paper shortages made it necessary to find substitutes for matches, some friction lighters used a metal match containing a wick immersed in an inflammable fluid and struck in a serrated groove. Some munition workers and soldiers made crude types of petrol lighters with scrap materials. These first attempts helped to develop the first fully reliable lighters, which appeared after the war ended.

In 1922, the Dunhill lighter appeared, a pocket lighter that carried a substantial amount of fuel and that could be operated with one hand. Five years later, Mr. Louis V. Aronson produced the Ronson lighter operated by a thumb-piece that turned a flint wheel. When pressure was released, the flame was extinguished. Both the Dunhill and Aronson designs paved the way for lighters of countless shapes and sizes.

Litigation. *See* TOBACCO LITIGATION: FIRST, SECOND, AND THIRD WAVES

Little, Clarence Cook (1888–1971)

A geneticist and cancer specialist with a doctorate in biology from Harvard University, Clarence Cook Little was president of the University of Maine—at 34 years of age—and later at the University of Michigan. He was forced to resign from the Michigan post because his views on sterilization of "criminals and mental defectives" outraged university officials (Pringle, 1998, p. 121). Then in 1929 his friend Roscoe B. Jackson, an automobile executive, made him supervisor of a research institute Jackson funded and named the Roscoe B. Jackson Memorial Laboratory in Bar Harbor, Maine. Dr. Little's Bar Harbor laboratory became world-famous for breeding mice for laboratory experiments. Also in 1929, Little was appointed managing director of the American Society for the Control of Cancer (ASCC), renamed in 1944 the AMERICAN CANCER SOCIETY (ACS).

In 1944, the year Little was unseated as chief spokesman for the cancer society, he authored an ASCC pamphlet, "Cancer: A Study for Laymen." He wrote that although there was "no definite evidence" of the lung cancer–smoking link, "it would seem unwise to fill the lungs repeatedly with a suspension of fine particles of tobacco product . . . . It is difficult to see how such particles can be prevented from becoming lodged in the walls of the lungs and when so located how they can avoid providing a certain amount of irritation . . . (Kluger, 1996)." At the same time, during the 1940s, Dr. Little advocated his belief in the "constitutional hypothesis" that it was a person's genetic makeup, a damaged gene, for example, that was responsible for the basic cause of cancer. Even when statistical evidence grew for the link between lung cancer and smoking, he maintained genetic makeup determined whether a person developed cancer. At the end of 1953, when epidemiologist Ernst Wynder showed in his research that tobacco tars caused cancer on the shaved skin of laboratory mice (selected from Little's "mouse house"), Little said the data were not relevant to humans.

In 1954, tobacco industry chiefs chose Little for the post of scientific director of the newly founded TOBACCO INDUSTRY RESEARCH COMMITTEE.

Dr. Little, who frequently said that the tobacco-disease link was "premature," said the 18 major epidemiological studies demonstrating the link were "the opinion of a few statisticians." He also said that the problem was not tobacco, but the type of person who smokes. By 1960, many government agencies around the world had concluded that there was sufficient evidence to establish a cause-effect relationship between smoking

and lung cancer. Dr. Little rejected them all as "oversimplified and perhaps superficial conclusions . . . that concern themselves solely with suggestive or incomplete data." He claimed such studies "stifle or delay needed research to find the basic origins of lung cancer and cardiovascular diseases, which are most powerful, diversified and deadly enemies to our well-being" (Pringle, 1998, pp. 118–19). *See also* EYSENCK, HANS J.; WYNDER, ERNST

References: Richard Kluger, *Ashes to Ashes*, New York: Alfred A. Knopf, 1996, p. 142

Peter Pringle, *Cornered: Big Tobacco at the Bar of Justice*, New York: Henry Holt and Company, 1998, pp. 118–19, 121.

Lodi, California

In 1990, Lodi, a rural community in northern California, passed a landmark ordinance eliminating all smoking in restaurants. This ordinance, the first to receive national media attention, provoked the tobacco industry to develop strategies against the nonsmokers' rights movement. The tobacco industry tried and failed to repeal Lodi's ordinance by putting it on the ballot. In 1992, Lodi's 100 percent smoke-free restaurant ordinance was upheld by a state appeals court, which found the ordinance reasonable and also found "no constitutional right to engage in smoking."

Loews Corporation

Loews Corporation, headquartered in New York City, was founded in 1969. The corporation has a cigarette unit, LORILLARD COMPANY INC., that makes KENT, Newport, OLD GOLD, and True cigarette brands. Other types of businesses it owns include insurance, Loews hotels, oil and gas well drilling, and watches and clocks. Since 1959, Lawrence A. Tisch has been the chief executive officer of Loews Corporation.

London, England, Underground

In 1984, the London Underground decided to end smoking on all underground trains for a one-year trial period beginning July 9, 1984.

A study was conducted to measure the air quality before and after the end of smoking. Before smoking was ended on trains, levels of nicotine and particulates were higher in the smoking cars than in the nonsmoking cars, although all levels were below industrial safety limits. One month after the end of smoking, NICOTINE levels were lower than they had been in both smoking and nonsmoking cars, suggesting that some smoke had leaked into nonsmoking cars. The significantly elevated levels of air pollution when smoking was allowed were reduced as well.

Lonsdale. *See* CIGAR SIZE AND SHAPE

Loosies

Around the turn of the century, single cigarettes were sold in neighborhood groceries, tobacco shops, or candy stores to youngsters just starting to smoke or to cash-poor individuals. Loosies were popular among urban smokers by 1930. They went for a penny each to customers who could not afford a whole pack. "The poor man's cigarette case," an empty package of some leading brand into which loosies were placed, appeared around this time. Although the widespread use of the practice has halted, it is still possible to find loosies being sold to teenagers and adults.

Lorillard, Pierre (1742–c. 1781)

In 1760, French immigrant Pierre Lorillard set up his tobacco manufacturing business, P. Lorillard Co., the first tobacco company in the colonies. (His company later evolved into the LORILLARD COMPANY INC, making it the oldest tobacco firm in the nation.) P. Lorillard Co. was located on New York City's Chatham Street (now Park Row). Lorillard imported tobacco from Virginia growers in the form of puddings—stick-like forms of squeezed and twisted leaves wrapped in linen covers—and turned it into pipe tobacco and SNUFF. He packed snuff in bladders of slaughtered animals, dried and tanned like parchment. They were light, waterproof, and efficient as packages for bulk tobacco that he resold to wholesalers. Bladders were forerunners of the cellophane wrappers, which today protect and preserve the freshness of CIGARETTES, CIGARS, and smoking tobacco.

Lorillard's closely guarded recipes for a dozen varieties of snuff became celebrated, and competitors tried to guess their ingredients. In an old manuscript, one rival suggested that "by observing what kind of tobacco Lorillard buys at auction or at private sale, the right complexion of the leaf can be come at." Lorillard called the following recipe for black snuff "Paris Rappee," which suggests some of the exotic ingredients that went into the endless combinations designed to appeal to the taste of snuffers:

> Take a good strong virgin tobacco without stems. Cut this in pieces and make it wet in a barrel. Set it in sweet room at 100 degrees for 12 days. Make into powder, letting stand three to four months, adding 1½ pounds salmoniac, 2 pounds tamarind, 2 oz. vanilla bean, 1 oz. tonka bean, 1 oz. camomile flowers. (Fox, 1947)

Lorillard's business prospered until the American Revolution came to New York. Pierre and his young family fled from the Tory-occupied city to his parents' home outside of town, but Hessian soldiers invaded that area as well and killed Lorillard. His widow struggled to keep the business going until her two sons, Peter and George, were old enough to take over.

References: Maxwell Fox, *The Lorillard Story*, New York: The Lorillard Company, 1947, p. 19.

Lorillard Company Inc.

Now a subsidiary of LOEWS CORPORATION, the Lorillard Company evolved from the oldest tobacco company in the American colonies. After the American Revolution, PIERRE LORILLARD's sons, Pierre Lorillard II (or Peter) and George, took over the business. It was then called P. Lorillard Co., but Pierre and George renamed it P and G Lorillard. They expanded manufacturing operations between the American Revolution and the Civil War.

Following the Treaty of Paris in 1783, Pierre Lorillard built a large wooden SNUFF MILL on the banks of the Bronx River in Westchester. The mill got waterpower from the Bronx River to turn its wheels. Over the years, workmen's cottages, a warehouse, facilities for packing smoking tobacco, and the Lorillard family mansion were added. The original wooden mill was replaced in 1840 by a stone structure, which is still standing in the Bronx Botanical Gardens. This landmark mill in tobacco history was dedicated in 1954 as a monument to the nation's oldest tobacco company.

On May 27, 1789, Lorillard's sons published the first known American advertisement for tobacco. It showed an American Indian smoking a long clay pipe while leaning against a HOGSHEAD marked "Best Virginia." The American Indian man recommends Lorillard products ranging from cut tobacco plug and SNUFF to ladies' twist (strips of tobacco leaves woven together). Since the American Indians were the first to grow and smoke tobacco, and P. Lorillard the first tobacco company to sell it, the early brand names manufactured by the Lorillards were American Indian in origin. The Lorillard trademark depicts two American Indians beneath the inscription "Established 1760."

In 1860, in honor of its 100th anniversary, Lorillard brought out its Century brand, a fine-cut tobacco. Into one package of each day's production, the company put $100 in currency or a combination of bills totaling $100. The distribution of money with the tobacco kept up for about a year and lured customers to buy Lorillard's tobacco until the practice was curtailed as being too similar to a lottery.

After George died in 1832 and Pierre in 1843, the business, producing chewing and smoking tobacco at the time, was carried on by Pierre III, who returned to the old business name of P. Lorillard. In 1860, Pierre IV was admitted to the firm.

As snuff was superseded by CHEWING TO-BACCO, the Lorillard company shifted its emphasis from the snuff mill to a new giant factory located in Jersey City. There the company got a head start in the era of mass-produced national brands, which began after the Civil War. During the late 1870s, the huge Jersey City plant made nearly 10 percent of all manufactured tobacco in the United States.

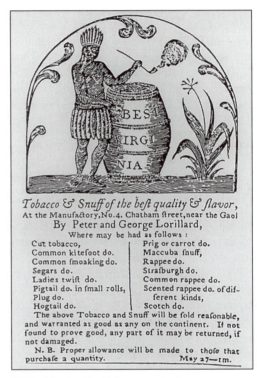

1789 ad for Lorillard tobacco products.

In 1885, *Leslie's Weekly,* one of the country's outstanding magazines, carried a story about Lorillard and the way the company operated. Readers learned that the Jersey City factories covered five acres and included a 15,000-volume library and 350-child schoolroom "for the free use of the army of about four thousand persons employed in their immense tobacco establishment" (Fox, 1947). The company published a house magazine for employees and customers. In the 1880s, the magazine was called *Puffs of Wisdom.* Decorated with woodcuts that advertised Lorillard brands, the text told facts about the company, such as the number of Lorillard customers (five million), as well as offering homely wisdom and etiquette tips.

During the postbellum years, Lorillard's line reflected the trend in smoking tobaccos as well as the increase in plug. By 1894, the Lorillard firm was producing 20 million pounds of plug tobacco a year. One of the brands was called Tin Tag, the first Lorillard plug to wear a novel identification. The company branded each of its plugs with a distinctive tin tag that it developed around 1870 when imitators put up plug tobacco in packages that looked like Lorillard's at bargain prices. At that time, the company sent out warnings that it had patented the tin tag for tobacco plugs. Anyone caught selling a non-Lorillard plug tagged with tin would be punished by the law. The metal tags, stuck into the tobacco by two pronged edges, stopped the widespread frauds. The tags were stamped in all kinds of designs and colors. In 1885, when Lorillard brought suit for infringement of patent, the court ruled that tin tags were not patentable.

Lorillard briefly made CIGARS when they replaced plug in popularity, but abandoned them to focus on CIGARETTES. Lorillard cigarettes started using TURKISH TOBACCO, so brand names like Egyptian Deities, Gods of the Nile, Harem Beauties, Helmar, MURAD, and Turkish Trophies appeared on the market.

Between 1898 and 1911, Lorillard was part of the tobacco combination. When the trust was dissolved, the company emerged without its snuff brands, but received the rights to 38 brands of cut plug and 29 brands of little cigars. It also got back 15 brands of scrap tobacco, 20 brands of plug tobacco, 8 brands of granulated tobacco, 56 brands of fine cut, and 5 brands of Virginia cigarettes of the Anargyros plant in New York City—Mogul, Murad, Helmar, Egyptian Deities, and Turkish Trophies.

In 1926, Lorillard introduced Old Golds, a blended cigarette that became the foundation of the company. "A Voice from the Sky" was one of the innovations used in 1927 to advertise the new cigarette. The company outfitted a Fokker airplane, the exact duplicate of the plane that carried Commander Richard Evelyn Byrd to the North Pole, with a loud speaker, piano, and microphones and flew it over New York broadcasting songs and commercials for OLD GOLD CIGARETTES. Before the plane left New York to visit 26 other cities in the nation, it flew up and down Broadway broadcasting the story of Old Golds.

Cartoon strip advertising was another Old Gold "first." The strips for Old Golds were by Clare Briggs, a world-famous cartoonist, and appeared across the country in 1,500 newspapers. With the advent of television, the famous Old Gold Dancing Pack became one of the outstanding commercials.

In the early 1950s, FILTERED CIGARETTES appeared on the scene. Lorillard, taking note of the growing trend in Switzerland and elsewhere towards filtered cigarettes, launched the Kent micronite filtered cigarette in March 1952, named for Lorillard executive Herbert A. Kent.

Since 1961, Alexander Spears, the chief executive officer of Lorillard, has been in different executive positions with Loews Corporation and then Lorillard. *See also* KENT CIGARETTES

References: Maxwell Fox, *The Lorillard Story*, New York: The Lorillard Company, 1947, p. 43.

Lucky Strike Cigarettes

About 1916, the AMERICAN TOBACCO COMPANY (ATC) introduced Lucky Strike cigarettes, an old brand name used on plug-cut CHEWING TOBACCO in 1856, the era of the California gold rush and Colorado silver strike. In 1871, it was introduced as a pipe tobacco. Its first advertising campaign showed a piece of toast with a fork through it. Ad copy said: "Lucky Strike, It's Toasted." A specially designed package with a bull's eye circle was created, and this initiated one of the most expensive and successful sales campaigns in the history of merchandising.

In 1928, GEORGE WASHINGTON HILL, president of the American Tobacco Company; advertising executive ALBERT LASKER; and public relations counselor EDWARD L. BERNAYS launched the campaign "Reach for a Lucky Instead of a Sweet." It was one of the most successful and profitable themes in the history of advertising, which increased profits of the American Tobacco Company from $21 million in 1925 to $46 million in 1931. The ad suggested to women that CIGARETTE smoking would help them slim down by showing fit and trim young women with shadows of double chins and fat bodies in the background. One story goes that the ad evolved from a chance moment when Hill saw two women, one slender and smoking a cigarette, the other stout and eating a big piece of candy. Noticing the contrast, Hill figured the stout woman should have been smoking instead of eating sugar. Furious candy companies sent out literature praising candy and condemning cigarettes. Hill shot back with literature saying sugar undermined the nation's health. The FEDERAL TRADE COMMISSION (FTC) ended the war of words by telling tobacco companies not to sell cigarettes as weight-reducing devices.

In the 1930s, women were not attracted to the forest green *Lucky Strike* packages. Surveys showed that the color green clashed with women's wardrobes. Since George Washington Hill had already spent millions of dollars to advertise the green package, he turned over the problem to Edward L. Bernays, a master at influencing public opinion. He developed a strategy to make green the fashion color of the 1934 season. Within six months, he made green the hot new color. Lucky Strikes sales did not climb, nor did they drop, during the Depression years.

During WORLD WAR II, Lucky Strike's green color made news again; but this time green was out. Cigarette ads pronounced: "Lucky Strike Green has gone to war!" According to the American Tobacco Company, war shortages of copper and chromium made it difficult for the American Tobacco Company to get the dyes for its gold and green Lucky Strike package. The tobacco company adopted its white package, patriotic slogan, and reported that it saved enough copper to provide bronze for 400 light tanks. There never was a shortage of green pigment. Critics believed the war was used as a cover-up to switch the unpopular green color to white because women simply didn't like the color.

Lynchburg, Virginia

Lynchburg, Virginia, a small town in the Blue Ridge foothills known as "The Tobacco City," became a tobacco center of first rank after 1840. A picturesque trumpeter summoned buyers to the leaf markets, or "breaks," so called because HOGSHEADS were opened for inspection so purchasers could sample the leaf on which they based their bids. The leaf markets were also in the middle of the tobacco fields as an experiment with the loose-leaf type of selling.

Lynchburg was comparable to RICHMOND, VIRGINIA, and Danville, Virginia, in antebellum importance because it turned out notable smoking tobaccos. Although it had 40 plug and twist factories, almost as many as Richmond, outside Lynchburg there were few firms devoted solely to smoking mixtures. Manufacturers like Maurice Moore, who started from scratch, concentrated on producing granulated tobacco for pipe smoking and captured half the market by the outbreak of the Civil War. Another manufacturer of pipe tobacco, John W. Carroll, prospered with his product, "Lone Jack."

M

Maccabee, Paul (1955–)

In the spring of 1991, Minneapolis-St. Paul, Minnesota, *Reader* reporter Paul Maccabee added a list of jazz greats who died of lung cancer to an article he wrote about BROWN AND WILLIAMSON TOBACCO CORPORATION's annual Kool Jazz festival. He was fired the next day. Mark Hopp, publisher of the 100,000-circulation *Reader* felt Maccabee had editorialized too much and he conceded that he feared losing the paper's cigarette ads because of the article. The paper's national sales manager wrote to all its cigarette advertisers apologizing for the story and informing them that Mr. Maccabee had been fired.

Machen, Arthur (1881–1937)

English novelist and essayist Arthur Machen wrote *The Anatomy of Tobacco* in 1884. In this excerpt, he extolled PIPE smoking:

> Firstly, it is good to smoke one pipe, and one only, before breakfast, at which time the body being empty of food is most amenable to the nicotinic energy. Secondly, fail not to smoke three pipes at the least immediately after breakfast. And these should be performed in the open air, and if it is possible, while sauntering about a fair garden or pleasaunce, off which the dew has not yet gone, and odorous with the scents of flowers. Thirdly, in the afternoon smoke not less than three pipes, but not immediately after eating lest they breed heaviness

> and black choler. Fourthly, and lastly, in the evening, and far into the night, when hanging over your books, smoke as many pipes as possible, at the least not less than four. This I propound not as a maximum but a minimum, and necessary to be discharged by all. For any one who smokes less than eleven pipes per diem is not so much to be accounted a smoker as one who smoketh. And if at any time the student should feel his mouth to be, as it were, cloyed and brackish with much smoking, let him by all means pause for while, and drink a strong decoction of tea without either sugar or milk. For nothing is more recuperative and invigorant than this same black tea, and altogether a drink mightily to be commended. And thus in constant smoking and meditation passeth the life of the Pipe Philosopher. (Infante, 1985)

References: G. Cabera Infante, *Holy Smoke*, London: Faber and Faber, 1985, p. 260.

Maddox, Roland (1930–1997)

On June 10, 1998, a state court jury awarded the family of Roland Maddox $500,000 in compensatory damages and $450,000 in punitive damages as well as $52,249 to Blue Cross and Blue Shield as repayment for Maddox's medical expenses. This was the third time a jury awarded damages in a tobacco liability case.

After smoking two packs of cigarettes a day for almost 50 years, grocery store owner Roland Maddox quit in 1995. He was diagnosed with lung cancer in 1996 and died in 1997. His family sued BROWN AND WILLIAMSON TOBACCO CORPORATION, arguing that the company was negligent, made a defective product, and conspired with other tobacco companies to hide the health risks of smoking from the public.

NORWOOD "WOODY" WILNER represented the Maddox family. In August 1996, he won $750,000 in compensatory damages for ex-smoker GRADY CARTER, also against Brown and Williamson, but it was overturned on appeal.

Two months after the verdict, the First District Court of Appeals in Tallahassee, Florida, ruled that the trial should have been moved to another city where the relatives of Roland Maddox lived, but it did not formally set aside the June 10 verdict. The trial took place in Jacksonville where Wilner had law offices. Brown and Williamson petitioned the court to set aside the verdict, and on January 29, 1999, the appeals court threw out the landmark $1 million jury verdict against the tobacco company, clarifying its earlier ruling that the suit had been tried in the wrong county. *See also* CIPOLLONE, ROSE; TOBACCO LITIGATION: FIRST, SECOND, AND THIRD WAVES

Mainstream Smoke

The portion of smoke pulled into the smoker's lungs from the butt end of the burning CIGA-RETTE is known as mainstream smoke. Before it is lit, the unburned cigarette is composed of many organic materials: (tobacco leaves, paper products, sugars, and NICOTINE) and inorganic materials (water, radioactive elements, and metals). When tobacco is lit and burns, more than 4,000 known compounds are created or transferred into the ash or smoke. The following list of the chemicals smokers take in from mainstream smoke is excerpted from the 1992 EPA report *Respiratory Health Affects of Passive Smoking: Lung Cancer and Other Disorders*:

- Carbon monoxide [auto exhaust poison]
- Carbon dioxide
- Benzene*
- Toluene [industrial solvent; in explo-

sives]
- Formaldehyde ** [embalming fluid]
- Acrolein [aquatic herbicide]
- Acetone [poisonous solvent]
- Pyridine [poisonous solvent]
- 3-Methylpyridine [insecticide solvent]
- Hydrogen cyanide [rat/insect poison]
- Hydrazine [rocket fuel chemical]
- Ammonia [poisonous gas, cleaning agent]
- Methylamine [tanning agent]
- Dimethylamine [tanning accelerator]
- N-Nitrosopyrrolidine**
- Formic acid [caustic solvent]
- Acetic acid [caustic solvent]
- Methyl chloride [poisonous refrigerant]
- Nicotine [insecticide]
- Phenol [toilet disinfectant]
- Catechol [tanning, dyeing agent]
- Hydroquinone [photographic developing agent]
- Aniline** [industrial solvent]
- 2-Toluidine [agent in dye manufacture]
- 2-Napthylamine*
- 4-Aminobiphenyl*
- Ben[a]anthracene***
- Benzo[a]pyrene**
- Cholesterol
- y-Butyrolactone***
- Quinoline [specimen preservative]
- Cadmium**
- Nickel*
- Zinc [anti-corrosion coating for metals]
- Polonium-210* [eadioactive element]
- Benzoic acid [tobacco curing agent]
- Lactic acid [caustic solvent]
- Glycolic acid [metal cleaning agent]
- Succinic acid [agent in lacquer manufacture]
- PCDDs and PCDFs (dioxins, dubenzofurns)

---

* Known Human Carcinogen
** Probable Human Carcinogen
*** Animal Carcinogen

The activity of these chemical substances, many of which initiate and promote cancer, was confirmed in the 1950s as a result of laboratory tests on animals conducted in Scandanavia, Germany, France, Great Britain, and the United States. *See also* ENVIRONMENTAL TOBACCO SMOKE (ETS); SECONDHAND SMOKE; SIDESTREAM SMOKE

Mann, Thomas (1875–1955)

In the 1924 novel *Magic Mountain* by Thomas Mann, the character Hans Castorp has the following to say about smoking cigarettes:

> I never can understand how anybody can *not* smoke—it deprives a man of the best part of life, so to speak—or at least of a first-class pleasure. When I wake in the morning, I feel glad at the thought of being able to smoke all day, and when I eat, I look forward to smoking afterwards; I might also say I only eat for the sake of being able to smoke—though of course that is more or less of an exaggeration. But a day without tobacco would be flat, stale and unprofitable, as far as I am concerned. If I had to say to myself to-morrow: "No smoke to-day"—I believe I shouldn't find the courage to get up—on my honour, I'd stop in bed. But when a man has a good cigar in his mouth—of course it musn't have a side draught or not draw well, that

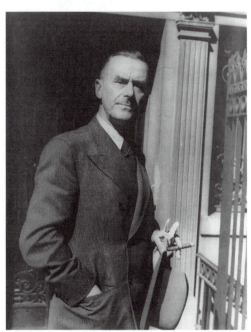

Author Thomas Mann holding a cigar. *Library of Congress.*

is extremely irritating—but with a good cigar in his mouth a man is perfectly safe, nothing can touch him—literally. It's just like lying on the beach: when you lie on the beach, why, you lie on the beach, don't you? You don't require anything else, in the line of work or amusement either. People smoke all over the world, thank goodness; there is nowhere one could get to, so far as I know where the habit hasn't penetrated. Even polar expeditions fit themselves out with supplies of tobacco to help them carry on. I always felt a thrill of sympathy when I read that. You can be very miserable: I might be feeling perfectly wretched, for instance; but I could always stand it if I had my smoke.

Marlboro Cigarettes

In 1924, PHILIP MORRIS USA introduced Marlboro cigarettes with its "Mild as May" slogan. Originally aimed at women, they were available with a red "fashion" tip designed to blend in with a smoker's lipstick. In 1954, Philip Morris reintroduced Marlboro with a filter tip.

Philip Morris hired Leo Burnett, an advertising genius in Chicago, who turned Marlboro from what he called a "sissy" CIGARETTE into a cigarette that appealed more to men. A designer named Frank Gianninoto created a new package design, much like the Campbell's soup can—red on top, white on the bottom. He changed the package Marlboro had used for the past 30 years to cardboard with a flip-top box. When Burnett wanted a tougher image for the new Marlboro ads, he decided on cowboys and hired real ones to be models. By 1975, Marlboro cigarettes were the number one selling brand in the United States and, in the 1990s, the number-one brand in the world. *See also* MARLBORO MAN

Marlboro Man

In January 1955, the cowboy Marlboro Man appeared for the first time in ads. For a time, however, the ad agency included the Marlboro Man in a mix of other rugged individualists including skin divers, football play-

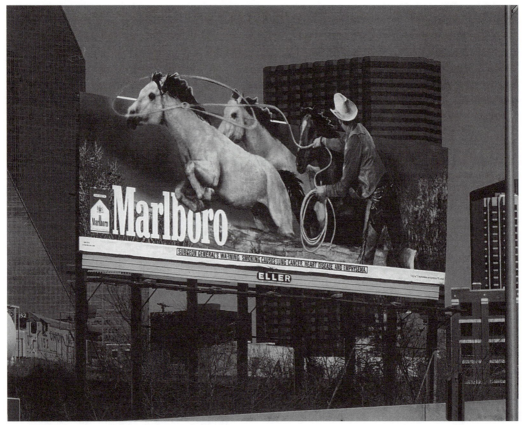

This Marlboro tobacco billboard depicting the Marlboro Man was photographed in downtown Dallas, Texas, in February 1998, only months before all tobacco advertising was to disappear from Texas billboards as part of the state's historic settlement with the tobacco industry. *AP/Wide World Photos.*

ers, military officers, pilots, and race-car drivers, all of whom wore tattoos.

In 1963, Philip Morris decided to concentrate on the cowboy as the only Marlboro Man. By that time, research showed that smokers liked the cowboy image the best. The advertising agency hired real cowboys, not models, to appear in televised and magazine ads. Then, the company created its "Come to where the flavor is. Come to Marlboro Country" theme. *See also* MARLBORO CIGARETTES

Marquette, Jacques (1637–1675)

Jesuit missionary and explorer Father Jacques Marquette accompanied Louis Jolliet in 1673 on a voyage down the Wisconsin and Mississippi Rivers, to the mouth of the Arkansas River and back to Lake Michigan via the Illinois River. In the journal he kept that was published in 1681, he observed the many ritual and ceremonial uses of pipes by the Illinois Indians.

[T]he Indians, having recognized them as Europeans, sent four old men to speak with them. Two of them carried pipes to smoke tobacco in; they were highly ornamented and adorned with feathers of different sorts. They walked solemnly and raised their pipes toward the sun; they appeared to present it to him to smoke . . . . The Father, reassured by this ceremony, spoke first to them and asked who they were; to which they answered they were Illinois, and to guarantee peace they presented their pipes to smoke . . . . One should not refuse the pipe unless we would be taken for an enemy, but it is enough to make out he is smoking. It is sufficient if one carries the calumet with him to show it, by which means he may walk in safety among enemies who, in the midst of fighting, will lower their arms to one who shows it . . . . There is a calumet for peace and one for war. They use them to end their differences, for strengthening alliances, and to communicate with strangers. [The] calumet dance . . . is not performed except on serious occasions; sometimes for making peace, or to reunite them for a great war, or for public rejoicing; sometimes for a nation's assistance; at times they use it at the reception of a person of considerable importance . . . . (Seig, 1971)

See also NATIVE AMERICANS; PIPE; PIPE SMOKING AND NATIVE AMERICANS

References: Louis Seig, *Tobacco Peace Pipes, and Indians*, Palmer Lake Co., Filter Press, 1971, p. 16.

Marsee, Sean (1965–1984)

On February 25, 1984, Sean Marsee, a 19-year-old Talihina, Oklahoma, high school track star, died from mouth cancer. Sean lifted weights, watched his diet, didn't drink, didn't smoke, and ran five miles a day six months of the year. A winner of 28 medals for running anchor leg on the 400-meter mile relay, he was voted Talihina High's outstanding athlete for 1983.

Since 1977, when he was 12 years old, Sean had been dipping SNUFF. A tobacco company had handed him free samples at a rodeo near his home. Snuff had no warning labels, and sports figures Sean admired promoted it on television. Five years later, Sean developed cancer of the mouth. In 1983, part of Sean's tongue was removed. During his second operation, he had radical neck surgery. His third operation cost him his jawbone. But none of the operations stopped the cancer from spreading. Before he died, a friend asked Sean if he would like to share something about his ordeal with young athletes. He penciled (he could no longer speak) "Don't dip snuff."

A year after Sean died, his mother filed a suit against the UNITED STATES TOBACCO COMPANY (UST), manufacturer of Copenhagen Snuff, the brand Sean used. She asked for

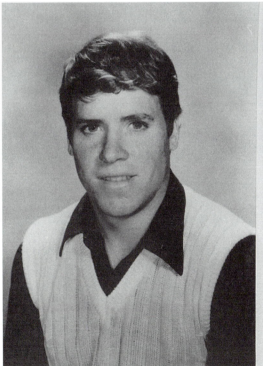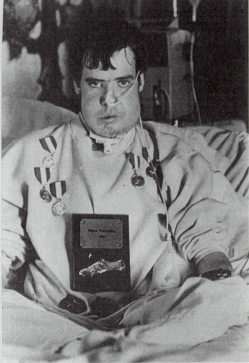

Sean Marsee before and after he developed oral cancer. His mother unsuccessfully sued the U.S. Tobacco Company, claiming that his death was caused by his use of snuff manufactured by the company. *AP/Wide World Photos.*

millions in punitive damages. Expert medical testimony linked SMOKELESS TOBACCO with oral cancer. The tobacco company that said there was no evidence proving its products caused cancer. The jury agreed with the tobacco company.

Before Sean died, he told his mother that smokeless tobacco "should carry a warning similar to that now required on cigarette packages and advertisements." In 1986, two years after Sean Marsee died, the U.S. Congress passed a law requiring the rotation of three warning labels on smokeless tobacco products and advertisements. The law also stopped the advertising of smokeless tobacco on TV and radio. The Smokeless Tobacco Council supported the legislation. Smokeless tobacco companies now claim that users are adequately warned and are responsible for any harmful effects they suffer from using their product.

The details of Sean's illness were presented in *Big Dipper,* an award-winning videotape. The videotape, narrated by teenagers, also includes interviews with teens who chew and users who have contracted cancer, as well as discussions with medical and dental experts. *Big Dipper* also explores advertising, peer pressure, and the history of snuff. *See also* HEALTH WARNINGS ON CIGARETTE PACKS AND ADVERTISEMENTS AND SMOKELESS TOBACCO; *MARSEE V. UNITED STATES TOBACCO COMPANY*

Marsee v. United States Tobacco Company

In June 1986, the UNITED STATES TOBACCO COMPANY (UST), the nation's largest manufacturer of SMOKELESS TOBACCO, won a trial in a suit brought against it in 1984 by Betty Marsee. Called a "classic David and Goliath story," reporters for several newspapers, wire services, financial analysts, and attorneys for cigarette companies closely followed the case.

UST joined the elite Fortune 500 group in 1985 when it was listed as the 476th largest industrial corporation in the U.S. The company manufactures Copenhagen and Skoal, the world's best-selling brands of SNUFF. The snuff business began to boom in the 1970s, especially among young people who turned to it as a safe alternative to CIGARETTES, oblivious to its dangers.

Betty Marsee, Sean Marsee's mother, came from a small town family that migrated from Ohio to the Dakotas to Talihina, Oklahoma. Her husband died of a heart attack in 1982. In 1984, at the age of 19, her son died of oral cancer at home. After he died, Betty Marsee, a registered nurse, sued the UST of Greenwich, Connecticut, which makes Copenhagen, the snuff Sean used, claiming damages of $147 million.

In her complaint filed on March 21, 1985, with the U.S. District Court in Oklahoma City, she said the company knew that its tobacco could cause cancer and that it had purposely concealed that knowledge. The case began shortly after Sean's death. George and Dania Braly, Betty Marsee's husband-and-wife team of lawyers, alleged that UST had failed to warn SEAN MARSEE of the deadly danger of its tobacco and that the law required the company be held strictly liable for the resulting injuries. The lawyers asked for punitive damages because of the "willful, wanton, or reckless disregard for the safety of the deceased and the public in general." The punitive damages requested were $136.54 million, UST's net earnings for 1983. "Such punitive damages are sought for the purposes of punishment, to set an example, and to deter other manufacturers from similar conduct" (Kluger, 1996). *Marsee v. United States Tobacco Company* was the first tobacco case in which the issue of punitive damages was allowed to go to the jury.

The Bralys went to court twice to ask federal district court judge David Russell for the western district of Oklahoma to order the tobacco company to answer more fully. The company delayed handing over subpoenaed documents from its files. Two days before the trial began, the company delivered to the Bralys 80,000 documents.

During the proceedings, UST officials noted that they had not looked into the dangers of nitrosamines, a likely carcinogen formed by nitrogen oxides and nitrogen bases, until 1984; Dr. Richard Manning, UST's vice president in charge of research, claimed not to know what a carcinogen was or the meanings of the words "safety" and "danger" in the context of how tobacco might relate to health. The former chief executive of UST remarked, "I am not aware that anyone has said that snuff causes cancer" (Kluger, 1996).

The lawyers for the defense presented a week's worth of medical experts, two of whom were doctors. They argued that the cause of tongue cancer in young people was not yet known; that it was an extremely rare and obscure disease.

The jury, composed of four women and two men and three alternates, was not convinced that Sean Marsee had died from using snuff and decided UST's Copenhagen snuff did not cause the cancer that killed him.

Resources: Richard Kluger, *Ashes to Ashes*, New York: Alfred A. Knopf, 1996, p. 564.

Marshall, Thomas Riley (1854–1925)

Vice president of the United States during the administration of Woodrow Wilson, Thomas Riley Marshall was a noted CIGAR smoker. Once while presiding over the Senate, and listening to a Republican senator ramble on about the country's needs, he uttered the now-famous remark "What this country needs is a really good 5¢ cigar" (Conrad, 1996).

Marshall's remark contained an economic truth. Cigar manufacturers knew only a 5¢ cigar could compete in the mass market with CIGARETTES.

References: Barnaby Conrad III, *The Cigar*, San Francisco: Chronicle Books, 1996, p. 38, 40.

Matches

Matches were known long before the end of the nineteenth century. The Greeks and Romans used tapers tipped with sulfur and animal fats that, if temperature and humidity were correct, could be ignited by friction. In the early seventeenth century, "tinder pistols," using flints and gunpowder, appeared in France. These contraptions required time and skill, otherwise explosions occurred.

After phosphorus was discovered accidentally in 1670, the word "match" (from the French *mèche*—a wick) referred to a prepared length of wick that would burn sufficiently and steadily to fire a cannon or flintlock gun. In the late eighteenth century, French inventors came up with "phosphoric candles" consisting of phosphorus-soaked paper sealed in a glass tube. When the tube was crushed, the paper would burst into flame. By 1800, "pocket luminaries" were introduced into London. These bottles lined with phosphorous oxide were kept tightly sealed until fire was needed. When the bottle was opened, a sulfur-tipped wooden match was rubbed against the interior and then quickly removed. If done correctly, when the match made contact with air, a flame was produced. If not, the bottle exploded, and a person suffered first-degree burns. Various matches prepared with phosphorus were tried out in the first decades of the nineteenth century, and in 1823 the "Dobereiner Lamp" appeared. This device generated hydrogen gas so that it impinged upon a small quantity of platinum; through chemical action the platinum became incandescent and ignited the gas.

Despite these attempts at match making, nothing more practical surpassed the tinderbox until about 1827 when John Walker, an English chemist and apothecary, created a match called a "Congreves." It was a wooden match dipped into a mixture of potassium chlorate, antimony sulfide, gum arabic, and water. When a fire was required, the matches were rubbed between sheets of sandpaper for friction heat, then withdrawn sharply, causing them to ignite. The Congreves was explosive in nature and unpredictably dangerous to handle.

Another chemist-apothecary, Samuel Jones, obtained a patent for the "Lucifer Match" in 1829, but the inventor worried that the gas that escaped from the match could cause harm to delicate lungs. These early attempts at phosphoric matches were dangerous because, on occasion, they lit too readily and the white phosphorous caused serious disease among the workers who made them.

These matches were followed by "Fuzees," especially designed for lighting pipes and cigars, "Vestas," with a stem of long-burning wax taper, and "Vesuvians." By the middle of the century, a harmless red form of phosphorous was discovered. It was incorporated into Safety Matches in which the rubbing surface was on the side of the box, not on the match head. "Strike Anywhere Matches" used a dangerous yellow phosphorus later forbidden by law. In 1898 a substitute was found so that matches like "Vestas" or "Safety" were rendered harmless and could be struck on any rough surface.

In the United States, inventors developed matchbooks rather than wooden matches. In 1836, Alonzo Dwight Phillips, a Massachusetts powder maker, patented a phosphorus match. It contained white phosphorus and sulfur, both dangerous unless used correctly.

In the post–Civil War era, matches were big business, and in 1881 a "match trust" was organized. Several manufacturers united to form Diamond Match Company, which immediately dominated the field. Diamond showed little interest in developing safe matches, although in 1882 it came out with a "drunkard's match," a splint that self-extinguished at midpoint.

In 1892, JOSHUA PUSEY, a Lima, Pennsylvania, lawyer announced his invention of matchbooks containing cardboard matches. The invention failed technologically because the striking surface was on the inside and the sparks created by the friction often ignited the remaining matches. Pusey sold his invention to Diamond in 1895. Henry C. Traute, a company salesman easily solved the problem by placing the striking surface on the outside to prevent flare-ups. Diamond's chemists also came up with a new formula that was far less toxic than phosphorus, and in making the flame less dangerous they placed more of the chemicals on the striking surface and less on the match itself. By 1912, the truly safe match was everywhere.

The invention of safe, inexpensive matches packed into small matchbooks and often given away free with the purchase of a pack of cigarettes meant that smokers could easily

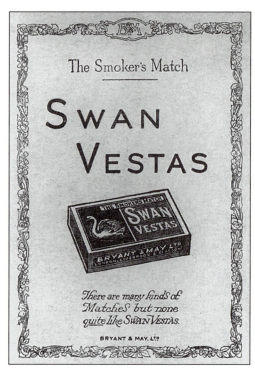

Box of Swan Vesta matches.

light up any time, any place, in all kinds of weather. Indeed, matches encouraged the consumption of more cigarettes. None of this was as important to cigar smokers who were accustomed to smoking indoors, protected from winds that carried away the smoke's aroma.

Matchbooks also became advertising vehicles. The earliest known commercial advertising on matchbooks was created in 1895 and distributed by the Mendelson Opera Company. The ad read "A cyclone of fun—powerful cast—pretty girls—handsome wardrobe—get seats early." The opera company purchased several boxes of blank matchbooks from Diamond Match and cast members pasted photos of the star of the company onto the cover.

Traute, who was promoted to vice president at Diamond, marketed matchbooks to Pabst Brewery, JAMES BUCHANAN DUKE's tobacco empire, and William Wrigley's chewing gum company. Soon businesses, large and small, and services advertised their products on the covers. Advertisers used matchbook covers to promote airlines, banks, beer, cigars and cigarettes, gas stations, hotels, movies, radio stars, restaurants, and soft drinks.

Through the 1920s, matchbooks earned money for every aspect of the industry. Thousands of advertisers used matchbooks, which had become the most popular form of advertising in the United States. When the Depression came in the 1930s, advertising budgets of businesses, services, and product manufacturers tightened and large production matchbook orders dwindled. Diamond Match saved the industry by producing and selling matches to the public for a penny. The matchbook covers, the smallest BILLBOARDS in the world, were printed with national celebrities like movie stars and sports figures. The sets continued until the late 1930s, and during WORLD WAR II matchbook companies produced matches for the U.S. military with patriotic and military advertising. After the Office of Price Administration (OPA) insisted that a free book of matches accompany every pack of cigarettes, free matchbooks became a mainstay. They were so much a part of every cigarette purchase that the OPA saw this practice as mandatory and regulations ensured continued free matchbooks with cigarette and cigar purchases. After the war, match production grew steadily until threats of disease from cigarette smoking became widely known and impacted the match industry, leading to a commercial decline of matchbook sales.

Despite the decline of matchbook sales, matchbook collecting is alive and well in the United States and rivals stamp collecting in popularity. Although once pegged to cigarette smoking, match-cover collecting has separated itself from that habit. *See also* CIGAR; CIGARETTE; LIGHTERS

Mather, Cotton (1663–1728)

American congregational clergyman Cotton Mather wrote the following about tobacco:

Taking the Use of TOBACCO under Consideration . . . . O! Had the *Religion* of our SAVIOUR near so many Disciples, as a silly and nasty *Custome,* in which so many Pro-

fessors of *His Religion,* have *Learnt the Way of the Heathen!* . . . . Tis a most *Vile Abuse* of Tobacco, for People by the *Daily Smoking* thereof, to Hurt themselves, and throw away their *Precious Hours,* and make a *Chimney, or a* Dunghil, *of the* brain, where the *Soul* should have a most Noble Habitation . . . .

III. I must and will insist upon it; That a *Slavery* to the *Custome of Smoking Tobacco,* is a Thing, by no means Consistent with the Dignity of a *Rational Creature;* and much less, of a *Vertuous Christian* . . . .

IV. If it were to be wish'd, That many who Should *know Better,* and particularly, the *Ministers* of the Gospel; were less *Excessive* this Way, than too many of them are . . . . Lett not your *Smoke* so blind your Eyes, as to hinder your discerning, *Whether it be not become a Lust that are you Serving of?* . . . .

X. I don't Suppose, that many Captives of the Pipe, will Easily Emancipate themselves; Lett 'em not Reform *All at once,* but leave off by *Degrees* . . . .

Parents, Tutors, Teachers of all sorts; Advise your children against it. Young, Be not rashly drawn into it. *My son, Be wise for thyslf. And, if thy Entice thee, Consent thou not* . . . .

Away with it! If you would act like People of Reason; *Away with it!* Yea, If you Love your lives. *Away with it!* (Jones, 1972)

References: Gordon W. Jones, ed. *The Angel of Bethesda: An Essay upon the Common Maladies of Mankind,* Barre, MA: American Antiquarian Society & Barre Publishers, 1972, pp. 301-11.

Maxim, Hudson (1853–1927)

Explosives expert Hudson Maxim, who invented the highly explosive maximite, a smokeless powder, predicted the effects of smoking when he said: "cigarette smoking will be responsible for a larger number of deaths than the poisonous gases of the Germans . . . because while the German gases affect the body, they do not, like the cigarette, impair the mind" (Gehman, 1943).

References: Dr. Jesse Mercer Gehman, *Smoke Over America,* Patterson, NJ: Beoma Publication House, 1943, p. 21.

Maximilian, Alexander Philip (1782–1867)

Prince Alexander Philip Maximilian of Wied was a naturalist, an anthropologist, and an explorer. He went on an expedition in 1832 to explore North America with the Swiss artist Karl Bodmer; they made their way to present-day North Dakota. Maximilian kept a journal of his travels and made an extensive study of the Northern Plains people, especially the Mandans, with whom he and Bodmer spent the winter of 1833–1834. He wrote at length about the Mandans' tribal life and reported thoroughly on their use of tobacco and pipes.

> Their pipes are made of the red-stone, or of black clay. They obtain the red pipe-heads, chiefly from the Sioux; sometimes they have wooden heads lined with stone; the tube is plain, long, round or flat, on the whole, of the same shape as among the Sioux, but they are not so fastidious about ornamenting their pipes as other tribes. They smoke the leaves of the tobacco plant, which is cultivated by them; the bark of the red willow (*Cornus sericea*), which they obtain from the traders, is sometimes mixed with the tobacco, or the latter with the leaves of the bearberry (*Arbutus uva ursi*). The tobacco of the Whites, unmixed, is too strong for the Indians, because they draw the smoke into their lungs; hence they do not willingly smoke cigars.
>
> The tobacco cultivated by the Mandans, Manitaries, and Arikkaras, attains a great height, and is suffered to grow up from seeds, without having any care whatever bestowed upon it. It is not trans-planted. When it is ripe the stalks are cut, dried, and powdered; or the leaves, with the small branches, are cut into little pieces. The taste and smell are disagreeable to an European, resembling camomile rather than tobacco. The plant is not now so much cultivated as formerly, being superceded by the more pleasant tobacco of the Whites; but the species is still preserved. It is used only on solemn occasions, for instance, in negotiations for peace, that this tobacco is still smoked; the seed is, therefore, preserved in the medicine bag of the nation, that the plant may never be lost. When they mean to smoke this tobacco, a small quantity of fat is rubbed on it. (Seig, 1971)

See also NATIVE AMERICANS; PIPE; PIPE SMOKING AND NATIVE AMERICANS

References: Louis Seig, *Tobacco, Peace Pipes, and Indians*, Palmer Lake, Co: Filter Press, 1971, p. 18.

Mayans

Antedating the birth of Christ the priest-dominated Mayan cultures of the Yucatan and Central America used tobacco of the *NICOTIANA TABACUM* variety. They smoked it in tubular pipes, elbow pipes with upright bowls, and self-burning tube pipes. The first "picture" of ceremonial tobacco smoking is thought to be the *Old Man of Palenque,* a bas relief carved on a large stone slab that formed one of a pair set in the wall on either side of the Temple of the Cross by the Mayans in what is now the state of Chiapas in the extreme south of Mexico. Although the date of the temple is about 114 A.D., the custom of making smoke offerings was believed to be already hundreds of years old. The old man, presumed to be a priest, holds a simple straight tubular or "cane" pipe tapering towards the mouthpiece. The early Mayan priests used tobacco as an incense accompanying worship.

CIGAR smoking was also part of Mayan culture, and they may have originated the "smoke-filled rooms" of politics, since cigars were smoked in council chambers.

It is believed that migrating Mayans brought the tobacco plant and pipe to the more northerly Toltec and Aztec tribes. *See also* NATIVE AMERICANS; PIPE; PIPE SMOKING AND NATIVE AMERICANS

McAlpin, D.H.

One of the most important New York tobacco manufacturers was D.H. McAlpin, who started out as a retailer-manufacturer and had a shop on Catherine Street before he founded his tobacco business prior to the Civil War. He concentrated on two specialties, a fine-cut chewing tobacco called "Virgin leaf" and a line of smoking tobaccos including "Virginia Killickinick" brand. His brand names were not original but they were shrewdly selected. "Virginia" was a synonym for fine tobacco and "killickinick" suggested an American Indian term *kinnikinnick* signifying tobacco blend. *See also* NEW YORK CITY

McCain Senate Tobacco Bill

On March 30, 1998, Senator John McCain, Republican from Arizona, offered a comprehensive tobacco bill that would toughen provisions of the tobacco settlement of June 1997 that the tobacco industry reached with state attorneys general and public health groups. McCain's bill would cost the tobacco industry more than $506 billion over 25 years, with the money going into a government trust fund. The bill called for the industry to restrict their advertising and marketing to youths and stiffened the industry's penalties if targets for reducing youth smoking were not reached. The cost of cigarettes would increase to $1.10 a pack over five years and civil damages tobacco companies would be forced to pay were capped at $6.5 billion yearly. The industry would receive no other protection from liability, and class-action suits would be permitted. The bill also gave full authority over tobacco products to the FOOD AND DRUG ADMINISTRATION (FDA). The McCain bill would have added a $28.5-billion tobacco bailout package including compensation for tobacco farmers, guaranteed prices for sales under tobacco quotas, economic development funds for adversely affected states, and education and retraining funds for tobacco workers.

The McCain bill was stronger than the agreement worked out between the tobacco industry and the state attorneys general and plaintiffs' attorneys in June 1997. The proposed $368.5-billion tobacco settlement was repudiated by every major anti-smoking and medical organization as well as by 23 public health organizations represented by the Advisory Committee on Tobacco Policy and Public Health, chaired by former surgeon general C. EVERETT KOOP and former Food and Drug Administration commissioner DAVID KESSLER. After the committee issued a report on July 9, 1997, to President Bill Clinton and Congress, highly critical of elements of the settlement proposal, Senator McCain proposed his tobacco bill (S. 1415).

On April 1, 1998, the Senate Commerce Committee passed—by an overwhelming, 19 to 1 margin—McCain's tobacco control bill. But the bill soon faced opposition and it was killed in the Senate on June 17, 1998. It was seen as too tough by the tobacco industry, which ran a $40-million campaign on television and radio to criticize the McCain bill as heavy-handed government regulation rather than a bill designed to discourage teenage smoking. It was seen as not tough enough by anti-smoking groups. Republican opponents of the bill argued the bill was a tax increase to pay for government programs. Amendments added to the McCain bill included a big tax cut for many married couples, anti-drug money, and grants for child care programs. Senators confronted one another over how to spend the billions of dollars that would be raised by the $1.10 price increase on cigarettes. Some senators objected to the expanded role of government. Opponents of the bill argued for removal of annual liability caps, larger penalties against the industry, and higher per-pack price increases. *See also* TOBACCO SETTLEMENT—JUNE 1997, TOBACCO SETTLEMENT—NOVEMBER 1998

Mele, Paul. *See* DENOBLE, VICTOR

Miami, Florida

Miami, Florida, is one of three important CIGAR manufacturing markets in the United States. The hand-rolled cigar industry existed in Miami for at least 100 years before the revolution in CUBA. But once Cubans left their homeland for Miami's Little Havana, that section of town became a dynamic center of economic activity. The new arrivals preferred freshly rolled cigars, which helped to drive up production levels.

Many of the cigar blends produced by *chinchals* (a Cuban term meaning "sweatshop," but not as derogatory in the world of cigars) in Miami are strong, fast-burning cigars made from Dominican seed tobacco as filler, a Mexican binder, and either Ecuador-grown Sumatra seed wrapper or U.S.-grown Connecticut shade tobacco. *See also* BINDER; CIGAR WRAPPER; CONNECTICUT TOBACCO; FILLER; KEY WEST, FLORIDA; YBOR CITY, FLORIDA

Minnesota Clean Indoor Air Act

In 1975, legislators from both parties in Minnesota passed a Clean Indoor Air Act aimed at protecting clean indoor air. Persons irritated by smoke headed for no-smoking zones while smokers looked for smoking sections before lighting up. The act, the first of its kind, became a model for other states. In 1980, the *Minneapolis Tribune* conducted a public opinion poll and found that 92 percent of nonsmokers and 87 percent of heavy smokers favored the law. Some legislators who voted against the bill became ardent supporters after conversations with constituents.

According to the law's chief sponsor, the honorable Phillis L. Kahn, it had an interesting effect on smokers. As smoking became considered socially and legally unacceptable, and also as it became more difficult to smoke, people smoked far less. Legislators who smoked told Kahn that with the passage of the nonsmoking rule on the floor of the Minnesota House, their CIGARETTE consumption went down because of the additional effort it took to go somewhere else to smoke.

Minnesota Medicaid Case

Of the 40 states suing the tobacco companies over the costs of health care for residents on Medicaid and public assistance, Minnesota's lawsuit was the first to go to trial and the fourth to be settled, after Mississippi, Florida, and Texas. In August 1994, Minnesota's state attorney general, Hubert "Skip" Humphrey III (the son of the former vice president), filed a lawsuit against tobacco companies to recover Medicaid expenses. Minnesota also charged the companies with consumer fraud in promoting and selling a product it knew to be harmful. The state alleged that the industry had engaged in a "de-

cades-long combination of conspiracy and of willful and intentional wrongdoing." Further, Minnesota charged violation of the state's anti-trust law, which prohibited "unreasonable restraint of trade and commerce." It was the industry's suppression of research into smoking and health, especially the healthier cigarette, that "had the purpose and effect of restraining competition in the market for cigarettes" (Pringle, 1998). Minnesota was the only state to bring the suit jointly with its largest purchaser of health care, Blue Cross and Blue Shield. Minnesota, the second state to file a Medicaid suit against tobacco companies (Mississippi filed in May 1994), had been one of the country's leading anti-tobacco states since the 1970s. It also refused to join in settlement talks with tobacco companies.

Humphrey picked a single law firm in Minneapolis, Robins, Kaplin, Miller and Ciresi (RKMC), one of the biggest in the Midwest, to be the sole representative of the state. The firm has over 200 lawyers, offices in every American city, and a reputation for taking on and winning complicated civil litigation. In response to the request from the law firm for internal company documents on smoking and health, the tobacco companies sent truckloads of reports, some of which had nothing of value in regard to the Minnesota lawsuit. Looking for a shortcut through the documents, the Minnesota lawyers presented a motion to the court asking for an index to the 30 million pages from tobacco company internal files. Sixteen months after the state's first request, in February 1995, after eight orders from the judge and two appeals, the tobacco companies sent index lists that enabled the lawyers to copy less than 2 percent of the material sent by the industry. Judge Kenneth Fitzpatrick, the state's chief judge, permitted other lawyers around the country access to the documents found by Minnesota. The documents, however, could not be made public before the Minnesota trial with one exception. If a document was used as an exhibit in arguing a motion before the court, it was automatically public unless sealed by the judge. Out of 40 states that eventually filed suit against tobacco companies, only

Connecticut and Washington helped RKMC lawyers with the task of sorting important documents from the mass of irrelevant papers.

Minnesota began the most thorough inquiry into the industry's past, but the search had its problems. To complete the document phase of their document hunt, RKMC lawyers needed to search the files of international affiliates of PHILIP MORRIS USA. The tobacco company did not respond to discovery requests and it claimed privilege over more than half a million pages. Eventually, Judge Kilpatrick ruled that "privileged" documents were to be reviewed by a special master of the court. Eventually, the tobacco companies, which fought all the way to the U.S. Supreme Court to block disclosure of 39,000 highly sensitive internal documents, were forced to turn them over to lawyers representing Minnesota. The Supreme Court refused to back the industry's claim of attorney-client privilege.

During the trial, the state's lawyers produced hundreds of industry documents in which tobacco company executives spoke about the need to entice minors to begin smoking to assure the industry's financial viability.

On May 8, 1998, the Minnesota lawsuit was settled for $6.5 billion as jurors were hearing closing arguments. The state of Minnesota was to receive $6.1 billion over 25 years. The settlement was also the industry's first with a health insurer, Blue Cross and Blue Shield of Minnesota, which will receive $469 million. The industry also paid $427 in attorneys' fees, which was not part of the $6.5 billion. The five tobacco companies sued by Minnesota agreed to disband the COUNCIL FOR TOBACCO RESEARCH, a nonprofit research group that the state accused the industry of using as a public relations front.

For the first time, the tobacco companies entered into a consent decree, enforceable in Minnesota courts, promising not to misrepresent the health hazards of smoking and agreeing to pay $100 million over 10 years for programs to reduce youth smoking. The companies also agreed to take down cigarette advertising on BILLBOARDS, buses, taxis, and bus stops in the state; ban marketing to minors in the state; stop paying for placement of tobacco products in movies and television nationwide (a practice the industry contends it stopped in 1989); and stop the sale of promotional merchandise with tobacco logos, such as caps and jackets, in Minnesota. The industry must disclose the amount it pays tobacco lobbyists in Minnesota, as well as amounts paid to third parties to testify at legislative hearings in the industry's defense. The companies also agreed not to mount legal challenges to Minnesota's existing laws against selling cigarettes to minors, the state's Clean Indoor Act, a state law against the free distribution of cigarettes and an ingredient-disclosure law enacted in 1997. Finally, the companies agreed to maintain for 10 years the state's depository of 33 million industry documents used in the trial. (The 39,000 documents were not covered by this part of the settlement.) *See also* FLORIDA MEDICAID CASE; MINNESOTA CLEAN INDOOR ACT; MISSISSIPPI MEDICAID CASE; TEXAS MEDICAID CASE

References: Peter Pringle, *Cornered: Big Tobacco at the Bar of Justice*, New York: Macmillan Company, 1998, p. 202.

Mississippi Medicaid Case

In May 1994, Mississippi was the first of 40 states to sue the tobacco companies, and the first to settle, on July 3, 1997, for $3.4 billion. The state used a new cause of action: recovery of monies the state had spent paying for the care of victims of smoking-related illnesses.

In the spring of 1993, the Mississippi Medicaid case was born when MICHAEL T. LEWIS, a University of Mississippi Law School graduate who practices in Clarksdale, Mississippi, contacted MICHAEL C. MOORE, the state's attorney general, about his desire to sue the tobacco industry to recoup state Medicaid monies that paid for the care of his bookkeeper's mother who died from lung cancer after a lifetime of smoking.

The tobacco companies first tried and failed to get the case dismissed in the chancery court and then challenged the central defense in the suit by saying the case was a personal injury action by the state on behalf of smokers. Moore argued the state was suing in its own right to protect its interests and to recoup funds it had no choice to provide under the federal Medicaid system. The "injury," he argued, was to the Mississippi taxpayer, not to the smoker. Mississippi claimed the tobacco companies had been "unjustly enriched" because the state paid bills that were the consequence of them selling cigarettes to Mississippi citizens. Based on a claim of indemnity, this called for shifting the loss incurred by the state onto the tobacco companies because the state was an innocent third party and had no choice but to pay the medical bills. The state also acted to abate a public nuisance created by the tobacco industry by providing health care to keep its citizens from dying sooner from smoking-related illnesses. Finally, Mississippi's claim was based on injunctive relief to protect the interests of minors. On February 21, 1995, Judge William Myers of the Jackson County Chancery Court officially endorsed Moore's arguments.

In March 1997, the Mississippi Supreme Court rejected a challenge by Governor Kirk Fordice to stop the lawsuit. The governor argued Moore overstepped his authority by trying to collect Medicaid funds, a program handled through the governor's office, without consulting Fordice. The governor said he would not have agreed to the lawsuit.

The state trial, the first in the nation, was scheduled to open on July 7, 1997. The defendants in the case included 13 tobacco companies, several distributors, tobacco research organizations, and a public relations company. Four days before Mississippi was scheduled to take its case to trial, the four largest cigarette makers (PHILIP MORRIS COMPANIES INC.; RJR NABISCO HOLDINGS CORPORATION, the parent company of R.J. REYNOLDS TOBACCO COMPANY; BAT INDUSTRIES PLC, the parent company of the BROWN AND WILLIAMSON TOBACCO CORPORATION; and the LOEWS CORPORATION, the parent company of the LORILLARD COMPANY INC.) settled and agreed to pay Mississippi $3.4 billion over 25 years and $136 million a year for every year that cigarettes continue to be sold in the United States. The settlement did not give Mississippi the public health benefits spelled out in the proposed tobacco settlement of June 1997 or those received by Florida, Texas, and Minnesota when they settled their lawsuits with tobacco companies. *See also* FLORIDA MEDICAID CASE; MINNESOTA MEDICAID CASE; TEXAS MEDICAID CASE; TOBACCO SETTLEMENT—JUNE 1997

Mohammed IV (1641–1691)

Mohammed IV, sultan of Turkey from 1648 to 1687, was a smoker who, when he found Turkey to have an ideal soil and climate for the cultivation of tobacco plants, established the growing of tobacco as one of the main enterprises and sources of revenue for the country. Tobacco remains an important crop and source of revenue in Turkey. *See also* TURKEY

Moore, Michael C. (1952–)

Mississipi's attorney general, Michael T. Moore, a graduate of the University of Mississippi Law School, is a leader in the national fight to make the tobacco industry liable for smoking-related medical expenses paid by states. Moore began his career as a district attorney in his hometown of Pascagoula. He stunned Jackson County by winning corruption convictions against several county supervisors in his first year of office.

Elected in 1987 as Mississippi's youngest attorney general in more than 75 years, Moore, a Democrat, was reelected in 1991 with 75 percent of the vote. In 1988, he and other state politicians were profiled in the *New York Times Magazine* in an article entitled "The Yuppies of Mississippi: How They Took Over the Statehouse."

Between 1988 and 1997, Moore, a longtime tobacco foe, made more than 2,000 appearances in schools to talk about the evils of drug abuse and smoking. When he became attorney general, Moore added the state of Mississippi to the nationwide lawsuits against the asbestos companies to recover the cost of removing asbestos from public buildings.

In 1993, one of Moore's classmates at law school, a lawyer named MICHAEL T. LEWIS, called him about suing the tobacco industry. The intent was to recoup state Medicaid funds that paid for the care of his bookkeeper's mother, who died from lung cancer after a lifetime of smoking. Moore put Lewis together with RICHARD F. SCRUGGS, a Republican country lawyer who had come up with a similar idea. Their legal theory worked; they teamed up and successfully persuaded the state to sue.

On May 23, 1994, Moore filed his four-count landmark lawsuit against the tobacco industry (13 tobacco companies as well as wholesalers, trade associations, and industry public relations consultants) in Pascagoula. He contended that the "tobacco cartel" reaped billions of dollars from Mississippi's citizens by selling them cigarettes without informing them of the "true carcinogenic, pathologic and addictive qualities" of those cigarettes. The complaint said

> Instead of honestly disclosing the genuine risks of smoking cigarettes, the tobacco companies have spent billions in slick, sophisticated marketing techniques designed to make smoking appear to be glamorous to our youngsters. In equity and fairness, it is the defendants, not the taxpayers of Mississippi, who should pay the costs of tobacco-related diseases.

Moore did not use state resources or employees to pursue the tobacco case. He enlisted a team of trial lawyers, most of them from Mississippi, who agreed to be paid only if a judge awarded damages and lawyers' fees. *See also* FLORIDA MEDICAID CASE; MISSISSIPPI MEDICAID CASE; MINNESOTA MEDICAID CASE; TEXAS MEDICAID CASE

Morbidity and Mortality Weekly Report (MMWR)

The *Morbidity and Mortality Weekly Report,* better known as *MMWR,* a series of publications and "surveillance summaries" prepared by the CENTERS FOR DISEASE CONTROL AND PRE-VENTION (CDC) of the PUBLIC HEALTH SERVICE, U.S. DEPARTMENT OF HEALTH AND HUMAN SERVICES, periodically contains articles about tobacco topics. The data in the weekly *MMWR* are provisional, based on weekly reports to CDC by state health departments.

Some of the various topics covered in the 1980s included "Cigarette Smoking among Public High School Students—Rhode Island" (1986); "Passive Smoking: Beliefs, Attitudes, and Exposures—United States"(1986); "Smokeless Tobacco Use in the United States—Behavioral Risk Factor Surveillance System" (1986); "Survey of Worksite Smoking Policies—New York City" (1987); and "Prevalence of Oral Lesions and Smokeless Tobacco Use in Northern Plains Indians" (1988).

Some of the various topics covered in the 1990s included "Cigarette Smoking among Reproductive-Aged Women—Idaho and New York" (1990); "Differences in the Age of Smoking Initiation between Blacks and Whites—United States" (1991); "Establishment of Smoke-Free Office Worldwide—U.S. Peace Corps" (1991); "Cigarette Smoking Bans in County Jails—Wisconsin, 1991" (1992); "World No-Tobacco Day, 1992" (1992); "The Great American Smokeout, November 18, 1993" (1993); "Green Tobacco Sickness in Tobacco Harvesters—Kentucky, 1992" (1993); "Influence of Religious Leaders on Smoking Cessation in a Rural Population—Thailand, 1991" (1993); "Minors' Access to Tobacco—Missouri, 1992 and Texas, 1993" (1993); "Smoking Cessation During Previous Year among Adults—United States, 1990 and 1991" (1993); "Cigarette Smoking among American Indians and Alaskan Natives—Behavioral Risk Factor Surveillance System, 1987–1991" (1992); and "Cigarette Smoking among Chinese, Vietnamese, and Hispanics—California, 1989–1991" (1992).

Examples of CDC surveillance summaries were "Surveillance for Selected Tobacco-Use Behaviors—United States, 1900–1994" and "Surveillance for Smoking-Attributable Mortality and Years of Potential Life Lost, by State—United States, 1990."

MMWR is available on a paid subscription basis from the superintendent of documents. *See also* OFFICE OF SMOKING AND HEALTH

More Cigarettes

In 1975, R.J. REYNOLDS TOBACCO COMPANY came out with More cigarettes, a brown CIGARETTE 120 mm in length that looked like a long, thin CIGAR. More, with its high content of both TAR and NICOTINE, was a success with urban white males as well as black urban males. Reynolds also created a mentholated version of More that did almost as well as the original.

In 1980, when sales lagged, R.J. Reynolds decided to "reposition" the brand to make it appeal to women. One promotion involved the Ebony Fashion Flair, which traveled around the country showing the latest fashions to women and at the same time promoting More cigarettes. The October 6, 1986, issue of the *Wall Street Journal* reported that "As model Kym Thomas makes her exit in a Jackie Rogers black and gold backless evening dress, she stops to take a puff. 'She smokes More cigarettes,' intoned a commentator in one of several plugs throughout the show." The *Journal* also reported that free More cigarettes were given out to spectators. More had spectacular growth among women. The company also produced a beige cigarette called More Light and targeted the advertising at young women. *See also* VIRGINIA SLIMS CIGARETTES

Morris, Philip (d. 1873)

In the late 1850s, a London tobacco merchant named Philip Morris, whose business had been established in the early part of the decade, took advantage of the demand for "Russian-style" cigarettes by British soldiers returning from the war in the Crimea. He began manufacturing hand-made cigarettes using Latakia, a smoke-cured variety of TURKISH TOBACCO. He imported a group of expert rollers from RUSSIA, TURKEY, and Egypt who, in a 10-hour day, turned out 3,000 cigarettes. On Philip Morris' death in 1873, his widow,

Margaret, and brother, Leopold, took over the business located on Bond Street. In 1880, after Leopold bought out his sister-in-law, Joseph Grunebaum joined him in ownership. In 1881, after a successful public offering of stock ownership, the company opened manufacturing facilities at Poland and Marlborough streets. By 1894, however, the company had slipped into the hands of creditors. It emerged from receivership in the hands of William Curtis Thomson and his family who revitalized the small company. In 1902, the firm of Philip Morris Ltd. was appointed royal tobacconist adding to its prominence in England and abroad. An upturn in the company's cigarette sales in the United States during the first decade of the twentieth century led the Thomson family to open a small American branch. Philip Morris & Company, Ltd. was incorporated in New York in April 1902. Seventeen years later, the PHILIP MORRIS COMPANIES INC. was founded which has evolved into the largest consumer packaged-goods company in the world. Its subsidiary, Philip Morris Inc. (or PHILIP MORRIS USA) is the largest U.S. cigarette company.

Mosaic

Mosaic is a virus, one of the most widespread maladies of the tobacco plant, and causes mottling of the tobacco leaves; parts of the leaves become a lighter green color than the rest of the leaf. The disease is highly infectious and may be carried by workers or communicated from one plant to another by direct contact. *See also* BLACK SHANK; BLUE MOLD

Moss, Frank E. (1911–)

A Democratic senator from Utah from 1958 to 1976, Frank E. Moss served as a member of the Senate Commerce Committee and as chairman of the Consumer Subcommittee. He consistently demonstrated an interest in protecting the public from a variety of health hazards including those that are the consequences of the inhalation of cigarette smoke. Senator Moss authored the 1970 amendment to the FEDERAL CIGARETTE LABELING AND AD-

VERTISING ACT OF 1965, which banned broadcast advertising of little cigars.

Motley, Ronald (1944–)

A key attorney representing states suing tobacco companies for reimbursement of Medicaid expenses as well as smokers in product liability cases, Ronald Motley is a trial lawyer of the plaintiffs' bar from Charleston, South Carolina. Motley is the son of a gas station owner who was the first of his family to go to college, at the University of South Carolina. A senior partner in Ness, Motley, Loadholt, Richardson and Poole, Motley had a national reputation in the 1980s as one of the leading litigators of asbestos-related personal injury claims and served as lead trial counsel in a number of consolidated asbestos cases. Since 1984, when his mother, a longtime smoker, lay dying of emphysema, Motley vowed to go after tobacco companies. He joined forces with Mississippi lawyer RICHARD F. SCRUGGS and the attorney general of Mississippi MICHAEL C. MOORE.

In 1994, Motley represented BUR BUTLER, a non-smoking barber who was diagnosed with lung cancer. Motley wanted to use several of the documents stolen by MERRELL WILLIAMS from BROWN AND WILLIAMSON TOBACCO CORPORATION's files. Motley argued in his brief that he should be able to use the documents because they had already been distributed by the media and by the University of California at San Francisco, which had placed a full set in its library. This was the first mention of the copy in the university's archives, and his argument eventually led to the documents becoming available to be used as evidence against the tobacco industry.

In 1994, Motley joined a group of lawyers in the Castano lawsuit and the MISSISSIPPI MEDICAID CASE. On November 29, 1995, he deposed JEFFREY WIGAND, former research chief at Brown and Williamson. Wigand accused his former boss, THOMAS E. SANDEFUR, JR., of perjuring himself in April 1994 before the House Subcommittee when he said NICOTINE was not addictive. Motley took part in negotiations in the Liggett settlement in 1996,

and beginning in 1997 he represented 30 states suing tobacco companies for reimbursement of Medicaid expenses.

In 1997, Motley teamed up with NORWOOD "WOODY" WILNER to represent JEAN CONNOR in a smoker's liability case won by R.J. REYNOLDS TOBACCO COMPANY. *See also* BROWN AND WILLIAMSON TOBACCO CORPORATION— MERRELL WILLIAMS DOCUMENTS; *CASTANO V. AMERICAN TOBACCO COMPANY*

Mulford v. Smith (1939)

The constitutional validity of the marketing quota provisions of the AGRICULTURAL ADJUSTMENT ACT OF 1938 (AAA) were upheld by the U.S. Supreme Court in the case of *Mulford v. Smith.*

The appellants, producers of FLUE-CURED TOBACCO, asserted that the AAA was unconstitutional because it affected their 1938 crop. They based their belief on three propositions: (1) that the AAA was a statutory plan to control agricultural production and, therefore, beyond the powers delegated to Congress; (2) that the standard for calculating farm quotas was uncertain, vague, and indefinite, resulting in an unconstitutional delegation of legislative power to the agriculture secretary; and (3) that the AAA took their 1938 crop, or property, retroactively, which amounted to taking property without due process, violating the Fifth Amendment.

The case was decided on April 17, 1939, when Justice Owen Roberts delivered the opinion of the court. On the first point, he ruled that the statute did not purport to control production and set no limits on the acreage that may be planted or produced and imposed no penalty for the planting and producing of tobacco in excess of the marketing quota. The Court said the AAA regulated interstate commerce "at the throat where tobacco enters the stream of commerce, the marketing warehouse." The Court had recently ruled that sales of tobacco by growers through warehousemen to purchasers for removal outside the state constituted interstate commerce. It also said that any rule, such as that embodied in the AAA that was intended to foster, protect, and conserve that commerce or to prevent the flow of commerce from working harm to the people of the nation, was valid and within the "competence of Congress."

On the second point, the court ruled that definite standards were laid down for the agriculture secretary in fixing the quota and in allotting it among states and farms. The secretary was directed to adjust the allotments so as to allow for specified factors that abnormally affected the production of the state or the farm in question in the test years. Congress, to protect against arbitrary action, afforded both administrative and judicial review to correct errors. Therefore, the court concluded that the AAA was valid respecting delegation to administrative officers.

On the third point, the court ruled that the statute operated not on farm production, as the appellants insisted, but on the marketing of their tobacco in interstate commerce. It also ruled that the AAA, enacted on February 16, 1938, affected marketing that was to take place the following August, and therefore was prospective in its operation, not retroactive. The court noted that the AAA did not prevent any producer from holding over the excess tobacco produced, or processing and storing it for sale in a later year.

References: *Mulford v. Smith*, 307 U.S. 38 (1939), Decided April 17, 1939.

Murad Cigarettes

During the summer of 1918, an advertising campaign for Murad cigarettes, manufactured by P. Lorillard, showed patriotic posters with a doughboy (the nickname for the World War I soldier) in a trench. Between his lips was a lit CIGARETTE and the message underneath: "Murad—After the Battle, the Most Refreshing Smoke is Murad 20¢-20." Other Murad ads showed upper-class women in fashionable clothes standing near uniformed soldiers.

Starting in 1919, the LORILLARD COMPANY pitched Murad to females. Models never had a cigarette in their hands or mouths and few ads showed pictures of the cigarette or the pack. In one ad, a brunette reclined against a silk-covered wall, her right arm behind her head. Close by her toe is an open box of Murad with the message: "Be Nonchalant. Light a Murad Cigarette."

Murad IV (1609–1640)

Murad IV, sultan of TURKEY and an anti-tobacco monarch, took special steps to stamp out the tobacco habit in Turkey. In 1633, smoking was declared a violation of the precepts of the *Koran* and the act punishable by death. It is recorded that he executed smokers regularly—as many as 18 in a day. Murad's tactics did not stamp out tobacco. Ironically, LORILLARD COMPANY INC. named a cigarette Murad.

After Murad died, his nephew succeeded him and continued the prohibition against tobacco as well as the punishments. In 1687, De Thevenot recorded that the sultan walked through the streets in disguise to see if his orders were obeyed and executed violators.

> He caused two men in one day to be beheaded in the streets of Constantinople, because they were smoking tobacco. He had prohibited it some days before, because, as it was said, when he was passing along the street where Turks were smoking tobacco, the smoke had gone up his nose. But I rather think it was in imitation of his uncle Sultan Amurat [Murad IV], who did all he could to hinder it so long as he lived. He caused some to be hanged with a pipe through their nose, others with tobacco hanging about their neck, and never pardoned any for that. I believe that the chief reason why Sultan Amurath prohibited tobacco, was because of the fires, that do so much mischief in Constantinople when they happen, which most commonly occasioned by people that fall asleep with a pipe in their mouth, that sets fire to the bed, or any combustible matter, as I said before. He used all the arts he could to discover those who sold tobacco, and went to the places where he was informed they did, where having offered several chequins for a pound of tobacco, made great entreaty, and promised secrecy, if they let him have it; he drew out a scimitar under his vest, and cut off the shopkeeper's head.

See also BUCKLEY, CHRISTOPHER; MURAD CIGA-RETTES

References: de Thévenot, *Travels Into the Levant*, 1687, p. 60.

Myers, George S. *See* LIGGET AND MYERS TOBACCO COMPANY

Myers, Matthew (1947–)

A one-time counsel to the COALITION ON SMOKING AND HEALTH, Matthew Myers, became vice president of Campaign for To-bacco-Free Kids, a group aimed at curbing under-age smoking. With his encyclopedic knowledge of the tobacco industry, he became the media spokesman for the public health community and one of the architects of the proposed tobacco settlement of June 1997 negotiated by state attorneys general, plaintiffs' lawyers, health advocates, and tobacco executives. In 1999, Myers became president of the National Center for Tobacco-Free Kids after Bill NOVELLI's departure. *See also* NATIONAL CENTER FOR TOBACCO-FREE KIDS; TOBACCO SETTLEMENT—JUNE 1997

N

National Association of Insurance Commissioners (NAIC)

The National Association of Insurance Commissioners (NAIC) adopted a resolution at its annual meeting in December 1984 calling for different health insurance rates for smokers and nonsmokers. Under this proposal, nonsmokers could save over $200 a year in health insurance costs and smokers could be forced to pay 50 percent more than they were already paying. The proposal adopted by NAIC applied to all types of health insurance providers, including health maintenance organizations (HMOs).

> BE IT RESOLVED, that the National Association of Insurance Commissioners encourages all segments of the health-care prepayment and insurance industry to provide financial incentives such as premium differentials under group and individual health-care programs designed to encourage individuals to bring these health risk factors under control and BE IT FURTHER RESOLVED, that the basis for such financial incentives include for example non-use of tobacco products, attainment of proper weight, and maintenance of blood pressure within proper limits.

The NAIC is made up of commissioners in each state who are charged with regulating rates and other aspects of the insurance industry. Its members are therefore in a uniquely powerful position to encourage, and in some cases compel, health insurance companies to provide differential rates based on smoking habits. ("Ash Wine," 1985) *See also* INSURANCE COVERAGE AND SMOKING

References: "ASH Wins Major Health Insurance Victory for Nonsmokers." *ASH Review*, March 1985, p. 3.

National Cancer Institute (NCI)

A component of the National Institutes of Health, the National Cancer Institute (NCI), established under the National Cancer Act of 1937, is the federal government's principal agency for cancer research and training. Within the Bethesda, Maryland-based NCI, the Smoking and Tobacco Control Program continually monitors the consumption of all forms of tobacco products and supports and coordinates research projects.

In 1983, the NCI developed its first annual report on the Smoking, Tobacco, and Cancer program (STCP) after Dr. Vincent DeVita announced the Institute's goal to reduce cancer mortality 50 percent by the year 2000. That report codified the change in direction for STCP outlining an approach that was in keeping with the intervention research strategy for NCI's cancer control program in general. The prevention and control of smoking and other forms of tobacco use became one of the top priorities for cancer prevention within the NCI.

Since 1991, the NCI has published a series of monographs to provide a mechanism for the rapid, systematic, and timely dissemination of information important to the research and public health communities about emerging issues in smoking and tobacco use control. The following Smoking and Tobacco Control monographs have been published:

- *Strategies to Control Tobacco Use in the United States. A Blueprint for Public Health Action in the 1990s.* Monograph No. 1
- *Smokeless Tobacco or Health. An International Perspective.* Monograph No. 2
- *Major Local Tobacco Control Ordinances in the United States.* Monograph No. 3
- *Respiratory Health Effects of Passive Smoking. Lung Cancer and Other Disorders. The Report of the U.S. Environmental Protection Agency.* Monograph No. 4
- *Tobacco and the Clinician. Interventions for Medical and Dental Practice.* Monograph No. 5
- *Community-based Interventions for Smokers. The COMMIT Field Experience.* Monograph No. 6
- *The FTC Cigarette Test Method for Determining Tar, Nicotine, and Carbon Monoxide Yields of US Cigarettes. Report of the NCI Expert Committee.* Monograph No. 7
- *Changes in Cigarette Related Disease Risks and Their Implications for Prevention and Control.* Monograph No. 8
- *Cigars: Health Effects and Trends.* Monograph No. 9.

In 1993, the National Cancer Institute and American Cancer Society teamed up as partners to create a large, comprehensive, non government-funded, health-based smoking control project. Called ASSIST (American Stop Smoking Intervention Study for Cancer Prevention), this program operated until September 1999 in 29 states plus Tucson, Arizona (originally 17 states) and relied on state and local tobacco-control coalitions to attack smoking from every possible angle. *See also* DEPARTMENT OF HEALTH AND HUMAN SERVICES (DHHS)

National Center for Tobacco-Free Kids

Founded in 1996, the National Center for Tobacco-Free Kids, based in Washington, D.C., was created to sponsor, coordinate, and encourage efforts to keep children from smoking, sniffing, and chewing tobacco and to protect them from exposure to SECOND-HAND SMOKE. The organization, the country's largest non-governmental initiative ever launched to decrease tobacco use, was set up with a $20 million grant from the Robert Wood Johnson Foundation, $10 million from the AMERICAN CANCER SOCIETY (ACS), and several smaller donations from other foundations and health groups such as the AMERICAN MEDICAL ASSOCIATION (AMA) and the AMERICAN HEART ASSOCIATION (AHA).

The center's mandate is to change the social, political, and economic environment regarding tobacco; change public policies at the federal, state, and local levels to reduce tobacco use by children; increase the number of organizations and individuals involved; and actively counter the tobacco industry and its special interests. The center serves as a resource and partner for more than 130 health, civic, corporate, youth, religious, and community organizations dedicated to reducing tobacco use among American children. It works with a bipartisan coalition of political leaders to serve as a communications and media center to counter the tobacco industry's marketing and sales practices that appeal to children. It disseminates information and implements media campaigns and events, assists state- and community-level programs, provides technical assistance to state- and community-level tobacco control education efforts, undertakes research and analysis, conducts outreach to broaden the base and depth of national support to reduce tobacco use by children, engages in advocacy for supportive public policies, and coordinates with international organizations and activists in other countries.

The center sponsors "Kick Butts Day," an annual nationwide event in April that encourages leadership and activism among youth. Thousands of elementary, middle, and high school students in hundreds of towns and cities across the country organize activities to counter the tobacco industry's advertising and promotional strategies aimed at children and teens. The Youth Advocates of the Year Awards recognize and celebrate outstanding young tobacco control activists who are leaders in their communities. The organization has placed advertisements in newspapers intended to sway public opinion towards the tobacco control effort. *See also* MYERS, MATTHEW; NOVELLI, BILL

National Clearinghouse for Smoking and Health

Shortly after Congress passed the FEDERAL CIGARETTE LABELING AND ADVERTISING ACT OF 1965, it created the National Clearinghouse for Smoking and Health. A unit added to the U.S. PUBLIC HEALTH SERVICE, it was created to be a repository for all data, studies, and articles dealing with smoking and to serve as a reference service for researchers everywhere. The technical information provided the basis of the updated surgeon general's reports to Congress.

Another function of the clearinghouse was to educate the public about the possible health hazards of smoking. It produced pamphlets on quitting; posters distributed to the public school classrooms, with captions such as "If you smoke, you're a turkey"; placards attached to the sides of U.S. mail trucks and placed in New York subways and other public transit systems; and unpaid anti-smoking commercials in the late 1960s. Congress appropriated $2 million so it could carry out educational campaigns and collect data on smoking-and-health research.

In 1974, the clearinghouse was absorbed into the CENTERS FOR DISEASE CONTROL AND PREVENTION (CDC) and moved from the Washington area to Atlanta, Georgia.

The clearinghouse, under the directorship of DANIEL HORN from 1965 to 1974, turned out anti-smoking tracts for civic groups and financed several local anti-cigarette projects. In 1969, it gave teenagers in Bakersfield, California, a grant of $47,000 to see if they could get anti-smoking messages across to their peers more effectively than adults could. The high school students set up their own advertising agency and created "Smoke Out," an advertising campaign against smoking. First, they surveyed the smoking habits of students in three Bakersfield schools. Then they asked ad agency professionals for information on planning and running the campaign. The student ad agency came up with bumper stickers, posters, BILLBOARD messages, decals, buttons, book covers, and school and local newspaper public service ads—all produced by the Smoke Out crew. Everything carried the Smoke Out logo, designed by a seventh grader who won a student contest. One radio commercial said: "Don't smoke in bed. You might burn a hole in your lungs." Another one said: "He: 'Have a cigarette.' She: 'I thought you said you love me.'" One TV spot showed a shot of an elegantly dressed woman: "She smokes," a voice says. Then there is a shot of burning trash: "So does the city dump," says the voice.

The youngsters launched their media campaign on March 1, 1969. Three TV stations in the area started running their filmed spots and radio stations broadcast their tapes. Outdoor signboards carried the same message as the 25,000 bumper strips "Smoke . . . Choke . . . Croak!" The Associated Press carried the story, and NBC and CBS sent TV news crews to Bakersfield. *Teen Magazine, Newsweek, Advertising Age*, and other magazines covered the story as did San Francisco's educational TV station. *See also* ANTI-SMOKING MESSAGES, 1967–1970

National Interagency Council on Smoking and Health

In the summer of 1965, as a result of meetings between Surgeon General Luther L. Terry and the voluntary health agencies, the first broad campaign to discourage smoking was launched. Called the National Interagency Council on Smoking and Health, it was a coalition of government agencies and virtually every national health organization except the AMERICAN MEDICAL ASSOCIATION (AMA). Its first chairman was EMERSON FOOTE, former chairman of the McCann-Erickson ad agency in New York. Foote, who took the job without pay, believed in eliminating advertising as a curb to smoking.

National Smokers Alliance (NSA)

The National Smokers Alliance (NSA) is a nonprofit membership organization that supports the accommodation of smokers and nonsmokers in public places and in workplaces. The NSA is dedicated to fighting discrimination against smokers. It represents the interests of its three million members, some 20 percent of whom are nonsmokers, and all of whom have certified themselves to be 21 years of age or older.

The NSA provides a voice for adult consumers of tobacco products as well as those who do not consume these products but support those who do in opposing unwarranted government intrusion. The NSA believes cigarettes are and must continue to be a legal product and opposes any federal regulations that attempt to curtail the rights of 50 million people to purchase and enjoy a legal product.

The NSA opposes government-imposed smoking bans and believes business owners should have the right to determine their own smoking policies. It opposes excessive taxation or regulation of tobacco products.

The NSA believes minors should not use tobacco products, a belief held by most adult Americans, including smokers. Since all 50 states and the District of Columbia have laws that prohibit the sale of cigarettes to minors, the NSA believes enforcing those laws is the most effective solution to preventing youth access to tobacco products. The NSA believes parents, teachers, and prominent role models can most effectively deter youth from smoking.

On August 11, 1995, the FOOD AND DRUG ADMINISTRATION (FDA) published proposed regulations restricting the sale, distribution, and promotion of tobacco products. The sole purpose of the regulations, the FDA says, is to reduce the incidence of tobacco product use by minors.

The NSA believes the FDA has no jurisdiction over tobacco and Congress has specifically precluded the FDA from jurisdiction. It believes proposed FDA regulations to restrict the sale and distribution of cigarettes and SMOKELESS TOBACCO products to protect children and adolescents violate the First Amendment and other constitutional protections. Since tobacco, a legal product, is regulated by a dozen other federal agencies and a myriad of state and local regulations, the NSA believes the FDA has no useful role in further regulating it. The NSA believes the classification of NICOTINE as an addictive drug is a subterfuge to gain control over tobacco, especially since the FDA makes no such claims of jurisdiction over other substances such as caffeine and alcohol commonly available in consumer products.

The NSA argues against each of the proposed FDA regulations.

1. The proposed FDA regulations state that cigarette sales be permitted only in direct face-to-face transactions between retailers and purchasers eliminating self-service displays, vending machines, mail-order sales, and mail-order redemption coupons. According to the NSA, prohibition would eliminate incentive payments for self-service displays retail stores receive. The face-to-face provision will also cause an increase in personnel costs because retailers will need to hire more personnel.

2. FDA proposed regulations state that tobacco products be sold only from a "controlled area of the store." This will limit the number of brands and the quantity that a retailer may stock. As a result, the NSA argues, the regulation will limit the choice of consumers in

brand, taste, length, quality, and price. Therefore this regulation will raise prices of tobacco products to adult consumers already burdened by discriminatory, and in some cases confiscatory, taxation. Indeed, some retailers might discontinue cigarette sales altogether.

3. The proposed FDA regulations prevent tobacco product manufacturers from offering premiums at point of sale or from redeeming proof of purchase for premiums. If the FDA bans mail order redemption, this imposes a new cost on consumers who now take advantage of these savings.

4. The FDA regulation proposes to limit the number of cigarettes per pack to no fewer than 20. This precludes the possibility of packs with reduced quantity, and, thus, reduced cost, in times of recession and depression where demand by less affluent adult consumers is sufficient to warrant tobacco manufacturers to provide such products. This also limits consumer choice.

5. If the FDA bars manufacturers of tobacco products from brand sponsorships, adult smokers and nonsmokers alike will be denied the reduced-cost and sometimes no-cost access to sports, entertainment, and cultural activities currently sponsored or partially sponsored by tobacco manufacturers.

6. FDA proposed regulations would ban all vending machines and make no provision for vending machines even in "adults only" or "adult supervised" locations, although the stated purpose of the regulation is solely to prevent minors from obtaining cigarettes. Cigarette and multi-product vending machines in factories and office buildings, in bars, restaurants and recreational facilities which cater to adults or to families would be banned, denying adult consumers the convenience to purchase tobacco products that exists for other legal products. This severely limits the options of adult consumers with regard to where and when they may purchase tobacco products.

7. The proposed FDA regulations outlaw mail order sales and redemption of coupons. This regulation makes no allowance for the adult consumer who cannot physically go to a retail outlet to engage in a face-to-face transaction. This penalizes disabled veterans and elderly smokers who rely on mail order transactions.

8. The proposed FDA restriction regarding the advertising of tobacco products would infringe upon the free speech rights guaranteed by the First Amendment. It will make advertising in publications less desirable to tobacco product advertisers, and their expenditures for advertising will decrease. The NSA argues that when advertising pages and revenue decrease, so does editorial content, which is unquestionably protected. The proposed regulations would prohibit the sale or distribution of T-shirts, hats, jackets, coffee mugs, and all other promotional items bearing the brand name, logo, symbol, motto, or other identifiable characteristics of cigarettes. To deny adult consumers the right to acquire or accept the products and to wear or use them as they see fit also violates the First Amendment freedom of expression.

The NSA concludes that the proposed FDA regulations would impose extremely heavy additional burdens on adult consumers who are already burdened by the high cost of taxation and by excessive limits on their ability to enjoy smoking. Higher costs to smokers, highly restricted access to legal products, less information, and restrictions on expression are completely unwarranted and will do little or nothing to achieve the FDA's stated objective of deterring youth from smoking. On behalf of its three million members, the National Smokers Alliance pledged to fight the adoption of the FDA regulations in every legal and appropriate venue. If the regulations had become law, the NSA pledged to fight them in every legal and appropriate venue to see them overturned. *See also* CIGARETTE; FOOD AND DRUG ADMINISTRATION (FDA) 1995 PROPOSAL FOR REGULATING TOBACCO

Native Americans

For thousands of years, tobacco has been used among the hundreds of tribal groupings in both North and South America. Researchers have concluded that pre-contact tobacco use originated among native peoples of South America, then spread through Central America, and later to North America.

Some forms of tobacco grew wild, and others were cultivated. In times prior to European contact, the most commonly used species of tobacco was *NICOTIANA RUSTICA*, used primarily by American Indians in the eastern United States and throughout the Great Plains. Often native peoples mixed tobacco with other substances such as parts of the bark of willow, dogwood, sumac, bearberry, rose bushes, and leadplant. In addition to the leaves and small stems of these plants, they also added herbs and oils to form a milder substance called *kinnikinnik* in the Algonquian language and *chan sha'sha* in the Siouan language. In most languages, the term applied to the mixture meant "mixed" or "mixed by hand."

Aboriginal tobacco was in small supply and was sacred. There were gender differences in the treatment of tobacco. Women generally were not allowed to participate in its cultivation, although they were responsible for other crops, thus affirming its distinctive sacred status. Among the Plains tribes, there were tobacco societies. Initiation into their ranks was required before members could sow tobacco. Duties of initiates included sweat lodge rituals, the selection of medicine, and the planting of sacred tobacco, all of which were executed with the greatest ritual and care.

Tobacco was used in agricultural rites. It was used in the harvesting of crops and to bless the harvest. The rising tobacco smoke was regarded as a means of communicating with the spirit world. Tobacco smoke was also an important visual symbol of contact with the supernatural world. The Haudenosaunee (Iroquois) believed the ascending smoke carried their petitions to the "Creator." Tobacco was commonly used to bind agreements between tribes and it often accompanied invitations to individuals or families. Tobacco was also given as payment to a sacred practitioner.

In addition to its ceremonial use, many different tribes used tobacco, especially its active component NICOTINE, medicinally and in medical ceremonies. It was chewed as a remedy for toothaches and was used to treat earaches. Open wounds and insect or snake bites were treated with tobacco because of its presumed analgesic properties. It was also used to treat ailments such as asthma, rheumatism, convulsions, intestinal disorders, childbirth pains, and coughs. Healers used tobacco as a fumigation to drive disease away from a patient's body.

Native American people believe that tobacco, used at the right time, the right place, and in the right way, helps in the spiritual development of a good person. Some tribes still have sacred people who know the proper way to plant, pick, prepare, and use tobacco. Today traditional native people use tobacco as a sign of respect and as an offering when praying to the Creator. By placing tobacco in a fire while praying, the smoke that rises carries their prayers to the Creator. Sometimes tobacco is smoked in a pipe, used in crumbled leaf or seed form, or as a paste. Sometimes it is sprinkled around young corn plants. When someone wishes to show respect to a healer or elder, tobacco is given. Traditional healers use tobacco to help cure illnesses. When a person travels to a foreign area and wishes to pay respect to the ancestors of that land, he or she offers tobacco to the earth. No matter what form it takes, this kind of tobacco use is sacred to native people. *See also* KINNIKINNICK; PIPE; PIPE SMOKING AND NATIVE AMERICANS

Natural American Spirit Cigarettes

In 1985, the Santa Fe Natural Tobacco Company in Santa Fe, New Mexico, introduced Natural American Spirit, an additive-free cigarette made from premium Virginia tobacco. The cigarettes come in three versions—filtered, unfiltered, and the ceremonial "Pow Wow Blend" of tobacco and herbs like red willow bark, bearberries, sage, and Yerba Buena. The package states: "Made From 100% Chemical-Additive-Free, Whole leaf, natural Virginia Tobacco and nothing else." While Spirits do not contain synthetic flavor enhancers, preservatives, moisteners, preservatives, and other agents called "burn accelerators," they contain, like all tobacco products, TAR and NICOTINE, substances considered highly addictive and harmful to health. They also contain 25 percent more tobacco than most other brands of the same size. The packs don't list tar and nicotine levels.

The Natural American Spirit logo depicts the silhouette of an American Indian man's head in a feathered headdress smoking a long-stemmed pipe along with the company's thunderbird symbol. The package also carries the surgeon general's warning. The company literature states: "Our package design was chosen because tobacco is a plant native to America and was introduced to 'Western civilization' by American Indians. We feel tobacco is a powerful herb worthy of the respect it has been shown in American Indian tradition" (Humphrey, 1997).

Santa Fe Natural Tobacco Company was not part of the tobacco settlement of November 1998. New Mexico attorney general Tom Udall, who accepted the settlement, sued the tobacco company along with the big national cigarette makers. Santa Fe Natural asked in court that it be dropped from Udall's suit, but the request was rejected.

The company faced two options, either to sign onto the agreement or face continued litigation from the state. A Santa Fe Natural Tobacco Company vice president said the company would not be affected by many of the cigarette advertising restrictions in the settlement because it does not use BILLBOARDS or cartoon figures in its advertising. If it became part of the settlement, Santa Fe Natural would not have to pay settlement dollars to the state as the major companies must, unless the company's sales jumped 125 percent after the settlement was in place.

References: Kay Humphrey, "Groups Fight Tobacco Firm with Boycott," *Indian Country Today*, July 28–August 4, 1997, p. D2.

Neuberger, Maurine B. (1906–)

Wife of Oregon Senator Richard Neuberger, Maurine Neuberger emerged as a leading anticigarette spokesperson in 1960. In March of that year, her husband died of lung cancer at the age of 48. Maurine Neuberger won the election to fill his seat in the Senate. Almost immediately on joining the Senate in November, she became involved in the issue of banning cigarette advertising.

In the spring of 1961, the AMERICAN CANCER SOCIETY, American Public Health Association, AMERICAN HEART ASSOCIATION, and National Tuberculosis Association (now called the AMERICAN LUNG ASSOCIATION) called for the establishment of a presidential commission to study "the widespread implications of the tobacco problem." When President John Kennedy ignored the request, Senator Neuberger brought it to the Senate floor by asking for passage of a resolution in favor of a commission. The various associations urged the public to flood Washington with letters and petitions supporting the Neuberger motion. In the end Kennedy accepted the Neuberger position and announced the White House would form the Surgeon General's Advisory Committee on Smoking and Health.

In April 1962, Senator Neuberger, who believed cigarette packages should have clear warnings about the health hazards of smoking, wrote the FEDERAL TRADE COMMISSION (FTC) chairman Paul Rand Dixon proposing that any cigarette ad that did not carry a health warning should be found deceptive. She also asked why the FTC couldn't require all cigarette advertising to carry a health warning. Neuberger wrote FOOD AND DRUG ADMINISTRATION (FDA) commissioner George P. Larrick and suggested the FDA had authority to control cigarette labels under the federal Hazardous Substances Labeling Act of 1960, but the FDA commissioner disagreed. *See also* HEALTH WARNINGS ON CIGARETTE PACKS AND ADVERTISEMENTS AND SMOKELESS TOBACCO

New Jersey Group against Smoking Pollution (GASP)

Founded in 1974 by REGINA CARLSON and other citizens, the New Jersey Group against Smoking Pollution (GASP) is one of the world's oldest and most successful nonprofit citizen nonsmokers' organizations and is recognized internationally as a pioneer in the smoke-free advocacy movement. Its goal is to secure smoke-free air for nonsmokers and tobacco-free lives for children.

New Jersey GASP has vigorous education and advocacy programs. It provides counsel and legal advice to legislators, policy makers, and citizens each year through its Tobacco Control Policy and Legal Resource Center. A research organization as well, New Jersey GASP tracked tobacco industry political contributions and lobbying in New Jersey from 1982 to 1995. The data, analyzed by the Institute for Health Policy Studies of the University of California School of Medicine, showed the tobacco industry was the number one contributor to New Jersey legislators.

A force for local, state, and federal legislation, regulation, and litigation, New Jersey GASP participated in obtaining the first court injunction banning smoking at work, *Shimp v. New Jersey Bell* (1976); helped more than 165 municipalities enact ordinances controlling tobacco sales to minors; helped pass more than a dozen smoke-free air laws in New Jersey since the early 1970s; helped most of New Jersey's large malls go smoke free; and helped Newark Airport create a smoke-free policy.

New Jersey GASP has published lists of smoke-free workplaces, malls, airports, and restaurants. Its newsletter, "The Smart Restaurateur," gives success stories of diverse smoke-free restaurants. It also bolsters smoke-free restaurants by giving them free signs about the policy and by doing statewide press releases on smoke-free dining. Besides publishing a newsletter plus action alerts, it has published *Smokefree Air Everywhere*, a how-to manual that looks beyond the workplace and has special sections for schools, governments, restaurants, landlords, and others.

New York City

New York has been a prime consumer of tobacco ever since the pipe-smoking Dutch defied a 1639 no-smoking edict by WILHEMUS KIEFT, director-general of New Amsterdam from 1637 to 1647, who thought smoking was a waste of time.

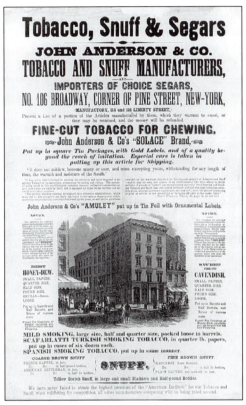

Ad for John Anderson & Co. manufacturer of snuff and tobacco products in New York City. *Library of Congress.*

After the city became English in 1664, the city rivaled Philadelphia in tobacco manufacture, including SNUFF and CIGAR production. These business were of little consequence compared with the mammoth exports of the tidewater planters of the southern colonies.

In 1760, PIERRE LORILLARD, a French Huguenot emigre, established a tobacco business in New York City. (The present-day P. Lorillard Company traces it origins to this beginning.) It was one of only two pre-revolutionary SNUFF MILLS in the colonies to survive British opposition to colonial manufacture.

After the American Revolution, retail tobacco shops added factories to their businesses. During the early 1800s, their principal manufactured product was CHEWING TOBACCO. Later, there was a shift to cigars, pipe tobaccos, and, after 1880, to CIGARETTES. A typical pre–Civil War factory was the nine-story factory, Lilienthal Tobacco and Snuff Manufactory located at "Nos. 217, 219, & 221 Washington and 78, 80, & 82 Barclay Sts." in lower Manhattan. It turned out many types of tobacco products including varieties of chewing and smoking tobacco as well as snuff.

Early in the nineteenth century, an import trade in cigars made of Dutch and German leaf sprang up. New Yorkers, dissatisfied with their quality, began cigar rolling, using better leaf from Connecticut Valley farms. An early rivalry with Philadelphia in snuff was replaced by competition in cigars, both cities using immigrant labor. By the outbreak of the Civil War, Philadelphia was still the leading cigar city. But by 1880, New York produced four times as many cigars as its rival.

New York manufacturers of the 1880s were almost completely uninterested in chewing tobacco. Virtually all their production was in straight smoking tobacco or "fine cut chewing" suitable for either mouth or pipe. Cigarettes were not yet important and cigars were made in hundreds of small shops, not factories.

Despite its prominence in all types of tobacco-making and as the country's distribution headquarters for tobacco, New York's principal contribution to the industry was its selling, not manufacturing, power. The arts of communication were quickly put to commercial use. New York attracted the best-selling talent. As a shipping and manufacturing center, New York was well placed to supply salesmen, especially cigar and cigarette salesmen, with quantities of premiums.

The earliest cigarette manufacturing of any consequence was done by hand in New York shops operated by Greek and Turkish immigrants. One such shop, run by the Bedrossian brothers, blended Virginia Bright tobacco with Turkish leaf in cigarettes at some time before 1870. Another New York City manufacturer, Goodwin and Company, employed Russian immigrants who had experience in London cigarette factories. *See also* CONNECTICUT TOBACCO PRODUCTION; LORILLARD COMPANY INC., TURKISH TOBACCO

Nicot, Jean (c. 1530–1600)

In 1559, Jean Nicot, Lord of Villemain and French ambassador at the Court of Portugal, became interested in the tobacco plant after a kinsman of one of Nicot's staff told him about its medicinal properties. He purchased some tobacco seed in Lisbon and planted it in the garden of the embassy. In a 1560 letter to Cardinal de Lorraine, he wrote about the plant's curative powers: "I have acquired an Indian herb of marvellous and proved worth against the Noli me tangere and fistulas given up as incurable by the physicians. As soon as it gives its seeds, I will send some of them to your gardener at Marmoustier in a barrel with instructions for replanting and cultivating it" (Corina, 1975).

Nicot sent samples of the herb to several people of importance in France, including the Grand Prior of France, and for a while the tobacco was known by the name *Herbe du Grand Prieur.* Returning to France in 1561, Nicot presented some tobacco plants to the queen, Catherine de Medici, and the name of the plant changed to *Herbe de la Reine* or *Herbe Medicea.* After 1570 in Europe, tobacco was named after Nicot himself, *Nicotiana.* Not only was he Europe's first importer of tobacco, he was instrumental in encouraging its use, although ANDRÉ THEVET, a Protestant missionary to Brazil, claimed the distinction of having first introduced tobacco to France.

In 1961, the *Confrèrie de Jean Nicot* was founded in France, a smoker's academy composed of 800 friends of tobacco. Despite this homage to Nicot, no evidence exists that Nicot ever smoked, sniffed, or chewed tobacco.

References: Maurice Corina, *Trust in Tobacco*, New York: St. Martin's Press, 1975, p. 43.

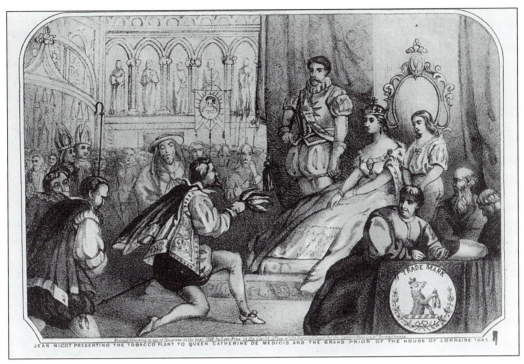

Jean Nicot presents the tobacco plant to French Queen Catherine de Medici. *Library of Congress.*

Nicotiana Attenuata

One of the 60 species of tobacco within the genus *Nicotiana, Nicotiana attenuata* is a species that was used in California and in the Great Basin and to a lesser extent in the Plains and Plateau regions of North America.

Nicotiana Petunoides

The truly wild tobacco, *Nicotiana petunoides,* flourished only in the temperate zones of both North and South America west of the continental divide.

Nicotiana Rustica

One of the 60 species of tobacco within the genus *Nicotiana* in widespread human use, the native tobacco *Nicotiana rustica* grew in the temperate zone east of the Rockies from northern Mexico through southern Canada. Because this plant with small leaves was not wild, it required cultivation.

Prior to European contact, *Nicotina rustica* was the most commonly used species of tobacco by American Indians in the eastern United States, throughout the Great Plains, and in parts of the eastern sub-Arctic. It is believed that this species originated in South America and spread throughout Central America and Mexico to the North American continent. Because of *Nicotiana rustica's* strength and bitterness, it was generally smoked in a pipe, often blended with milder leaves of various plants. This tobacco was gradually replaced by the West Indian variety NICOTIANA TABACUM. *See also* PIPE SMOKING AND NATIVE AMERICANS

Nicotiana Tabacum

Nicotiana tabacum, a plant with large leaves that originated and was extensively grown and used across the upper half of South America and in Central America, is one of 60 species of tobacco within the genus *Nicotiana* within widespread human use. Noted for its rich taste, aroma, and higher potency (i.e., the ability to produce hallucinations and supernatural visions), Central Americans have smoked it for more than 1,500 years. Used at first for personal use, then for trading, this species of tobacco was popularly cultivated for commercial use by Europeans and the rest of the world.

It was reported that *Nicotiana tabacum* was initially too strong for North American Indians and that they preferred *Nicotiana rustica* smoked in a pipe. In 1843, Prince Alexander Philip Maximilian of Wied, who spent much time with the Mandans in the early nineteenth century, reported "The tobacco of the Whites, unmixed, is too strong for the Indians, because [the whites] draw smoke into their lungs; hence [the Indians] do not willingly smoke cigars" (Seig, 1971).

Nicotiana tabacum, the commercial leaf, was transplanted from the Yucatan to Cuba and to Haiti during the 1550s. The transplant of this milder species into the West Indies was more for the convenience of Spanish sailors and slaves than for commercial exploitation. But after the middle of the sixteenth century, the Spanish were trafficking in tobacco, and other Europeans responded by planting tobacco in their own countries. Tobacco cultivation spread to Belgium in 1554, France in 1556, Germany in 1559, the Netherlands in 1561, and England in 1570. The rapid expansion of *Nicotiana tabacum* to the European market proved crucial to the survival of the first American colonies.

In the Chesapeake region, two main types of *Nicotiana tabacum* were cultivated: sweet-scented, which predominated in the James and York River regions, and the orinoco (also spelled oronoko, aronoko, oronoko), which predominated in the Maryland district. *See also* Pipe Smoking and Native Americans

References: Louis Seig, *Tobacco, Peace Pipes, and Indians.* Palmer Lake Co: Filter Press, 1971, p. 18.

Nicotianae

A member of the *Solanaceae,* all tobacco species of the genus *Nicotianae* are kin to peppers, petunias, the deadly nightshades, the poisonous datura, belladonna, as well as eggplants, potatoes, and tomatoes.

Nicotine

Nicotine, an active ingredient in tobacco, belongs to a class of compounds called alkaloids that also includes cocaine and morphine.

Tobacco plants produce nicotine as a toxic chemical defense against insects.

Nicotine is a potent drug that occurs naturally in the leaves of *Nicotiana tabacum*. It is one of the most harmful poisons known. One drop of it in a concentrated state is enough to kill a dog. Eight drops of nicotine will kill a horse in four minutes. One drop of the pure substance placed on a man's tongue will kill him within minutes. Nicotine does not kill the smoker because it is absorbed over a period of time. The body breaks it down and eliminates it in urine. Most cigarettes sold in the United States contain about 8 to 9 milligrams of nicotine. The smoker typically takes in 1 to 2 milligrams per cigarette.

Nicotine is absorbed by the body at remarkable speed. After a smoker inhales smoke, nicotine transfers directly from the tiny air holes in the lungs into the bloodstream. From there inhaled nicotine rushes to the brain in less than 10 seconds and reaches the big toe in 15 to 20 seconds. Since it is also well absorbed through the very thin skin of the nose and mouth, which are dense with capillaries, chewing tobacco and snuff are effective ways to take in nicotine.

Nicotine is an addictive drug. Some experts believe it is the most addictive drug there is—more so than heroin or alcohol. It affects mood, feeling, and behavior by entering the brain and causing some effect. A number of cells in the brain have receptors that are highly sensitive to nicotine. This unique sensitivity causes the drug to provide a real "hit" when it reaches the brain. Repeated exposure to nicotine through smoking results in rapid tolerance. Smokers get used to it and need increasing doses to achieve the "hit." As cigarettes are smoked, the smoker gets less and less of a psychological and physical effect. As the day wears on, and more cigarettes are smoked, people often smoke more out of habit or to avoid discomfort than for pleasure. There seems to be an internal sensing system, like a thermostat, that knows when nicotine levels are too low. Most smokers require a minimum of about 10 cigarettes a day to maintain a so-called comfort zone. If too many cigarettes are smoked, the person may experience nausea and other symptoms of nicotine poisoning. The younger people start smoking cigarettes, the more likely they are to become strongly addicted to nicotine. *See also* CARBON MONOXIDE; CIGARETTE; TAR

References: Institute of Medicine, *Growing Up Tobacco Free: Preventing Nicotine Addiction in Children and Youth*, Washington, D.C., National Academy Press, 1994.

U.S. Surgeon General, *Preventing Tobacco Use Among Young People*. Washington, D.C.: Public Health Service, 1994.

Nicotine Replacement Products

Nicotine replacement products are a major breakthrough in treating smokers who want to ease their nicotine cravings while trying to quit smoking. After 20 years of research, products were developed to provide an alternative and less harmful source of nicotine and alleviate some of the acute symptoms associated with withdrawing from tobacco use—cravings, anxiety, irritability, hunger, restlessness, decreasing concentration, drowsiness, and sleep disturbance. The products enable smokers to taper off gradually or act as a substitute for the nicotine "rush" experienced by smoking a cigarette. The products are now available either over the counter or by prescription.

Nicotine Gum

Once researchers realized that there were other ways to deliver nicotine to the body, they set about looking for ways to administer it in a controlled manner with the goal of reducing its intake. Nicorette®, a nicotine gum, was one of the first replacement products developed. Approved for smoking cessation by the FOOD AND DRUG ADMINISTRATION (FDA) on January 13, 1984, it was first made available by prescription in the United States. When chewed, the gum, which contains nicotine bound to an ion exchange resin, releases small amounts of nicotine that are absorbed through the lining of the mouth. This produces blood levels of nicotine sufficient to help reduce the withdrawal symptoms experienced by many smokers trying to quit smoking.

One advantage of nicotine gum is that it allows the user to control the nicotine doses. The gum can be chewed as needed or on a fixed schedule during the day. With an as-needed schedule, the smoker can chew more nicotine during a craving.

Nicorette gum has not been entirely successful because smokers use the gum improperly, chewing it too quickly and swallowing most of the nicotine. The gum must be chewed slowly and parked against the cheek on and off for about 20 to 30 minutes.

In early 1996, the FDA removed the prescription requirement for Nicorette, manufactured by SmithKline Beecham Consumer Healthcare. Its sale was restricted to people 18 years or older.

Nicotine Patches

The next nicotine replacement product came in 1992 when the nicotine transdermal delivery system, known as the "nicotine patch" was developed. Approved by the Food and Drug Administration, the patch was considered to be the most effective pharmacological agency available to combat CIGARETTE addiction. It was designed to decrease withdrawal symptoms without the shortcomings of the gum.

Patches release a measured dose of nicotine through the skin, where the drug is absorbed into the bloodstream. As the nicotine doses are lowered over a course of weeks, the smoker is weaned away from nicotine. Applied in the morning, patches require little attention while they produce steady serum levels of nicotine over a 16- or 24-hour period. Different types and different strengths of patches are available over the counter.

Nicotine Nasal Spray

A third alternative source of nicotine is the nasal spray, available by prescription only. It delivers nicotine quickly to the bloodstream as it is absorbed through the nose. Smokers squirt it into their nostrils whenever they feel the urge to light a cigarette. The drug is absorbed in five minutes. Nasal spray gives immediate relief of withdrawal symptoms and offers the smoker a sense of control over nicotine cravings.

Nicotine Inhaler

Smokers can inhale nicotine vapor through a nicotine inhaler, a fourth alternative source of nicotine, available by prescription. Resembling a fat plastic cigarette with a plastic mouthpiece, the inhaler provides something for the smoker to hold and satisfies the hand-to-mouth ritual. Absorbed within 15 to 30 minutes, the chemical delivers the sensation smokers get in the back of the throat.

Chewing nicotine gum or using a patch, spray, or inhaler does not provide the satisfaction of smoking a cigarette. But in addition to relieving the physical discomfort of smoking cessation, nicotine replacements offer a health advantage because they are free of TAR, CARBON MONOXIDE, and chemicals—cancer-causing and lung-damaging substances created during the burning process. Also, because replacement products deliver nicotine more slowly, they produce a less intense effect on the heart and blood vessels. *See also* NICOTINE; SMOKING CESSATION; ZYBAN

Night Riders

During the first decade of the twentieth century, the tobacco growers of Tennessee and Kentucky, in an area known as the Black Patch, were receiving low prices for their tobacco, a situation they blamed on the tobacco trust and foreign monopolies. The Dark Tobacco District Planters' Protective Association was organized in Guthroe, Kentucky, in 1906 by 5,000 to 6,000 tenant farmers of the Black Patch region.

The tenant farmers sought remedy by forming cooperative marketing groups that jointly sold their pooled tobacco to manufacturers, tobacco brokers, and overseas agents. Buyers from the AMERICAN TOBACCO COMPANY and foreign monopolies tried to woo with high prices the farmers that did not join the association. Farmers who were aloof or spoke out against the association, known as "Hill Billies," were attacked at night by groups of masked horsemen called the "Night Riders," the militant element of the association.

Eventually, about 10,000 men joined the Night Riders, who organized formally as a secret fraternal order under the name "The Silent Brigade" or "The Inner Circle." Their chief interest was beating up or lynching the non-member farmers, burning their crops, and dynamiting or burning down barns and processing factories that handled non-pool leaf.

The first exhibition of Night Rider power occurred on December 1, 1906, when a small army of masked men captured the town of Princeton, Kentucky, and destroyed two factories. On December 7, 1907, they took Hopkinsville, Kentucky, burning a tobacco factory and large warehouse operated by Italian American independent tobacco dealers. Troops were sent in and local communities organized law-and-order leagues. The Night Riders, who controlled the state courts in the tobacco district, were never convicted. Night Riders, who were most active during 1907 and 1908, saw membership decline by 1909. By 1915, the association was dissolved.

No Net Cost Tobacco Program Act of 1981

The No Net Cost Tobacco Program Act of 1981 substantially revised the provisions of the AGRICULTURAL ADJUSTMENT ACT OF 1938 relating to tobacco. It mandated that loses on the tobacco loan program be paid for by tobacco growers instead of the federal government. Among other things, it made the marketing of tobacco subject to the same penalties that are imposed for selling tobacco in excess of a farm's quota.

The law was the first to authorize owners of flue-cured and Burley tobacco allotments and quotas to sell these rights separately from the farms to which allotments were attached. The allotments and quotas had to be sold to actual producers for use on other farms in the same county. The law also required corporations, utilities, educational and religious institutions, and other entities owning tobacco allotments, but not involved in farming, to sell their allotments or forfeit them. The law required the adjustment of the national average goal for FLUE-CURED TOBACCO in 1983 and at five-year intervals, and also required that producers of dark AIR-CURED

TOBACCO and FIRE-CURED TOBACCO be given in 1983 (and in subsequent years if the agriculture secretary determined that there was sufficient interest) the opportunity in a referendum to choose whether they favor or oppose the establishment of farm marketing quotas on a poundage instead of an acreage allotment basis. *See also* AGRICULTURAL ADJUSTMENT ACT OF 1933; CONSOLIDATED OMNIBUS BUDGET RECONCILIATION ACT (COBRA) OF 1995; DAIRY AND TOBACCO ADJUSTMENT ACT; OMNIBUS BUDGET RECONCILIATION ACT (OBRA) OF 1993; SOIL CONSERVATION AND DOMESTIC ALLOTMENT ACT

Nonsmokers' Rights Movement

In the 1970s, the nonsmokers' rights movement emerged at the state and local levels. The goal of the movement was to protect nonsmokers from the effects of tobacco smoke by restricting smoking in public places. *See also* ANTI-TOBACCO MOVEMENTS, UNITED STATES; ENVIRONMENTAL TOBACCO SMOKE (ETS); STEINFELD, JESSE

Northwest Airlines

As of April 23, 1988, Northwest Airlines announced it would become the first airline to voluntarily ban smoking on all its domestic flights in North America regardless of length. The decision was based on marketing surveys that showed the overwhelming majority of the passengers were in favor of an end to smoking on flights. *See also* ANTI-TOBACCO MOVEMENTS, UNITED STATES

Novelli, Bill (1942–)

President, until 1999, of the Washington, D.C.-based NATIONAL CENTER FOR TOBACCO-FREE KIDS, a privately funded organization established in 1996 to focus the nation's attention and action on reducing tobacco use among children, Bill Novelli began his career as a Rinso salesman. From there, he made his way to the New York office of Lever Brothers, a package goods marketing company, where he became product manager. After a stint in a Manhattan advertising agency and working on President Richard Nixon's 1972 reelection campaign, he linked up with Jack Porter to found their own public relations agency, Porter/Novelli, the fourth largest public relations firm in the United States. The firm, founded to apply marketing to social and health issues, was named the best public relations agency in America for 1995 by the industry's leading trade publication. In 1990, Novelli retired from Porter/Novelli and launched a career as executive vice president of CARE, the international relief and development organization.

Then, in 1995, he began working with the Robert Wood Johnson Foundation (RWJF), the AMERICAN MEDICAL ASSOCIATION, the AMERICAN CANCER SOCIETY, and others to found a tobacco-control coalition to help the FOOD AND DRUG ADMINISTRATION assert its jurisdiction over tobacco. In 1996, the RWJF committed up to $20 million for a five-year period for a project that was named the NATIONAL CENTER FOR TOBACCO-FREE KIDS.

Novelli holds a B.A. and M.A. in communications from the University of Pennsylvania and pursued doctoral studies at New York University. He taught marketing management for 10 years in the University of Maryland's M.B.A. program and also taught health communications there. He taught social marketing in the School of Public Health at Emory University. *See also* MYERS, MATTHEW

O

Ochsner, Alton (1896–1981)

Renowned thoracic surgeon and medical teacher, Dr. Alton Ochsner [1896–1981] was named chairman of surgery at Tulane University at the age of 30. He first became interested in the causes of lung cancer in the 1930s and made a presentation to the Clinical Congress of the American College of Surgeons in 1938 in which he said that "the increase in smoking with the universal custom of inhaling is probably a responsible factor in the case of lung cancer" (Wagner, 1971, p. 103).

Dr. Ochsner persisted in the belief that cigarette smoking was the principal cause of the growing epidemic of lung cancer, a theory he publicized throughout the 1940s in the face of ridicule and attacks even from within the medical profession. On October 23, 1945, at Duke University, he stated, "there is a distinct parallelism between the incidence of cancer of the lung and the sale of cigarettes, and it is our belief that the increase is due to the increased incidence of smoking and that smoking is a factor because of the chronic irritation that it produces" (Wagner, 1971, pp. 70–71).

In 1951, at the annual meeting of the AMERICAN MEDICAL ASSOCIATION, Dr. Ochsner said: "It is frightening to speculate on the possible number of bronchogenic cancers that may develop because of the tremendous numbers of cigarettes consumed in the two decades from 1939 to 1950" (Wagner, 1971, p. 104). By 1952, Dr. Ochsner; Michael deBakey, a famous heart surgeon; and two other colleagues wrote in the *Journal of the American Medical Association (JAMA)* that "There is a distinct parallelism between the sale of cigarettes and the incidence of bronchogenic carcinoma" (Blum, 1983). They predicted the death rate from lung cancer would escalate as long as smoking continued to exist and that lung cancer would be the leading cause of death from cancer. So controversial was Ochsner that prior to his appearance on "Meet the Press" in the mid-1950s, he was told he could not mention on air the causal relationship between cigarette smoking and lung cancer. In the 1960s and 1970s, Ochsner pointed out that cigarette-related deaths from heart attack and emphysema would outnumber those from lung cancer.

Besides criticizing insurance companies for not giving preferential rates to nonsmokers, Ochsner debunked the government's research effort to develop a SAFE CIGARETTE. Whenever Dr. Ochsner was asked if FILTERED CIGARETTES had any value, he would reply: "Yes, for the tobacco industry. They help sell more cigarettes."

Dr. Ochsner testified in the 1960 FRANK LARTIGUE case that he examined the autopsy report and concluded the husband of the plaintiff (Mrs. Lartigue) had died of epidermoid cancer caused by smoking. During the hour he was questioned on his qualifications, it was brought out that he had seen about 2,000 lung-cancer patients and operated on half that amount, the other cases far too advanced for surgery to make any difference. He testified that more than 400 of his scientific papers had been published, 50 of which dealt with lung cancer. In 1964, Dr. Ochsner also authored a book entitled *Smoking and Your Life.*

References: Alan Blum, M.D., "Alton Ochsner, MD, 1896–1981," *New York State Journal of Medicine*, December 1983, p. 1251.

Susan Wagner, *Cigarette Country: Tobacco in American History and Politics*, New York, Praeger Publishers, 1971, pp. 70–71, 103–04.

Office on Smoking and Health (OSH)

The Office on Smoking and Health (OSH), located in Atlanta, Georgia, is a focal point for the U.S. DEPARTMENT OF HEALTH AND HUMAN SERVICES smoking and health activities. It is a division of the National Center for Chronic Disease Prevention and Health Promotion, CENTERS FOR DISEASE CONTROL AND PREVENTION (CDC), PUBLIC HEALTH SERVICE, U.S. Department of Health and Human Services. Since 1986, when OSH became part of the CDC, it has targeted tobacco-related diseases, the nation's primary preventable health problems.

OSH develops and distributes the annual surgeon general's report on the health consequences of smoking, coordinates a national public information and education program on tobacco use and health, and coordinates tobacco education and research efforts. OSH distributes information about the health risks of smoking and how to stop smoking in a variety of forms including brochures, pamphlets, posters, scientific reports, and public service announcements. It keeps track of smoking-related deaths each year and epidemiological information on who smokes, broken down by age, income, and race. It serves as a WORLD HEALTH ORGANIZATION (WHO) collaborating center for tobacco and health and collaborates with CDC's toxicology laboratory on the analysis of tobacco

products. OSH provides financial assistance to 32 state health departments, the District of Columbia, and eight national organizations. It puts out the *Smoking and Health Bulletin,* a quarterly.

The predecessor of OSH was the NATIONAL CLEARINGHOUSE FOR SMOKING AND HEALTH created by the U.S. Congress when it passed the FEDERAL CIGARETTE LABELING AND ADVERTISING ACT OF 1965. *See also MORBIDITY AND MORTALITY WEEKLY REPORT (MMWR)*; SURGEON GENERAL'S REPORTS, 1964–1998

Old Gold Cigarettes

In 1942, P. Lorillard launched an advertising campaign claiming that Old Gold cigarettes contained less NICOTINE and TAR than six competing brands. The claim was based on an article in *Reader's Digest* that showed, on the basis of laboratory tests, that Old Gold cigarettes had a trace less nicotine and tar, an insignificant difference. The *Digest* article concluded: "The differences between brands, are, practically speaking, small, and no single brand is so superior to its competitors as to justify its selection on the ground that it is less harmful" (Littell, 1942). Nevertheless, Lorillard launched a mammoth campaign urging readers to buy "this highly respected magazine" and see for themselves how Old Golds did in the test.

After several years, the FEDERAL TRADE COMMISSION (FTC) ordered Lorillard to cease and desist "from representing by any means directly or indirectly" that Old Gold cigarettes or the smoke from them contained less nicotine, tars, and resins and were less irritating to the throat than six other leading brands.

Lorillard appealed the FTC order to the Fourth Circuit Court of Appeals, basing its defense on a claim that it reported truthfully what the *Reader's Digest* article said. The court, however, did not agree:

An examination of the advertisements . . . shows a perversion of the meaning of the *Reader's Digest* article which does little credit to the company's advertising department—a perversion which results in the use of the truth in such a way as to cause the reader to believe the exact opposite of what was intended by the writer of the article . . . .

The table referred to in the article was inserted for the express purpose of showing the insignificance of the difference in the nicotine and tar content of the smoke from the various brands of cigarettes . . . . The company proceeded to advertise this difference as though it had received a citation for public service instead of a castigation from the *Reader's Digest* . . . . ("Old Golds Lose," 1951)

The court faulted Lorillard for not printing all of what the *Digest* said, but rather for printing

a small part thereof in such a way as to create an entirely false and misleading impression . . . . To tell less than the whole truth is a well-known method of deception; and he who deceives by resorting to such method cannot excuse the deception

by relying on the truthfulness per se of the partial truth by which it has been accomplished. ("Old Golds Lose," 1951)

See also LORILLARD COMPANY INC.

References: Robert Littell, Cigarette Ad Fact and Fiction," *Reader's Digest*, vol. 41, July 1942, p. 5.

"Old Golds Lose a Court Battle," *Consumer Reports*, April 1951, pp. 187–88.

Old Joe Camel

Old Joe Camel, one of the most controversial—and oldest—images in cigarette advertising, first appeared in 1913. R.J. REYNOLDS TOBACCO COMPANY had introduced CAMEL CIGARETTES, a new brand of cigarettes that featured a "modern" blend of home-grown and Turkish tobaccos. The company chose the name "Camel" to suggest the Middle Eastern origin of the tobacco leaf. Just as R.J. Reynolds package designers were looking around for a model of a camel to copy for

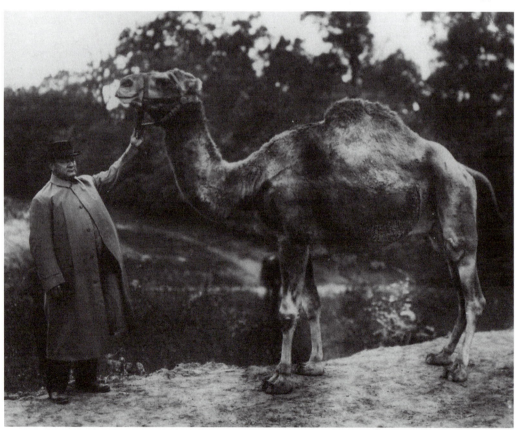

"Old Joe," a Barnum & Bailey circus camel, supplied the likeness on packs of Camel cigarettes, which were introduced by R.J. Reynolds Tobacco Company in 1913, the year this photo was taken. *AP/Wide World Photos.*

the package, the Barnum and Bailey Circus came to Winston-Salem, North Carolina, the home of R.J. Reynolds. One of the stars of the circus was "Old Joe," a one-humped camel from Arabia. After a tobacco company employee took a photo of the camel, a package designer used its likeness to make a drawing for the cigarette pack. Old Joe's profile has been featured on every pack of Camels ever since.

In 1974, the modern Old Joe, also known as Joe Camel, was born when Nicholas Price, a British illustrator for a French advertising campaign depicted his head bursting through a pack of unfiltered Camels in a French poster. The caricature had a face dominated by an enormous nose. Over the next decade, Old Joe appeared in promotions around the world. Then in 1987, when Reynolds was redoing Camel's image in cigarette advertising, it pitched him with the slogan "Smooth Character," and dressed the camel in a suit and sunglasses.

In 1988, in materials created by Trone Advertising in Greensboro, North Carolina, for the 75th anniversary of the Camel brand, RJR Nabisco launched the "smooth character" advertising campaign featuring "Old Joe," a cartoon James Bond–like camel. McCann-Erickson in New York came up with the first ads featuring Old Joe Camel, with the theme "75 years and still smokin'!" The character's appeal led Reynolds to make it the focal point of all Camel advertising campaigns, under the theme "Smooth Character."

Old Joe and his cronies appeared in T-shirts, leather jackets, sunglasses, and other garb. The character appeared in ads, catalogs, and on promotional merchandise like caps and lighters even when the account switched from McCann-Erickson to Young and Rubicam Advertising to Mezzina/Brown, both located in New York.

R.J. Reynolds built on the Joe Camel campaign in 1991 with the "Camel Cash" promotion, offering coupons resembling $1 bills in every pack of filtered Camel cigarettes. These "Camel C-notes" pictured Joe Camel, in sunglasses and smoking, dressed as George Washington. Consumers could redeem Camel Cash for "smooth stuff" like flip-flops, insulators for beverage cans, jackets, towels, T-shirts, and hats that all featured images of Joe Camel.

Health professionals who worried that "Old Joe" caught the attention of children began to do research. A landmark study by Dr. PAUL FISCHER in the December 11, 1991, issue of the *Journal of the American Medical Association (JAMA)* showed that 30 percent of three-year-olds correctly matched the "Old Joe" cartoon camel with a picture of a CIGARETTE. The study also showed that 91 percent of six-year-olds recognized "Old Joe." The cartoon camel was as familiar to the six-year-olds as the Mickey Mouse silhouette.

After the "Old Joe" cartoon character was introduced in 1988, the number of teens who started smoking Camels jumped dramatically. The proportion of smokers under 18 years of age who chose Camels rose from 0.5 percent to 32.8 percent, according to data supplied by a coalition of health groups. Among smokers aged 18 to 24, Camel's share rose from 4.4 percent to 7.9 percent. R.J. Reynolds insisted that the camel mascot was used only to entice adult smokers to switch brands. But according to researcher JOSEPH DIFRANZA, whose study also appeared in the December 1991 *JAMA*, a survey of high school students showed they were far more likely than adults to recognize Camel ads. When teenagers were shown the Old Joe Camel ads, 98 percent correctly identified the brand, compared with only 67 percent of adults. A 1998 study by the CENTERS FOR DISEASE CONTROL AND PREVENTION said the number of youngsters who took up smoking as a daily habit jumped 73 percent between Joe Camel's debut in 1988 and 1996.

In 1992, Surgeon General Antonia Novello called on Reynolds to withdraw the Joe Camel campaign. In 1993, the FEDERAL TRADE COMMISSION (FTC) staff recommended banning Joe Camel ads because they appealed to children. The full FTC rejected the recommendation in 1994, but on May 28, 1997, the FTC filed a complaint that the Joe Camel campaign illegally promoted cigarettes to minors. R.J. Reynolds retired Joe Camel from its domestic marketing in July 1997. *See also* FEDERAL TRADE COMMISSION; FEDERAL TRADE COMMISSION (FTC) AND JOE CAMEL ADVERTISING; TURKISH TOBACCO

Olmstead, Frederick Law (1822–1903)

Frederick Law Olmstead, a journalist vigorously opposed to slavery and known as the father of American landscape architecture, took a 14-month journey through the southeastern states. He reported on "the influence of Slavery as a mode of employing labor, on the development of the general resources of the South." He wrote approximately 50 long letters about life in the South that were published in the *New York Times*. His observations were also published in an edited and expanded version of his earlier *Times* articles. *A Journey in the Seaboard Slave States with Remarks on Their Economy* (1856) contained a description of a Virginia tobacco plantation. The following excerpt deals with a plantation owner whose land is wearing out from cultivating tobacco, but who feels the crop returns enough money for the "negroe labor" to make it worthwhile.

> Mr. W was one of the few large planters of his vicinity who still made the culture of tobacco their principal business. He said there was a general prejudice against tobacco in all the tidewater region of the State, because it was through the culture of tobacco that the once fertile soils had been impoverished; but he did not believe that, at the present value of negroes, their labor could be applied to the culture of grain with any profit, except under peculiarly favorable circumstances. Possibly the use of guano might make wheat a paying crop, but he still doubted. He had not used it himself. Tobacco required fresh land, and was rapidly exhausting, but it returned more money for the labor used upon it than anything else, enough more, in his opinion, to pay for the wearing out of the land. If he was well paid for it, he did not know why he should not wear out his land.
>
> His tobacco-fields were nearly all in a distant and lower part of his plantation;

land which had been neglected before his time in a great measure, because it had been sometimes flooded, and was, much of the year, too wet for cultivation. He was draining and clearing it, and it now brought good crops.

> He had an Irish gang training for him, by contract. He thought a negro could do twice as much work in a day as an Irishman. He had not stood over them and seen them at work, but judged entirely from the amount they accomplished: he thought a good gang of negroes would have got on twice as fast. He was sure they must have "trifled" a great deal, or they would have accomplished more than they had. He complained much, also, of their sprees and quarrels. I asked why he should employ Irishmen, in preference to doing the work with his own hands. "It's dangerous work, and a negro's life is too valuable to be risked at it. If a negro dies, it's a considerable loss, you know." (Olmstead, 1959)

References: Frederick Law Olmsted, *The Slave States*, edited by Harvey Wish, New York: Capricorn Books, 1959, p. 19.

Olympic Games of Calgary, Canada (1988)

The 15th Winter Olympic Games held in Calgary, Canada, in 1988 were the first to have a smoke-free program. The objectives of this program were to protect athletes, officials, and spectators from secondhand tobacco smoke; to enhance the dignity and healthy image of the games by ensuring that there was no connection with tobacco; and to promote the idea of a smoke-free life.

Under the provisions of the Olympic Charter, tobacco promotion was not allowed at the Olympic venues or on "equipment used in the Olympic Games nor on the uniforms or numbers worn by contestants or officials." After a letter-writing campaign was organized by health groups, the chairman of the Olympic Organizing Committee (OOC) received over 60 letters from Canada, Europe, and the United States supporting a program free of any connection with tobacco.

The final program included a ban on tobacco advertising and sponsorship, smoking permitted in designated areas, information packages and press releases sent to all participating countries, extensive use of the red and green international no-smoking signs, monitoring of both no-smoking and smoking spaces by evaluation teams, and education programs for the community.

The clean air policy applied to the three Olympic villages housing athletes and support staff; all transportation operated by the OOC, as well as all waiting areas at ski vents and access lifts to and within sports facilities; medical facilities under the direction of the medical service program; Olympic venues near competition areas except in designated smoking areas; all restaurants serving athletes, coaches, and officials; bars with separate smoking areas; and press centers and lodges with designated smoking areas.

The policy was popular with athletes. Of 262 athletes and coaches who responded to a survey, an overwhelming majority favored the policies to restrict smoking. Two-thirds of those surveyed said they had been bothered by tobacco smoke at other athletic events. Of the spectators interviewed, 71 percent said they were nonsmokers, but 87 percent agreed the policy was appropriate. Of the 825 staff and volunteers who were interviewed, 70 percent agreed with the restrictions. *See also* SECONDHAND SMOKE

Olympic Games of Lillehammer, Norway (1994)

An ingrained smoking culture exists in politics and sport in Norway, so a campaign to arrange a smoke-free Olympics at Lillehammer, Norway, in 1994 took more than two years. A petition calling for a smoke-free Olympics was signed by the top people in the environment and public health administration, chief municipal executives in the five Olympic municipalities, and the heads of almost 30 Norwegian voluntary health agencies. The petition demanded that the indoor Olympic arenas should be smoke free, Olympic staff should not smoke on duty, spectators should be encouraged not to smoke at outdoor arenas, and tobacco articles should not be sold at Olympic arenas. The petition

also recalled that Norwegian law bans all tobacco advertisements and requires working areas and meeting rooms, and premises and means of transport frequented by the general public to be smoke free.

The petition was handed over to the president of LOOC (the Olympic organization) at a press conference one year before the games were due to be held. Speed skater Johann Olav Koss promised the journalists four new world speed-skating records if the indoor arena in Hamar was declared completely smoke free.

An agreement was signed at a press conference in the National Sports Center in Oslo to underscore the connection with the athletes. Posters with the Olympic mascot and the smoke-free slogan in six languages underscored the international aspect of the campaign. The LOOC stated that it had been the most smoke-free Olympics to date.

Omnibus Budget Reconciliation Act (OBRA) of 1993

Section 1106, "Tobacco Program," of Title 1 of the Omnibus Budget Reconciliation Act (OBRA) of 1993, Public Law 103-66 of August 10, 1993, amended the AGRICULTURAL ADJUSTMENT ACT OF 1938 by requiring a domestic manufacturer of cigarettes to use at least 75 percent U.S. grown tobacco (flue-cured and Burley) in their cigarettes during each calendar year whether for domestic consumption or for export.

If a domestic manufacturer failed to certify to the agriculture secretary the percentage of U.S. tobacco used to produce cigarettes, the manufacturer was presumed to have used only imported tobacco in manufacturing cigarettes and was subject to penalties. The penalties could be waived during natural disasters or because of low reserve stocks.

The law gave the agriculture secretary and Office of Inspector General the power to examine records, books, and other materials of manufacturers of domestic cigarettes to ensure compliance with the law. If drought, insect, or disease infestation, or other natural disaster beyond the control of producers substantially reduced a crop of burley or flue-cured tobacco, and pool inventories for the kind of tobacco involved were depleted as well, the law allowed the secretary of agriculture to reduce the minimum percentage of domestic tobacco to a percentage below 75 percent. *See also* AGRICULTURAL ADJUSTMENT ACT OF 1933; AGRICULTURAL TOBACCO POLICY OF THE U.S. GOVERNMENT; BURLEY TOBACCO; CONSOLIDATED OMNIBUS BUDGET RECONCILIATION ACT (COBRA) OF 1995; DAIRY AND TOBACCO ADJUSTMENT ACT; FLUE-CURED TOBACCO; NO NET COST TOBACCO PROGRAM ACT; SOIL CONSERVATION AND DOMESTIC ALLOTMENT ACT

Oral Health America (OHA)—National Spit Tobacco Education Program (NSTEP)

The National Spit Tobacco Education Program (NSTEP) is administered by Oral Health America (OHA), a national nonprofit organization headquartered in New York City. NSTEP, a public education anti-spit tobacco initiative, is dedicated to promoting oral health and educating youth, parents, and coaches about oral cancer prevention and the dangers of spit tobacco use.

Following the unprecedented success of NSTEP's first two years of existence, the Princeton, New Jersey-based Robert Wood Johnson Foundation (the nation's largest philanthropy devoted to health and health care) awarded in 1996 a three-year grant to OHA. According to Dr. Stephen Corbin, a former chief of staff to the U.S. Surgeon General, "The combined and pooled efforts of NSTEP with the baseball community, tobacco control groups, and members of the Oral Health 2000 Consortium have created an alliance unique in the history of public health in the United States" (Oral Health America, 1997).

Through NSTEP, OHA has forged a special relationship with baseball—from Major League baseball down to Little League. Hall of Fame broadcaster Joe Garagiola, all-time home run and RBI hitter Hank Aaron, and

1994 National and American League Most Valuable Players Jeff Bagwell and Frank Thomas, among others, have lent their names and support to NSTEP's goals.

As a result of the Robert Wood Johnson Foundation's support during the 1997 Major League baseball season, every fan who attended a game, read a game program, listened to a game on radio, or watched one on television encountered a message from NSTEP. All-Stars like Lenny Dykstra, Alex Rodriguez, Paul Moliter, and the Peanuts Gang delivered a message warning of the dangers of spit and emphasizing prevention and cessation.

References: Oral Health America, Press Release, July 17, 1997, p. 1.

"Oriental" Tobaccos

For years, tobacco manufacturers have used names of "Oriental" tobaccos to increase the mystique of their blends. Oriental tobaccos are identified by the topographical areas in which they are grown. The regions that supply American and English manufacturers with the "Oriental" tobaccos are Western Turkey, where Smyrna tobacco is grown in the vicinity of Izmir; Cyprus, where Smyrna is also grown; North-Central Turkey, where Samsun-Bafra tobacco is grown; Thrace, where Xanthian leaf is grown; and Macedonia, where a medium-bodied tobacco is grown.

Latakia and Périque are categorized as condiment, or flavoring tobaccos. Latakia, with the richest and most pungent aroma of all tobaccos used in blending, gets its name from the Syrian port of Al Ladhiqiyah. Today, Latakia comes from Cyprus. Périque, unique to the St. James Parish of Louisiana, was perfected by a French colonist, Pierre Chemot. Chemot observed Choctaw and Chickasaw Indians of Louisiana pressing local tobacco leaves in logs to release their natural juices in which they steeped; he developed the fragrant tobacco to which he gave his nickname, Périque.

In the 1800s and early 1900s, Périque was used to a large extent in chewing tobaccos, cigarettes, and some smoking mixtures. Its major role is in high-grade pipe mixtures.

Orinoco. *See* NICOTIANA TABACUM

Osteen, William L. (1931–)

On April 25, 1997, Federal District Court Judge William L. Osteen dealt tobacco companies their biggest legal blow when he ruled that the FOOD AND DRUG ADMINISTRATION (FDA) had jurisdiction under the FOOD, DRUG, AND COSMETIC ACT OF 1938 to regulate NICOTINE-containing CIGARETTES and SMOKELESS TOBACCO. The judge rejected industry arguments that the FDA lacked congressional authorization to regulate cigarettes and that tobacco did not fit the agency's definition of a "drug" or "medical device." But Judge Osteen also ruled that the agency exceeded its power when it ordered the tobacco industry to curtail advertising intended for minors. The decision left in effect the agency's separate new rules to restrict actual sales to minors, including a national ban on tobacco sales to anyone younger than 18.

After President Bill Clinton's August 1995 news conference empowering the FDA to regulate cigarettes and smokeless tobacco, the nation's five biggest tobacco companies filed a lawsuit to block the proposals in Federal District Court in Greensboro, North Carolina, the heart of tobacco country. The companies contended that the FDA had no jurisdiction over these tobacco products, When Judge Osteen was assigned to decide the tobacco industry's legal challenge, tobacco control activists were angry because they insisted he would not give the issue a fair hearing. In 1974, Osteen, then a private attorney in Greensboro, worked as a paid lobbyist for a group of North Carolina tobacco farmers. The farmers hired him to go to Washington, D.C., to lobby Secretary of Agriculture Earl Butz not to proceed with a plan to scrap the federal tobacco production/ quota program. As a federal judge, Osteen ruled that tobacco companies had legal standing to bring a lawsuit challenging the Environmental Protection Agency's 1993 classification of SECONDHAND SMOKE as a carcinogen.

Judge Osteen, who grew up on a farm outside Greensboro and attended high school and college in the area, received his law degree from the University of North Carolina. A staunch Republican, he was elected in 1960 to the state general assembly; he was the first Republican to hold elective office in Greensboro's Guilford County since the Depression. He quit the legislature in 1964, and in 1968 he ran unsuccessfully for Congress. In 1969, President Richard Nixon appointed him U.S. attorney for the middle district of North Carolina. In 1973, Judge Osteen returned to private practice until his 1991 appointment to the bench.

The tobacco industry challenged the FDA's bid to regulate cigarettes and Judge Osteen's ruling was overturned on August 14, 1998, by the U.S. Court of Appeals for the Fourth Circuit in RICHMOND, VIRGINIA. *See also* FOOD AND DRUG ADMINISTRATION (FDA) REGULATIONS: FEDERAL DISTRICT COURT RULING; FOOD AND DRUG ADMINISTRATION (FDA) REGULATIONS : U.S. COURT OF APPEALS FOR THE FOURTH CIRCUIT

Oviedo, Gonzalo Fernandez de (1478–1557)

In his 21-volume work *General and Natural History of the Indies,* published from 1526 to 1535, Spanish chronicler Gonzalo Fernandez de Oviedo described native use of tobacco as follows:

> Among other evil practices, the Indians have one habit especially harmful: the inhaling of a certain kind of smoke which they call tobacco, in order to produce a state of stupor. The *caciques* [Indian chiefs] employed a tube shaped like a Y, inserting the forked extremities in their nostrils and the tube itself [filled] with the lighted weed; in this way they would inhale the smoke until they became unconscious and lay sprawling on the ground like men in a drunken slumber. Those who could not procure the right sort of pipe took their smoke through a hollow reed; and this is what the Indians call *tabaco,*

not the weed nor its effect, as some have supposed. (Infante, 1985)

Oviedo, the first European to give a record of tobacco being planted, finished his description of tobacco by observing: "They [the Indians] prize their herb very highly and plant it in their orchards or on their farms for the above-mentioned purpose."

References: G. Cabera Infante, *Holy Smoke*, London: Faber and Faber, 1985, pp. 10–11.

P

Pall Mall Cigarettes

When GEORGE WASHINGTON HILL managed Butler-Butler Inc., a subsidiary of AMERICAN TOBACCO COMPANY (ATC) manufacturing various tobacco products, he made up his mind that the CIGARETTE was the future of the tobacco business. He persuaded his father, PERCIVAL SMITH HILL, who headed American Tobacco, to let him concentrate on Pall Mall. The cigarette brand is a Turkish blend with a sophisticated constituency and the firm's leading brand. Hill turned it into a money maker with dealer displays, advertising on magazine back covers, and the first of many slogans: "a shilling in London, a quarter here."

In 1939, the American Tobacco Company relaunched Pall Mall cigarettes with a new blend of tobaccos. Most of the Turkish leaf was eliminated and replaced with bright and flavored Burley. Pall Mall was lengthened to a king-sized brand, a length of 85 mm, 15 mm longer than a standard cigarette. *See also* BRIGHT TOBACCO; BURLEY TOBACCO; TURKISH TOBACCO

Palmer v. Liggett Group

An example of a cigarette case litigated during the second wave of tobacco litigation (1983–1992) was the case of *Palmer v. Liggett Group*. It was argued under the theory of failure to warn.

Joseph C. Palmer (1931–1980) died at the age of 49, allegedly from lung cancer. He had smoked three or four packs of Liggett's cigarettes per day until his death. On August 19, 1983, Ann M. Palmer, individually and as administrator of the estate of her late husband, and her mother-in-law, Daphne S. Palmer, filed a suit in the U.S. District Court for the District of Massachusetts. The Palmers contended that liability should be imposed on Liggett because of the inadequacy of the warning label on Liggett's cigarette packs and advertisements. They complained that the tobacco company negligently gave inadequate warnings about the dangers of cigarette smoking and that this negligence caused Palmer's death.

Liggett filed a motion to dismiss all inadequate warning claims on the grounds that they were preempted by the FEDERAL CIGARETTE LABELING AND ADVERTISING ACT OF 1965. After reviewing the record, the judge denied Liggett's motion to dismiss. The court noted Congress's express purpose in enacting the act was to strike a balance between a concern for national health and protection of trade and commerce in the tobacco industry. The court looked to this congressional intent and found the 1965 act preempted the plaintiff's suit. *See also* HEALTH WARNINGS ON CIGARETTE PACKS AND ADVERTISEMENTS AND SMOKELESS TOBACCO; LIGGETT AND MYERS TOBACCO COMPANY; TOBACCO LITIGATION: FIRST, SECOND, AND THIRD WAVES

Panama

Tobacco has been grown in Panama for centuries. The country's tobacco is grown mostly on small farms in the northern province of Chiriquí. Farmers grow many varieties including BURLEY TOBACCO, creole type, Sumatra, and Copán.

Growers sell approximately 95 percent of their crop to several cigarette manufacturing companies operating in Panama, two of which are controlled by multinational tobacco companies. Tabacalera Nacional S.A. is controlled by PHILIP MORRIS USA and Tabacalera Istmeña is a subsidiary of BRITISH-AMERICAN TOBACCO COMPANY LTD. Panamá Cigar has both domestic and foreign backing and produces mainly dark tobacco for cigars.

Panetela. *See* CIGAR SIZE AND SHAPE

Parson's Cause

From the early days of settlement, the services of the clergy in Virginia (and Maryland and some other southern colonies) were paid for in tobacco. By the early eighteenth century, Virginia clergymen received 16,000 pounds of tobacco annually as salary. When tobacco became scarce in 1755 because of a drought, Virginia law passed the Option Act allowing payment in money or tobacco at the rate of two pence per pound. The legislation, reenacted in 1758, became known as the "Two Penny Act." Because the drought caused a scarcity of tobacco with a resultant rise in market price, all creditors, especially clergy, wanted to be paid in tobacco, not currency.

The clergymen resisted and obtained an Order of Council from the Crown declaring the Two Penny Act null and void. Some of the clergy brought suit against Virginia for their "losses," the difference between two pence per pound and the higher market price. A famous case, known as the Parson's Cause, followed during which 27-year-old lawyer Patrick Henry successfully defended the Two Penny Act against the plaintiff, Reverend James Maury. Henry based his argument on the right of Virginia to manage its own affairs and pay clergy cash instead of tobacco, a right not recognized by the British king.

Partagas Cigar

The oldest CIGAR brand still being manufactured today and the second largest premium cigar sold in the United States, the Partagas cigar was "born" in 1843 in CUBA when Don Jaime Partagas put his family name on each cigar made in the Royal Partagas Cigar Factory. The factory that manufactured these cigars from tobacco grown in the VUELTA ABAJO and Semi Vuelta was built in 1827 in the heart of Havana's Old Town. Although it is a commonly accepted fact that the factory began manufacturing cigars in 1843, the cigars manufactured today by General Cigar have "1845" on the label, and a sign on the Habanos-owned factory that makes Partagas cigars in Cuba also reads "1845."

Almost 30 years after Don Jaime Partagas died in 1861, the factory was purchased by Don Ramon Cifuentes, the head of a prominent Cuban family who controlled the factory up until the Cuban revolution. In 1959, the Cifuentes family and all other families who owned large tobacco factories fled Cuba for the DOMINICAN REPUBLIC. Ramon, the grandson of the man who bought the factory in 1889, eventually went to the United States and entered into a joint venture with General Cigar to market and distribute the Partagas cigars he manufactured.

Both the Partagas company in Cuba, operated by the Cuban government's tobacco monopoly Habanos S.A., and the General Cigar company hosted galas in honor of the 150th anniversary of the Partagas cigar with each company producing an Aniversario cigar. At the Habanos party, held in mid-September, 1995, in New Havana, Cuba, dignitaries, celebrities, Habanos distributors, and journalists from around the world attended. An auction of HUMIDORS filled with 150 limited-edition Partagas Aniversario cigars signed twice by Fidel Castro raised thousands for the Cuban Medical Fund. *See also* CUBAN TOBACCO HISTORY

Pearl, Raymond (1879–1940)

In his article entitled "Tobacco Smoking and Smoking" published in the March 4, 1938, issue of *Science*, Professor Raymond Pearl, an eminent scientist and professor of biological statistics at Johns Hopkins University, made a pioneering statistical study of the effect of smoking on life span. He reported that heavy smokers (who smoke more than 10 cigarettes a day) did not live as long as light smokers and that nonsmokers outlived both. He concluded that "Smoking is associated with a definite impairment of longevity" (Kluger, 1996).

Time magazine reported Professor Pearl's findings and suggested they would "make tobacco users' flesh creep." Most major newspapers refused to publish the findings and others buried the Pearl report in places where people barely noticed it. According to George Seldes, an ex-newspaper man, articles about Pearl's study ran in small-town papers, while large metropolitan newspapers ducked the report because they depended on tobacco advertising.

References: Richard Kluger, *Ashes to Ashes*, New York, Alfred A. Knopf, 1996, p. 106.

Périque. *See* "Oriental" Tobaccos

Perkins, Frances (1880–1965)

Frances Perkins became the first woman to serve in a presidential cabinet when President Franklin Delano Roosevelt appointed her secretary of labor. She served in that position from 1933 to 1945. Before she took that position, Perkins had investigated the horrible conditions under which women and children worked. She never forgot the tragic fire in 1911 at the Triangle Shirtwaist Company in New York City. Locked inside and unable to escape the blaze, 147 women and girls died.

Perkins especially detested CIGARETTES because they were known to cause the most fires in the United States. She blamed department stores for allowing women to smoke while they shopped. And she blamed women for flicking ashes around flimsy dresses that could easily ignite. She vented her feelings about women smoking in an article published in the May 7, 1930, issue of the *New Republic*.

> The most common cause of fire of all classes in the United States is cigarettes. Our carelessness with them is proverbial and, now that women are smoking, the big mercantile establishments which have heretofore been free of great disasters in this country are subject to a new hazard. (Perkins, 1930)

References: Frances Perkins, "Can They Smoke Like Gentlemen?" *New Republic*, May 7, 1930, p. 320.

Pertschuk, Michael (1933–)

Codirector of the ADVOCACY INSTITUTE, headquartered in Washington, D.C., Michael Pertschuk, has practiced, written about, counseled, strategized, and taught public interest advocacy. Born in London, England, he received his bachelor's and law degrees from Yale University. He has taught law at Georgetown Law Center, American University Law School, and New York University Law School.

From 1965 to 1977, Pertschuk acted first as staff counsel and then as chief counsel and staff director of the Senate Commerce Committee, which "chaperoned" the first cigarette labeling bill through Congress in 1965. Pertschuk helped guide landmark consumer protection legislation through Congress, including the broadcast ban on CIGARETTE advertising. He also was an assistant to anti-tobacco fighter Senator MAURINE B. NEUBERGER.

Pertschuk was appointed chairman of the FEDERAL TRADE COMMISSION (FTC) by President Jimmy Carter in March 1977. In his first days at the FTC, one of his top priorities was to take action against cigarette advertising and promotion activities, but Senator Wendell Ford, Democrat from Kentucky, authored legislation crippling the FTC's power to restrain cigarette advertising.

At the FTC until 1984 when he left to found the Advocacy Institute, Pertschuk's efforts to restrain advertising and marketing provoked much controversy. *See also* FEDERAL CIGARETTE LABELING AND ADVERTISING ACT OF 1965

Pharmacoepia of the United States (USP), 1890 Edition

The 1890 edition of the *Pharmacoepia of the United States (USP),* an official reference work on drugs periodically updated since its first appeared in 1820, classified tobacco as a drug. Pharmacists today primarily use the book to check whether a substance is considered a drug, a device intended for use in the cure, treatment, or prevention of a disease. A drug is also defined as an article—other than food and cosmetics—intended to affect the structure or function of the body.

In 1906, Congress passed the PURE FOOD AND DRUG ACT OF 1906, the first food and drug law intended to ensure the safety of products sold as food or drugs. The act defined "drugs" narrowly to include only articles listed in the *USP.* On June 30, 1906, tobacco was removed from the book, so it was no longer considered a drug and was no longer subject to FOOD AND DRUG ADMINISTRATION jurisdiction. *See also* FOOD, DRUG AND COSMETIC ACT OF 1938

Philip Morris Companies Inc.

Founded in 1919, Philip Morris Companies Inc. is the largest consumer packaged-goods company in the world. Its five principal operating companies are Philip Morris Incorporated or PHILIP MORRIS USA, the largest U.S. cigarette company; PHILIP MORRIS INTERNATIONAL INC., the leading U.S. cigarette exporter; Kraft Foods Inc., the largest U.S. processor and marketer of retail packaged goods; Miller Brewing Co., the second largest U.S. brewer; and Philip Morris Capital Corporation.

Headquartered in New York City, its cigarette division Philip Morris USA makes Basic, Cambridge, MARLBORO, Merit, Parliament, and VIRGINIA SLIMS cigarette brands. In late 1998, Philip Morris bought Lark, L and M, and CHESTERFIELD from the Liggett

Group. Philip Morris Companies Inc. owns Kraft Foods Inc., Jacobs Suchard and Miller Brewing Co., financial services, and real estate. Since 1994, GEOFFREY BIBLE has been chief executive officer of Philip Morris Companies Inc.

For 40 years, the Philip Morris family of companies has supported the arts. Its first grant, made by Philip Morris USA, was in 1958 for an outdoor concert in its hometown of Louisville, Kentucky. Since then, the companies have developed the leading corporate arts support program in the world. It also gives general operating support to a variety of music, theater, and opera organizations. It also has sponsored international and cultural exchanges including support for the U.S. tour of China's first modern dance company, performances of Alvin Ailey in Prague, and an exhibition of emerging Mexican artists in Puerto Rico.

Philip Morris International Inc.

Philip Morris International Inc. makes and sells cigarettes worldwide for its giant cigarette parent PHILIP MORRIS COMPANIES INC. Headquartered in Rye Brook, New York, the company sells about 710 billion CIGARETTES a year and controls approximately 15 percent of the world market. Philip Morris International's MARLBORO CIGARETTES alone hold almost 6 percent of the world market. The company's other brands include Basic, Bond Street, Cambridge, CHESTERFIELD, Lark, L and M, Merit, Parliament, Philip Morris, and VIRGINIA SLIMS.

Philip Morris International makes cigarettes in 52 facilities in 29 countries for major markets including Australia, FRANCE, Hong Kong, Italy, JAPAN, Poland, and TURKEY.

Philip Morris Magazine

Philip Morris Magazine, launched in late 1985 with a free circulation of 125,000, grew into a glossy four-color, 48-page bimonthly, with a claimed circulation of 13 million at its peak. Devoted to such subjects as smokers' rights and smoking issues, the magazine had lively graphics and name writers and a cheery tone celebrating the outdoor American lifestyle. The magazine was discontinued in 1992 because, according to the tobacco company, it was "redundant." *See also* PHILIP MORRIS COMPANIES INC; PHILIP MORRIS USA

Philip Morris/Tobacco Institute— "It's the Law" Program

To demonstrate its commitment to prevent CIGARETTE sales to minors, the TOBACCO INSTITUTE created the "It's the Law" program in 1989, which encourages enforcement of minimum age requirements that have been passed into law. "It's the Law" provides retailers, free of charge, the following tools they need to effectively enforce these laws:

- Information outlining each state's age and licensing requirements for the sale of cigarettes. The information includes information about penalties for sales to minors.
- Educational materials instructing retail employees how to verify purchasers' ages and enforce minimum-age laws.
- A selection of "It's the Law" decals for posting on windows, displays, and cash registers. The use of these materials tells the public that retailers and the tobacco industry are working together to prevent minors from obtaining cigarettes.

As far back as 1963, Philip Morris announced that it would not advertise cigarettes in youth publications or even in college newspapers, even though most college students are 18 years or older. All models appearing in Philip Morris advertising must be and must look at least 25 years of age. The company insists on signed certification that an individual is both 21 years of age or older and a smoker to be eligible to receive Philip Morris promotional materials. *See also* DIFRANZA, JOSEPH

Philip Morris USA

One of the oldest names in the CIGARETTE manufacturing business, Philip Morris USA is the largest tobacco company in the United States and first in sales. Its MARLBORO CIGARETTES account for one out of three cigarettes sold in the United States and one out of 15 sold elsewhere.

Philip Morris has twice the combined value of its four principal U.S. competitors (including BAT INDUSTRIES PLC). Philip Morris is the 10th largest company on the Fortune 500. It is the only cigarette maker in the Standard and Poors Tobacco Index with 15 times the capitalization of the index's other firms (SMOKELESS TOBACCO maker UNITED STATES TOBACCO COMPANY (UST) and cigarette-paper maker Schweitzer-Mauduit.

Philip Morris and its subsidiaries employ about 152,000 people worldwide, not including those who sell or advertise the product or make the paper and filters for cigarettes. In 1992, the company paid $4.5 billion in taxes on revenues of $59 billion, paid billions more in employee and excise taxes, and contributed more than $50 million to tax-exempt organizations.

Philip Morris sells much more than cigarettes, however. After it acquired the Miller Brewing Company and General Foods in 1985 and Kraft Foods in 1988, Philip Morris amassed 72 brands of consumer products that each generate more than $100 million in annual sales. Still, Philip Morris derives more than half of its revenues and nearly two-thirds of its profits from cigarette sales.

The company traces its origin back to "Philip Morris, Esq., Tobacconist and Importer of Fine Seegars" in Victorian London. After the CRIMEAN WAR (1853–1856), Philip Morris turned out expensive hand-rolled cigarette brands—such as Philip Morris Cambridge, Oxford Blues, and Ovals—made by expert "rollers" from RUSSIA, TURKEY, and Egypt. Later, the Philip Morris firm introduced a cork tip.

When PHILIP MORRIS died in 1873, Leopold Morris bought the business from his brother's widow, sold stock to the British public, and managed the company for 20 prosperous years. In 1893, the company went bankrupt when competitors offered customers free cigarette samples and lower prices. In 1894, an industrialist named William Thomson took control and began exporting Philip Morris cigarettes to the United States. Thanks to Gustav Eckmeyer, who had been the exclusive importer of the Bond Street cigarettes of Philip Morris in New York since 1872, smokers were already familiar with the reputation of Philip Morris brands. In 1902, he helped organize the first Philip Morris Corporation in New York. Listed among its assets was a top-selling brand sold in London called Marlboro, named after Marlborough Street in London, where the home company's factory was located.

In 1919, a new U.S. concern, Philip Morris and Company was formed in Virginia. In 1929, Philip Morris opened its first factory in the United States in RICHMOND, VIRGINIA.

During the Depression, when U.S. cigarette makers raised their prices, partly to pay for new cellophane wrappers on cigarette packs, Philip Morris introduced inexpensive brands and its sales took off. By 1940, the company's Philip Morris and Marlboro cigarettes commanded 10 percent of the market. Philip Morris expanded in 1954 when the company bought Benson and Hedges, the cigarette manufacturer that made Parliament. Benson and Hedges President Joseph Cullman stayed on as an executive vice president and eventually became president of the company three years later. Under Cullman, Philip Morris moved into other international businesses.

From the 1950s until the broadcast ban on cigarette advertising in 1971, Philip Morris used the power of advertising on radio and television and after the ban the print media to boost its cigarette sales. MARLBORO MAN ads are the most widely recognized advertising image in the world. Since 1975, Marlboros have been the number-one cigarette brand in the United States and today they are the number-one brand in the world. *See also* PHILIP MORRIS COMPANIES INC.; ROVENTINI, JOHN

Philip Morris USA—Action against Access Program

On June 27, 1995, PHILIP MORRIS USA announced the most comprehensive and expensive program in the company's history to prevent children and teens from having access to cigarettes. Costing $5 million, Philip Morris's voluntary program called Action against Access entailed a number of initiatives, including placing a notice on Philip Morris packs and cartons reading "Underage sale prohibited"; discontinuing free samples of cigarettes to consumers; discontinuing distribution of cigarettes to consumers through the mail; preventing use of Philip Morris brand names and logos on items marketed to minors, especially video games and toys; and supporting posting of minimum-age signs in all retail outlets.

Philip Morris promised to deny merchandising benefits to retailers who were fined for or convicted of selling cigarettes to minors as well as to assist retailers in complying with minimum-age laws by providing our "Ask First/It's the Law" materials and by funding retailers education programs. The tobacco company also promised to join with others to seek state legislation requiring that all cigarettes be sold in sight of, or under the direct control of, a sales clerk; to prevent minors' access to cigarettes in vending machines; and to call for reasonable cigarette retail licensing requirements in all 50 states. *See also* PHILIP MORRIS COMPANIES INC; PHILIP MORRIS—"IT'S THE LAW" PROGRAM

Philip Morris USA—"We Want You to Know Where We Stand"

In 1994, PHILIP MORRIS USA created an informational booklet, "We Want You to Know Where We Stand," that informed people where the tobacco company stood on various smoking issues, based on facts as well as on common sense. The following six issues were discussed in detail:

- **Accommodation:** Philip Morris believes accommodation is the way for smokers and nonsmokers to work out their differences. It opposes the small but vocal minority that advocates the view that the only way to accommodate nonsmokers is to enact laws banning smoking altogether. The tobacco company created a program to help owners of businesses, such as restaurants, bars and hotels, bowling alleys, and shopping malls, to accommodate smokers and nonsmokers alike. The Accommodation Program provides welcome signs, employee training materials, technical materials on ventilation, and a "Source Book" showing how to create separate areas to effectively accommodate both smokers and nonsmokers.

- **Choice:** Philip Morris believes people should be able to make the choice to smoke or not to smoke, but underscores people should have the right to their individual choice. The role of the government is to provide responsible information about smoking, from which adults can decide whether or not to smoke.
- **Courtesy:** Philip Morris believes common courtesy and mutual respect are the best ways for smokers and nonsmokers to resolve their differences, without the need for government-imposed rules and regulations. Smokers can ask "Do you mind if . . . ?" before they light up. And nonsmokers bothered by cigarette smoke can say "Would you mind . . ." as well as respect the right of smokers to smoke a cigarette in separate, designated smoking areas.
- **Minors:** Philip Morris believes minors should not smoke nor should anyone be allowed to sell cigarettes to them. The tobacco company developed a program called "It's the Law," that tells retailers and their employees that it is illegal to sell cigarettes to minors. The company also explained that all models appearing in Philip Morris advertisements must look at least 25 years of age. Individuals receiving promotional materials from the company must sign a certificate that he or she is at least 21 years old and a smoker. Philip Morris also has strongly supported legislative initiatives in all 50 states that establish minimum age requirements for the sale of cigarettes.

- **Secondhand Smoke:** After the Environmental Protection Agency (EPA) declared in its report that SECONDHAND SMOKE was a Group A carcinogen, Philip Morris raised questions about the validity of the report. The tobacco company believes that the EPA disregarded established scientific methods to arrive at its conclusions and believes that secondhand smoke has not been proven to cause disease in nonsmokers.
- **Smokers:** Philip Morris believes that smokers have the right to make a personal choice and that the rights of one group should not supersede the rights of the other. The company supports the creation of smoking and nonsmoking areas that take into account the rights and preferences of nonsmokers and smokers alike.

See also PHILIP MORRIS COMPANIES INC.; PHILIP MORRIS/TOBACCO INSTITUTE—"IT'S THE LAW" PROGRAM; PHILIP MORRIS USA—ACTION AGAINST ACCESS PROGRAM

Pierce, John P.

A cancer researcher at the University of California at San Diego, John P. Pierce has authored numerous studies that link tobacco advertising and smoking increases. In 1992, he published a study in the *Journal of the American Medical Association (JAMA)* that demonstrated a sharp increase in the choice of CAMEL CIGARETTES by teen-age smokers after R.J. REYNOLDS TOBACCO COMPANY launched the OLD JOE CAMEL advertising campaign in 1988. In 1994, he directed a study, published in the February 23, 1994, issue of *JAMA*, that linked a sharp increase in smoking by teen-age girls in the late 1960s and early 1970s to the soaring sales and advertising of widely advertised CIGARETTES for women.

In 1996, Dr. Pierce published a study, in the October 1996 *Journal of the National Cancer Institute* that showed that an interest in tobacco advertising and promotional gifts from tobacco companies was a strong predictor of whether a child would go on to smoke. He showed that children who are receptive to advertising are two to four times as likely to start smoking as are those who are not receptive. He concluded that receptivity to tobacco advertising is twice as good an indicator of whether a child will smoke as whether peers or family members smoke. Marketing has an effect on children before they begin to smoke.

Pipe

A pipe is an apparatus, usually a small bowl with a hollow stem, for smoking tobacco. Pipes have varied from simple tubes to elaborate smoking devices such as the Hookah (water pipe) and Nargileh (Persian water pipe made of coconut).

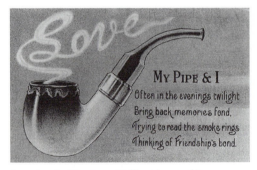

My Pipe & I
Often in the evenings twilight
Bring back memories fond,
Trying to read the smoke rings
Thinking of friendship's bond.

A postcard with verses extolling pipe smoking.

Pipe, Briar-Root

Briar was introduced as material for pipes and eventually became the major and most successful pipe material. Not until the 1850s were briar pipes introduced on a large scale, but they competed with the intricately designed meerschaums. Despite their design, which was similar to meerschaums, briar pipes were considered poorer in quality. After the invention of power equipment for mass production of pipes in the early 1900s, the machinery enabled pipe makers to design more functional pipe shapes from briar. The smaller, lighter, durable briar pipes overtook meerschaums. During WORLD WAR I, briar pipes were popular with soldiers in the field because they were so convenient to smoke.

The pipe maker works with the burl, or knotty section, that forms the root of the heath tree, *Erica arborea*. The plant is one of several hundred species of *Erica* that grows largely in South Africa and the Mediterranean region. Briar is harvested primarily in Spain, southern France, Corsica, Sardinia, Albania, Dalmatia, Greece, and Algeria. The burl of the plant is a section lying just below the surface of the ground that acts as an anchor for the main roots and trunk that stems from it. The older the plant, the larger the burl. It takes 50 to 100 years of growth to produce a prime burl. A prime burl produces at least 30 or 40 blocks from which pipes are cut.

The freehand pipe, the most expensive of all briar pipes, is designed by hand by the most highly skilled craftsmen in the factory; standard shapes are cut from blocks by machine. Although large and intricately designed pipes are the most expensive, the grain of the wood determines its value. Pipes made of dense, straight-grained wood, cut and styled by hand, are the most desirable. *See also* PIPE, MEERSCHAUM

Pipe, Calabash

The calabash is a lightweight pipe made from a club- or bottle-shaped gourd, which has been scooped out and dried. A brown clay, in most cases, is connected to the top of the bulbous portion of the gourd by means of a tube. The pipe then is fitted at the neck with a long wooden or gourd stem. The pipe is generally two to three feet in length.

In the early 1900s, the pipe was refined and became popular in England, Europe, and the United States. The particular gourd used by the pipe-making industry is a single species of *Lagenaria*. Virtually all the gourds used by pipe makers come from Africa where the ideal amount of heat and sunlight mature these hard-shelled fruits. Since nature forms the gourd from which the calabash is made, no two are alike.

Pipe, Clay

Based on published reports in England at the end of the sixteenth century, the English saw clay pipes in use among native Virginians and brought them home for their own use in 1586. Owing to the rapid spread of smoking, especially among courtiers, manufacture of clay pipes on a large scale began. In 1598, Paul Hentzer, a visitor to England, mentioned the use of clay pipes by the English.

> [T]he English are constantly smoking tobacco and in this manner: They have pipes on purpose made of clay, into the further end of which they put the herb, so dry that it may be rubbed into powder, and putting fire to it they draw the smoke into their mouths, which they puff out again, through their nostrils, like funnels, along with it plenty of phlegm and defluxtion from the head. (Dunhill, 1969)

By 1615, William Camden, a contemporary historian commented that tobacco shops in England were as ordinary as taverns and tap-houses.

By the early 1600s, England was a major manufacturer of clay pipes. The earliest clays, sometimes known as fairy, elfin, or Roman pipes were small owing to the expense of smoking tobacco.

When King JAMES I ascended the throne in 1603, pipe makers, like others who trafficked in tobacco, found their lives made miserable by the king's distaste for the plant. When SIR WALTER RALEIGH, the passionate pipe smoker, was charged with treason and executed, English pipe makers, who incorporated in 1619, championed their hero posthumously with pipes that had his effigy molded into the bowls. After 1620, the king, angered by the defiant pipe makers, set up a pipe-makers' guild in London and made any practice of the trade outside the guild unlawful. As a result, great numbers of pipe makers left the county for the Netherlands and the Dutch and immigrant English controlled the clay-pipe industry.

The pipe makers produced short-, medium-, and long-stemmed models. Their trademark was the art work molded into the bowls and stems in relief. Mythological characters, heroes, and designs of all types were created. In the Dutch city of Gouda, which gained preeminence for the quality and quantity of its clay pipes, approximately 500 marks were registered in the year 1660, the year the pipe makers incorporated in the Netherlands.

The smoking of clay pipes became so popular that a pipe cleaner's trade was established. It was important to have a clean pipe.

Although the popularity of clay pipes began to decline after WORLD WAR I, they lend a satisfying, earthy taste to tobacco. Today's clay pipes are virtually identical in materials and methods of manufacture to those of 200 years ago. The Dutch eventually became the leading producers of clay pipes, even though the English originated the form of clay pipe that began the pipe-making industry.

References: Alfred Dunhill, *The Pipe Book*, New York: Macmillan Company, 1924, 1969, p. 164.

Pipe, Meerschaum

It is believed that in the early eighteenth century, Count Andrassy, a noble from Hungary who was an envoy to TURKEY, brought home two blocks of meerschaum, a mineral used in pipe making. The story goes that the count gave the blocks to a skilled wood carver who fashioned a pair of tobacco pipes from them. After 1750, pipes of this mineral were in heavy demand.

Meerschaum, a German word meaning "sea foam," takes its name from the mineral often seen floating on the Black Sea. Meerschaum is a soft, porous hydrous silicate of magnesia found in pockets within clay or serpentine deposits. Its geological name, sepiolite, comes from the Greek "Sepio," or cuttlefish bone, which it resembles. The German term, however, has been used for the pipe because German-speaking people controlled the meerschaum-pipe industry until WORLD WAR II.

Meerschaum deposits are found in many areas of the world, but the finest grades of meerschaum used by the pipe industry come mainly from Turkey and, to a lesser degree, from Tanzania. Meerschaum from England, Greece, Spain, Morocco, and Arizona and

South Carolina in the United States is of poorer quality.

Unlike clay, which was available to everyone, meerschaum was restricted to the rich and titled who could afford to commission the hand work of a carver. In the 1850s, as more artisans and wood carvers turned to pipe making in factories, thousands of meerschaums made their way into the hands of middle-class smokers. The majority of the pipes were carved in Vienna, Austria, a city linked with amber, which provided the mouthpiece for the meerschaum pipe. Great skill is required to carve a bowl of meerschaum.

A new meerschaum pipe is generally either pure white or a pale creamy yellow. As it is smoked, tars and oils color the base until it approaches black-brown or dark-cherry.

Pipe, Mound

Excavations of earth mounds made by Algonquian and Muskogean Indians in North America have revealed pipes buried with the dead. Since the pipe was sacred as well as a valued possession, many pipes were buried in graves. The characteristic shape of the unornamented grave mound pipe is a bowl mounted on a base curved slightly downwards projecting equally in either direction. The front portion serves for the smoker to hold the pipe; the back portion is both stem and mouthpiece. More elaborate mound pipes had carved animal totems, human heads, and figures mounted on the base.

Pipe, Porcelain

In the eighteenth century, porcelain pipes became as standard as clay pipes. The bowls of the two were shaped very much the same, but the porcelains were larger. The bowls were made to fit vertical wood or wood-and-bone stems that reached 3 or 4 feet in length. More elaborately decorated than standard clays, porcelain bowls often had hand-painted scenes, portraits of monarchs, and religious symbols. The standard-shaped porcelain pipes come principally from the Royal Goedewaagen factory in Gouda, the Netherlands. They are offered in a variety of finishes, from pure white to reddish-brown. This factory also makes the famous Baronite pipe, which is a double-walled porcelain pipe. One disadvantage of a porcelain pipe, as with clays, is that they become extremely hot, making them difficult to hold. The Baronite has air space between the inner and outer bowl walls and acts as an insulator, keeping the bowl cooler and more comfortable to hold in the hand. *See* PIPE, CLAY

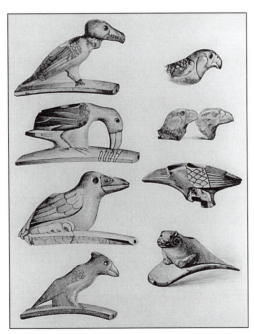

Examples of mound pipes.

Pipe, Straight or Tube

Because the literal meaning of the Spanish word *cañuto* (pipe) and the English word "pipe" is a hollow tube, the name was first given to a smoking apparatus of a simple tubular construction. The word was later extended to all types of pipes. Tobacco was likely to fall out of the simple pipes, a difficulty overcome by pressing in a little pebble or lying in a recumbent position. In English literature, according to the *New English Dictionary*, the word "pipe," in the sense of "tobacco pipe," appeared for the first time in 1594.

What is believed to be the earliest written description of a tobacco pipe used by natives in the West Indies was by GONZALO FERNANDEZ DE OVIEDO in 1535. Another early account was by JACQUES CARTIER in 1536; he described pipe use by American Indians in the vicinity of the St. Lawrence River. In 1564, JOHN SPARKE, who accompanied JOHN HAWKINS on his first voyage to the Indies and Florida, described pipe smoking.

The principal areas where straight or tube pipes were used were North and South America and Southwest Africa where Bushmen and Hottentots, men and women, smoked.

Tubular pipes were made from fragile materials, such as reed or cane, as used in Mexico, or rolled from birch bark by the native peoples of Nova Scotia and Newfoundland. Bone, wood, sandstone or steatite, and pottery made a more satisfactory pipe.

Pipe, Water

The custom of cooling and cleansing the smoke of a tobacco pipe by drawing it through a vessel of water is almost universal in the Asian continent and also practiced in Africa, but it was never found in America nor was it customary among Europeans. Water pipes, which include the narghile, or *nargileh,* (the Indian word for coconut), hookah, or *kalian,* and hubble-bubble, had their origin in Africa where the dakka-pipe was used for smoking hemp.

After a visit in 1615 as ambassador to the Mogul's Court in India, Sir Thomas Roe documented the use of a water pipe.

Their way of taking it is something odd and strange, tho' perhaps they don't fire their mouths by it as we do; for they take a little narrow-necked Pot and fill it with water up to the lower part of the Spout; then they lay their tobacco loose in the top of the Pot, and upon it a Coal of fire, and so with a Reed or cane of an Ell long they draw the Smoak into their mouths. They say it is much more cool and wholesome to do it thus than as the Europeans do, since all the smoak falls upon the surface of the Water before it passes into the Cane[sic]. (Dunhill, 1969)

In its original form, a water pipe was composed of a coconut shell partially filled with water, two tubes or reeds, a stem, and a clay bowl. One tube from the clay bowl ran through a long, 2- to 3-foot stem down into the coconut shell below the water line. A second reed or tube was fitted into the side of the shell above the water line. The smoker drew in smoke from the second tube; the smoke traveling from the bowl, where the tobacco burns; down the first tube, through the water where it was cooled and made softer; and then, ultimately, into the smoker's mouth. The base of the water pipe changed when it spread beyond African villages, but the bulbous water-holding base of the pipe has always remained, even though other materials, such as terra cotta or clay, are used.

The hookah, with a fancy glass bottle or vase as a base, evolved from the basic water pipe. In the Middle East and India, the base was made from brass.

References: Alfred Dunhill, *The Pipe Book*, New York: Macmillan Company, 1924, 1969, p. 119.

Pipe, Wood

In the nineteenth century, wood carvers in Europe started making elm, oak, and walnut pipe bowls similar in design to porcelain bowls used in long, wood-stemmed pipes. Pipes are also made from cherry and apple wood, hickory, and rosewood. *See also* PIPE, PORCELAIN

Pipe Smoking and Native Americans

Among native tribes up and down the hemisphere, pipe smoking was the universal form of consuming tobacco. Hardly a culture in North or South America did not have some kind of pipe made from clay, stone, or wood.

The pipe was and continues to be a sacred object central to belief, ritual, and ceremony for natives across North America. The pipe is of considerable antiquity; some tribal groups trace its spiritual origins back to the time of creation or to the period of a great deluge, as spoken of in their oral traditions. Early European observers, as well as archaeological evidence dating some pipes back thousands of years, corroborate this sacred object's long history in native religious life. JACQUES CARTIER gave an account in 1535 of pipe smoking in the St. Lawrence region. Samuel Champlain reported being passed a pipe as a welcome by the Montagnais after he arrived among them in 1603. Father Andrew White described a pipe ritual in Maryland in 1633. Father JACQUES MARQUETTE noted in 1673 that through the pipe's use, tribal differences were ended, alliances formed or strengthened, travelers safeguarded in distant or foreign territory, weapons deflected, and strangers greeted.

The native origins, traditions, and types of pipes are extensive. Among the most sacred are those that originated as spiritual gifts to the entire tribal nation. The well-being or the very existence of the group is linked to the supremely holy pipes of this nature. They are generally ritually cared for by qualified individuals or keepers and are rarely exposed to view. Individual sacred pipes may also be associated with certain venerated leaders, particular religious ceremonies or movements, and historic events. Their origins may sometimes be traced to holy beings who bestowed them upon the people, to spiritual instructions given to individuals during visions, and to particular animals, feathered creatures, and other beings. Some are believed to have such spiritual power that only a particular medicine person may safely use them.

The origins and instructions for particular sacred pipes generally determine their rituals and other elements of their use and care as well as their ownership or keepership by individuals, families, clans, societies, bands, or by the entire tribal group. In the Plains region, for example, a number of pipes are used only for specific ceremonial purposes. These include a pipe used for praying with the people, the Sun Dance pipe, the preamble pipe used by one individual before council meetings, the peace pipe smoked during council meetings, the sweat lodge pipe or the medicine man pipe, the eagle pipe, and the woman's pipe.

The shapes and types, including the separate-stemmed pipe, reflect differing religious use. The bowls of the pipes are generally made from black or red stone and the stems from wood. Much of the stone used to make pipes came from a PIPESTONE quarry in Minnesota. Other materials and colors are also used. The bowls sometimes include inlay decorations or carved figures. The stems, usually made of wood, may be plain or wrapped with porcupine quills, horsehair, animal fur, feathers, beadwork, cloth fabric, or other materials. The stems may also have feathers or other sacred objects attached to them. Among some tribes, the decoration of pipe stems had great ceremonial significance; even the attachment holding the pipe to the stem was fixed with special care. A pipe may be made a particular way according to spiritual instructions received in a vision or dream.

The bowl of the sacred pipe generally symbolizes the life-giving and life-sustaining female, the woman and the Earth. Its colors, shapes, hollows, and other features are also linked to this symbolism. The substance of the bowl, often stone or clay, comes from Mother Earth. The stem of the sacred pipe is also symbolic. Representations attributed to it include male energy, all growing things, a person's voice, the road or path of life, and life itself. When the male stem and female bowl are joined, the sacred pipe becomes ritually active and powerful. The two components only come together in religious use; otherwise they are kept separate.

Although ceremonial pipes were used to some extent in the East, their greatest use was in the Prairies and Plains. Among the American Indians in these two cultural areas, the pipe took a variety of shapes. The tube pipe, made of bone or stone, was the simplest, and perhaps the oldest. Pipes with an L-shaped stone bowl and separate wood stem were popular over the Plains country in historic times. Although many kinds of stone were used for making pipe bowls, on occasion wood and pottery were used to make the bowls.

Like the American Indians in the Plains region, the Western Eskimo used a pipe with a small bowl carved from stone and lashed with rawhide to the stem made from wood. Their practice of deeply inhaling a few whiffs, which smoked out of the bowl, produced a condition of intoxication. The Eastern Eskimo and Greenland Eskimo, on the other hand, used large-bowled pipes, also carved from stone with stems of wood, smoked in the ordinary way. Although Eskimos worked in wood and stone, they made pipes and other precious possessions using walrus ivory, their favorite medium, onto which hunting scenes were carved.

Tobacco, including *Nicotiana* varieties and varieties made from the inner bark of particular trees, is a sacred plant fundamental to the pipe and its rituals. It is offered to the spirit world not only through ceremonial smoking but by direct placement on the earth, in the water, in the fire, or in other places. During a sacred pipe ceremony with the people, each participant becomes part of a sacred circle of prayer. The ritual is conducted by a qualified person who makes the necessary preparations and offers the pipe to the four directions (or semi-cardinal directions), the earth, and the sky. The leader then passes it to each person taking part in the ceremony, generally in a sunwise (clockwise) direction. Among some tribes, the pipe, in being passed from one individual to another during a ceremony, was differently grasped and held, according to the nature of the ceremony or to the taboo obligation of the individual.

Smoking the pipe equated taking an oath and the act also sealed an agreement, whether public or private. Pipes were used on occasions of war and peace conferences and used in the ratification of treaties and alliances. The peace pipe of any particular tribe was as easily recognizable to other tribes as was the banner or the coat of arms of a European feudal lord. The pipe often served as a pass or safe conduct for a messenger through hostile country. *See also* HENNEPIN, LOUIS; NATIVE AMERICANS; PIPE; PIPE, CLAY; *NICOTIANA RUSTICA*; SMOKING; WHITE BUFFALO CALF WOMAN

Pipe Tobacco Council (PTC)

Headquartered in Washington, D.C., the Pipe Tobacco Council (PTC) is the national trade association of pipe tobacco and roll-your-own tobacco manufacturers and importers, as well as suppliers to those industries. Founded in 1988, the purpose of the council is to advance and foster the economic interests of its members, the general welfare of the pipe and smoking tobacco industries, and the nation's economy and society. The PTC also provides statistical reporting programs for its members.

Pipestone

Pipestone is a soft red stone that is sacred to the Dakota and other Native American groups. Used in making sacred pipes, pipe bowls, and other objects, the principal source of the stone is at a quarry in Pipestone, Minnesota. One account of the origin of the stone states that during a great flood members of various tribal groups went into highland areas in an effort to escape the rising water. Unable to survive the deluge, all but one person perished, and the bodies of those who had died, from many tribal groups, turned to stone. The young woman who managed to escape later gave birth to twins, beginning the repopulation of the land. The sacred site became a neutral territory where the stone could be quarried in peace.

Archaeological evidence indicates a long history of Native American use of the pipestone quarry. The area first came to the attention of Euro-Americans in the nineteenth century, primarily through the work of the artist GEORGE CATLIN. Although not the first non-American Indian visitor, Catlin publicized his visit in the 1830s through his paintings and writings. He also took samples of the stone, later called "catlinite" by Euro-Americans, to Boston for chemical analysis.

The pipestone quarry's long history of occupancy saw numerous changes in jurisdiction. In 1851, the Sisseton, Wahpeton, Mdewakanton, and Wahpekute bands of Dakota lost the site as well as other lands in Minnesota territory in treaties at Traverse des

Sioux and Mendota. In an 1858 treaty, the Yankton people relinquished millions of acres of land but retained unrestricted use of the quarry. Two years later a Minnesota survey created a reserve around the site, an action that did not deter homesteaders from encroaching on the land. In 1891, Congress authorized the construction of a government boarding school in the area, a decision challenged by the Yankton people. After a 1926 ruling by the United States Supreme Court, the tribal band later received monetary compensation for land taken for the school. The federal government then held title to the site, and the Yankton people retained rights to its use.

Eventually, Pipestone National Park Association was created, renamed in 1932 the Pipestone Shrine Association. Its members sought federal protection for the site and enough land for a park. In 1937, Congress created the Pipestone National Monument. Native pipe makers continue to mine the sacred stone from the quarry on a permit basis. *See also* NATIVE AMERICANS; PIPE SMOKING AND NATIVE AMERICANS

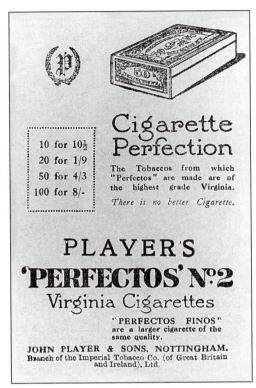

Ad for John Player & Son cigarettes.

Player, John Dane (1865–1950) and Player, William Goodacre (1866–1959)

Two brothers, John Dane Player and William Goodacre Player, inherited their father's tobacco manufacturing business in England. The company, John Player and Sons, introduced in 1886 Player's Gold Leaf Navy Cut cigarettes. In 1883, John Player commissioned an artist to draw the legendary trademark—the head of a bearded sailor wearing a Royal Navy uniform. The head was circled in 1888 with a lifebuoy, with the brand title Player's Navy Cut superimposed. In 1901, two ships were added.

Point-of-Purchase (P-O-P) Tobacco Advertising

Point-of-Purchase (P-O-P) CIGARETTE ads and displays where tobacco products are sold in drugstores, supermarkets, gas stations, and so on grab attention and influence an individual to buy because the product is there or nearby.

P-O-P includes tobacco product logos on neon signs, banners, clocks, awnings, floor and counter mats, dividers (long bars used to separate grocery orders), signs attached to display racks, signs hung from ceilings, in-store decal ads on doors, windows, shopping carts and baskets, and checkout counters.

Premier

In the early 1980s, R.J. REYNOLDS TOBACCO COMPANY developed a "SAFE CIGARETTE," a device called Premier that featured a hollow aluminum cylinder filled with alumina pellets coated with NICOTINE and glycerin plugged in at the far end with a piece of charcoal and insulated from the mouth with two mouthpieces, one of tobacco paper and one of polypropylene.

The device was sheathed in a tiny bit of "reconstituted tobacco" (about 5 percent of the tobacco in a conventional cigarette) and the charcoal tip was clad in a fiberglass insulator. Wrapped in cigarette paper, Premier looked like a typical cigarette. When the charcoal tip of Premier was lit, the burning charcoal heated the coated alumina beads, which, in turn, produced a nicotine-laden aerosol. The mouthpiece was designed to cool the aerosol without filtering it. Premier delivered about 0.4 mg of nicotine, along with CARBON MONOXIDE. It cost Reynolds $300 million to develop its "smokeless" cigarette.

Without making any explicit health claims, company lawyers told federal officials the device would prevent cancer. Reynolds published a monograph comparing the toxicology of Premier prototypes with conventional cigarettes.

The public health community did not feel Premier was a safe alternative to conventional cigarettes, The device maintained addiction to nicotine while delivering large amounts of carbon monoxide. Carcinogens also remained in the aerosol.

Researchers at the National Institute on Drug Abuse showed that Reynolds's unqualified assertions that Premier could not be used to smoke crack cocaine were untrue. They put crack into the device and showed that cocaine vapor evolved from the user's end in a smoking machine. Public health groups called on the FOOD AND DRUG ADMINISTRATION to regulate Premier as a drug. Before the agency could decide whether to classify it as a cigarette, Reynolds took it off the market after five months. The company said Premier was withdrawn because of poor consumer acceptance. Besides complaints about its bad taste, a special lighter was required to light it. *See also* ARIEL; ECLIPSE

Prince Albert Pipe Tobacco

In 1907, RICHARD JOSHUA REYNOLDS, anticipating an increase in the popularity of smoking tobacco, introduced a smoking tobacco using Kentucky Burley and named it after Prince Albert of Wales who had become the British monarch, Edward VII. He wrote instructions to the printer regarding the wording of the label, sending along a photograph he had torn from a newspaper. It showed

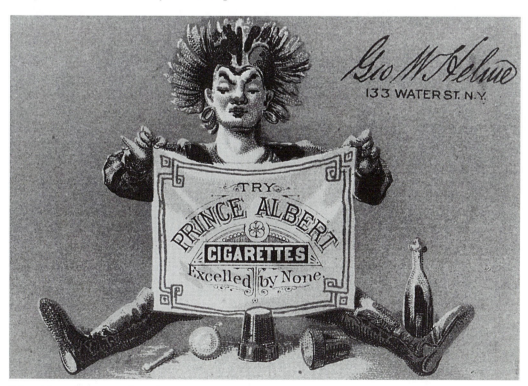

Prince Albert cigarettes trade card.

MARK TWAIN at a Windsor castle tea party with the royal family. The king wore a coat he had originated years before as Prince Albert.

The new product caught on, and was a national favorite by 1912. Packing, wrapping, stamping, and labeling smoking tobacco on a large scale forced Reynolds into finding machinery that could increase production. The pipe tobacco first came in 5¢ cloth bags and 2-ounce tins, then in half-pound and 1-pound hermetically sealed HUMIDORS conceived by Reynolds.

The introduction of Prince Albert pipe tobacco was a turning point for the R.J. REYNOLDS TOBACCO COMPANY. In 1918, Reynolds hired an agency, N.W. Ayer and Son, to mount a national advertising campaign. Ads that read Prince Albert "can't bite the tongue" ran in the *Saturday Evening Post, Collier's Weekly, Literary Digest,* and other magazines. On a huge electric signboard overlooking New York City's Union Square, blinking lights revealed a tall man and the words: "Prince Albert—The Nation's Joy Smoke, R.J. Reynolds Tobacco Company."

Pritchard v. Liggett and Myers Tobacco Company

An example of a cigarette case litigated during the first wave of tobacco litigation (1954–1973) was the case of *Pritchard v. Liggett and Myers Tobacco Company.* It was argued under the theory of a breach of express warranty based on statements made by a tobacco company in magazine and newspaper advertisements. The ads extolled the healthful benefits of cigarettes based on research and the opinion of medical specialists and physicians.

Otto E. Pritchard, a Pittsburgh, Pennsylvania, carpenter who smoked CHESTERFIELDS for 20 years and lost his right lung to cancer, alleged that Chesterfield's advertising statements expressly warranted that the defendant's cigarettes were not harmful to a smoker's health. Pritchard smoked cigarettes since he was 15 years old. He was a habitual cigarette smoker for several years prior to 1924, when he began smoking Chesterfields. Thereafter, and during the period between

1924 and the latter part of 1953, he smoked Chesterfields regularly, consuming "at least a carton" per week. The alleged warranties were contained in a series of advertisements published periodically in both newspapers and magazines. These ads featured in bold type such factual affirmations as "A Good Cigarette Can Cause No Ills," "Nose, Throat and Accessory Organs Not Adversely Affected by Smoking Chesterfields," "Chesterfields Are as Pure as the Water You Drink and the Food You Eat," and "Play Safe Smoke Chesterfields." Many of the ads contained assurances that the affirmations were based upon extensive research and the opinion of medical specialists. Implicit in these assurances was a strong suggestion that while other brands of cigarettes might be harmful, Chesterfields were not.

The trial court instructed the jury that for the defendant to be liable, the plaintiff had to show reliance on the express warranty in buying the cigarettes. The jury found for the defendant finding that the defendant made no "express warranties upon which the plaintiff relied and by which he was induced to purchase" the cigarettes. Pritchard appealed.

The Third Circuit Court of Appeals held that Pritchard did not need to show reliance on the express warranty. The plaintiff did, however, have to demonstrate that the ads tended to induce the purchase of goods. However, because this was nearly impossible to prove, the plaintiff never tried the case on remand. *See also* TOBACCO LITIGATION: FIRST, SECOND, AND THIRD WAVES

Promotions and Tobacco Products

Promotions of tobacco products have included free CIGARETTE samples or SMOKELESS TOBACCO products or gifts that come wrapped with the purchase of tobacco products (T-shirts, coffee mugs, lighters, ash trays, key chains). Promotions can include the appearance of a tobacco product name on television (the Marlboro Grand Prix) or the sponsorship of community and cultural events. Promotions can be "2 for the price of 1" specials, a third pack for free when you buy two or coupons for free packs with the next purchase or $1 or $2 off a purchase.

Another type of promotion involves offering catalog merchandise in exchange for coupons retrieved from cigarette packs. More and more companies adopted this form of advertising because it did not require that merchandise carry the surgeon general's health warning. CAMEL CIGARETTES offered "Camel Cash" coupons resembling dollar bills. The "Camel C-notes" pictured Joe Camel in sunglasses with a cigarette in his mouth, dressed as George Washington, the first president of the United States. The only way to get "the smooth stuff" pictured in Camel Cash catalogs was to collect and mail in coupons packed in Camel cigarette packs. In 1994, Hard Pack T-shirts cost 35 C-Notes; in 1995, Camel Leather Backpacks cost 185 C-Notes; in 1996, "Camel's Rockin Road CDs and Cassettes" cost 70 C-Notes each; and Joe's Denim Biker Jacket cost 490 C-Notes. All the merchandise featured Joe Camel and carried no health warnings.

In 1993 and 1994, MARLBORO CIGARETTES offered merchandise through its "Adventure Team" promotion. PHILIP MORRIS COMPANIES INC. reported that four million people participated, sending in coupons (called "miles") for 14 million promotional items like team caps (115 miles), sweatshirts (395 miles), towels (140 miles), original Swiss Army knives (210 miles), Series 2000 watches (1,200 miles), and rain gear (500 miles). Analysts figured that the company spent $250 million on the campaign. Philip Morris also paid for a Marlboro Country Store campaign (more gear) and distributed catalogs in English and Spanish. The company also sent vans around to store parking lots so customers could redeem their "Marlboro miles" on the spot. In 1996, Philip Morris launched the "Marlboro Unlimited" campaign. Starting in August 1996, a multimillion-dollar, 20-car specially built train (with cinemas, dance club, hot tubs, and Marlboro logos) was scheduled to take 25-day trips through the West. On board were 100 winners of a sweepstakes contest who testified they were smokers over 21 years old.

Tobacco companies have aimed promotions at women. VIRGINIA SLIMS CIGARETTES entered the catalog program in 1992 with the VWear collection of "free" merchandise sent to smokers who collected and mailed Philip Morris UPCs (bar codes/proofs of purchase) from their cigarette packs. Catalogs contained merchandise geared towards young women and girls, including "Totally Temporary Tattoo" kits, backpacks, choker necklaces, and charm bracelets. A VWear leather jacket cost 400 UPCs, a cost in real dollars of over $800 in cigarettes. Virginia Slims also offered a daily planner, including coupons (money off cartons or packs) for their product. Ads reminded women to "start saving UPCs today." Camel Cash catalogs also carried merchandise specifically for women, including robes, scarves, silk pajamas, and charm bracelets. Benson and Hedges offered women "a black leather cigarette holder with a gold tone clasp and two convenient pockets for credit cards and lighters" and unisex pea coats.

Cigarette advertising expenditures for promotional items in catalogs quadrupled from $184 million to $756 million between 1991 and 1993. Many of the catalog items made their way into the hands of young people under 21. They got them from relatives or friends or directly from a tobacco company. A 1992 Gallup survey found that half of the smokers (12 to 17 years old) and one quarter of nonsmokers (12 to 17 years old) owned at least one tobacco item such as a T-shirt, cap, or lighter.

Mail-order promotions have enabled tobacco companies to build huge direct-mail lists of smokers. A nationwide phone survey of children ages 12 to 17 found that 7.6 percent of teens had received cigarette companies' mail addressed directly to them. Based on the survey, it is estimated that the names of over one million teens are on the mailing lists of tobacco companies.

Public Health Cigarette Smoking Act of 1969

In April 1970, President Richard Nixon signed the Public Health Cigarette Smoking Act of 1969. The law banned cigarette ads from television and radio as of midnight January 1, 1971. Congress gave tobacco companies an extra day to air their commercials during New Year's Day football bowl games. All the cigarette makers spent heavily on their final TV fling. PHILIP MORRIS COMPANIES INC., maker of MARLBORO CIGARETTES, poured $1.2 million into commercials that aired between 11:30 P.M. and midnight on all three networks.

The law strengthened the health warning on CIGARETTE packs, but not on SMOKELESS TOBACCO products. The cigarette package warning had to read: "WARNING: The Surgeon General Has Determined That Cigarette Smoking Is Dangerous to Your Health." The law temporarily preempted the FEDERAL TRADE COMMISSION (FTC) requirement of health labels on advertisements. States and localities were prevented from regulating or prohibiting cigarette advertising or promotion for health-related reasons.

The law required a yearly report on the health consequences of smoking. Since 1971, the surgeon general has released reports that give detailed information about the health hazards of smoking. *See also* HEALTH WARNINGS ON CIGARETTE PACKS AND ADVERTISEMENTS AND SMOKELESS TOBACCO

Public Health Service (PHS)

Created in 1798, the Public Health Service (PHS) is the primary health agency of the national government and has the responsibility, through its surgeon general, to inform the public and health professions on all matters relating to public health problems and issues. *See also* APPENDIX 2: SURGEON GENERAL'S REPORTS, 1964–1998

Puritan Anti-Tobacco Statutes. *See* ANTI-TOBACCO MOVEMENTS, UNITED STATES; CONNECTICUT GENERAL COURT

Pusey, Joshua (d. 1916)

Joshua Pusey, a patent attorney from Lima, Pennsylvania, is credited with making the first portable cardboard matchbook in 1889. No record exists of the number of match sticks in that first book, an invention he called "flexibles." After Pusey announced his invention towards the end of 1892, he spent three years defending it in various lawsuits. After winning the patent battle, he sold the rights to Diamond Match Company for $4,000 in 1896. He accepted a job the company offered him and remained with Diamond until his death 20 years later.

Pusey's invention failed because he put the striking surface on the inside. Sparks created by the friction from one match often ignited the others. Henry C. Traute, a salesman at the Diamond Match Company fixed the problem by putting the striking surface on the outside, thus preventing one match from igniting the others. Traute lobbied to protect the customer by insisting that the phrase "Close cover before striking" be included on the front flap. Once the matchbook was safe to use, it made it possible for smokers to light up whenever and wherever they wished. *See also* MATCHES

R

Radio and Cigarette Advertising

During the Depression years, radio grew and flourished. In 1929, more than 10 million households owned radios; by 1939, 27.5 million houses had them. By the 1930s, radio listeners were accustomed to hearing commercials interrupt their radio programs. CIGARETTE manufacturers were among the most enthusiastic pioneers in using radio for coast-to-coast advertising. After magazines, it was the second greatest national advertising medium. In the depth of the Depression, tobacco companies spent around half their advertising budgets on radio commercials to boost sales.

By 1930, the AMERICAN TOBACCO COMPANY (ATC), BROWN AND WILLIAMSON TOBACCO CORPORATION, LORILLARD COMPANY INC., and R.J. REYNOLDS TOBACCO COMPANY were all buying radio time. In 1931 alone, tobacco companies poured an estimated $75 million into advertising cigarettes, cigars, and pipe tobacco. The American Tobacco Company's LUCKY STRIKE brand sponsored many radio comedies and musical shows. The Lucky Strike Hit Parade, a popular music program that appealed to a young audience, started on radio in 1928 and ran into the 1950s on television. It featured teen idols like Frank Sinatra. The "Lucky Strike Hit Parade" was so popular in 1938 that when its producers introduced a sweepstakes promotion offering free cartons of "Luckies" for correctly guessing each week's three most popular tunes, nearly seven million entries were sent in each week.

By the early 1930s, R.J. Reynolds was sponsoring radio programs that were popular with youth, such as the "Camel Pleasure Hour," the "All Star Radio Revue," and the "Camel Caravan." In the late 1930s, Lorillard (OLD GOLD) hired Artie Shaw and Brown and Williamson (Kool, Raleigh) signed up Tommy Dorsey. Liggett and Myers (CHESTERFIELD) hired the Andrew Sisters. It also put Bing Crosby on the payroll, but he didn't last long. He was fired because he refused to say on the air: "Don't forget to buy your mother a carton of Chesterfields on Mother's Day." His mother hated smoking. *See also* BROADCAST BAN ON CIGARETTE ADVERTISING; TELEVISION AND CIGARETTE ADVERTISING

Raleigh, Sir Walter (c. 1552–1618)

English navigator and merchant adventurer, Sir Walter Raleigh, who sailed up the Orinoco River (Guiana region) in 1595 recounted that the natives of the region "make the most and fairest houses, and sell them into Guiana for golde, and into Treinedado for Tobacco, in the excessive taking wereof, they exceed all nations . . ." (Heimann, 1960).

Raleigh acquired the habit of smoking tobacco in America and introduced *NICOTIANA TABACUM* in England. Numerous Englishmen had been smoking for 30 or 40 years before Raleigh puffed his PIPE in the Elizabethan court, but, because of his popularity and eminence as a national hero and the effects which smoke produced, Raleigh popularized pipe smoking at the English court.

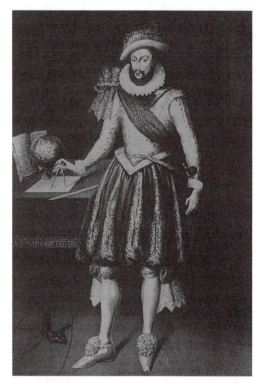

English explorer, courtier, and colonizer Sir Walter Raleigh was among the first Elizabethan Englishmen to use tobacco. *Library of Congress.*

King JAMES I, of England persecuted Raleigh for making smoking fashionable. Charged with treason for allegedly plotting to make peace with Spain, he was imprisoned in the Tower of London for 13 years during which time he wrote about his explorations and smoked tobacco. Released in 1616, Raleigh was beheaded on October 29, 1618. Always accompanied by his pipe, Raleigh took one with him to the scaffold.

References: Robert K. Heimann, *Tobacco and Americans,* New York: McGraw-Hill Book Company, 1960, p. 37.

Raleigh Cigarettes

In 1929, BROWN AND WILLIAMSON TOBACCO CORPORATION introduced Raleigh cigarettes, an English blend. It was an expensive brand, and sales dropped during the Depression. In 1931, Raleighs were revamped, given a new blend of tobaccos and a competitive price. To attract buyers, Raleighs offered coupons that could be exchanged for merchandise, one per pack and four extras in each carton. Coupons helped push up sales, and in 1939 Raleighs were the nation's fifth best-selling cigarette.

Reader's Digest

DeWitt and Lila Wallace, editors and publishers of *Reader's Digest,* were long interested in the anti-smoking movement. Because their magazine, with the largest circulation in the nation, carried no advertising, the Wallaces said this made them more independent than other magazines that had to rely on liquor and CIGARETTE ads for their well-being.

Since November 1924, when *Reader's Digest* ran an article entitled "Does Tobacco Injure the Human Body?" by Dr. JOHN HARVEY KELLOGG who called tobacco a "heart poison," the magazine has been running articles about the dangers of smoking ever since. Well over 100 articles on the issue of smoking and health have appeared.

Repace, James L. (1938–)

A physicist who suffers from asthma, James L. Repace became a clean-air and anti-smoking activist in his off-hours. Over a 10-week period in 1978, Repace undertook field research into pollution levels in restaurants, bowling alleys, and other public spaces and found the risk of exposure to lung cancer from the ENVIRONMENTAL TOBACCO SMOKE (ETS) levels he obtained to be 250 to 1,000 times above the acceptable level as set down by federal guidelines for carcinogens in air, water, and food.

Repace and Alfred Lowrey, a theoretical chemist and a friend, submitted an article to *Science.* Published in May 1980, it was Repace's first article in a major journal. Another article published in *Environment International* in1985 by the two men about lung cancer risk and passive smoking withstood a stringent peer-review process. The TOBACCO INSTITUTE issued a 43-page rebuttal pamphlet entitled *Tobacco Smoke in the Air* a few months after the article's early 1985 publication, charging it with too many theoretical or unwarranted assumptions.

Repace, who had a job in the air policy office of the Environmental Protection Agency (EPA), spoke out in his free time on the ETS problem. A conservative Tennessee congressman, Representative Don Sundquist, who was a member of the House subcommittee that controlled the EPA's budget, mounted an investigation into every phase of Repace's ETS studies. Repace was exonerated.

Reynolds, Patrick (1949–)

A grandson of the founder of R.J. REYNOLDS TOBACCO COMPANY, Patrick Reynolds is one of the most influential advocates of a smoke-free United States. He saw his father, oldest brother, and other relatives die from cigarette-induced emphysema and lung cancer. Concerned about the mounting health evidence against tobacco, he turned his back on his family's tobacco business and began to campaign in 1986 for a smoke-free nation.

Since starting his campaign, he has spoken before numerous state and municipal legislatures in support of proposed smoking ordinances that became law. In 1988 in California, he helped pass the 25¢-per-pack state cigarette tax increase. Mr. Reynolds has testified in Congress in favor of an end to all cigarette advertising and to help bring about the six-hour smoking ban on U.S. domestic flights. He also has asked Congress to limit the export and advertising of U.S. tobacco brands abroad and has lobbied for a new law banning cigarette sales to those under 21 years of age.

In addition to addressing corporations, universities, associations, and medical conferences, Reynolds has been interviewed in hundreds of television, radio, and print venues to remind millions of people of the dangers of smoking.

In 1989 in Los Angeles, California, Reynolds founded the Foundation for a Smokefree America, a charitable organization whose mission is to help bring about a smokefree society.

Reynolds's work has been recognized. In 1988, the United Nation's WORLD HEALTH ORGANIZATION honored Reynolds with a special award. In 1989, Chicago's Mt. Sinai Hospital awarded him its Humanitarian of the Year award. *See also* REYNOLDS, RICHARD JOSHUA

Reynolds, Richard Joshua (1850–1918)

The son of Hardin W. Reynolds, a slave owner, farmer, and factory owner in Patrick County, Virginia, Reynolds founded R.J. REYNOLDS TOBACCO COMPANY that eventually became the world's largest producer of flat goods, or loosely compressed plugs, used

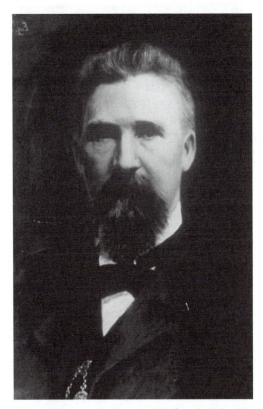

Richard Joshua (R.J.) Reynolds founded the R.J. Reynolds Tobacco Company in 1875 and began manufacturing Camel cigarettes in 1913. *AP/Wide World Photos.*

chiefly for chewing before he launched CAMEL CIGARETTES, the first modern CIGARETTE.

Like his rival JAMES BUCHANAN DUKE, founder of the AMERICAN TOBACCO COMPANY (ATC), Reynolds had broken away from a partnership with his father in tobacco. In 1873, he set up a small factory in Winston, North Carolina, and expanded it in 1875, employing two full-time employees and seasonal labor to make twist on a contract basis for workers. After two brothers joined him, the firm incorporated in 1890. As the Reynolds company grew, so too did Richard Joshua Reynolds's reputation in Winston. He helped get roads built, established a savings bank, and served as city commissioner.

Although Reynolds reportedly told a friend that "If Buck Duke tries to swallow me, he'll get the bellyache of his life," he gave in to JAMES BUCHANAN DUKE's proposal to become part of the tobacco trust. Later, Reynolds, who hated Duke, openly cooperated with government trust busters and anti-trust journalists. He told Josephus Daniels, North Carolina newspaper editor, that more than anything else, he wanted to be free of Buck Duke.

Reynolds, who had not been awarded any cigarette brands in the dissolution of the Tobacco Trust, had to start from scratch. He first created a new cigarette, Red Kamel, a Turkish cigarette. He discarded it in 1909, but in 1913 launched his famous Camel brand of BURLEY TOBACCO cigarettes. He did this even though he vowed never to produce cigarettes (he considered them a prostitution of fine leaf that catered to decadent tastes of the worst elements in society) and vowed R.J. Reynolds and Company would never market a brand containing Burley. Reynolds was capable of adjusting to new circumstances, however, and he entered the cigarette field in hopes of profiting from the product as well as competing with his arch enemy. By an unprecedented advertising and promotion campaign, Reynolds made Camel a national brand offered in all the states. He bested James Buchanan Duke, but only by accepting Burley and cigarettes.

Reynolds not only organized a sales force that aggressively marketed Reynolds products, he brought in new machinery to boost production of chewing and smoking tobacco. He also had enough capital to buy out his competitors. Shortly after the turn of the century, Reynolds was making a quarter of the nation's flat plug. He also introduced Prince Albert smoking tobacco, a product that rapidly became popular with the public.

Little is known about Richard Joshua Reynolds. When he died, only the *New York Times* carried an obituary, and it was 12 lines long. Although many articles have been written about his company, little has been written about the man who created it. *See also* PRINCE ALBERT PIPE TOBACCO; REYNOLDS; PATRICK

Richmond, Virginia

Richmond, Virginia, is a city rooted in tobacco history. It was the site of America's first mass farming of tobacco. In 1612, British settler JOHN ROLFE cultivated the plant, which he then shipped to London. The English and others around the world liked the taste of Rolfe's tobacco and demanded it. Money poured into Richmond, which became a commercial boomtown and the first tobacco manufacturing capital of the nation by 1860. Along the James River, huge tobacco farms and plantation homes sprang up, worked by slaves.

Richmond had all the requisites—leaf markets, transportation, and banks as well as shrewd businessmen like James Thomas, Jr., and Robert A. Mayo. Home to over 50 factories employing 3,400 workers, the manufacturers produced goods valued at almost $5 million per year.

During the Civil War, Richmond's tobacco warehouses were converted into hospitals and prisons. One brick tobacco plant, occupied at the war's outbreak by Libby and Sons, ship chandlers, became known as Libby Prison. Because Virginia's tobacco manufacturing was affected, production shifted southward to small towns in leaf areas of North Carolina. On the night of April 2, 1865, Confed-

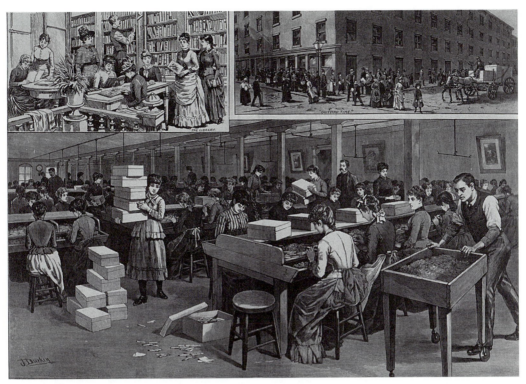

Cigarette rollers in Richmond, Virginia, c. 1887. *Library of Congress.*

erate troops burned the city's remaining to-bacco warehouses to deny valuable leaf stores to Ulysses S. Grant's advancing army. Out of control, the fire raged for days and was still burning when Robert E. Lee sent his flag of truce to Grant at Appomattox on April 9.

Richmond revived after the war. A make-shift tobacco leaf exchange was set up, but one reporter observed that "the growth and sale of this staple in Virginia is just now a mockery of what it was at the outbreak of the war, though still of sufficient importance to be one of the leading items in the commerce of the State, if not its most important one" (Heimann, 1960). Although Virginia tobacco planting and manufacturing regained an im-portant place, the center of Bright-leaf culti-vation shifted to North Carolina.

Richmond, still striving to regain its former top position on tobacco, moved into newer tobacco products like the hand-rolled CIGARETTE even though CHEWING TOBACCO was still the chief product. Production was slow because the best cigarette girls rolled only four to five per minute. In 1886, the Kinney Com-pany of New York built a sizeable Richmond factory to make smoking tobacco and ciga-rettes.

In Richmond, where manufacturing re-quirements and leaf sales both mounted into big-volume totals, the custom of "breaks," opening HOGSHEADS to inspect tobacco leaf, took too long. In an "exchange," which took the place of an AUCTION WAREHOUSE, leaf samples instead of whole hogsheads were inspected to save time and space.

In 1929, Philip Morris, a British company, opened its first factory in the United States. It chose Richmond because of its rich tobacco history. Today, the Philip Morris facility turns out 400 billion-plus cigarettes a year. *See also* BRIGHT TOBACCO LEAF; PHILIP MORRIS COM-PANIES INC.

References: Robert K. Heimann, *Tobacco and Ameri-cans,* New York: McGraw-Hill Book Company, 1960, p. 167.

R.J. Reynolds Tobacco Company

R.J. Reynolds Tobacco Company, the second largest tobacco company in the United States, manufactures nearly one out of every four cigarettes sold in the nation. It is a subsidiary of RJR Nabisco Inc, and is headquartered in New York City. The company's product line includes four of the 10 best-selling U.S. CIGARETTE brands. Reynolds Tobacco has about 9,000 full-time employees, and it operates two of the world's most modern cigarette manufacturing facilities—Whitaker Park, located in Winston-Salem, North Carolina, and the Tobaccoville Manufacturing Center, located near Winston-Salem, which is one of the largest manufacturing plants in the world. In addition to its two cigarette-manufacturing facilities, RJR houses leaf tobacco in 166 storage facilities across North Carolina.

RJR Reynolds also operates a packaging division—RJR Packaging. It produces flexible packaging materials printed by gravure process, aluminum foil, and laminated and coated products for a variety of external customers. This operation grew out of the Reynolds Tobacco unit that historically supplied packaging materials for the company's cigarette operations.

Founded in 1875 in Winston, North Carolina, R.J. Reynolds Tobacco Company incorporated in North Carolina in 1890 with RICHARD JOSHUA REYNOLDS as president and his brother Will as vice president. A third brother, Walter, joined the firm later. From 1875 until the 1890s, all Reynolds Tobacco products were chewing tobaccos.

From 1899 until 1911, Reynolds Tobacco was part of JAMES BUCHANAN DUKE's tobacco trust and the company was the vehicle by which Duke gained control of the American chewing tobacco industry. When the trust was broken up in 1911, Reynolds tobacco was independent once again and owned the rights to an estimated 1,500 CHEWING TOBACCO trademarks. By 1906, Reynolds was producing one-seventh of the nation's chewing tobacco, and by 1912, one-fourth.

Between 1895 and 1910, R.J. Reynolds also introduced several smoking tobacco products. Although they did well in the market, Reynolds wanted something different In 1907, the company introduced PRINCE ALBERT

PIPE TOBACCO, a product that rapidly became popular with the public. Made from Kentucky BURLEY TOBACCO, it was named after the popular Prince Albert of Wales who had become the British monarch, Edward VII in 1901. Soon after it was introduced, it became one of the nation's best-selling tobacco products. In its first four years of operations, production rose from 250,000 pounds annually to more than 14 million.

By 1913, Reynolds Tobacco Company had introduced four brands of cigarettes, Reyno (discontinued), Osman (a failure), Red Kamel (discontinued, but revived in the 1990s), and the now-famous CAMEL CIGARETTES, which grew to be the nation's best-selling cigarette. The Camel label's background of temples, minarets, an oasis, and pyramids resembled the one on the pack today. The camel itself was modeled after a one-humped dromedary in the Barnum and Bailey circus. Through an innovative advertising and sales campaign created by N.W. Ayers advertising company, Camels became a hugely successful cigarette. When Reynolds died in 1918, the company he had begun employed 10,000 people in 121 buildings in Winston-Salem.

Over the next 40 years, a combination of new methods of storing, packaging, and shipping tobacco; improvements in cigarette-making machines; large-scale marketing and lively radio and televised advertising campaigns; better living and working conditions for workers; company philanthropy; and wise planning made Reynolds Tobacco Company the nation's leading tobacco company in 1958 with sales of more than $1 billion. The company has since dropped to second place, overtaken by PHILIP MORRIS COMPANIES INC., the largest tobacco company in the United States.

Reynolds Tobacco has established virtually every tobacco industry packaging standard. The 20-cigarette pack was developed by RJR in 1913, and in 1915 the company introduced the one-piece, 10-pack carton. In 1931, RJR became the first company to package its cigarettes with a moisture-proof, sealed cellophane outer wrap—dubbed the "Humidor pack" when first introduced—to preserve freshness. In 1991, Reynolds Tobacco trademarked FlavorSeal,™ which retains tobacco moisture, critical to cigarette quality, 10 times better than the clear film wrap.

In 1954, Reynolds introduced Winston filter-tip cigarettes. By 1966, it was the best-selling cigarette in the nation. In 1956, Salem, the first filter-tipped menthol cigarette was introduced. It eventually dominated not only the menthol field but also became one of the world's top-selling brands.

Reynolds researchers pioneered a significant advance in tobacco processing when they developed a method of removing stems from tobacco leaves. They also fabricated reconstituted leaf, making possible the economical use of the entire tobacco leaf. In the late 1960s, Reynolds perfected a process to expand shredded tobacco, cutting cigarette manufacturing costs. Experimenting with filters and tobacco led researchers to develop Vantage, introduced in 1970, and Doral. Both provided low TAR and NICOTINE.

On April 22, 1970, shareholders approved a plan to create a new parent company, R.J. Reynolds Industries Inc., that signaled the investment of the tobacco company in non-tobacco enterprises. R.J. Reynolds Tobacco Company became a wholly owned subsidiary. Later, in 1985, the company name changed to RJR NABISCO HOLDINGS CORPORATION when R.J. Reynolds acquired Nabisco. *See also* DIVERSIFICATION; OLD JOE CAMEL

RJR Nabisco Holdings Corporation

The RJR Nabisco Holdings Corporation, headquartered in New York City, is the parent company of RJR Nabisco Inc. RJR Nabisco Inc. was an international consumer products company with subsidiaries engaged in domestic and international tobacco businesses and an 80.7 percent interest in Nabisco Holding Corporation (Oreo, Ritz, and Snackwells), an international food company.

The cigarette division of RJR Nabisco Holdings Corporation was RJR TOBACCO COMPANY, which makes CAMEL, Doral, Magna, Salem, and Winston cigarette brands.

Since 1996, the chief executive officer of RJR Nabisco has been STEVEN GOLDSTONE. In March 1999, RJR Nabisco announced that it was splitting its food and tobacco businesses and selling its foreign tobacco company to JAPAN TOBACCO INC. The domestic tobacco business will become a separate company.

Robusto. *See* CIGAR SIZE AND SHAPE

Rogers, Richard (1935–1987)

An Indianapolis, Indiana, lawyer, Richard Rogers smoked two to three packs of cigarettes a day and died at 52 years of age from lung cancer. Rogers's case was filed in the Marion County Superior Court shortly before his death by lawyers who contended NICOTINE is addictive and that smoking caused his cancer. His wife, Yvonne, claimed that four tobacco companies that made the brands he smoked had sold a defective product and had failed to warn of the health risks and addictive qualities of cigarettes. She sought $2 million in compensatory damages and an unspecified amount in punitive damages.

There were two trials. The first, in 1995, ended in a mistrial. In the second trial, on August 23, 1996, the jury ruled in favor of the cigarette companies, finding them not responsible for Rogers's death and barring damages. The judge limited evidence to what had been admitted at the first trial. Internal BROWN AND WILLIAMSON TOBACCO CORPORATION documents on the addictiveness of nicotine were not allowed into evidence by the judge. In Indiana, juries cannot rule for the plaintiff if they think the plaintiff bears more than 50 percent of the blame. The jury foreman said: "under the laws of Indiana we felt that Richard Rogers bore a greater responsibility for the conditions that caused his death than did the actions of the defendants" (Collins, 1996). The tobacco companies hailed the verdict as confirmation that the Grady Carter case was "an aberration." *See also* CARTER, GRADY; CIPOLLONE, ROSE; CONNOR, JEAN; MADDOX, ROLAND

References: Glen Collins, "Jury in Indiana Lawsuit Bars Damages in Lawsuit Over Lung Cancer," *New York Times*, August 24, 1996.

Rolfe, John (1585–1622)

John Rolfe, a pipe-smoking Englishman from Norfolk, Virginia, has been credited with the success of Jamestown's tobacco crop. In 1612, the colony of JAMESTOWN in Virginia (the first permanent English settlement in North America) was near financial collapse and looking for a crop that would make it economically viable. Rolfe, who shunned NIC-OTIANA RUSTICA, the harsh-tasting product grown by American Indians, managed to obtain from the Spanish "enemy" seeds of their prized tobacco. Several stories tell how he got his hands on the valuable seed. Some say when he was shipwrecked in the Bermudas, Rolfe gathered seeds from the coveted NIC-OTIANA TABACUM strain then being grown in Trinidad and South America and brought some of the plants back to the Jamestown settlement—though Spain had declared a penalty of death to anyone selling such seeds to a non-Spaniard. Another story has it that Rolfe bribed sailors on a Dutch trading ship to bring the seeds back to him. Whatever the story, in the sandy soil of Virginia, the Spanish tobacco thrived.

Rolfe found better ways of growing and curing tobacco. Some scholars feel he was guided in the techniques by Pocahontas, daughter of American Indian chief Powhatan. Rolfe married Pocahontas in April 1614. The marriage helped engineer eight years of peace with the Powhatan Indians, a period when the energies of the colonists could be devoted to the growing of their new cash crop–which soon became the "New World's" currency.

In June 1614, Rolfe shipped his first cargo of Virginia tobacco, called "Orinoco," to England. (Rolfe undoubtedly named the brand to evoke the mystery and adventure of Sir WALTER RALEIGH, who led expeditions up the Orinoco River in Guiana in search of the legendary city of gold, El Dorado.) The tobacco, with its excellent aroma, was an immediate success in the London market. Two years later, Rolfe, his wife Rebecca (Pocahontas's Christian name), and other leaders of the colony went to London to discuss tobacco, the colony's major export. *See also* JAMES I

Roper Organization

In the 1970s, the tobacco industry was worried about the emerging nonsmokers' rights movement that focused on SECONDHAND SMOKE. In 1978, the Roper Organization conducted a secret study for the tobacco industry on the attitudes of the public towards smoking. The FEDERAL TRADE COMMISSION eventually obtained the report and made it public. The study concluded that

- A majority of Americans believe it is probably hazardous to be around people who smoke, even if they are not smoking themselves.
- A steadily increasing majority of Americans believe that the tobacco industry knows that the case against cigarettes is true.
- More than 9 out of 10 Americans believe that smoking is hazardous to a smoker's health.
- A majority of people want separate smoking sections in public places.

The Roper study concluded with a statement that was notable for a time when little evidence had accumulated proving smoking did long-term damage to nonsmokers.

What the smoker does to himself may be his business, but what the smoker does to the nonsmoker is quite a different matter . . . . This we see as the most dangerous development to the viability of the tobacco industry that has yet occurred. (Taylor, 1984)

The Roper report recommended that the industry engage in research to discredit the evidence that passive smoking is dangerous to nonsmokers.

The strategic and long run antidote to the passive smoking issue is, as we see it, developing and widely publicizing clear-cut, credible, medical evidence that passive smoking is not harmful to the non-smokers' health. (Taylor, 1984)

References: Peter Taylor, *The Smoke Ring*, New York: Pantheon Books, 1984, pp. 190–92.

Rosenblatt, Stanley and Rosenblatt, Susan. *See Broin v. Philip Morris Companies Inc.; Engle v. R.J. Reynolds*

Ross, Alexander (1783–1856)

In 1818, Alexander Ross, a Scottish trader and explorer, explored the Columbia River to the mouth of the Snake River in what is now southeastern Washington. In 1823–1824, he explored the Snake River region of present-day Idaho. In his journals, he frequently mentions tobacco as an essential tool of trade with native people. The principal use of smoking, he noted, was "the introductory step to all important affairs, and no business can be entered upon with these people before the ceremony of smoking is over." When Ross and his trappers made their way into the Rockies, they encountered the Snake nation. Ross thought they were "perhaps the only Indian nation on the continent that manufacture and smoke their own tobacco."

> The Snake tobacco plant grows low, is of a brownish colour and thrives in most parts of the country, but is a favourite of sandy or barren soil . . . it is weaker than our tobacco, but the difference in strength may be owing to the mode of manufacturing it for use. For this purpose their only process is to dig it and then rub it fine with the hands or pound it with stones until it is tolerably fine. In this state it almost resembles green tea. In smoking it leaves a green taste or flavour in the mouth.
>
> Our people however seemed to like it very well . . . yet with all their fondness for the Snake tobacco, I observed that the moment they reached the fort the Snake importation was either bartered away or laid aside; one and all applied to me for good old twist!
>
> The Snakes would often bring it to our people for sale; but generally in small parcels, sometimes an ounce or two, sometimes a quart, and sometimes as much as a gallon. In their bartering propensities, however, they would often make our friends smile, to see them with a beaver skin in one hand and a small bag containing perhaps a pint of the native tobacco in the other: the former they would offer for a

paper looking glass worth two pence; while for the latter they would often demand an axe worth four or five shillings! (Heimann, 1960)

References: Robert K. Heimann, *Tobacco and Americans*, New York: McGraw-Hill Books, 1960, p. 125.

Ross v. Philip Morris and Company

An example of a cigarette case litigated during the first wave of tobacco litigation (1954–1973) was the case of *Ross v. Philip Morris and Company*. It was argued under the theory of breach of implied warranty. The plaintiff, John T. Ross, alleged he developed throat cancer as a result of smoking cigarettes manufactured by the defendant.

Ross began smoking cigarettes when he was 28 or 29 years old, became a confirmed smoker in 1934, and smoked Philip Morris brand cigarettes almost exclusively. Ross increased his consumption of smoking cigarettes from the early 1930s and within four to five years was smoking two packs a day. Again, he increased his intake to the point where in 1939 and 1940 he smoked as many as three and sometimes four packs a day. He did not reduce his smoking until he went to Mayo Clinic in 1952 for surgery to remove cancer. Since the operation, Ross has had to breathe through an opening in his neck and can speak only with the aid of an electric device attached to his throat.

The plaintiff maintained that the defendant breached an implied warranty that the cigarettes it provided were not harmful. Philip Morris asserted that an implied warranty did not cover substances in cigarettes that could not be detected with the exercise of reasonable skill. Therefore, the manufacturer argued it should be held liable only for breach of implied warranty for injuries it knew or should have known existed in its cigarette.

The case was tried in the United States District Court for the Western District of Missouri in 1962 where a judgment was entered for the defendant. Ross appealed and the Eighth Circuit Court of Appeals agreed with the defendant and found that an implied warranty does not cover harmful substances within a product that could not be detected through reasonable skill or knowledge. Because Ross and Philip Morris agreed that human skill could not have foreseen the cancer-smoking relationship, the manufacturer was not held liable for breach of implied warranty. *See also* PHILIP MORRIS COMPANIES INC.; TOBACCO LITIGATION: FIRST, SECOND, AND THIRD WAVES

Roventini, Johnny (1912–1998)

When Philip Morris Tobacco Company introduced Philip Morris cigarettes, the company hired Johnny Roventini, a 22-year-old, 43-inch-tall Hotel New Yorker bellhop from Brooklyn. Credit for hiring Johnny goes to two advertising men, Milton Biow and Kenneth Goode, who in 1933 asked a bellhop at the New York Hotel to page Philip Morris. The bellhop was Johnny Roventini who went through the lobby singing out in a clear voice the words printed on a card handed him by the men: "Call for Phil-lip Mor-ris." The two advertising men, taken by the reaction of people in the lobby who responded with smiles, hired him to become the voice of Philip Morris cigarettes.

From the time Mr. Roventini first went on the air on April 17, 1933, on the "Ferde Grofé Show" until the cigarette company phased him out as a radio and television spokesman in the early 1950s, he had one of the most recognizable voices in the United States. The radio voice for Philip Morris, his famous line "Call for Phil-lip Mor-ris" rang out on top radio programs, at conventions, and ball games during the 1930s and 1940s.

Dressed in a bright red, gold-trimmed uniform, Johnny Roventini appeared in most of the ads that appeared in newspapers and quality magazines such as *Vogue* and *Town and Country*. His picture also showed up in store windows, making him one of the most recognizable figures in the nation.

Roventini retired in 1974, but he had a lifetime contract with Philip Morris.

Royal College of Physicians (RCP)

In 1959, the British Royal College of Physicians (RCP) established a committee that reviewed the scientific literature and considered all the alternative explanations put forth for the rise in lung cancer in people who smoked. At a press conference on March 7, 1962, Sir Robert Platt, president of RCP, issued the first major report reviewing the data on cigarettes and disease. The major conclusions of the report were as follows:

> Cigarette smoking is a cause of lung cancer and bronchitis, and probably contributes to the development of coronary heart disease and various other less common diseases . . . . The number of deaths caused by diseases associated with smoking is large. (Corina, 1975)

References: Maurice Corina, *Trust in Tobacco: The Anglo-American Struggle for Power*. New York: St. Martin's Press, 1975, p. 244.

Rush, Benjamin (1745–1813)

Around 1798, Dr. Benjamin Rush, the most prominent American physician of the late eighteenth century, wrote a famous and arguably the first significant anti-tobacco document published in the United States. Entitled "Observations upon the Influence of the Habitual Use of Tobacco upon Health, Morals, and Property," it appeared in Rush's 1798 book *Essays, Literary, Moral, and Philosophical.* Dr. Rush described the disastrous effects of tobacco on the stomach, nerves, and oral cavity. Besides being expensive, he said tobacco led to idleness, uncleanliness, poor manners, and drinking.

> One of the usual effects of smoking [sic] and chewing is thirst. This thirst cannot be allayed by water, for no sedative or even insipid liquor will be relished after the mouth and throat have been exposed to the stimulus of the smoke, or juice of Tobacco. A desire of course is excited for strong drinks, and these when taken between meals soon leads to intemperance and drunkenness. One of the greatest sots I

knew, acquired a love for ardent spirits by swallowing cuds of Tobacco, which he did, to escape detection in the use of it, for he had contracted the habit of chewing, contrary to the advice and commands of his father. He died of Dropsy under my care in the year 1780. (Wagner, 1971)

References: Susan Wagner, *Cigarette Country: Tobacco in American History and Politics*, New York: Praeger Publishers, 1971, p. 26.

Russia

In the seventeenth century, Russia ended a long period of isolation from European influences. Italian, Spanish, and Portuguese sailors introduced tobacco into eastern Europe. In northeast Europe, Turkish ships carried it to the coastal cities of the Black Sea, English sailors to the Baltic, and travelers from Germany and Poland to inland Russia. The habit of smoking began to permeate Eastern Europe. By the mid-seventeenth century, people openly smoked in churches, even during services. Russian smokers, who made heavy use of water pipes, inhaled so deeply that the combination of hyperventilation and intoxication produced unconsciousness.

In 1634, Tsar Michael issued an edict that smoking was to be regarded as a deadly sin. Nobody, national or foreign, was allowed to smoke, take SNUFF, or trade in tobacco. First offenders, whether users or vendors, were to be punished by having their noses slit. A special court for dealing with smokers was established. Persistent offenders were exiled to Siberia and their property confiscated. Nevertheless, tobacco use continued. Financial pressures led the tsar to violate his own laws when he established a fiscal monopoly of tobacco.

In 1649, Tsar Alexis (1645–1676) published an edict forbidding smoking. Punishments remained severe, including torture and exile. Criminals were racked and publicly tortured. Special vigilantes were appointed to search for contraband tobacco in Moscow. In 1655, an ordinance confirmed the death penalty, but still tobacco use continued.

Tsar Theodore III (1676–1682) inaugurated a period of milder restraints, and tobacco use spread from the court and foreign circles to other parts of the population. In the last years of the tsar's reign, tobacco use was widespread.

In 1689, Peter the Great (1689–1725) became sole ruler of Russia. He inaugurated a program of modernization, relying on Western models. In his travels to Europe in 1697, he picked up the habit of pipe smoking and decided the Russian clergy's ban was oppressive. He issued an edict permitting open sale and consumption of tobacco because of its wide use and ubiquitous secret trade in which the state did not share.

The Russian Church feared modernization and other "Western" influences, and disliked tobacco as much for being a symbol of foreign influence as a health hazard. The Church resisted Peter the Great's attempts to "modernize" society and his acceptance of tobacco use, which ultimately prevailed. The Church, like other critics, also blamed smoking for the increase in fires in Moscow. Negligent smokers who fell asleep set their houses on fire. *See also* PIPE, WATER

S

Sackman, Janet (1931–)

Janet Sackman, for years a top cigarette model for Liggett and Myers's Chesterfields and AMERICAN TOBACCO COMPANY's Lucky Strikes, was urged by an executive of a tobacco company to smoke at 17 years of age so she would look authentic in television ads. Soon she smoked two packs a day and, in 1983, was diagnosed with throat cancer. She had her larynx removed and learned to talk again by forcing air through her esophagus. Seven years later, in 1990, she found the cancer had spread to her right lung. Sackman decided to devote what was left of her life to warning children not to be taken in by glamorous cigarette ads like the ones she appeared in, still found in magazines and on BILLBOARDS. She appeared in anti-smoking ads in the Massachusetts campaign to stop teen smoking.

In 1993, Sackman instituted a lawsuit against the Liggett Group, charging the company had sold a defective and addictive product, had failed to warn her of the health consequences, had fraudulently denied that smoking was a hazard, and had conspired with other tobacco companies to conceal evidence of the health threat posed by smoking. She ended her lawsuit in 1997 for an estimated multimillion-dollar settlement. Under the terms of the settlement, she and her lawyers were forbidden from discussing details. Today Sackman, an outspoken opponent of smoking, gives speeches across the country. *See also* CHESTERFIELD CIGARETTES; LIGGETT AND MYERS TOBACCO COMPANY; LUCKY STRIKE CIGARETTES

Safe Cigarettes

Since the 1950s, scientists on both sides of the Atlantic have debated whether a "safe cigarette" could be developed or whether it could exist at all, because it is not known what levels of carcinogens are safe or how the dozens of toxic compounds in CIGARETTE smoke interact in the body. Cigarette smoke contains more than 4,000 compounds including 40 to 50 substances scientists believed to be carcinogens. In general, these cancer-causing substances are generally contained in TAR, a term referring to the solid compounds produced when tobacco burns. Nitrosamines are the biggest group of carcinogens found in tobacco and cigarette smoke. Smoke also contains CARBON MONOXIDE, suspected to have a role in heart disease. In theory, a cigarette with reduced levels of carcinogens would still give smokers the NICOTINE they crave. While nicotine has physiological effects, it is not considered as dangerous as tar.

By the end of the 1960s, tobacco industry researchers hoped to produce a safer cigarette. In the early 1970s, they had succeeded in identifying what the hazards were, and they were finding methods of counteracting them. By the late 1970s, however, after sponsoring research and work on filters, additives, and safe cigarettes, R.J. REYNOLDS TOBACCO COMPANY, PHILIP MORRIS USA, and BROWN AND WILLIAMSON TOBACCO CORPORATION closed their laboratories on the advice of company lawyers. The research by the scientists into less dangerous cigarettes was dropped because industry lawyers argued that such research could produce an onslaught of lawsuits and imply that a company's other products were hazardous. Companies also feared that smokers would not buy safer cigarettes that did not smell or taste good. By the mid-1980s, when lawsuits were accumulating, legal departments worried about what would happen if years of studies on biological hazards of cigarettes became available to plaintiffs in court cases.

In the 1960s, the Brown and Williamson Tobacco Corporation, a division of BAT INDUSTRIES PLC, started and dropped work on a cigarette project called ARIEL that heated, rather than burned, tobacco. This procedure would have reduced tar. The company, which was granted a patent in 1966, never brought the product to the market. According to company documents and interviews with scientists working on the project, the company decided against moving the safer products to the marketplace because they would make their other products look bad. The documents also suggested that smokers might not find the cigarettes satisfying and would not buy them.

For 13 years, Brown and Williamson also conducted a series of more than 40 separate biological experiments called Project Janus, after the Roman god of two faces, one facing the future, the other facing the past. Its aim was to isolate the biological effects of cigarette smoke and to help identify which parts of the smoke were dangerous, so they could be removed. Reports from Project Janus were negative, as more and more toxic compounds were found in smoke.

Another safe cigarette was made by Dr. Thomas Mold, assistant director of research for LIGGETT AND MYERS TOBACCO COMPANY, and his colleagues. The research began in 1955 and the product was ready for the market by 1979. Company executives voted, on the advice of lawyers, not to produce a safer cigarette that used palladium, a heavy metal, in the filter to eliminate the carcinogenic activity of cigarettes, as measured by skin-painting tests.

During the late 1980s, tobacco companies continued their research into manufacturing a safe cigarette. RJR NABISCO HOLDINGS CORPORATION, parent company of R.J. Reynolds Tobacco Company, test-marketed PREMIER, a smokeless cigarette that heated, rather than burned, tobacco. The product failed because it was difficult to keep the cigarette lit and it tasted bad. In 1996, Reynolds introduced an updated and improved version of Premier called ECLIPSE and tested it in Chattanooga, Tennessee. The product cut down on tar and SECONDHAND SMOKE, but smokers took in a full dose of nicotine and high levels of carbon monoxide.

In 1989, Philip Morris introduced Next cigarettes, promoted as a low-nicotine cigarette, but it was dropped in 1991 because of lack of consumer demand. WILLIAM A. FARONE, a Philip Morris researcher from 1976 to 1984, said the company's Next cigarette "should have had extremely low levels of tobacco-specific nitrosamines."

In 1968, the federal government organized a task force, including NATIONAL CANCER INSTITUTE researchers, to work with the tobacco industry on developing a less hazardous cigarette. After more than 10 years and an outlay of tens of millions of dollars, no product was developed. According to Dietrich Hoffman, associate director of the AMERICAN HEALTH FOUNDATION, a research institute headquartered in New York that studies tobacco and health issues, the U.S. government shared the blame with cigarette makers for not making a less hazardous cigarette.

The federal government has minimally regulated cigarettes because tobacco products are not classified as drugs, which fall under the FOOD AND DRUG ADMINISTRATION jurisdiction. However, in 1987, when a tobacco company in Texas marketed a cigarette-like plastic tube called Favor that contained a nicotine vapor, federal officials objected and it was pulled from the market.

In the landmark proposed $368.5 billion tobacco settlement of June 1997 between tobacco companies and state attorneys generals, plaintiffs' lawyers, and others, one provision encouraged manufacturers to develop and market "less hazardous tobacco" products. The settlement negotiators did not define the term. Star Tobacco and Pharmaceuticals, a small producer of discount cigarettes in Petersburg, Virginia, said it developed a way to reduce cancer-causing nitrosamines in tobacco. *See also* TOBACCO SETTLEMENT—JUNE 1997

Sandefur, Thomas E., Jr. (1939–1996)

Thomas E. Sandefur was chairman and chief executive of the BROWN AND WILLIAMSON TOBACCO CORPORATION. He became a national figure when the tobacco industry's highest-ranking defector, JEFFREY WIGAND, accused his former boss in late 1995 of lying under oath to Congress when he testified in 1994 that NICOTINE was not addictive.

Sandefur began his career in the early 1960s selling CIGARS and CHEWING TOBACCO for the R.J. REYNOLDS TOBACCO COMPANY in North Carolina. For 18 years, he worked for the company's European operations, rising to executive vice president. In 1982, Sandefur joined Brown and Williamson, whose British parent, BAT INDUSTRIES PLC, is the world's second biggest cigarette maker. As a marketing executive, he became chairman and chief executive in 1993 and retired in 1995.

Mr. Sandefur played a major role in developing Brown and Williamson's full-price brands and positioned the company in the discount-brand sector of the American cigarette market. As chief executive officer, he integrated Brown and Williamson's operations with those of the AMERICAN TOBACCO COMPANY after BAT's 1994 merger of the two companies.

In April 1994, Mr. Sandefur became a national figure, along with the chairmen of six other major tobacco companies, when he testified at Henry Waxman's House subcommittee that he believed nicotine was not addictive. He did acknowledge that the company controlled nicotine levels in cigarettes, but he said it was only to maintain the cigarettes' taste.

Towards the end of January 1996, Alix Freedman of the *Wall Street Journal* published key sections of a transcript of sealed testimony of Jeffrey S. Wigand, who headed Brown and Williamson's research department from 1989 until 1993 when he was fired by Sandefur. Deposed by RONALD MOTLEY, a Charleston, South Carolina, trial attorney, on November 29, 1995, Wigand accused Sandefur of lying under oath to Congress about his views on nicotine addiction. Sandefur never took the witness stand to defend himself. He died on July 15, 1996.

After Sandefur's death, Nick Brookes, the chairman and chief executive officer of Brown and Williamson, said Sandefur "was a strong leader who not only saw opportunities before most, as in the growth of value-for-money brands, but was quick to take advantage of those opportunities" (Collins, 1996). *See also* WAXMAN HEARINGS

References: Glenn Collins, Thomas Saudefur, "Tobacco Leader, Dies at 56," *New York Times*, July 16, 1996, p. B18.

Santa Fe Natural Tobacco Company.
See NATURAL AMERICAN SPIRIT CIGARETTES

Schwartz, Tony (1923–)

Tony Schwartz, often called a media guru and an advertising genius, has been making radio and television commercials since the 1950s. In 1988, the WORLD HEALTH ORGANIZATION awarded him a Tobacco or Health Medal, given to people who have made an outstanding contribution towards a tobacco-free society.

In 1964, Schwartz produced the first anti-smoking public service announcement for the AMERICAN CANCER SOCIETY (ACS). The message, which has won many prizes, showed two small children trying on grown-up clothes. The voice-over said: "Children love to imitate their parents. Children learn by imitating their parents. Do you smoke cigarettes?" The girl then looked at the camera and giggled while on the screen came the words "American Cancer Society." This commercial has been credited with striking the first blow in getting CIGARETTE advertising off the air in the United States. Since 1964, Schwartz has created more than 200 anti-smoking messages, most of them radio spots narrated by Bob Landers, his longtime associate in San Diego, California.

In a 1991 interview about countering tobacco ads published in *World Smoking and Health*, a journal of the American Cancer Society, Schwartz was asked "Do you think that ads should focus on the tobacco industry, not the smokers?" He answered as follows:

> The smokers are victims. There's no one thing that makes people stop smoking. Some people are affected by hypnotism; some people by commercials they hear; some by stories about people who have just died, some by family members who died. But the real thing these people are not aware of is that the cigarette companies are only interested in one aspect of them, and that's their wallet, their money.
>
> Make fun of the tobacco companies if you can. Make them look ridiculous. Make them look vicious. ("An Interview," 1991)

See also ADVERTISING AND CIGARETTES AND SMOKELESS TOBACCO; RADIO AND CIGARETTE ADVERTISING; TELEVISION AND CIGARETTE ADVERTISING

References: "An Interview with Tony Schwartz." *World Smoking and Health*, vol. 16, no. 3, 1991, p. 4.

Scruggs, Richard F. (1946–)

A lead negotiator in the 1996 landmark settlement between BENNETT LEBOW's Liggett Group and five states as well as co-counsel to states suing tobacco companies for reimbursement of medical expenses, Richard F. Scruggs is a Mississippi lawyer living in the port town of Pascagoula. In 1984, Richard Scruggs began handling and winning asbestos cases. A master at cutting deals, he settled for lower awards and consolidated thousands of claims into a single trial. When the attorney general's office decided to litigate asbestos companies, close friend and Mississippi Attorney General MICHAEL C. MOORE hired Scruggs, a fellow law school classmate at the University of Mississippi, to represent the state.

In the summer of 1993, Scruggs turned his attention to suing tobacco companies. His experience in pursuing asbestos cases had taught him a great deal about lungs and the effects of tobacco smoke. Many of the victims of asbestosis also smoked and the two agents worked synergistically. In 1993, Scruggs and DON BARRETT tried a case on behalf of Anderson Smith, a paranoid schizophrenic who began smoking while hospitalized. After lending cash to Barrett in the second NATHAN HORTON trial, Scruggs concluded a new theory was needed to sue tobacco companies because they defended themselves by pinning individuals with responsibility choosing to smoke. When MICHAEL T. LEWIS suggested to Scruggs that they file a suit against the tobacco industry to recoup the Medicaid costs incurred by the state for treating poor people sick from smoking, they teamed up and successfully persuaded the state to sue. In 1994, after thousands of hours of preparation, Scruggs and his colleagues went public with their lawsuit.

In 1995, Scruggs took on a client pro bono—JEFFREY S. WIGAND, former head of research at BROWN AND WILLIAMSON TOBACCO CORPORATION and the tobacco industry's highest-ranking defector. When Brown and Williamson tried to silence Wigand, Scruggs got Attorney General Moore to subpoena Wigand for the state of Mississippi's lawsuit against tobacco companies. Scruggs deposed Wigand for the Mississippi case. As a result, Brown and Williamson accused Scruggs of compromising Wigand's legal interests to benefit his client, the state of Mississippi.

Scruggs, deputized by Attorney General Moore, helped assemble a team of law firms, both Democratic and Republican, that would sue tobacco companies on behalf of the state. Besides being a lead negotiator in the settlement between Bennett LeBow's Liggett Group and five states, he also was involved in settlement talks with tobacco company executives and their lawyers in 1997. *See also* MISSISSIPPI MEDICAID CASE

Secondhand Smoke

Until the mid-1970s, concern about tobacco was limited to how smoking harmed smokers. But increasingly people were becoming concerned about air pollution from cars, incinerators, power plants, and secondhand smoke from cigarettes. Nonsmokers argued that cigarette smoke smelled bad, irritated their eyes, burned their noses, and gave them headaches. People with allergies were bothered by cigarette smoke. Yet little was known about the effects of secondhand smoke on nonsmokers. Scientists were not ready to say for certain that exposure to tobacco smoke caused serious illness in nonsmokers.

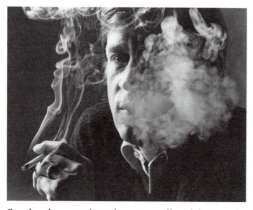

Smoke that can be taken secondhand by nearby nonsmokers wreathes a smoker's face and hand. *American Cancer Society.*

The medical community and health groups did not focus on the passive smoking issue, but as early as November 1971 Surgeon General Jesse Steinfeld called for a national Bill of Rights for the Nonsmoker. He wanted bans on smoking in public places such as restaurants, public transportation, and theaters. Besides Steinfeld receiving thousands of letters, people began writing letters to

newspaper editors demanding smoke-free air. Gradually, people began to support the idea that nonsmokers had a right to clean air. Steinfeld's 1972 surgeon general's report examined the harmful ingredients of tobacco smoke and "public exposure to air pollution from tobacco smoke." The report identified CARBON MONOXIDE, NICOTINE, and TAR as smoke constituents likely to produce health hazards. The report said tobacco smoke may worsen allergies in the nonsmoker and carbon monoxide in smoke-filled rooms may harm the health of people with chronic lung or heart diseases.

The passive smoke issue was largely carried by small grassroots citizen groups. Group Against Smoking Pollution (GASP) was one of the first to demand clean air free of secondhand smoke. *See also* ENVIRONMENTAL TOBACCO SMOKE (ETS); MAINSTREAM SMOKE; NEW JERSEY GROUP AGAINST SMOKING POLLUTION; SIDESTREAM SMOKE

Seldes, George (1890–1995)

George Seldes was a noted foreign correspondent in the 1920s who turned press critic in the 1930s. In 1940, he began publishing *In Fact: An Antidote to Falsehoods in the Daily Press,* a weekly four-page newsletter devoted to press criticism and investigative reporting. *In Fact* reached a peak circulation of 176,000 subscribers, making it the largest liberal periodical of its time. It outsold the *Nation* and the *New Republic* combined, but its circulation and reach fell far short of mainstream dailies and periodicals. *In Fact* discontinued publishing in December 1952.

In the January 13, 1941, issue of *In Fact,* Seldes published his first cigarette story about the 1938 study by Dr. RAYMOND PEARL of Johns Hopkins University that showed that heavy cigarette smoking severely limited one's life span. While several scientific journals had published Pearl's study at the time it came out, Seldes pointed out that almost no mainstream American daily carried the story despite the fact it had been carried on the Associate Press (AP) wire. He argued the reason for the widespread omission was that newspapers did not want to offend tobacco advertisers, one of their biggest sources of revenue.

Over the next decade, in more than 50 stories published between January 1941 and October 1950, Seldes covered five areas: (1) scientific studies, (2) the failure of most of the press to carry news of these studies, (3) the relationship of the tobacco companies and the press, (4) false advertising claims by the tobacco industry and the FEDERAL TRADE COMMISSION reports citing those ads, and (5) public policy concerning cigarettes.

Seventh Day Adventist Church

The Seventh Day Adventist Church, headquartered in Silver Spring, Maryland, has long preached against the harmful effects of smoking, and has created a world-famous plan to stop using tobacco. In 1959, a Seventh Day Adventist physician, Dr. J. Wayne McFarland, and Reverend Elman J. Folkenberg combined efforts to pilot a project in Denver, Colorado, called the Five-Day Plan to Stop Smoking. The clinic was so successful that it was extended to many other cities throughout the United States and into the international arena as well. Their efforts were also combined into book form.

Certain elements of the Five-Day Plan were based on techniques used for many years by the Adventist denominations to help people break the smoking habit. The plan involves a series of five consecutive 90-minute sessions designed to show smokers how to beat the habit in four dimensions of life: physical, mental, social, and spiritual. The program is usually presented by a team consisting of a Seventh Day Adventist physician and clergyman. It is often conducted in cooperation with, or cosponsored by, other civic or church groups.

The Five-Day Plan urges participants to quit "cold turkey" and make a strong decision not to relapse. The techniques it advocates during withdrawal from tobacco include warm baths, increased fluid intake, regular eating and sleeping habits, extra exercise, avoiding alcohol and caffeine, extra vitamins,

and prayer. *See also* AMERICAN CANCER SOCIETY; AMERICAN LUNG ASSOCIATION; NICOTINE REPLACEMENT PRODUCTS; SMOKING CESSATION

Seville, Spain

The world's great CIGAR manufacturing center, Seville, Spain, is identified with fine cigars made with the best tobaccos. Indeed, Spanish cigars are known as *Sevilles*. The first cigar factories in Seville appeared in 1676; by 1731 the royal cigar factories were established there. The Spanish king rigidly controlled leaf culture in his colonies and prohibited export except to Seville. The renowned opera CARMEN was set in Seville. *See also* SPAIN

Shew, Joel (1816–1855)

A prominent American physician and anti-tobacco crusader, Dr. Joel Shew attributed 87 ailments to tobacco including insanity, cancer, epilepsy, sexuality, impotency, and delirium tremens.

Shields, Brooke (1965–)

In 1981, the PUBLIC HEALTH SERVICE contacted an ad agency to develop a hard-hitting anti-cigarette commercial. The agency suggested creating an ad with 15-year-old Brooke Shields, a famous nonsmoking teen, one of the most sought-after models in the world, and star of the movie *Blue Lagoon*. Shields agreed to do the commercial at no charge not only because she and her mother both disliked smoking, but also because both of Shields's grandfathers died from smoking-related diseases.

The young model made hard-hitting TV spots and ads for magazines. One TV ad showed the model stretched out on a studio bed saying:

> There was this guy who I thought was terrific, was self-assured and I really liked that in a guy. Anyway, one night I saw him at a party and got up the nerve to say hello. He took out this cigarette—blew my whole image of him. I know I make some people nervous, but I thought he had it all to-

gether. Smoking! It's a dead giveaway. I think people who smoke are real losers. ("Brooke Shields Take a Stand," 1981).

The Public Health Service cancelled the campaign. Reagan administration officials claimed Shields was not the "most appropriate model" for teens, nor did they feel the spots would do an effective job of curbing teen smoking. Almost immediately, the AMERICAN LUNG ASSOCIATION (ALA) secured the rights to sponsor the ads and TV spots. In June 1981, Shields's mother testified before a congressional subcommittee: "I think it is sad that our government, which professes to be for the people would cancel an anti-smoking campaign which is, naturally, for the people" (Testimony of Teri Shields, 1981).

References: "Brooke Shields Takes a Stand Against Smoking, But the Government Didn't Want Her Message," *American Lung Association Bulletin*, June–July 1981, p. 14.

Testimony of Teri Shields before Subcommittee on Oversight and Investigation of the House Energy and Commerce Committee, 99th Congress, June 25, 1981.

Shimp v. New Jersey Bell (1976)

In the 1976 landmark case, *Shimp v. New Jersey Bell*, a nonsmoking telephone company representative who was allergic to tobacco smoke won a permanent injunction banning smoking in the office where she worked. It was the first lawsuit to win such an injunction. Donna Shimp's lawsuit turned on the fact that New Jersey Bell, the employer, protected its electronic switches from smoke but did not show as much concern for its "human equipment." The court said that

> The evidence is clear and overwhelming. Cigarette smoke contaminates and pollutes the air, creating a health hazard not merely to the smoker but to all those around her who must rely upon the same air supply. The right of an individual to risk his or her own health does not include the right to jeopardize the health of those who must remain around him or her in order to perform properly the duties of their jobs. (Carlson, 1997)

References: Regina Carlson, *Smokefree Air Everywhere: Why and How for Decision Makers in Workplaces and Public Places*, Montclair, NJ: New Jersey Group Against Smoking Pollution, 1997, p. 25.

Shook, Hardy, and Bacon (SHB)

Since the 1950s, the largest law firm in Kansas City, Missouri, Shook, Hardy, and Bacon (SHB), has defended, counseled, and been chief trouble-shooter for the tobacco industry. An international enterprise with 175 lawyers (in 1998) and scores of specialist researchers, biochemists, oncologists, statisticians, radiologists, and veterinarians, SHB has branch offices in Houston, London, Milan, and Zurich. More than half of its annual revenues comes from tobacco.

The firm, famous for its relentless pursuit of any possible alternative explanation for a plaintiff's disease, has successfully represented five of the six biggest tobacco companies—AMERICAN TOBACCO COMPANY, BROWN AND WILLIAMSON TOBACCO CORPORATION, R.J. REYNOLDS TOBACCO COMPANY, PHILIP MORRIS USA, and LORILLARD COMPANY INC. as well as the TOBACCO INSTITUTE in Washington, D.C. More than half of the firm's lawyers work in the tobacco division.

SHB's association with tobacco companies began in 1954 when Philip Morris hired the law firm's legendary litigator, David R. Hardy, to represent the company in a lawsuit filed by a Missouri smoker who lost his larynx to cancer. Six years later when the case ended, in 1962, the jury took only one hour to find for the tobacco company. Mr. Hardy used the victory to build a national tobacco practice.

The role of SHB surfaced when 2,000 pages of internal documents of Brown and Williamson Tobacco Corporation were leaked from its files by JEFFREY WIGAND, a former company research vice president who turned against the tobacco industry. Brown and Williamson records showed that SHB chose recipients for grants from the COUNCIL FOR TOBACCO RESEARCH from 1976 until at least 1995, the last year covered by the documents.

Internal company memos and correspondence with SHB showed that the lawyers worked with tobacco companies to generate favorable science. In the 1990s, SHB's activities were the subject of investigations by federal prosecutors, and its records involving industry research were subpoenaed by plaintiffs' lawyers in the third wave of litigation. *See also* TOBACCO LITIGATION: FIRST, SECOND, AND THIRD WAVES

Shopland, Donald (1944–)

A federal employee who has devoted his life to fighting cigarettes, Donald Shopland quit smoking as soon as the 1964 surgeon general's report was issued. Shopland worked at the NATIONAL CLEARINGHOUSE ON SMOKING AND HEALTH, and later at its successor, the OFFICE ON SMOKING AND HEALTH, where he was a technical information specialist and later the acting director. Shopland oversaw the studies, articles, and data on smoking that provided the basis for the annual updated surgeon general's reports to Congress.

An aide to the original surgeon general's panel on smoking, Shopland stayed at the National Library of Medicine, became the keeper of the smoking and health archives when they were turned over to the Clearinghouse and Office on Smoking and Health, and made himself knowledgeable on the subject. In 1979, the 15th anniversary of the original surgeon general's report, he worked with Dr. DAVID BURNS to create a surgeon general's report that was accurate and comprehensive.

Shopland, who did not have the academic credentials required by the PUBLIC HEALTH SERVICE to become director of the Office on Smoking and Health, went to the NATIONAL CANCER INSTITUTE where he coordinates smoking intervention programs.

Sidestream Smoke

The portion of smoke that comes off the burning end of a CIGARETTE, PIPE, or CIGAR between puffs is called sidestream smoke. When a person breathes in sidestream smoke it is called passive or involuntary smoking. The components of sidestream smoke are somewhat different from the MAINSTREAM SMOKE that smokers exhale. Sidestream smoke contains higher concentrations of certain toxic substances than mainstream smoke, because it is not filtered and because cigarettes burn at a lower temperature when they are smoldering, leading to a less complete, dirtier combustion.

Because the organic material in tobacco doesn't burn completely, cigarette smoke contains more than 4,700 chemical compounds, including CARBON MONOXIDE, NICOTINE, carcinogenic TAR, sulfur dioxide, ammonia, nitrogen oxides, vinyl chloride, hydrogen cyanide, formaldehyde, radionuclides, benzene, and arsenic. Animal studies have shown these chemicals to be highly toxic. Many are treated as hazardous when emitted into outdoor air by toxic-waste dumps and chemical plants. *See also* SCONDHAND SMOKE

Simpson, Allan (1931–)

On October 29, 1987, the U.S. Senate resumed consideration of an amendment to a bill sponsored by Senator Frank Lautenberg (D-NJ) banning smoking on U.S. flights of less than two hours duration. During the deliberation, Senator Allan Simpson (R-WY) made the following statement:

> I strongly support the Senator from New Jersey's amendment to the transportation appropriations bill which would ban smoking on all scheduled domestic flights of 2 hours or less. Recent studies by the National Academy of Sciences and the surgeon general confirm that there is a significant risk taken by those who inhale passive smoke, or second-hand smoke. The surgeon general states the inhalation of this smoke does cause disease, including lung cancer and emphysema. . . .
>
> I do not in any way view this as an antitobacco issue. It is not to me a win-or-lose confrontation. I do not view this as a discriminatory issue either. I certainly do not need another test or study or white paper to tell me that my body physically reacts to the presence of any subsequent inhalation of another person's smoke.
>
> In your own home, the sky's the

limit—you can light a campfire in your own living room if you wish—but spare me the debilitating smoke on an aircraft—at least for 2 hours. (*Congrssional Record*, 1987)

References: *Congressional Record—Senate*, October 29, 1987, p. 29819.

60 Minutes

In November 1995, the CBS News program *60 Minutes* decided not to broadcast a planned interview with whistle blower JEFFREY WIGAND, a former vice president for research and development at BROWN AND WILLIAMSON TOBACCO CORPORATION because CBS lawyers felt the interview would expose the network to a multibillion-dollar lawsuit. Wigand, who was at Brown and Williamson, the nation's third-largest tobacco company, from December 1988 to March 1993, had a nondisclosure contract with his former employer. In place of the interview, the network broadcast a report on how tobacco companies block information from reaching the public.

Someone from CBS leaked a transcript of the Wigand interview to the *New York Daily News* that identified Wigand for the first time as the CBS industry source. In parts of the transcript published by the *Daily News,* Wigand accused his former employer of using coumarin, an additive in pipe tobacco that causes cancer in laboratory animals and of dropping plans to develop a safer cigarette. He also said that he believed the Brown and Williamson chief executive, THOMAS E. SANDEFUR, perjured himself before a congressional committee by denying knowledge of how cigarettes were used to deliver NICOTINE.

Much of the legal debate inside CBS over whether to broadcast the Wigand interview focused on the arrangements that *60 Minutes* made with the former research executive. He was paid a $12,000 fee as a consultant for an earlier *60 Minutes* report on fire-safe cigarettes, promised indemnity against a Brown and Williamson lawsuit for libel or breach of contract by CBS lawyers, and assured that the interview would not appear without his consent.

Freed by the disclosure of Wigand's testimony, CBS News broadcast on January 26, 1996, portions of the interview with Wigand. *See also* DAY ONE; SAFE CIGARETTES

Slade, John (1949–)

Dr. John Slade is a national leader in addiction medicine and tobacco control. He is also a professor of environmental and community medicine at the Robert Wood Johnson Medical School at the University of Medicine and Dentistry of New Jersey, and a practicing internist specializing in addiction medicine at St. Peter's Medical Center in New Brunswick. In the early 1980s, frustrated by the difficulty he had helping his patients stop smoking and by the lack of attention this problem received in medical education, he began studying the clinical and public health aspects of tobacco.

Dr. Slade coedited the first comprehensive clinical textbook on NICOTINE addiction, *Nicotine Addiction: Principles and Management,* and has helped organize seven annual national conferences on nicotine dependence for the Society of Addiction Medicine. He is an associate editor of *Tobacco Control: An International Journal,* published by the British Medical Association, and project director of *Nicotine Challenger.* He also served as president of STOP TEENAGE ADDICTION TO TOBACCO (STAT) in 1994 and 1995. Dr. Slade, who has published extensive analyses of internal documents from tobacco companies, coauthored *Cigarette Papers* and has worked for more than a decade on problems related to tobacco product regulation.

In 1995, Dr. Slade received the Goethe Challenge Trophy presented by the German Medical Association to recognize his outstanding achievements in the field of smoking prevention. The trophy is a full-sized, sterling silver bust of Johann Wolfgang von Goethe, the German poet and ardent campaigner against tobacco in the early 1800s. Usually given to an institution, on rare occasions the trophy is given to an individual.

Slavery

During the three-and-a-half centuries of the Atlantic slave trade, around 10 million African people were forcibly brought to North America. Before 1720, when the Virginia slave population began to grow faster from natural increase, only about 25,000 Africans had been brought to this region. Indeed, Virginia imported no more than 87,000 Africans during the whole of its history, less than 1 percent of all the Africans brought to the New World. The Virginia slave population almost doubled in size in the last three decades of the eighteenth century. Slavery spread rapidly from the colony's Tidewater region to its southern and western Piedmont, and became entrenched in large measure because of the great expansion of tobacco production. Tobacco farming required a large body of slave labor, But, by the end of the eighteenth century in Virginia, economic diversification caused a shift from tobacco planting to grain farming.

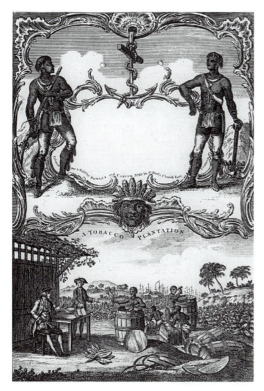

Slaves working on an American tobacco plantation. *Arents Collection, The New York Public Library, Astor, Lenox and Tilden Foundations.*

In Maryland's slavery-dominated southern counties, slaves were the backbone of the tobacco economy. Without them, there would have been no one to till the ground, plant the seeds, raise the plants, harvest, and cure the tobacco. In some areas, slave populations grew from 7 percent to 35 percent of the Chesapeake regions' population between 1690 and 1750.

Tobacco was extremely exhausting to the soil. After three years of being harvested, tobacco used up the soil nutrients, leaving much of the land depleted, forcing people to move on in search of acreage they could use to plant tobacco. Soil depletion led to a geographic shift westward into Tennessee and Kentucky and the introduction of the institution of slavery into these regions.

Many accounts of life under slavery appeared prior to the Civil War and as a result of the efforts of the Federal Writers' Project of the Works Progress Administration during the 1930s. In interviews, former slaves in Virginia (and 16 other states) gave personal accounts in their own words about what it felt like to be a slave.

Gabe Hunt, born in 1845 in Rustburg, Virginia, interviewed by William T. Lee, gave a graphic description of a slave's work in tobacco fields and in preparing the curing barn.

> You see, de fust pickin' come roun' de fust of August. You git de wheat in, den come de tobacco. Ole Marse go roun' pluckin' at de leaves, den one mornin' he say, "Come on, boys, git de smoke house in order." Den one go down an' clean out de barn. Got to rake out all de leavin's and dirt an' clean de mud an' dirt out whar de fire box is. Barns was built on hills, you see. Build dem on hills so's you kin lay de sticks way fum top to bottom. Pack de top fum de upper winder right level wid de groun' an' pack de bottom fum de do'. Spend one day gittin' de barn ready, den de nex' day you go to pickin'. Got to pick dem leaves what's jus' startin to brown. Pick 'em too soon dey don't cure, an' you pick 'em too late dey bitters. Got to break 'em off clean at de stem an' not twist 'em cause if dey bruised dey spile. Hands git so stuck up in dat old tobaccy gum it git so yo' fingers stick together. Dat old gum was

de worse mess you ever see. Couldn't brush it off, couldn't wash it off, got to wait tell it wear off. Spread de leaves on a cart an' drag it to de barn. Den de women would take each leaf up an' fix de stem 'tween two pieces of board, den tie de ends together. Den hand 'em all up in dat barn an' let it smoke two days an' two nights. Got to keep dat fire burnin' rain or shine, 'cause if it go out, it spile de tobaccy. Ev'ybody happy when de tobaccy curin' is done, 'cause den ole Marse gonna take it to market an' maybe bring back new clothes fo' de slaves. (Perdue, 1976, p. 148)

Simon Stokes, born in 1839 in Guinea, Virginia, interviewed by Lucille B. Jayne in 1937, remembered picking worms off tobacco leaves.

Me sho' didn't like dat job, pickin' worms off de terbaccer plants; fo' our ober-seer wuz de meanes ole hound you'se eber seen, he hed hawk eyes fer seein' de worms on de terbaccer, so yo' sho' hed ter git dem all, or you'd habe ter bite all de worms dat yo' miss into, or git three lashes on yo' back wid his ole lash, and dat wuz powfull bad, wusser dan bittin' de worms, fer yo' could bite right smart quick, and dat wuz all dat dar wuz ter it; but dem lashes done last a pow'full long time. (Perdue, 1976, p. 281)

References: Charles L. Perdue, Jr. et al, *Weevils in the Wheat: Interviews with Virginia Ex-Slaves,* Richmond: University Press of Virginia, 1976, pp. 148, 281.

Small, Edward Featherstone

In New York City in the mid-1880s, JAMES BUCHANAN DUKE, head of the AMERICAN TOBACCO COMPANY (ATC), needed "a road man" who could come up with new concepts. He hired Edward Featherstone Small, the son of an impoverished southern family, who began his career in the Atlanta, Georgia, market. That market was, at the time, dominated by Allen and Ginter brands.

Small, who discarded Duke's approach based on price competition and rebates, used his innate genius in sales and advertising when he created picture cards series based on "Famous Actresses." Until that time, none of the cigarette companies had used pictures of scantily dressed females on cigarette cards for the southern market, which was not considered as sophisticated as "racy" northern cities. After Small flooded Atlanta with free samples, especially pictures of Madame Rhea, a popular French actress with her arm on a pedestal containing a box of Duke's cigarettes, Atlanta became Duke territory. Rewarded with a higher salary, Small came up with his most famous card series, "Rags to Riches," portraits of businessmen who ascended from obscurity. Small guessed rightly that lower-class males would be attracted to these cards and purchase the smokes. Sex and power made Duke's cigarettes the best selling in the nation.

When several retailers in St. Louis ignored him, Small hired red-headed Mrs. Leonard, a pretty widow, to sell Duke's cigarettes. He called in reporters and cameramen for a press conference and got front-page coverage for the novelty of a woman selling cigarettes. Sales picked up in St. Louis.

Duke, who felt Small spent too much time talking with retailers and not enough time working and spreading the word to the general public, began questioning Small's expense accounts and rejected some of his ideas for picture card series. Duke also questioned Small's work, which seemed to be accomplished with little effort.

Although Small's district was in the West, he insisted on keeping his family in Atlanta and billed Duke's company expense money for trips back home to see them. In 1888, after Duke told Small to move his family to Cincinnati, Ohio, the heart of Duke territory, Small quit W. Duke Sons and took a position with ALLEN AND GINTER. When Allen and Ginter merged in 1890 with Duke to form the American Tobacco Company, Small left the cigarette business. *See also* CIGARETTE PICTURE CARDS, UNITED STATES

Smith, Lynn R.

Lynn R. Smith was publisher of the Monticello, Minnesota, *Times* and creator in 1974 of the first quit-smoking-for-a-day event that eventually evolved into the GREAT AMERICAN SMOKEOUT. He wrote a full-page editorial on the rights of a smoker, entitled "The Tyranny of Smoking." The piece was published in the *Congressional Record—Senate* on January 9, 1973. In the following excerpt, Smith discussed how smoking has a debilitating effect on sexual vigor:

> Yet possibly the most telling point of all is the disclosure that smoking has a debilitating effect on one's sexual vigor. Said one noted psychologist: "Cigarettes destroy sexual desire. Men who are heavy smokers can suffer from impotence."
>
> When you question a man's virility, you cut to the very core of his manliness. Cigarette advertising has long portrayed the smoker as a man of singular vigor. You know, the tattoo . . . or the western mien. But the truth lies otherwise.
>
> Advertising-wise, the smoker is often depicted hand-and-hand with his lover, cavorting through fields green or alongside waterfalls blue. But that purported "springtime freshness" of cigarettes provides in actuality an autumnal chill to the lovers' ardor.
>
> One sales pitch for these new little cigarette-like cigars is blatantly suggestive that smoking them will make one an alluring lothario. In his fantasy, this smoker is an over-believer; in reality, he is sexually an under-achiever.
>
> If both the husband and the wife are on the weed, one can only conclude that in such households, conjugal activity is quite congealed.
>
> Smokers may find some solace in the fact that one physician did report that some impotent men who had quit smoking "had their normal sexual function restored." (*Congressional Record*, 1973)

See also GREENFIELD, IOWA; IMPOTENCE AND SMOKING

References: *Congressional Record—Senate*, January 9, 1973, p. 678.

Smoke: Cigars, Pipes and Life's Other Burning Desires

Premiering in the winter of 1995/1996, *Smoke: Cigars, Pipes and Life's Other Burning Desires* reports on the tobacco industry with contemporary writing on cigars and pipes as well as the lifestyles of the young executives who smoke them. Published by Robert and George Lockwood, the sixth generation of the Lockwood family that has been part of the publishing industry since 1886, *Smoke,* a quarterly magazine, contains feature articles, columns on U.S. cigar manufacturers, photographs, cartoons, and illustrations that celebrate tobacco use in all its forms by men and women all over the world.

A feature article covered the Flores family, makers of Flor de Florez cigars, a premium brand that originated in CUBA around 1950 and is sold by mail and through the family's stores. Other features include cigar label history; Alfred Dunhill pipes; and how stars like Groucho Marx, Mae West, Humphrey Bogart, and YUL BRYNNER made smoking a part of their lives and careers. Other features cover travel, music, liquor, movies, fashion, collecting, cigar reviews, as well as celebrity and cigar Q and A. Kurt Russell, Mel Gibson, Elle MacPherson, Carmen Electra, and other celebrities have been pictured on past covers of *Smoke. See also* CIGAR; CIGAR LABELS; PIPE

SmokeFree Educational Services

In 1987, JOE CHERNER founded SmokeFree Educational Services, a nonprofit health advocacy organization headquartered in New York City. The goals of the organization are to win the right for nonsmokers to live and work in a smoke-free environment and to educate people about the disadvantages of tobacco addiction. The organization encourages legislation to prevent anti-health tobacco companies from targeting young people.

In 1988, Smoke Free Educational Services organized the first pro-health advertising contest for New York City school children. Poster designs had to stress the benefits of being tobacco free, the disadvantages of being addicted to tobacco, or the unhealthy consequences of breathing SECONDHAND SMOKE. In all, more than 100,000 entries came in from over 600 city schools. At the awards ceremony, which was held at City Hall, the winners, two each from grades 1 through 12, were awarded savings bonds. The contest received national and worldwide attention. In 1991, Workman Publishing Company published 46 full-color posters by the students who entered the annual SmokeFree Ad contest.

One of the winning posters, "Come to Where the Cancer Is" by Melissa Antonow, a fifth grader, appeared in 6,000 New York subway cars for the month of November 1990. Melissa and her poster made the NBC *Nightly News* twice, because at first Gannett Transit rejected the poster. Her poster appeared again for the month of May 1994 on bus shelters throughout New York City.

In 1991, the contest went national. With the help of *Scholastic Magazine,* the contest was opened to all schools in the United States and Canada. Invitations were mailed to 500,000 teachers and 71,000 principals. The SmokeFree American Ad Contest drew 100,000 entries from schools throughout North America.

SmokeFree Educational Services publishes *SmokeFree Air,* a newsletter that contains articles about smoke-free issues in New York City and the rest of the nation. It also maintains a website <www.smokescreen. org> and has established a fax tree and an e-mail tree to notify smoke-free advocates of important events on a timely basis. SmokeFree also produces brochures, stickers, posters, and other information.

SmokeLess States Program. *See* American Medical Association (AMA)

Smokeless Tobacco

Smokeless tobacco includes CHEWING TOBACCO and SNUFF. Most smokeless tobacco is grown in Kentucky, Pennsylvania, Tennessee, Virginia, West Virginia, and Wisconsin. Snuff is sold in cans and comes in three forms: moist, dry, and fine-cut. Chewing tobacco comes in several forms: loose-leaf, plug, and twist. Regardless of the form of smokeless tobacco, its use is generally called "chewing" or "dip-ping" and users are called "chewers" or "dippers." One portion is usually referred to as a "dip," a "pinch," or a "chew."

Moist snuff is by far the most popular form of smokeless tobacco, consisting of particles or strips of tobacco (or packets resembling tea bags) that may be treated with flavors such as mint, menthol, and wintergreen.

Loose-leaf chewing tobacco consists primarily of AIR-CURED TOBACCO and, in most cases, is heavily treated with licorice and sugars. Plug tobacco is the oldest form of chewing tobacco. Plug tobacco is produced from the heavier grades of leaves harvested from the top of the plant, freed from stems, immersed in a mixture of licorice and sugar, pressed into a plug, covered by a wrapper leaf, and reshaped. Twist tobacco is made from cured Burley, and air- and fire-cured leaves, which are flavored and twisted to resemble a decorative rope or pigtail. Dry snuff is processed into a powdered substance that may contain flavor and aroma additives, including spices.

People who chew tobacco place a wad of loose-leaf tobacco or a plug of compressed tobacco in their cheek. Snuff users place a small amount of powdered or finely cut tobacco (loose or wrapped in a pouch) between their gum and cheek. The user sucks on the moist mass of tobacco, called a "quid." Most "dippers" hold the quid in the same location in the mouth. Chew and its juices must be disposed of periodically, usually by spitting rather than swallowing because tobacco juice is not considered appetizing. Contrary to what smokeless tobacco users think, smokeless tobacco use can cause illness. A 1992 NATIONAL CANCER INSTITUTE monograph entitled *Smokeless Tobacco or Health: An International Perspective* discusses how animal studies suggest that the cancer-causing agents in smokeless tobacco can cause lung cancer, even though they do not enter the body through the lungs. Besides cancer of the mouth, pharynx, esophagus, and pancreas, smokeless tobacco causes gum disease and irreversible gum recession. Also, the 1994 surgeon general's report states that it might play a role in cardiovascular disease and stroke by increasing blood pressure and causing an irregular heart beat. *See also* ADDITIVES TO TOBACCO PRODUCTS; BURLEY TOBACCO; FIRE-CURED TOBACCO; HEALTH WARNINGS ON CIGARETTE PACKS AND ADVERTISEMENTS AND SMOKELESS TOBACCO; MARSEE, SEAN

Smokeless Tobacco Council (STC)

The Smokeless Tobacco Council (STC), headquartered in Washington, D.C., is a tobacco industry-sponsored research organization that focuses on smokeless tobacco. Supported by contributions from individual tobacco companies, the STC funds research. *See also* TOBACCO INDUSTRY RESEARCH COMMITTEE (TIRC)

Smoking

For more than a century after the discovery of America, nearly all the early voyagers remarked on a practice described as "a fumigation of a peculiar kind" that they found prevailing in some form almost everywhere in North America. Narrations stated that the Spaniards were honored as though they had been deities. Cortés was reported to have been received with incense, and one chronicler said that he was "met by persons carrying vessels with lighted coals to fumigate him." The natives were said to burn incense to or to fumigate their idols, and the priests to "prepare themselves by smoking to receive the devil's oracles."

These and many similar expressions indicate that the practice of smoking was not understood by Europeans. The CIGAR or the CIGARETTE was used throughout Spanish America. Montezuma and other chiefs of Mexico were said "to compose themselves to sleep by smoking." In 1540, Alarcon found the natives on the lower Colorado using "small reeds for making perfume" likening them to "the Indian *tobagos* of New Spain." JACQUES CARTIER found the practice of smoking to prevail on the lower St. Lawrence. Champlain referred to the native assemblies as *tabagies*. THOMAS HARIOT said the natives took the fumes of smoke as a cure for disease, and that they knew nothing of many

ailments "wherewith we in England are oftentimes afflicted."

Tobacco or some mixture was invariably smoked in councils with the whites and on other solemn occasions. No important undertaking was entered into without deliberation and discussion in a solemn council at which the PIPE was smoked by all present. The remarkable similarity in smoking customs throughout the continent proved the great antiquity of the practice.

The custom of offering incense was not restricted to men; women, in certain locations, were said to have offered incense to idols. It was not necessarily a religious act; it was also observed as a compliment to "lords and ambassadors." The women of Cartagena in 1750 could offer no higher courtesy to a person than to light his tobacco for him.

Smoking was early introduced from America into Europe and spread to the most distant parts of the world with astonishing rapidity until it encircled the globe, returning to America by way of Asia. But the act of inhaling and exhaling smoke through a tube for medicinal purposes was known to the ancients in Europe and Asia from a time antedating the Christian era. The fear that smoking would cause degeneration of the race or affect injuriously the revenues of the government caused stringent edicts to be passed against the use of tobacco, the violation of which was punished sometimes with death. *See also* MURAD IV; NATIVE AMERICANS; PIPE SMOKING AND NATIVE AMERICANS

Smoking Cessation

Smoking cessation is determined by the balance between two opposing forces: the motivation to stop and the level of NICOTINE dependence. Treatment is irrelevant for smokers who have little motivation to stop, and strong motivation is sufficient for smokers who are not highly dependent. In 1990, the surgeon general's report stated that more than 38 million Americans had quit smoking and almost half of all living adults in the United States who ever smoked had quit. Since then, it has been estimated that each year approximately one million smokers quit successfully.

Many smokers, men and women, who are strongly motivated and not highly dependent on the effects of nicotine are able to quit without formal help or treatment. For those who need help, however, there are many methods to help smokers quit.

Smoking cessation programs have evolved significantly since the release of the 1964 Report of the Surgeon General on Smoking and Health. Voluntary health organizations and commercial providers offer formal cessation programs that are primarily behavioral and cognitive in nature. The oldest of the nonprofit programs is a five-day plan sponsored by the SEVENTH-DAY ADVENTIST CHURCH. Now called "Breathe-Free Plan to Stop Smoking," more than 14 million smokers in more than 150 countries have been estimated to have entered the plan. The AMERICAN CANCER SOCIETY (ACS) and the AMERICAN LUNG ASSOCIATION (ALA) have offered smoking cessation clinics for years. Several commercial smoking cessation programs, including Smokenders, Smokeless, and Smoke Stoppers, are available.

Self-help interventions for smoking cessation include written materials explaining coping strategies, audio tapes and videotapes, and self-help manuals.

Since the early 1970s, the smoking control policies of Western countries have focused on strategies that are predominantly motivational. These include education and publicity about the health risks of smoking and passive smoking, high tobacco taxes, restrictions on smoking in public places, and bans on advertising and promotion of tobacco products. These strategies, however, do not help reduce the difficulties of overcoming dependence on nicotine.

The landmark 1988 report of the U.S. surgeon general concluded that the processes underlying addiction to nicotine are similar to those of other addictive drugs such as alcohol, heroin, and cocaine. It said more rapid progress in efforts to promote cessation is hampered by smokers' addiction to nicotine. It suggested one way to reduce the difficulties of giving up smoking is to provide nicotine from an alternative and less harmful source.

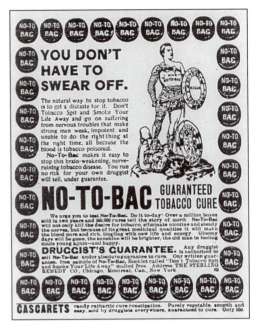

Ad for NO-TO-BAC, a product that claimed to help smokers quit smoking in the early 1900s.

After 20 years of research, NICOTINE REPLACEMENT PRODUCTS have been a major breakthrough in treatment for smokers to ease their nicotine cravings while breaking the habit. Nicotine gum, the transdermal nicotine patch, the nicotine nasal spray, and nicotine vapor puffer effectively reduce the severity of withdrawal symptoms. Other smokers have used hypnosis and acupuncture to quit, while some use behavioral counseling that teaches smokers how to break their associations with cigarettes and how to find effective substitutes for the benefits they derived from smoking, including relaxation, weight control, and mental stimulation.

Most smokers require several serious attempts, sometimes over a number of years, before quitting permanently. But quitting provides major and immediate health benefits for former smokers of all ages, with or without smoking-related diseases. People who quit smoking, regardless of age, live longer than people who continue to smoke. Quitting smoking substantially decreases the risk of lung, laryngeal, esophageal, oral, pancreatic, bladder, and cervical cancer. Quitting smoking decreases the risk of heart disease, stroke, chronic lung diseases, and respiratory illnesses. Ex-smokers also have reduced rates of bronchitis and pneumonia. Besides improving one's health and reducing the risk of disease, stopping smoking also improves personal appearance. Cessation prevents premature wrinkling of the skin, bad breath, clothes and hair that smell bad, and nails that turn yellow. *See also* APPENDIX 2: SURGEON GENERAL'S REPORTS, 1964–1998

Smoking Tobacco

There have been four basic types of smoking tobacco for pipes. The first, plug cut, was sliced from a compressed, flavored cake of tobacco. In later years, the porous Burley lent itself to a wide variety of textures: cube cut, curve cut, straight cut, wavy cut, Cavendish cut, and granulated plug cut. The second type, granulated tobacco was worked through toothed cutters and sieved for uniform fineness. Usually, the tobacco was straight, naturally sweet bright leaf, cased lightly or not at all. The third type, long cut, or ribbon cut, was shredded strip leaf. Usually the leaf was dipped Burley or a Burley blend, and could be made in a variety of strand widths. (Cigarettes are a variety of long-cut.) The fourth type, scrap, was a byproduct of cigar manufacture. These cigar cuttings (leaf ends) and clippings (cigar ends) were both chewed and smoked. *See also* BURLEY TOBACCO; BRIGHT TOBACCO LEAF; CHEWING TOBACCO; SNUFF

Smyth, J.F.D.

An Englishman, J.F.D. Smyth, published in *A Tour in the United States of America* an account of tobacco growing in Virginia in 1784. He provided a valuable guide to the methods of cultivating a plant he called narcotic that had become essential to commerce. His description began in the fall when beds were prepared for the planting of seeds in rich, moist, but not too wet, plots of ground about a quarter of an acre or more, according to the number of plants to be planted.

Smyth explained that experienced planters had several of those plant beds in different stages of growth so that if one failed there were others that might succeed. The plots, which were generally in the woods, were cleared and covered with 5 to 6 feet of brush or timber until the tobacco was sowed, usually within 12 days after Christmas. Tobacco seed, which is exceedingly small, was mixed with ashes, sown, raked in lightly, and covered immediately with brush to keep it warm. When the frosts were gone, the brush was removed, and the young plants exposed to the sun, which, according to Smyth, "quickly invigorates them in an astonishing degree" so they become strong and large enough to be removed for planting.

Once the ground was broken up and rendered soft and light, the field was "made into hills, each to take up the space of three feet and flattened on the top." In the first rains after the vernal equinox, Smyth described how "negro children" carefully pulled the tobacco plants out while the ground was soft, carried them to the field where they were planted, and dropped one on every hill. Then the most skilled slaves began planting them by making a hole with their finger in each hill, inserting the plant with the tap-root carefully placed straight down, and pressing the earth close on each side of it. This continued as long as the ground was wet enough to enable the plants to take root, and it required several periods of rain to enable them to complete planting their crop until the operation was finished in July.

After the plants took root and began to grow, the ground was carefully weeded and worked either with hand hoes or the plough. After the plants began to shoot up, the tops were pinched off, and only 10, 12, or 16 leaves remained. When the tops were nipped off, a few plants were left untouched for seed. On the plants that had been topped, young sprouts sprang out, which were called suckers. These were carefully and constantly broken off because they drew too much of the nourishment and substance from the leaves of the plant. This operation, performed from time to time, was called suckering tobacco.

Two species of worms that prey on tobacco were carefully picked off and destroyed. One was the short, dark-brown colored ground-worm, which cuts the plant off just

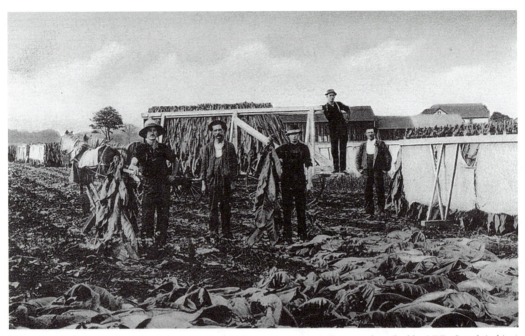

This postcard shows men cutting tobacco, part of the harvesting process that was described by J.F.D. Smyth in his *A Tour in the United States of America*.

beneath the surface of the earth. The other was the bright-green horn-worm, several inches in length, which devours tobacco leaves. Smyth reported that it was discovered that turkeys were particularly dexterous at finding the worms and eating them. Every planter kept "a flock of turkeys, which he has driven into the tobacco grounds every day by a little negroe that can do nothing else; these keep his tobacco more clear from horn-worms, than all the hands he has got could do, were they employed solely for that end."

Smyth wrote that when tobacco ripened, it was cut in mid-day when the sun was powerful. If the plant was large it was split down the middle three or four inches and cut off two or three inches below the extremity of the split; then it was turned directly bottom upwards for the sun to kill it more speedily, and to enable the slaves to carry it out of the field. Otherwise the leaves would break off in transporting it to the scaffolds.

After the tobacco plants were cut, they were placed in outdoor scaffolds to dry, or cure. As the plants cured, they were removed from the scaffolds and taken into the tobacco house and placed on other scaffolds. Inside,

tobacco curing was frequently promoted by making fires on the floor below. Smyth explained that to take down the cured tobacco, workers had to wait for rainy or moist weather when the plants could be handled, because in dry weather the leaves would crumble.

Smyth explained the process of packing tobacco in HOGSHEADS and taking them to public warehouses. Every night slaves were sent to the tobacco house to strip the leaves from the stalk, and tie them up in "hands" or bundles. In stripping they were careful to throw away all the ground leaves and faulty tobacco, binding up only tobacco that was merchantable. The tied bundles were laid in what was called a "bulk," and covered with the refuse tobacco or straw to preserve their moisture. After this the tobacco was carefully packed in hogsheads and pressed down with a large beam, at one end of which weights were suspended and at the other inserted with a mortise in a tree, close to which the hogshead was placed. The vast pressure was continued for some days, and then the cask was filled again with tobacco. Then the hogshead was carried to the public warehouse for inspection. The cask was taken off and the tobacco opened by means of long iron wedges. After being examined, if the tobacco was found to be good and merchantable, it was replaced in the cask, weighed at the public scales, and stowed away in the public warehouses. A note was given to the proprietor, which he gave to the merchant. If the tobacco was found to be totally bad, and refused as unmerchantable, the whole lot was publicly burned in a place set apart for that purpose. *See also* SLAVERY

References: Susan Wagner, *Cigarette Country: Tobacco in American History and Politics*, New York: Praeger Publishers, 1971, p. 20.

Snuff

Snuff, powdered tobacco that is sniffed into the nostrils, held against the lip, or chewed, became fashionable at the turn of the eighteenth century. Pulverized and perfumed, tobacco was inserted into the nostrils in pinches and the excess removed with a tiny snuffspoon.

At first snuffing was crude, prepared by grating tobacco. After factory mills ground the tobacco much finer, snuff making became a thriving business in cities of Western Europe, especially Glasgow, Scotland. The Scotch imported leaf from the Chesapeake colonies, manufactured and exported snuff, selling the most in London and in Virginia.

Although varieties of snuff were infinite, three basic types were made in Europe from Virginia leaf. Scotch snuff was a dry, strong, virtually unflavored product that was finely ground. Maccaboy snuff was moist and heavily scented. Rapee snuff (from the French word râpé meaning rasped or grated), also known as Swedish, was grated to a coarse consistency. A snuff seller in 1740 made a list of prices for some 18 different kinds of "rappee," including English, best English, high-flavored, low-scented, composite, and

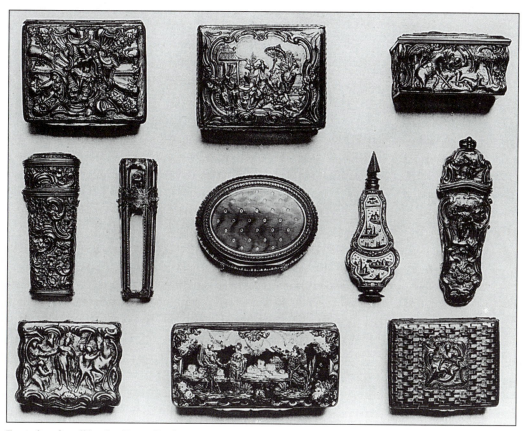

Examples of snuff bottles. *Brown Brothers.*

so on. None of these equalled the quality of Seville or Spanish snuff, ground from Havana leaf and known as "Musty."

Tobacco powder was sold by the ton, not only to the well-born and the clergy, but also among the ordinary subjects of Portugal, Spain, France, and England.

By the nineteenth century, CIGARS, PIPES, and CHEWING TOBACCO eclipsed snuff. *See also* FRANCE

Snuff Equipment

People in innumerable countries prized not only the snuff but the vessels in which it was contained. The Chinese hand-painted exquisite designs on snuff bottles, Tibetans made boxes from Yak horn, Africans used gourds, and West Indians worked with shell.

In the early eighteenth century, the French developed snuffing into an elaborate social ritual imitated by the upper classes of Great Britain. Fashionable ladies and gentlemen in London and the rest of the European continent "wore" elegant and elaborate snuff bottles. In them they stored colored, bleached, perfumed, and spiced snuff.

Since it was customary for English dandies to grate their own snuff, they carried a collection of equipment: the roll or twist of hard tobacco, a wooden grater, and a snuffbox. These boxes were jewelled, sometimes with diamonds, or inlaid with silver, hand-painted, or decorated. Even an ordinary wooden box had perfectly fitted hinges and lids. Some were small, but the majority were 4 or 5 inches in length and fit well into a pocket of a waistcoat. Snuff-boxes contained pins, usually of silver, for pricking holes in the grater; a hammer for tapping it; a rake for separating the coarse and fine snuff; and a spoon for taking it from the box. Some carried a hare's foot for wiping surplus snuff from the upper lip. *See also* COHAUSEN, JOHANN; SNUFF; SNUFF MILLS

Snuff Mills

Although snuff was associated with an aristocratic way of life Americans despised, colonists took to snuffing. Several snuff mills were created in America, one by French Huguenot emigre, PIERRE LORILLARD, in NEW YORK CITY around 1760. The present-day P.

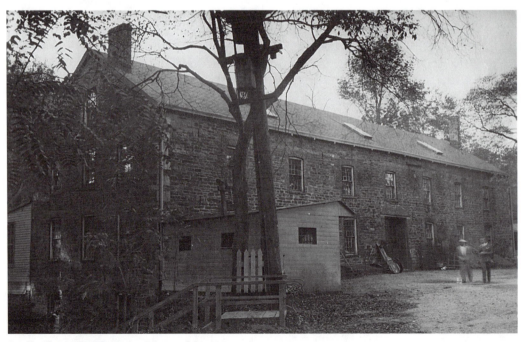

Snuff mill, Lorillard Company. *Library of Congress.*

Lorillard Co., the nation's oldest tobacco manufacturer, traces back to that beginning.

One of the first important snuff mills was built in Rhode Island around 1750 by Gilbert Stuart, a millwright and native of Perth, Scotland. (His son, born in 1755, became famous for his portraits, particularly that of George Washington.) Stuart wanted to use the nearby Connecticut Valley leaf as a source of supply, but he was hampered by the unavailability of glass bottles. Like early Spanish sailors, he tried to use animal bladders as containers. Because the crude packaging discouraged sales, his factory closed down. Snuff made from New England tobacco was said to have equaled the Scottish varieties. *See also* CONNECTICUT TOBACCO; LORILLARD COMPANY INC.; SNUFF; SNUFF EQUIPMENT

Soil Conservation and Domestic Allotment Act

In February 1936, Congress enacted the Soil Conservation and Domestic Allotment Act replacing the AGRICULTURAL ADJUSTMENT ACT OF 1933 that offered payments to farmers who volunteered not to grow tobacco and other crops that were in oversupply. Congress passed the 1936 law to conserve national resources; prevent the wasteful use of soil fertility; and to preserve, maintain, and rebuild farm land by encouraging soil-building and soil-conserving crops and practices.

In this new version, farmers were urged to stop growing soil-depleting crops such as cotton, tobacco, corn, and wheat on their land. Farmers who participated in the program through their county agricultural associations leased to the government land they withdrew from use. In return, they received payments depending on the number of acres they withdrew from soil-depleting crop production and the number they planted with soil-conserving crops. However no limits were set on what farmers could produce.

In February 1938, the voluntary agreement by farmers to restrict tobacco production broke down and farmers planted thousands more acres of tobacco and flooded the market. Economic disaster resulted again. To stabilize crop prices and farmers' incomes, Congress tried to cure overproduction by passing the AGRICULTURAL ADJUSTMENT ACT OF 1938. The law set farm marketing quotas on the number of acres farmers could plant and prevented prices from collapsing. *See also* AGRICULTURAL TOBACCO POLICY OF THE U.S. GOVERNMENT; CONSOLIDATED OMNIBUS BUDGET RECONCILIATION ACT (COBRA) OF 1995; DAIRY AND TOBACCO ADJUSTMENT ACT; NO NET COST TOBACCO PROGRAM ACT OF 1981; OMNIBUS BUDGET RECONCILIATION ACT (OBRA) OF 1993

Spain

Within 40 years after CHRISTOPHER COLUMBUS's first voyage to America in 1492, the Spanish were cultivating tobacco crops commercially in the West Indies. By the mid-sixteenth century, the Spanish government trafficked in *NICOTIANA TABACUM* brought from its colonies, the Spanish West Indies. By the late sixteenth century, the Spanish had a monopoly on the markets in England and Western Europe. Spanish leaf was smuggled into southern England in the 1590s to avoid the queen's penny-a-pound duty.

Because the English soil was not suitable for *Nicotiana tabacum,* the tobacco grown by English settlers at JAMESTOWN was far inferior to the Spanish leaf. The Spanish continued to sell thousands of pounds of it to England until the middle of the seventeenth century. Counterfeit and adulterated tobacco was so common in England that "Spanish tobacco" was all the more prized.

In 1614, the Spanish king ordered that all export tobacco from his colonies was to be shipped to SEVILLE, SPAIN, under penalty of death. The edict made Seville a repository for the choicest tobaccos grown in the Americas and a famous cigar-manufacturing city.

The Spanish empire, still mighty in the mid-eighteenth century, controlled almost every West Indian source of choice cigar leaf.

From the beginning, the Spanish were architects of the cigar industry. The first cigars made in similar fashion to those of today were produced by the state tobacco monopoly, Tabacalera, in Seville in the early eighteenth century. At this time, the idea of constructing a cigar with FILLER, BINDER, and CIGAR WRAPPER was invented. The booming cigar industry encouraged the Spanish to perfect the process of growing, fermenting, and curing a leaf flexible and strong enough to hold the cigar, or *puro,* together, while blending it with the burning tobacco.

Spain was quickly challenged by French, German, and Italian cigar manufacturing industries in the mid-eighteenth century. The British also competed with Spain when Connecticut, one of its colonies in North America, began rolling cigars in 1810. During this period, the leaf grown in Cuba, a Spanish colony, was shipped to Spain to be made into cigars. When it became clear that cigars survived the trans-Atlantic voyage better than the tobacco leaves, cigar factories were born in Cuba. They sprang up from eighteenth-century plantations, each offering its own brand of cigars. The Cuban cigar industry was therefore created by the Spanish.

On June 23, 1817, King Fernando VII of Spain signed a royal decree that allowed free trade for the island of Cuba. The port of Old HAVANA was filled with ships that distributed Cuban cigars all over the world. As steamships further ensured rapid distribution of Cuba's superior brands, the once-dominant Spanish factories diminished in importance. After King Fernando decreed that Cubans had the right to produce and sell tobacco in their homeland, new producers emerged throughout the island. From then on, the Spanish Crown obtained its entire supply of cigars from Cuba. By the mid-nineteenth century, the demand for cigars from Cuba outstripped the demand for *Sevilles,* as the Spanish version is called. To this day, Spain remains the world's largest importer of Cuban cigars. Every year, King Juan Carlos of Spain receives a gift of Cuba's premier cigars from Fidel Castro. *See also* CIGAR; CONNECTICUT TOBACCO FARMING; CUBA; CUBAN TOBACCO HISTORY

Sparke, John

In 1564, John Sparke, who accompanied John Hawkins on his voyage to the Indies and Florida, described a pipe without using its name.

The Floridians have a kinde of herbe dried, who with a cane and an earthen cup in the the end, with fire, and the dried herbs put together, doe sucke throw the cane the smoke thereof, which smoke satisfieth their hunger, and therewith they have four or five days without meate or drinke, and this all the Frenchmen used for this purpose. (Dunhill, 1969)

References: Alfred Dunhill, *The Pipe Book,* New York: Macmillian Company, 1924, 1969, p. 43.

State Regulation of Tobacco

Under the American federal system of government, the protection of the public health is largely a responsibility of state and local governments. Although there has been little regulation of tobacco products at the state level, states do have a variety of powers to protect their citizens.

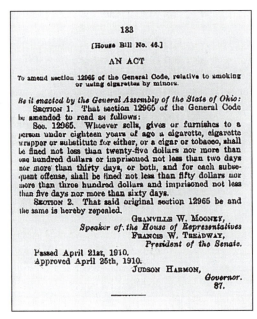

A 1910 Ohio law regulating the sale of tobacco.

During the 1890s, state legislators in at least 21 states prohibited the sale or distribution of cigarettes to minors. "Minor" meant different things to various state legislatures and ranged anywhere from "under 16" to "under 21." New York legislators made it a misdemeanor for under-16-year-olds to smoke in public. In September 1890, the *New York Times* reported that an officer arrested Edward McGrath and George Ryan, both under 16, who pleaded they did not know about the new law making it illegal for them to smoke. The boys got off with a warning. State laws forbidding the sale of cigarettes to minors were unenforceable and fairly useless.

Between 1893 and 1921, 15 states banned the sale, manufacture, possession, advertising, or use of cigarettes. But by 1927, each of these states had repealed their prohibitory laws against cigarettes.

- **Washington:** The sale and manufacture of cigarettes were banned in 1893, repealed in 1895, and reenacted in 1907. The sale, manufacture, and possession of cigarettes were banned in 1909 and repealed in 1911.
- **North Dakota:** The sale of cigarettes was banned in 1896 and repealed in 1921.
- **Iowa:** The sale and manufacture of cigarettes were banned in 1896 and repealed in 1921.
- **Tennessee:** The sale and giving away of cigarettes were banned in 1897 and repealed in 1919.
- **Oklahoma:** The sale and giving away of cigarettes were banned in 1901 and repealed in 1915.
- **Indiana:** The sale, manufacture, and possession of cigarettes were banned in 1905 and repealed in 1909.
- **Wisconsin:** The sale, manufacture, and giving away of cigarettes were banned in 1905 and repealed in 1915.
- **Arkansas:** The sale and manufacture of cigarettes were banned in 1907 and repealed in 1921.
- **Illinois:** The sale and manufacture of cigarettes were banned in 1907; the law was declared unconstitutional six

months after enactment but remained on the books until it was finally repealed in 1967.
- **Nebraska:** The sale, manufacture, and giving away of cigarettes were banned in 1909 and repealed in 1919.
- **Kansas:** The sale of cigarettes was banned in 1909; the law was amended to ban advertising and possession as well as sale in 1917, and repealed in 1927.
- **Minnesota:** The sale, manufacture, and giving away of cigarettes were banned in 1909 and repealed in 1917.
- **South Dakota:** The sale, manufacture, and giving away of cigarettes were banned in 1909 and repealed in 1917.
- **Idaho:** The sale of cigarettes was banned in 1921 and repealed two weeks later.
- **Utah:** The sale and advertising of cigarettes were banned in 1921 and repealed in 1923.

Cigarette prohibition laws were also considered in Alabama, Arizona Territory, California, Colorado, Delaware, Georgia, Kentucky, Maine, Maryland, Massachusetts, Michigan, Missouri, Montana, Nevada, New Hampshire, New York, North Carolina, Ohio, Oregon, Pennsylvania, South Carolina, and Texas.

In the 1990s, all 50 states and the District of Columbia had laws banning sales of tobacco products to persons under the age of 18.

States also have consumer protection laws that are a major tool for tobacco product regulation at the state level. *See also* ANTI-TOBACCO MOVEMENTS, UNITED STATES; CIGARETTE; IOWA; TAXATION IN THE UNITED STATES

Steinfeld, Jesse (1927–)

Surgeon general of the U.S. PUBLIC HEALTH SERVICE from 1969 to 1973, Dr. Jesse Steinfeld was an outspoken foe of smoking. In 1968, Dr. Steinfeld went from the University of Southern California, where he was a cancer specialist, to the NATIONAL CANCER INSTITUTE (NCI) where he became deputy

NCI director. The Nixon White House made him deputy assistant secretary of the Department of Health, Education, and Welfare, with oversight of the National Institutes of Health and the FOOD AND DRUG ADMINISTRATION.

When he became surgeon general, he had pressing matters to deal with, including the hazards of pesticides, restrictions on phosphate detergents, and the effects of television on children. Without a mandate on the smoking issue, Dr. Steinfeld nevertheless allied himself with the NATIONAL CLEARINGHOUSE ON SMOKING AND HEALTH, which turned out the surgeon general's report to Congress. He ordered an upgrading of the report, which had amounted to little more than a synthesis of old and new studies and data issued under the surgeon general's signature.

In 1971, the 488-page document called attention to important new developments in smoking research including the retarding effects of maternal smoking during pregnancy on fetal growth and the possible effects of CARBON MONOXIDE in smoke as a promoter of heart disease. In Dr. Steinfeld's 1972 report, for the first time, the surgeon general discussed the hazards of SECONDHAND SMOKE on nonsmokers at a time when little scientific evidence supported the idea. He was convinced secondhand smoke was a factor in deaths due to lung cancer of nonsmokers.

Wherever he spoke, Dr. Steinfeld called for an investigation of the effects of secondhand smoke. He proposed a ban on smoking in restaurants, theaters, and mass transit systems. In testimony he gave in 1974 before the Minnesota legislature when it debated the passage of the MINNESOTA CLEAN INDOOR AIR ACT, he said the following:

> There is no doubt in my mind that in some future time a healthier group of humans will look back with horror and amazement on these three or four centuries when people voluntarily committed a slow form of suicide through smoking, and foisted a noxious environment upon their nonsmoking companions.

Dr. Steinfeld was not reappointed during Nixon's second term. He left to become head of oncology at the Mayo Clinic.

Stogie

A "stogie" is a general term for any CIGAR, especially an inexpensive one. The term also applies to a handmade cigar of uncertain shape and size. The stogie originated as the long thin hand-rolled cigar that drivers of Conestoga wagons smoked or chewed for their own consumption. The cigars became known as "stogies" from the name of the town where covered wagons were made—Conestoga. *See also* LANCASTER COUNTY, PENNSYLVANIA

Stop Teenage Addiction to Tobacco (STAT)

In 1985, Stop Teenage Addiction to Tobacco (STAT) was founded as a nonprofit corporation to focus on reducing the use of tobacco by children and teens. Now headquartered in Boston, Massachusetts, STAT has an experienced staff of community organizers and trainers who are available to support tobacco control organizing and counter-advertising efforts around the nation. Its annual conference was recognized as among the most important meetings in the international tobacco control movement.

STAT advocates banning unethical advertising by tobacco companies. It has spoken out against the OLD JOE CAMEL cartoon, cigarette smoking in movies, and other ads and

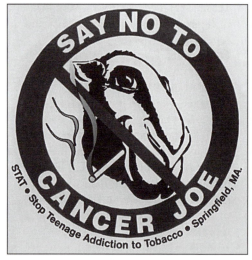

Stop Teenage Addiction to Tobacco (STAT) logo. *Courtesy of STAT.*

promotions aimed at children and teens. Teenagers work at STAT headquarters, participate in the annual conference, and help in community projects. From 1986 until 1995, STAT members received *Tobacco-Free Youth Reporter,* a newspaper filled with articles about tobacco and youth. *See also* ACTION ON SMOKING AND HEALTH (ASH); AMERICANS FOR NON-SMOKERS RIGHTS (ANR); DOCTORS OUGHT TO CARE (DOC); SMOKEFREE EDUCATIONAL SERVICES

Surgeon General's Report of 1964

On Saturday, January 11, 1964, the legendary surgeon's general report entitled *Smoking and Health* was released. Its bottom-line pronouncement "Cigarette smoking is a health hazard of sufficient importance to warrant appropriate remedial action" was broadcast, cabled, and telephoned around the world by the reporters who attended a carefully orchestrated press conference.

President John F. Kennedy, under pressure from the American medical establishment to create a commission on the medical-tobacco issue, handed the responsibility to Dr. LUTHER L. TERRY, U.S. surgeon general at the time. From the beginning, Terry made sure the tobacco industry had input into the formation of the Surgeon General's Advisory Committee of experts so it could not discredit the findings. Terry sent the tobacco industry a list of 150 outstanding medical scientists in the United States and asked it to delete any unacceptable names.

Eventually, 11 scientists were chosen whose names were acceptable to everyone. Dr. Terry acted as chairman and Dr. James M. Hundley, assistant surgeon general, acted as vice chairman. The other members of the committee were announced on October 27, 1962: Dr. Stanhope Bayne-Jones, former dean, Yale School of Medicine; Dr. Walter J. Burdette, head of the Department of Surgery, University of Utah School of Medicine; William G. Cochran, professor of statistics, Harvard University; Dr. Emmanuel Farber, chairman, Department of Pathology, University of Pittsburgh; Louis F. Fieser, professor of organic chemistry, Harvard University; Dr.

Jacob Furth, professor of pathology, Columbia University; Dr. John B. Hickam, chairman, Department of Internal Medicine, Indiana University; Dr. Charles LeMaistre, professor of internal medicine, University of Texas Southwestern Medical School; Dr. Leonard M. Schuman, professor of epidemiology, University of Minnesota School of Public Health; and Dr. Maurice H. Seevers, chairman, Department of Pharmacology, University of Michigan. One member was dismissed shortly after his appointment for telling a reporter that evidence "definitely sug-

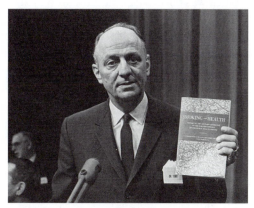

Surgeon General Luther Terry displays the 1964 report of the Surgeon General's Committee on Health and Smoking. *UPI/Corbis-Bettmann.*

gests that tobacco is a health hazard" (Taylor, 1984).

The committee worked over a year in absolute secrecy in a windowless basement office of the new National Library of Medicine in Bethesda, Maryland. Besides pouring over key information provided by the tobacco industry and some 6,000 articles in 1,200 publications, the committee questioned hundreds of witnesses. Despite efforts by journalists to break the secrecy of the committee's deliberations, security was maintained to the end. At the government printers, the report was treated with a security classification similar to military and state secrets.

The report was released in a dramatic manner. The press was invited to a Saturday morning press conference in a State Department auditorium affixed with signs announcing "no smoking." As 200 reporters walked in, they were given copies of the 387-page report and time to review it. Locked in the room so they could not leave until the news conference was over, Dr. Terry and his experts marched them through the document. The captive reporters were given 90 minutes to ask questions and then released.

The committee of experts had concluded that smoking was causally related to lung cancer in men, outweighing all other factors including air pollution. Evidence pointed in the same direction for women, even though information on smoking and lung cancer in women was not available because women had begun smoking in substantial numbers only 20 years before. The report also stated that cigarette smoking was a major cause of heart disease, chronic bronchitis, emphysema, and cancer of the larynx.

The committee found insufficient evidence that filter-tipped cigarettes did any good. The only good news reported was that smokers could reduce health risks by quitting. The same day, George V. Allen, Tobacco Institute spokesman said, "This report is not the final chapter. I endorse [the call] for more research." Howard Cullman, president of the Tobacco Merchants Association, and Philip Morris director said: "We don't accept the idea that there are any harmful agents in tobacco" (Whelan, 1984). Surgeon General Terry halted the free distribution of cigarettes to 16 public hospitals and 50 American Indian hospitals under the direction of the Public Health Service.

The surgeon general's report had an immediate but short-lived impact on cigarette sales. In 1963, the year before publication, 510 billion cigarettes were sold in the U.S. In 1964, cigarette sales fell to $495 billion. A year later, cigarette sales picked up again.

The major conclusions of the report are as follows:

- **Effects of Smoking: Principal Findings:** In view of the continuing and mounting evidence from many sources, it is the judgement of the Committee that cigarette smoking contributes substantially to mortality from certain specific diseases and to the overall death rate.
- **Lung Cancer:** Cigarette smoking is causally related to lung cancer in men; the magnitude of the effect of cigarette smoking far outweighs all other factors. The data for women, though less extensive, point in the same direction.
- **Chronic Bronchitis and Emphysema:** Cigarette smoking is the most important of the causes of chronic bronchitis in the United States, and increases the risk of dying from chronic bronchitis and emphysema . . . . Studies demonstrate that fatalities from this illness are infrequent among nonsmokers.
- **Cardiovascular Diseases:** It is established that male cigarette smokers have a higher death rate from coronary artery disease than non-smoking males . . . . Although a causal relationship has not been established, higher mortality of cigarette smoking is associated with many other cardiovascular diseases, including miscellaneous circulatory diseases, other heart diseases, hypertensive heart disease, and general arteriosclerosis.
- **Other Cancer Sites:** Pipe smoking appears to be causally related to lip cancer. Cigarette smoking is a significant factor in the causation of cancer of the larynx. The evidence supports the belief that an association exists between tobacco use and cancer of the esophagus.

See also Cigarette; Filtered Cigarettes

References: Peter Taylor, *The Smoke Ring: Tobacco, Money & Multi-National Politics*, New York: Pantheon Books, 1984, p. 9.

Elizabeth Whelan, *A Smoking Gun: How the Industry Gets Away with Murder*, Philadelphia: George F. Stickley Co., 1984, p. 102.

Sweda, Edward L. (1955–)

Senior staff attorney at the Boston, Massachusetts-based Tobacco Control Resource

CENTER, Edward L. Sweda is an expert on SECONDHAND SMOKE litigation and in confronting the tobacco industry tactics. In his third decade fighting the tobacco industry, he examines all aspects of secondhand smoke issues from workplace smoking policies to custody battles related to smoking. Mr. Sweda has been an anti-tobacco lobbyist and has represented individuals injured by secondhand smoke and maintains a separate criminal defense practice in Boston. *See also* DAYNARD, RICHARD; GOTTLIEB, MARK; KELDER, GRAHAM; TOBACCO LITIGATION: FIRST, SECOND, AND THIRD WAVES

Synar, Mike (1950–1996)

A United States congressman representing Oklahoma from 1979 until 1994, Mike Synar was known for his leadership in the fight against tobacco in Congress. He worked actively to pass legislation requiring rotating health-warning labels on cigarette packages and ads. He sponsored the law requiring health warnings on smokeless tobacco products and ads.

He introduced the first legislative proposal to ban all tobacco ads and sponsorships and the first proposal to ban all tobacco ads and sponsorships aimed at children. He introduced an amendment to a 1992 bill authorizing block grants to reduce drug abuse that became known as the "Synar Amendment," which required states to address the problem of youth access to tobacco. He played a key role in the congressional hearings that questioned tobacco company CEOs about the addictiveness of NICOTINE and the marketing of tobacco products to children. *See also* HEALTH WARNINGS ON CIGARETTE PACKS AND ADVERTISEMENTS AND SMOKELESS TOBACCO; SYNAR AMENDMENT

Synar Amendment

In 1992, Congress enacted and President Bill Clinton signed the Alcohol, Drug Abuse and Mental Health Administration Reorganization Act, which included the Synar Amendment. The amendment was a policy designed to discourage tobacco use among young people.

Written by MIKE SYNAR, a congressman from Oklahoma, the Synar Amendment was the first major anti-tobacco provision to emerge from Congress since it banned smoking on domestic airplane flights in 1989. Once enacted, the amendment was designed to put teeth into existing laws regarding the sale of tobacco products to minors.

On July 19, 1996, final Synar Amendment regulations were released by the DEPARTMENT OF HEALTH AND HUMAN SERVICES (DHHS) under the title Substance Abuse Prevention and Treatment Block Grants: Sale and Distribution of Tobacco Products to Individuals Under 18 Years of Age. The first requirement is that all states must have in effect a law prohibiting the sale or distribution of tobacco products to any individual under the age of 18. The law directly affected nine states that had no minimum age requirement or allowed sales to persons younger than 18. The second section of the regulation requires that states enforce such laws in a manner that can reasonably be expected to reduce the extent to which tobacco products are available to minors. The third provision calls for states to conduct annual random, unannounced inspections of both stores and vending machines to ensure compliance with the law. These inspections must be conducted in such a way as to provide a valid sample of outlets accessible to youth. States must report annually on their tobacco control efforts as well as on future plans for enforcement. In the event a state fails to comply with enforcement provisions, penalties affecting Substance Abuse Prevention Block Grants may be imposed by the DHHS.

The Synar rule requires states to demonstrate that they have reduced the percentage of children who successfully buy cigarettes at stores to 20 percent of those who try. States must develop a strategy and time frame for achieving an inspection failure rate of less than 20 percent of outlets. States risk losing up to 40 percent of their federal funds to fight abuse of alcohol and drugs if they cannot demonstrate that they have dramatically reduced illegal sales of cigarettes to children under 18 years of age by sales clerks and from vending machines. The rule, however, gives states latitude in determining when they must get illegal sales to minors down to the 20 percent figure and how to punish stores that sell cigarettes illegally.

In August 1995, proposed rules of the FOOD AND DRUG ADMINISTRATION (FDA), another DHHS agency, overshadowed the Synar regulation. Under the FDA's plan, cigarette vending machines would be banned altogether and tobacco advertising would be restricted to limit children's exposure to cigarette images. *See also* VENDING MACHINES

T

Talman, William (1915–1968)

William Talman, the actor who played the prosecutor Hamilton Berger on the *Perry Mason* television series, filmed a one-minute anti-smoking commercial at his own home in July 1968. At the age of 53, he was dying of lung cancer with only a few weeks to live. He approached the American Cancer Society (ACS), volunteering to tell his story so that it would serve as a reminder to television viewers of what smoking can do. In the commercial, viewers first saw Talman's wife and children, then Talman. He said:

> You know, I didn't really mind losing the courtroom battles. But I'm in a battle right now I don't want to lose at all, because if I lose it, it means losing my wife and those kids you just met. I've got lung cancer. So take some advice about smoking and losing from someone who's been doing both for years. If you haven't smoked—don't start. If you do smoke—quit. Don't be a loser. (Kluger, 1996)

Talman died August 30, 1968, before the commercial aired.

References: Richard Kluger, *Ashes to Ashes*, New York: Alfred A. Knopf, 1996, p. 309.

Tampa, Florida. *See* Ybor City, Florida

Tanton, Alice

Alice Tanton, a student at Michigan State Normal College in 1922, was expelled for smoking cigarettes and sent home by the dean of women, Bessie Leach Priddy. An investigation revealed Tanton was addicted to cigarettes before coming to college. The dean claimed that Alice was given warnings before the school forbade her to register for the spring term. Tanton brought suit against the college president, Charles McKenney, on the ground that her personal freedom was violated. On March 5, 1924, the Michigan Supreme Court upheld Tanton's expulsion. *See also* College Students and Cigarettes; Women, United States

Tar

Tar is the product of organic matter burned in the presence of air and water at a sufficiently high temperature. Tobacco products that are not burned, such as snuff and chew, do not deliver tar—but they still contain nicotine.

Tar is one of the major hazards in cigarette smoking. It causes a variety of cancers in laboratory animals. The minute separate particles fill the tiny air holes in the lungs and contribute to respiratory problems such as emphysema. Cigarette manufacturers have reduced the tar in their cigarettes in an effort to provide "safer" cigarettes. Because tar is important to the taste of cigarettes, when people smoke low-tar cigarettes, they have to inhale deeply to get maximum enjoyment. Ironically, cigarettes engineered to deliver low-tar results when smoked by machines deliver higher yields when smoked by people. *See also* CARBON MONOXIDE; MAIN-STREAM SMOKE; SAFE CIGARETTES

Taxation in the United States

Historically, the United States and other governments have levied tobacco taxes to generate revenues. Increasingly, however, taxing tobacco products is being recognized as a strategy to discourage tobacco use and enhance public health.

In the United States, tobacco is taxed by federal, state, and local governments. Tobacco products are taxed in two ways: the unit tax, which is based on a constant nominal rate per unit (that is, per pack of cigarettes), and the ad valorem tax, which is based on a constant fraction of either wholesale or retail price. Federal taxes on cigarettes, small cigars, and smokeless tobacco products are unit taxes; federal taxes on large cigars are ad valorem taxes.

All states and most localities use a unit tax for taxing cigarettes and ad valorem taxes for non-cigarette tobacco products.

Federal Taxation

To the federal government, tobacco has been a financial asset. It was one of the first consumer goods to be taxed in North America. The federal government began to tax tobacco products in 1794, when Alexander Hamilton proposed to Congress a bill with the first federal excise tax on refined sugar, tobacco, and SNUFF, much to the dismay of snuff manufacturers. The proposal engendered one of the first tax debates in the U.S. Congress over taxing manufactured tobacco and snuff, not leaf tobacco. Congress took the position that since snuff was a fad for the vain, it should be taxed while ordinary people who smoked a pipe or chewed should not be burdened. During the debate on this bill, James Madison delivered the following opinion opposing a tax on tobacco:

As to the subject before the House, it was proper to choose taxes the least unequal. Tobacco excise was a burden the most unequal. It fell upon the poor, upon sailors, day laborers, and other people of these classes, while the rich will often escape it. Much has been said about the taxing of luxury. The pleasures of life consisted in a series of innocent gratifications, and he felt no satisfaction in the prospect of their being squeezed. Sumptuary laws had never, he believed, answered any good purpose. (Heimann, 1960)

In 1794, Congress compromised with a tax on snuff and did not tax chewing and pipe tobacco; in 1796, the tax was repealed.

Following the War of 1812, a "war-cost" tax was imposed on all manufactured tobacco, but that, too, was repealed after only 10 months.

Tobacco was taxed during the Civil War because the federal government needed to raise funds for the government's military operations. On July 1, 1862, a tax was imposed on cigars for the first time. In 1864, the government levied the first federal tax on cigarettes as well as other tobacco products as a means of raising revenue for the Union war effort. In its first year of enforcement, the tax netted only $15,000. Taxes were increased; when producers and consumers opposed the taxes, they were repealed. Even the Confederacy wanted to levy a tax-in-kind on tobacco crops, but was precluded from doing so by the inspection system that required the inspector to deliver the full amount of tobacco specified in the warehouse receipt.

Taxes were raised again in 1865, 1866, and 1875. A temporary reduction followed, until the end of the nineteenth century when the Spanish-American War necessitated a steep increase in cigarette taxes as a way of financing the war. Taxes jumped from 50¢ to $1 per 1,000 cigarettes in 1897 and to $1.50 in 1898.

During the first half of the twentieth century, federal taxes were increased to help finance U.S. military involvement in various wars. Another increase took place on November 1, 1951, during the Korean War. The tax was increased from 7¢ to 8¢ per pack and remained at that level for the next 30 years. In 1986, the federal tax on cigarettes doubled to 16¢ per pack. Taxes were raised to deal with the increasing federal budget deficit. In 1991, the federal taxes on cigarettes were increased to 20¢ per pack and in 1993, these taxes rose to 24¢.

State and Local Taxation

To state governments, tobacco is a financial asset. All 50 states have enacted tax laws affecting cigarettes. IOWA led the way when, in 1921, it became the first state to impose an excise tax on cigarettes, followed in 1923 by Georgia, South Carolina, South Dakota, and Utah. By the end of the 1920s, six additional states had enacted cigarette excise tax laws. In the 1940s, more than half the states levied taxes on cigarettes. In 1969, North Carolina became the last state to impose an excise tax on cigarettes.

Like the federal government, state taxes on cigarettes have represented attempts to raise revenues rather than lower smoking rates. In 1985, however, Minnesota enacted the first state legislation to use cigarette taxes as a means of discouraging tobacco use. It earmarked a portion of the state cigarette excise tax to support anti-smoking programs. Other states like California (1988), Massachusetts (1992), and Arizona (1995) have used increases in cigarette taxes to fund anti-smoking campaigns and discourage people from smoking.

State Cigarette Tax Rates—January 1, 2000

State	Tax Rate (¢ per pack)	Rank
Alabama*	16.5	43
Alaska	100	1
Arizona	58	14
Arkansas	31.5	29
California	87	3
Colorado	20	37
Connecticut	50	19
Delaware	24	32
District of Columbia	65	12
Florida	33.9	27
Georgia	12	46
Hawaii	100	1
Idaho	28	31
Illinois*	58	14
Indiana	15.5	44
Iowa	36	24
Kansas	24	32
Kentucky	3	50
Louisiana	20	37
Maine	74	8
Maryland	66	11
Massachusetts	76	6
Michigan	75	7
Minnesota	48	20
Mississippi	18	39
Missouri*	17	41
Montana	18	39
Nebraska	34	26
Nevada	35	25
New Hampshire	52	17
New Jersey	80	5
New Mexico	21	36
New York	56	16
North Carolina	5	49
North Dakota	44	21
Ohio	24	32
Oklahoma	23	35
Oregon	68	10
Pennsylvania	31	30
Rhode Island	71	9
South Carolina	7	48
South Dakota	33	28
Tennessee*	13	45
Texas	41	23
Utah	51.5	18
Vermont	44	21
Virginia*	2.5	51
Washington	82.5	4
West Virginia	17	41
Wisconsin	59	13
Wyoming	12	46
U.S. Median		**34**

*Counties and cities may impose an additional tax on a pack of cigarettes: AL, 1¢ to 6¢; IL, 10¢ to 15¢; MO, 4¢ to 7¢; TN, 1¢; and VA, 2¢ to 15¢.

In addition to state taxes, the TOBACCO INSTITUTE reported in 1993 that over 440 cities and counties in nine states also levied taxes on cigarettes while 82 cities and counties levied taxes on non-cigarette tobacco products.

Differences in cigarette tax rates among states and localities can create problems in the enforcement of tax laws. There are a variety of tax evasion strategies, including casual smuggling (people buying cigarettes in neighboring states with lower taxes); buying cigarettes through tax-free outlets, such as military stores and American Indian reservations; commercial smuggling for resale; and illegal diversion of cigarettes within the distribution system by forging tax stamps and underreporting. *See also* CALIFORNIA'S PROPOSITION 99; CIGAR; CIGARETTE; CONFEDERATE GOVERNMENT; STATE REGULATION OF TOBACCO

References: Robert K. Heimann, *Tobacco and Americans*, New York: McGraw-Hill Book Company, Inc. 1960, p. 79.

Television and Cigarette Advertising

The cigarette industry was so successful using radio that it was one of the first businesses to move into television advertising. By 1950—when only 1 in 10 houses had a television set—cigarette sellers sponsored more than seven hours per week. That year, in an editorial in the industry's magazine, *United States Tobacco Journal,* the tobacco industry applauded itself for being the dominant factor in television advertising.

Tobacco companies spent record-setting money on television advertising, feeling certain that television advertising sold their products better than radio, magazines, and other mediums. Spending went from $40 million in 1957 to about $115 million in 1961 while cigarette sales and profits increased.

In 1971, cigarette advertising on television was banned. *See also* BROADCAST BAN; RADIO AND CIGARETTE ADVERTISING

Texas Medicaid Case

In January 1998, the state of Texas settled its lawsuit against the tobacco industry for at least $14 billion to be paid over 25 years, just as jury selection was about to begin. Texas became the third state, after Mississippi and Florida, to make a deal while preparing to fight the tobacco industry in court. In March 1996, Texas sued five large tobacco companies (PHILIP MORRIS COMPANIES INC.; RJR NABISCO HOLDINGS CORPORATION, the parent of R.J. REYNOLDS TOBACCO COMPANY; BAT INDUSTRIES PLC, the parent of BROWN AND WILLIAMSON TOBACCO CORPORATION; the LOEWS CORPORATION, the parent of LORILLARD COMPANY, INC.; and UNITED STATES TOBACCO COMPANY) and three groups affiliated with the industry (the TOBACCO INSTITUTE, the COUNCIL FOR TOBACCO RESEARCH, and Hill and Knowlton). The state wanted to recover $4 billion in Medicaid money spent on tobacco-related illnesses dating to 1968.

The suit, filed in U.S. District Court in Texarkana, made Texas the first state to file in federal court. The suit accused the tobacco industry of causing the addiction of millions of people to tobacco products by manipulating NICOTINE levels. It also alleged that tobacco companies aimed its advertising at children to replace adult smokers dying from tobacco-related illnesses and hired a public relations firm to organize a "propaganda campaign" to suppress information about the harmful effects of smoking.

Under an agreement with the state, the roughly 150 lawyers hired by Texas were to receive 15 percent of the settlement, or a little over $2 billion. These private lawyers underwrote the cost of the state's case against the cigarette companies in return for a share of the money. Some congressional leaders denounced the fees for the state's lawyers. Governor George W. Bush, calling the fees "outrageous," went to court to block payment to the lawyers who assisted Texas. A bipartisan group of seven Texan lawmakers, arguing that the fees were "excessive and unconscionable," filed a separate legal challenge against the settlement. *See also* FLORIDA MEDICAID CASE; MINNESOTA MEDICAID CASE; MISSISSIPPI MEDICAID CASE

Thackeray, William Makepeace (1811–1863)

In an 1897 issue of *Tobacco Talk*, a description appeared of English novelist William Makepeace Thackeray, who began his writing day with a cigar.

Thackeray always began writing with a cigar in his mouth. Every morning found him up and ready to begin work, though he sometimes was in doubt and difficulty as to whether he should commence operations sitting or standing, or walking about or lying down. Often he would light a cigar, and after pacing the room for a few minutes, would put the unsmoked remnant on the mantlepiece, and resume his work with increased cheerfulness, as if he had gathered fresh inspiration from the gentle odours of tobacco. (Infante, 1985)

In *Sketches and Travels in London* (1896), Thackeray wrote the following tribute to cigars:

Honest men, with pipes or cigars in their mouths, have great physical advantage in a conversation. You may stop talking if you like—but the breaks of silence never seem disagreeable, being filled up by the puffing of the smoke—hence there is no awkwardness in resuming the conversation—no straining for effect—sentiments are delivered in a grave easy manner—the cigar harmonizes the society, and soothes at once the speaker and the subject whereon he converses. I have no doubt that it is from the habit of smoking that Turks and American Indians are such monstrous well-bred men. The pipe draws wisdom from the lips of the philosopher, and shuts up the mouth of the foolish: it generates a style of conversation, contemplative, thoughtful, benevolent, and unaffected: in fact, dear Bob, I must out with it—I am an old smoker. At home I have done it up the chimney rather than not do it (the which I own is a crime). I vow and believe that the cigar has been one of the greatest creature-comforts of my life—a kind companion, a gentle stimulant, an amiable anodyne, a cementer of friendship. May I die if I abuse that kindly weed which has given me so much pleasure. (Conrad, 1996)

See also CIGAR

References: Barnaby Conrad III, *The Cigar*, San Francisco: Chronicle Books, 1996, p. 55.

G. Cabrera Infante, *Holy Smoke*, London: Faber and Faber, 1985, p. 256.

Thevet, André (1502–1590)

A chronicler of BRAZIL in 1555, André Thevet observed that Brazilians believed tobacco to be "wonderfully useful for several things."

They carefully gather this herb and dry it in the shade of their little cabins. When it is dry they enclose a quantity of it in a palm leaf which is rather large, and roll it up about the length of a candle. They light it at one end and take in the smoke by the nose and the mouth . . . . Even when they are taking counsel they inhale this smoke and then speak . . . . The Christians there today have become very attached to this plant and perfume . . . . (Heimann, 1960)

Thevet took Brazilian tobacco, *NICOTIANA TABACUM* to FRANCE in 1556 or 1557. It is ironic that Thevet is virtually unknown to history while the plant was named after JEAN NICOT, who sent tobacco to the French court later.

References: Robert K. Heimann, *Tobacco and Americans*, New York: McGraw-Hill Book Company, Inc., 1960, p. 14.

Thomas, James, Jr. (d. 1882)

The most famous of all mid-nineteenth century tobacco manufacturers was James Thomas, Jr. of RICHMOND, VIRGINIA. In the 1830s, he employed 150 hands and produced more than one million pounds of CHEWING TOBACCO per year. He got his start buying leaf for a French tobacco monopoly. After gold was discovered in California, he was among the first to ship quality chewing tobacco to California during the Gold Rush years, achieving a virtual stranglehold on the state's business.

On learning about the firing on Fort Sumter in April 1861, he shipped his tobacco to agents abroad and deposited his funds with the English J.K. Gilliat Company. He also stored as large a leaf inventory as his facilities could hold. In the years of the blockade and shortage that followed, he profited handsomely enough to equip a battery of Confederate artillery at his own expense, and became an unofficial adviser to Jefferson Davis's government. After the war, the Gilliat monies helped him get through the postbellum days. At the time of his death, he was reputed to be the wealthiest citizen of Richmond. *See also* CONFEDERATE GOVERNMENT

Tobacco

Tobacco is a member of a large family of plants—the *Solanaceae,* or potato family, which also includes the Irish potato, the tomato, belladonna, and nightshade. Tobacco belongs to the genus, *Nicotiana* that includes about 50 species including *NICOTIANA RUSTICA,* native to North America. Until *NICOTIANA TABACUM* was introduced, the production of tobacco was not profitable.

The following botanical description of tobacco appeared in *Gerard's Herball* in 1636:

> Tobacco, or henbane of Peru, hath very great stalks of the bigness of a child's arm, growing in fertile and well-dunged ground seven or eight feet high, dividing itself in sundry branches of great length, whereon are placed in most comely order very fair, long leaves, broad, smooth, and sharp pointed; soft and of a light green colour; so fastened about the stalk that they seem to embrace and compass it about. The flowers grow at the top of the stalks, in shape like a bell-flower, somewhat long and cornered; hollow within, of a light carnation colour, tending the whiteness towards the brim. The seed is contained in long, sharp-pointed cods, or seed vessels, like unto the seed of yellow henbane, but somewhat smaller and browner of colour. The root is great, thick, and of a woody substance, with some thready strings annexed thereunto. (Infante, 1985)

Tobacco leaves have differing characteristics that are important in the manufacture of tobacco products. These differences have been systematically classified by the U.S. Department of Agriculture. There are seven major classes of tobacco produced in the United States, with differences arising from the variations in soils and climate, in cultural practices, and in curing methods.

Tobacco is used in the CIGARETTE, CIGAR, CHEWING TOBACCO, SNUFF, and PIPE. Tobacco is the nation's sixth largest cash crop behind corn, soybeans, wheat, cotton, and hay. *See also* TOBACCO CLASSES

References: G. Cabrera Infante, *Holy Smoke*, London: Faber and Faber, 1985, p. 10.

Tobacco as Currency. *See* CURRENCY IN COLONIAL NORTH AMERICA

Tobacco Associates Inc.

Founded in 1947, Tobacco Associates Inc. promotes the use of U.S.-grown, FLUE-CURED TOBACCO throughout the world. With offices in Washington, D.C.; Raleigh, North Carolina; and Dillon, South Carolina, Tobacco Associates has represented the growers' interest in the development of export markets for American flue-cured tobacco. Exports are vital to the livelihood of American tobacco growers. More than half of the U.S. flue-cured crop is sold to overseas buyers each year, accounting for nearly $1 billion in export sales.

Tobacco Associates stimulates export demand by providing technical assistance in the use of U.S.-produced tobacco; communicating the unique quality, characteristics, and benefits of purchasing U.S. tobacco; and monitoring international tobacco trade trends and reporting developments to U.S. producers. The company trains overseas buyers and leaf exporters to evaluate the qualities of U.S.-grown tobaccos as described by U.S. Department of Agriculture official standards. Trade study missions to the United States give prospective customers the opportunity to see the U.S. tobacco industry first-hand from production through shipping, and to meet key U.S. farm, government, and industry leaders to gain a better understanding of the U.S. marketing system and requirements for purchasing, packing, and shipping.

Tobacco Associates participates in national and international trade fairs promoting the superior attributes of U.S. leaf, the expertise of U.S. growers, and the stability of U.S. supplies.

Tobacco Associate's policy objectives are determined by an annually elected board of directors composed of flue-cured tobacco growers and tobacco AUCTION WAREHOUSE operators. The organization is financed by tobacco auction warehouse operators and tobacco growers from the five flue-cured tobacco producing states—North and South Carolina, Virginia, Georgia, and Florida.

Tobacco Classes

The Department of Agriculture grades tobacco leaf by dividing it into seven classes, based on the methods of curing it as well as on the types of leaf groups. The first three classes are non-cigar leaf classes (tobacco used to make the CIGARETTE, SMOKING TOBACCO, CHEWING TOBACCO, and SNUFF); the next three classes are CIGAR leaf; and the seventh is a miscellaneous group. Non-cigar leaf classes are divided on the basis of curing methods: class one, FLUE-CURED TOBACCO (comprising the majority of varieties used in the cigarette industry); class two, FIRE-CURED TOBACCO; and class three, AIR-CURED TOBACCO. The cigar leaf classes (all air-cured) are determined on the basis of the uses of the product: class four, filler; class five, binder; and class six, wrapper. Class seven includes miscellaneous domestic leaf.

- **Class One: Flue-Cured.** Flue-cured (the official name for BRIGHT TOBACCO LEAF) is produced in Virginia, North Carolina, South Carolina, and Georgia, with scattered acres in Florida and Alabama. Most flue-cured is used to make cigarettes.
- **Class Two: Fire-Cured.** Fire-cured tobacco is grown in Virginia, Kentucky, and Tennessee. Most of the fire-cured tobacco is used to make snuff.
- **Class Three: Air-Cured.** Divided into light (BURLEY TOBACCO and Maryland) and dark types (used in chewing tobacco) air-cured tobacco is grown in Kentucky, Tennessee, Virginia and corners of North Carolina, Ohio, Indiana, West Virginia, and Missouri.
- **Class Four.** Cigar filler types include Pennsylvania seedleaf, Gebhardt, Zimmer, Dutch, and Georgia and Florida sun-grown.
- **Class Five.** Cigar binder types grown mainly in the Connecticut Valley include Connecticut Valley broadleaf and Havana seed, New York and Pennsylvania Havana, and Southern and Northern Wisconsin types of tobacco.
- **Class Six.** Cigar wrapper types, the most expensive of all types of tobacco to produce include Connecticut Valley shade-grown and Georgia and Florida shade-grown.
- **Class Seven: Miscellaneous Types**. Under this designation were NICOTIANA RUSTICA, the original tobacco used by American Indians, with a strong coarse leaf with high NICOTINE count used in the making of insecticides, and périque, grown in Louisiana and used in the manufacture of fine smoking tobacco.

Classes are further divided into types: flue-cured types 11–14; fire-cured types 21–24; air-cured types, 31–32, 35–37; cigar-filler types, 41–45; cigar-binder types, 51–55; and cigar-wrapper types, 61–62. *See also* BINDER; CIGAR WRAPPER; CONNECTICUT TOBACCO; FILLER

Tobacco Control: An International Journal

Launched in 1992, *Tobacco Control: An International Journal* reports on the nature and extent of tobacco use worldwide; the effects of tobacco use on health, the economy, the environment, and society; the efforts of the health community and health advocates to prevent and control tobacco use; and the activities of the tobacco industry and its allies to promote tobacco use.

The journal publishes research articles that have undergone rigorous peer review including the evaluation of smoking prevention and cessation programs, the tracking and evaluation of tobacco control policies and legislation, epidemiological and behavioral research on tobacco use, and the health effects of smoking, SMOKING CESSATION, passive smoking, and SMOKELESS TOBACCO use.

The journal also includes book reviews, obituaries of tobacco control activists, and anti-tobacco cartoons for comic relief.

When the journal was launched, the editor, deputy editor, and technical editor resided in the United States, Australia, and United Kingdom, respectively, because of the journal's international scope. Regional and associate editors and members of the Editorial Advisory Board represented 30 countries throughout the world.

The first issue of *Tobacco Control* (March, 1992) pictured stamps from eight countries encompassing all six regions of the world, according to the WORLD HEALTH ORGANIZATION's classification system. The stamps of Argentina, Niger Republic, Mali, Portugal, Indonesia, and Tunisia were all issued on World Health Day in 1980 to support the theme "Smoking or Health—The Choice Is Yours." *See also* ANTI-TOBACCO POSTAGE STAMPS

Tobacco Control Resource Center (TCRC)— Tobacco Products Liability Project (TPLP)

The Tobacco Control Resource Center (TCRC) was established in 1979 as a non-profit educational foundation focusing on legal and policy approaches to control and curtail morbidity and mortality caused by the use of tobacco industry products. The Tobacco Products Liability Project (TPLP), founded in 1984, is the legal subdivision of the TCRC focusing on tobacco litigation. Northeastern University School of Law professor RICHARD A. DAYNARD founded TPLP and serves as chairman as well as president of TCRC. The organizations are located on the campus of Northeastern University in Boston, Massachusetts.

For many years, TCRC has provided tobacco policy information to federal, state, and local officials throughout the United States. TCRC has also pioneered creative local tobacco control measures and drafted state legislation.

TCRC closely follows the progress of all innovative tobacco control policies around the nation in *Tobacco Control Update*, a quarterly magazine for public health officials and tobacco control activists; and in *Tobacco on Trial*, a newsletter focusing on tobacco litigation. TCRC personnel also publish the *Tobacco Products Litigation Reporter*, a loose-leaf law reporter published eight times a year.

Over the course of the past 17 years, TCRC has evolved into a national resource on tobacco control issues for attorneys, both public and private; the national press; and government officials and tobacco control activists. The national media regularly turn to Professor Daynard and other TCRC legal staff members for their reactions to and analysis of breaking news in tobacco litigation and tobacco control.

TPLP has hosted 14 conferences at Northeastern University on tobacco and law, which have attracted prominent figures in tobacco control. Attorneys from throughout the United States, as well as CANADA, Great Britain, Finland, ITALY, Israel, Australia, and a dozen other countries have also attended. *See also* TOBACCO LITIGATION: FIRST, SECOND, AND THIRD WAVES

Tobacco Documents

Since 1994, thousands of secret tobacco industry documents have emerged revealing how the companies suppressed research on the health hazards of smoking, fearing lawsuits, and sought to attract teenagers as "replacement" smokers.

In May 1994, 4,000 pages of documents stolen by a former employee of a law firm doing work for Brown and Williamson were described in the May 7, 1994, edition of the *New York Times*, the first of several high-profile stories based on the stolen documents. In district and state courts, BROWN AND WILLIAMSON TOBACCO CORPORATION tried unsuccessfully to have the documents, including memorandums, indexes, chronologies, and minutes of research meetings attended by company executives and researchers, suppressed. Courts noted that much, if not all, of the information in the documents had already been made available to the news media through leaks.

Eventually, all the Brown and Williamson documents were declared to be in the public domain, either by Congress or by the courts. On July 1, 1995, at 12:01 A.M. Pacific Standard Time, the University of California, San Francisco Library and Center for Knowledge Management posted the documents on the Internet making the papers available to the world. The library also made a CD-ROM.

The documents revealed that executives of the company struggled in the 1960s and 1970s about whether to disclose what the company knew about the hazards of the CIGARETTE. Documents show that executives talked about NICOTINE, its addictive qualities and beneficial effects. Research dealt with the tranquilizing or anxiety-reducing effects of nicotine and its role in controlling body weight.Brown and Williamson stopped work on a safer cigarette and pursued a legal strategy of admitting nothing.

Addison Yeaman was general counsel for Brown and Williamson, then became a vice president, and eventually became director of the industry's Council on Tobacco Research. In 1963, Mr. Yeaman wrote: "We are, then, in the business of selling nicotine, an addictive drug effective in the release of stress mechanisms" (Hilts, 1996). He suggested in July 1963 that the company "accept its responsibility" and disclose the hazards of cigarettes to Surgeon General Luther Terry, who was preparing a report on smoking and health that would be issued in 1964. Yeaman wanted the company to free itself so it could research openly to develop safer cigarettes. Although he acknowledged that accepting responsibility might worsen the industry's position in lawsuits, he thought the risk would be worth it. His proposal was turned down.

In June 1995, the *New York Times* described documents from PHILIP MORRIS COMPANIES INC. that showed the tobacco company had conducted 15 years of nonpublic research on nicotine, finding that it affected the body, brain, and behavior of smokers. From 1966 to 1981, the tobacco company scientists carried out extensive studies on nicotine and manipulated nicotine levels in test cigarettes and studied the effects of nicotine on smokers. The Philip Morris researchers wrote about the "pharmacologic" effects of nicotine. The company said the research was never used in creating products for the market.

In October 1995, the *Wall Street Journal* reported it had obtained two major confidential reports, both drafted in the 1990s by BROWN AND WILLIAMSON TOBACCO CORPORATION. The first was a 54-page handbook issued in 1991 for leaf and product developers laying out the rudiments of ammonia chemistry. It explains that ammonia scavenges nicotine from tobacco and converts it into a form with greater impact on smokers. The second report, dated October 23, 1992, was Brown and Williamson's competitive analysis of Marlboro's composition and design. The report concludes: "What . . . makes Marlboro a Marlboro? Looking at all of the technology employed in Marlboro on a worldwide basis, ammonia technology remains the key factor . . . Ammonia technology is critical to the Marlboro character, taste, and delivery" (Freedman, "Tobacco Firm," 1995).

In October 1995, documents leaked from R.J. REYNOLDS TOBACCO COMPANY files showed that, as early as 1973, the company was looking for ways to reach young potential smokers. Claude E. Teague, Jr., assistant director of research and development wrote in a 1973 memo: "The fragile, developing self-image of the young person needs all of the support and enhancement it can get." A 1976 memo states: "[T]he 14-18 year old group is an increasing segment of the smoking population . . . R.J. Reynolds *must* soon establish a successful *new* brand in this market" ("Where There's Smoke," 1995). The tobacco company said the documents were drafts and not the policy of the company then or now.

In December 1995, a confidential internal undated document from Philip Morris, first revealed in the *Wall Street Journal* and then available on the Internet, acknowledged that cigarettes were a nicotine delivery system and that the main reason people smoke is to get nicotine into their bodies.

The 15-page draft report likens nicotine to a drug in both its composition and its effects on the brain. In calling nicotine a "similar, organic chemical" to the drugs cocaine, morphine, quinine, and atropine, the document states: "while each of these substances can be used to affect human physiology, nicotine has a particularly broad range of influence." The memo reviewed attempts by other companies to develop "nicotine delivery devices" including patches, pills, inhalers, and PREMIER (Freedman, "Philip Morris," 1995).

Philip Morris said that it had never disputed that nicotine has "pharmacologic" effects. The company also said noting that nicotine is a member of a chemical family that includes addictive drugs like cocaine does not prove that nicotine itself is addictive.

In July 1996, an R.J. Reynolds secret 77-page report from 1984 revealed that the tobacco company needed to pitch its cigarettes to young adults to "replace" other smokers. "Younger adult smokers are critical to RJR's long-term performance and profitability. Therefore, RJR should make a substantial long-term commitment of manpower and money dedicated to younger adult smoker programs" ("R.J. Reynolds Saw Need," 1996). The report was filed by the tobacco company as part of the discovery process in the MINNESOTA MEDICAID CASE.

In September 1996, a Philip Morris memorandum said that if a study showed that nicotine produced the same withdrawal symptoms as highly addictive drugs like morphine, "we will want to bury it." A November 1997 memorandum about a researcher's efforts written by a Philip Morris scientist, William Dunn, suggested a cover-up of the results about nicotine's effects proved damaging. The documents were filed by the tobacco company as part of the discovery process in the Minnesota Medicaid case.

In August 1997, a Palm Beach, Florida, circuit court judge released eight secret tobacco industry documents that reflected decades of discussions among cigarette company lawyers to suppress scientific research, potentially destroy documents, and mislead the public about the health effects of smoking.

In December 1997, 834 documents from the files of the Liggett Group, which turned state's evidence in 1997 to settle lawsuits with states, were put on the Internet by the House Commerce Committee. The documents showed the role tobacco-hired lawyers played over the decades as the industry struggled to refute scientific evidence of smoking's dangers and play down the risks of smoking.

In January 1998, R.J. Reynolds documents were released. The documents indicated that top tobacco industry executives long believed that people under 18 were its most crucial customers because by that age, minors who smoked had chosen their brand. A marketing plan suggested placing ads in magazines read by young people and sponsoring sports events like auto racing. The documents, which date from 1973 to 1990, showed that for decades R.J. Reynolds commissioned or subscribed to surveys that tracked the smoking habits of teenagers, including those as young as 14. In 1973, a Reynolds marketing profile included a study of black smokers ages 14–20.

The documents were obtained in pretrial fact-finding in a California lawsuit over Joe Camel ads that was settled in 1997, and were released by U.S. Representative Henry Waxman.

In February 1998, more tobacco-industry documents were released that provided a detailed look at how Brown and Williamson and R.J. Reynolds marketed cigarette brands to blacks. The records show how the cigarette makers ran ad campaigns in magazines, on BILLBOARDS and buses, and in other media to attract blacks, especially to mentholated brands like Kool and Salem. The documents also showed that R.J. Reynolds, which makes Salem, and Brown and Williamson, which makes Kool, were locked in battle for African Americans, who smoked a greater percentage of mentholated cigarettes than whites.

The documents were made public at congressional hearings on the proposed—but defeated—$368.5 billion tobacco settlement in 1997.

In February 1998, thousands of internal memoranda were posted on the Internet by tobacco companies. The documents were initially collected by lawyers for Minnesota for use in the state's lawsuit against the nation's four largest tobacco companies. Although the cigarette makers initially resisted disclosing the papers, they finally agreed to do so. The documents showed tobacco companies focused on nicotine, its physiological and pharmacological effects and the different ways in which it might be controlled and altered while being delivered to the smoker.

In April 1998, some 39,000 secret tobacco industry documents were posted on the Internet by the House Commerce Committee after a lengthy fight by the tobacco companies to keep them confidential. The data revealed new details about some of the chemicals tobacco companies added to their products and how companies deliberately hid their potential perils from the public. While some of the records date as far back as the 1960s, hundreds of documents from the years 1993 and 1994 offered new insight into how the industry fought off regulatory and legal assaults, and they offered clues as to why five tobacco companies negotiated a $368.5 billion settlement in June 1997. *See also* BROWN AND WILLIAMSON TOBACCO CORPORATION— MERRELL WILLIAMS DOCUMENTS; LEBOW, BENNETT; MARLBORO CIGARETTS; OLD JOE CAMEL; SAFE CIGARETTES; TOBACCO SETTLEMENT—JUNE 1997; WAXMAN HEARINGS

References: Alix M. Freedman, "Tobacco Firm Shows How Ammonia Spurs Delivery of Nicotine," *The Wall Street Journal*, October 18, 1995, p. A14.

———, " Philip Morris Memo Likens Nicotine to Cocaine," *The Wall Street Journal*, December 8, 1995, p. B1.

Philip J. Hilts, *Smoke Screen: The Truth Behind the Tobacco Industry Cover-Up*, Reading, MA: Addison-Wesley Publishing Co., Inc., 1996, p. 36.

"R.J. Reynolds Saw Need to Target Young Adults," *The Record*, July 11, 1996.

"Where There's Smoke, There's . . ." *Newsweek*, October 30, 1995, p. 74.

Tobacco Drinking

The term "tobacco drinking" gained currency because of an early belief that tobacco smoke had therapeutic qualities. Smokers inhaled the smoke so that it would circulate and "fume the innerds"; then they exhaled the smoke as slowly as possible out their noses. Somehow, this manner of smoking came to be known as drinking. Midway through the seventeenth century the term faded out of use and "smoking" came to be the common term.

Tobacco Industry Cigarette Advertising Code

In 1965, following the release of the first surgeon general's report on smoking, the nation's largest tobacco companies began creating self-regulatory cigarette advertising and promotional codes. The standards related primarily to four areas: advertising appealing to the young, advertising containing health representations, the provision of samples, and the distribution of promotional items to the young. The code prohibited cigarette advertising in school and college publications, testimonials from athletes or other celebrities perceived to appeal to the young, the use of advertising through comic books or newspaper comics, and the distribution of samples at schools.

The code was administered by a former governor of New Jersey, Robert Meyner. Although Meyner was given power to fine violators up to $100,000, no record exists of a fine being levied. By the early 1970s, the position of administrator was terminated.

One of the code's provisions states that

> no one depicted in cigarette advertising shall be or appear to be under 25 years of age; cigarette advertising shall not suggest that smoking is essential to social prominence, distinction, success or sexual attraction; cigarette advertising may picture attractive, healthy-looking persons provided there is no suggestion that their attractiveness and good health is due to cigarette smoking; nor shall it show any smoker participating in, or obviously just having participated in, a physical activity

requiring stamina or athletic conditioning beyond that of normal recreation.

Four months after the code was formulated, VICEROY CIGARETTES ads pictured young tennis players lighting up after a game. Salem showed a young couple playing games next to a waterfall. A television commercial producer admitted he looked for older models who were over 25 years old, but who "looked young."

The advertising code also restricted promotional items, stipulating that "there shall be no mail distribution of non-tobacco premium items bearing cigarette brand names, logos, etc., without written, signed certification that the addressee is 21 years of age or older, a smoker and wishes to receive the premium." A 1993 study showed that more than two million youth aged 12 to 17 had promotional items such as T-shirts, caps, and key-chains; seven million, or 35 percent of those aged 12 to 17, had been active participants in that they had had catalogs or items or had saved coupons; and about a million-and-a-half youth were on tobacco company mailing lists.

Finally, the code prohibited cigarette advertising on shows whose audience was primarily under-age, that is with 45 percent or more viewers under 21 years old. The rule allowed for considerable interpretation. For example, R.J. REYNOLDS TOBACCO COMPANY continued to sponsor *The Beverly Hillbillies* even though the audiences for two selected individual episodes of the show exceeded the code requirement; a later intepretation by the tobacco industry held that the code would be applied to two successive months of audience analyses, rather than to selected specific shows. Later that year, after monthly data showed high levels of minors, R.J. Reynolds ceased sponsoring the show.

Tobacco Industry Research Committee (TIRC)

In 1954, in reaction to the investigations linking smoking and disease and a decline in cigarette sales, 14 leading tobacco manufacturers and allied groups established and financed the Tobacco Industry Research Committee (TIRC), which was renamed the COUNCIL FOR TOBACCO RESEARCH (CTR)—USA in 1964.

On January 4, 1954, the tobacco industry announced formation of the TIRC in a full-page advertisement titled "A Frank Statement to Cigarette Smokers." The ad, which appeared in 448 newspapers in 258 cities, told readers that although the TIRC believed the products the tobacco industry made were not injurious to health, the industry planned joint financial aid to research the health effects of smoking. It also planned to appoint "a scientist of unimpeachable integrity and national repute" to oversee the program; it hired CLARENCE COOK LITTLE, founder and retiring president of the Roscoe B. Jackson Memorial Laboratory in Maine and an internationally known cancer fighter.

The tobacco industry identified the TIRC as an independent research organization run by a board of scientists. During the decade 1954–1964, the committee awarded grants in excess of $7 million to some 230 scientists in more than 100 hospitals, universities, and research institutions around the country. In 1963, the research chief of LIGGETT AND MYERS TOBACCO COMPANY was quoted in a publication of Consumers Union as saying that the TIRC was mostly a publicity organization.

Tobacco Institute

In 1958, the major CIGARETTE, CHEWING TO-BACCO, and SNUFF manufacturers formed the Tobacco Institute, headquartered in Washington, D.C. It was created to take over the industry's lobbying and public relations needs as well as to counteract the possible adverse effects of health studies. The institute has worked to develop the case for smoking by emphasizing the inconclusiveness of the research evidence, the contribution of tobacco products to the national economy, and the individual rights of smokers. *See also* PHILIP MORRIS/TOBACCO INSTITUTE—"ITS THE LAW" PROGRAM

Tobacco Litigation: First, Second, and Third Waves

Dating back to the 1950s, smokers have sought recovery from the tobacco industry for smoking-related diseases. Cases seeking to hold the tobacco industry liable for smoking-related illnesses have been classified into three waves. The first wave, from 1954 to 1973, came after the lung cancer scare of the early 1950s; laboratory research linked smoking to cancer in mice and was first published, but doubts about the dangers of cigarette use persisted. In the second wave, from 1983 to 1992, when scientific evidence was more firmly established, the industry still defeated claims for damages by persuading juries that smokers know the risks when they choose to smoke. The third wave began in 1994.

In the first wave of cases, four theories were used to bring cigarette cases to trial. One theory under which recovery was sought was breach of implied warranty, or that it is implied by the manufacturer that the product being sold is fit for the buyer's intended use. Otherwise, a buyer would be forced to discover the dangers of the product. *Ross v. Philip Morris and Company* illustrates this theory.

A second theory under which recovery was sought against cigarette manufacturers was breach of express warranty, or that a promise is issued with a sale of goods in which the seller or manufacturer expressly assures the quality, description, or performance of its product. *Pritchard v. Liggett and Myers Tobacco Company* illustrates this theory.

A third theory for which recovery was sought was deceit. Deceit is the fraudulent misrepresentation of fact, opinion, or law for the purpose of inducing another to act. Liability for deceit arises when a fraudulent misrepresentation is made and the party perpetrating the fraud knows or believes a matter is misrepresented, does not possess confidence in the accuracy of the misrepresentation, or knows the misrepresentation is without basis. A party who deceives another is liable for damages if the other party detrimentally relies on the first party's representation. *Cooper v. R.J. Reynolds Tobacco Company* illustrates this theory.

The final theory under which recovery was sought in the first wave of cases was negligence. Negligence is the failure to use the care that a reasonable person would use in similar circumstances. To maintain a cause of action for negligence, the plaintiff must demonstrate that the defendant owed a duty to the plaintiff, that the defendant breached that duty, that the defendant's breach caused harm, and that the harm was a direct result of the defendant's conduct. Negligence claims against a tobacco company assert that the company owed its customers a warning about the detrimental health effects of smoking their cigarettes, and that they breached this duty by failing to inform. *Lartigue v. R.J. Reynolds Tobacco Company* illustrates this theory.

The second wave of cigarette litigation began in the 1980s. These cases were in part the result of medical studies finding a direct link between cigarettes and disease and a change in society's perception of smoking cigarettes. This wave of cases was brought under two new theories. The first, strict liability, is an outgrowth of the law of implied warranty. Strict product liability places an absolute burden on a manufacturer for any injuries by the user of a defective product. The liability applies regardless of whether the manufacturer has taken all possible care in preparing and selling its product. Holding manufacturers to a higher standard forces them to produce safer products. To be held strictly liable, the product must be unreasonably dangerous. *Gilboy v. American Tobacco Company* illustrates this theory.

The second theory in the second wave of cases was failure to warn. Failure to warn cases are based on the proposition that to make an informed decision whether to use a product, the consumer should be warned of the risks associated with it. The theory presupposes that the manufacturer is in the best position with its knowledge and expertise to know of the potential harmful effects of its product. *Palmer v. Liggett Group Inc.* illustrates this theory.

Throughout the first and second waves, although more than 800 claims were filed against the tobacco industry, nothing was paid in damages. The tobacco industry maintained that its products were not harmful at the same time it argued that smokers who chose to smoke assumed the risks of smoking and negligently contributed to their own harm. Rather than identifying the tobacco industry as the cause of the myriad tobacco-induced illnesses, jurors blamed plaintiffs who continued to smoke despite health warnings on cigarette packs that linked tobacco use and disease. In the first and second waves, the tobacco industry took deposition after deposition and filed and argued every motion. According to J. Michael Jordan, an attorney who successfully defended R.J. Reynolds in the 1980s, the strategy was "to make these cases extremely burdensome and expensive for plaintiffs' lawyers" (Pringle, 1988).

In the third wave of tobacco litigation in the 1990s, which comprises class actions like CASTANO V. AMERICAN TOBACCO COMPANY and state medical cost reimbursement suits in Florida, Minnesota, Mississippi, and Texas, plaintiffs overcame the tobacco industry's defenses. Success has been attributed to a number of factors: resources were expended on behalf of millions of plaintiffs in a class action rather than on behalf of a single individual; well-financed attorneys shared resources and information; there was an absence of blameworthy plaintiffs in class actions and medical cost reimbursement cases and an unavailability to the tobacco industry of two defenses—assumption of risk and contributory negligence in the medical cost reimbursement cases; a wealth of evidence existed of industry wrongdoing stemming from former industry researchers and internal documents; new facts surfaced concerning tobacco industry knowledge of the addictive and pharmacological properties of NICOTINE and the efforts of the industry to manipulate nicotine levels to addict smokers. The last factor absolves users of tobacco products of responsibility for their addiction.

Underlying many of the cases filed in the third wave of tobacco litigation are new claims that tobacco companies knew, but hid their knowledge that nicotine is pharmacologically active and highly addictive and that they manipulated nicotine levels in their products to hook smokers. *See also* BROIN V. PHILIP MORRIS COMPANIES INC.; ENGLE V. R.J. REYNOLDS TOBACCO COMPANY; FLORIDA MEDICAID CASE; MINNESOTA MEDICAID CASE; MISSISSIPPI MEDICAID CASE; TEXAS MEDICAID CASE

References: Peter Pringle, *Cornered: Big Tobacco at the Bar of Justice*, New York: Henry Holt and Company, 1988, p. 194.

Tobacco Manufacturers' Standing Committee (TMSC)

In 1956, the British tobacco companies formed the Tobacco Manufacturers' Standing Committee (TMSC), modeled on the American TOBACCO INDUSTRY RESEARCH COMMITTEE (TIRC). In 1962, it changed its name to the Tobacco Research Council, and later it was renamed Tobacco Advisory Committee.

Like the TIRC, the TMSC funded independent researchers to study issues related to smoking and health. Unlike the TIRC, it conducted in-house research at a jointly sponsored industry laboratory, opened in 1962 in Harrogate, England. The lab conducted several studies on the effects of tobacco smoke inhalation, and NICOTINE absorption.

Tobacco Merchants Association (TMA)

Founded in 1915 to manage information of vital interest to the worldwide tobacco industry, the Tobacco Merchants Association (TMA) is an important source for current, objective information on the worldwide tobacco industry. Headquartered in Princeton, New Jersey, TMA is dedicated to supplying factual information to a variety of companies, associations, and other organizations whose livelihoods depend on timely, comprehensive, and accurate data about the global tobacco business.

TMA is supported by tobacco product manufacturers, industry suppliers, financial institutions, leaf dealers, advertising agencies, consultants, distributors, and other industry sectors the world over who need the data that play an important role in decision making. TMA's data bank comprises more than 10,000 domestic and international sources and is maintained through a collection of computerized databases that yield daily, weekly, biweekly, monthly, quarterly, annual, and semi-annual reports.

TMA publishes three major compendiums: *Tobacco USA,* a 2,000-page compilation, updated annually, of everything one needs to know about the U.S. tobacco industry broken down nationally and by the 50 states and the District of Columbia. With data from 1975 to the present, *Tobacco USA* provides in-depth economic data and public policy information. It includes *Tobacco Tax Guide,* a summary of key provisions of all state tobacco product tax laws, and *International Tobacco Guide,* a 3,000-page reference source that breaks down tobacco by country and region, covering both manufactured products and unmanufactured leaf tobacco. Updated three times a year, this publication provides comprehensive economic data, public policy information, and media updates. TMA's "Alert/Electronic Bulletin Board," a daily annotated electronic clipping service that delivers worldwide news as it happens, features coverage of breaking industry news, full text of U.S. federal legislation and regulations, and transcripts of press conferences and television broadcasts. Finally, monthly "tobacco-on-a-disk" updates bring members up-to-date information on the worldwide tobacco industry. Members of TMA also receive the following publications:

- *Executive Summary:* A two-page weekly summary of the principal industry developments occurring over the past week around the world.
- *Tobacco Weekly:* A compilation of all key industry issues and events as they unfold across the United States including excise taxes, marketing and distribution, corporate finance, leaf and trade, anti-tobacco campaigns, product standards, use accommodations and restrictions, and legal issues.

- *World Alert:* A weekly country-by-county compilation of key industry issues and events as they emerge outside the United States.
- *Legislative Bulletin:* A bi-weekly report that analyzes U.S. congressional and state legislative activity that affects the tobacco industry.
- *Leaf Bulletin:* A bi-weekly report appearing during the U.S. tobacco marketing season that furnishes tobacco auction market statistics for all leaf types.
- *Trademark Report:* A monthly report that tracks all trademarks for tobacco products and tobacco accessory products in the United States.
- *Tobacco Barometer:* A monthly industry guide to manufactured production, taxable removals, and tax-exempt removals for all cigarettes, large cigars, little cigars, snuff, and chewing and pipe tobacco manufactured in the United States as reported by the U.S. Bureau of Alcohol, Tobacco, and Firearms.
- *Tobacco Barometer (Smoking, Chewing, and Snuff):* A quarterly industry guide to production, with invoices of U.S. sales, imports, and exports for chewing tobacco, snuff, and forms of smoking tobacco, including roll-your-own tobacco, manufactured in the United States.
- *Tobacco Trade Barometer:* A monthly publication detailing all U.S. imports and exports of all tobacco leaf, products, and smokers' accessories. The data are broken down by product and country providing quantities and dollar values on a monthly and cumulative basis comparing current data to the previous year.
- *China Watch:* A monthly publication that results from a cooperative information sharing agreement with the China National Tobacco Corporation (CNTC). Monthly, CNTC provides TMA with statistical information dealing with cigarette production and sales,

tobacco leaf and cigarette trade quantities and values, by trading partner, and cigarette filter material imports.

- *Japan Tobacco Trade Barometer:* A monthly publication providing statistical information dealing with tobacco leaf and product trade quantities and values.

- *Issues Monitor:* A semi-annual review of the principal issues facing the tobacco industry in the United States. It summarizes all economic, legislative, regulatory, and trade developments.

See also TOBACCO ASSOCIATES INC.

Tobacco Products Control Act of Canada (TPCA)

In 1988, the Canadian government passed the TOBACCO PRODUCTS CONTROL ACT (TPCA) whose key provision said: "No person shall advertise any tobacco product offered for sale in Canada." The new law, which came into force in January 1989, was struck down by the Canadian Supreme Court in 1995. That ruling was seen as a setback for anti-smoking groups in many countries, including the United States, which had held up the Canadian law as a model.

Broadcast advertising in Canada had been forbidden voluntarily since 1972, and print advertising was supposed to be limited in terms of dollar expenditures and minimum ages targeted. The tobacco industry adopted these voluntary restrictions to persuade the federal government that legislation was not necessary. However, by the mid-1980s, it was clear that the voluntary approach was not working, and the new law was passed in 1988.

The major provisions of the TPCA and its regulations included no advertising in the electronic and print media, no BILLBOARDS or transit posters after January 1993, no contests or free distribution of cigarettes, and no use of trademarks other than on tobacco products. Sponsorship of cultural and sporting events was limited to their 1987 dollar value and no use of tobacco product names

in association with the sponsored events was permitted.

Health warnings and toxic components had to be "legible and prominently displayed in contrasting colors" on all packages with leaflets inserted in undersize packages. Four health warnings had to rotate on cigarette packages: "Smoking Reduces Life Expectancy," "Smoking Is the Major Cause of Lung Cancer," "Smoking Is a Major Cause of Heart Disease," and "Smoking During Pregnancy Can Harm the Baby." Two health warnings had to rotate on cigar and pipe tobacco packages: "This Product Can Cause Cancer" and "This Product Is Not A Safe Alternative to Cigarettes." A health warning had to appear on all smokeless tobacco packages: "This Product Can Cause Mouth Cancer."

Tobacco companies had to report to the government the constituents of all tobacco products and their smoke, whether manufactured or imported; the volume of all tobacco products manufactured or imported; and the monetary value of sponsorships.

Almost immediately after the TPCA passed, RJR-Macdonald Inc., a subsidiary of RJR NABISCO HOLDINGS CORPORATION, and Imperial Tobacco Ltd., a unit of Imasco Ltd., challenged the law claiming the advertising ban violated their constitutional right to free expression. On July 26, 1991, Justice Jean-Jude Chabot of the Superior Court in the Province of Quebec declared the act to be contrary to the Canadian Charter of Rights and Freedoms and consequently null and void. In a 148-page judgment, Justice Chabot, who called the ad ban "social engineering" and "state moralism," said: "This form of paternalism or totalitarianism is unacceptable in a free and democratic society" (Good, 1991).

After a Quebec appeals court overturned the Superior Court ruling on September 21, 1995, the Canadian Supreme Court struck down key sections of the law. In a 5-4 ruling, the high court said the TPCA was unconstitutional. Limited restrictions on tobacco ads were permissible, but a comprehensive ban improperly prohibited a manufacturer from communicating with customers about a legal product. The decision left the advertising and promotion of tobacco products substantially unregulated in CANADA.

References: G. Pierre Good, "Canada's Tobacco-Ad Ban is Overturned by Judge," *The Wall Street Journal*, July 29, 1991, p. B.1.

Tobacco Settlement—June 1997

At 3:30 P.M. on Friday, June 20, 1997, a small group of state attorney generals, led by MICHAEL C. MOORE of Mississippi, announced "the most historic public health achievement in history" and the largest proposed industry payout in history. In this proposed landmark settlement between tobacco companies and state attorneys general, the tobacco industry would pay a total of $368.5 billion (covering the first 25 years) to smokers and states to cover medical costs for cigarette-related illnesses.

In the first year, it would pay $10 billion, with $7 billion going to the states and $3 billion going to the federal DEPARTMENT OF HEALTH AND HUMAN SERVICES to fund a SMOKING CESSATION campaign, enforce a ban on sales to minors, and set up a compensation fund for smokers who win court cases. After the first year, the industry would pay $8.5 billion rising to $15 billion annually in perpetuity.

Despite the efforts of CEO BENNETT LEBOW to exclude the Liggett Group, —he had made a settlement in March 1997 with 22 states— the settlement included LIGGETT AND MYERS TOBACCO COMPANY. Tobacco executives, especially GEOFFREY BIBLE, CEO of PHILIP MORRIS COMPANIES INC., despised him for his defection. There were no special rules for Liggett and no letter to the White House recommending that LeBow's company be exempted.

The proposal permitted the industry to raise prices, to make full use of tax deductions on the penalties, and to legitimize business expenses unless ruled otherwise by Congress. It also contained a clause allowing the companies to "jointly confer, coordinate, or act in concert" to achieve the goals of the settlement. A final provision included

amnesty for JEFFREY WIGAND and other whistle blowers to the fullest extent against any recriminations.

While the massive tobacco deal, negotiated hastily behind closed doors and without peer reviews, drew praise; it also drew virulent criticism. For various reasons, DAVID KESSLER, commissioner of the FOOD AND DRUG ADMINISTRATION (FDA); former surgeon general C. EVERETT KOOP (chosen by a bipartisan group of congresspeople to form an advisory committee on tobacco policy and public health to study the proposal); public health groups; and trial lawyers across the country called the deal flawed. Kessler said the settlement was far too lenient, especially for taking away from the FDA some of the regulatory control over cigarettes that the agency had won in Judge WILLIAM L. OSTEEN's District Court in April 1997. The agreement prevented the FDA from regulating NICOTINE levels in cigarettes for at least 12 years. Also troubling to Kessler and other health advocates was the series of hurdles written into the settlement that the FDA had to clear before it could regulate nicotine.

The FDA was required to create a scientific advisory board to study nicotine and health issues. In addition, it had to show, with substantial evidence, that before reducing nicotine levels such a move would result in a significant reduction of the health risks associated with smoking, and that it would not create a black market for U.S. cigarettes with a higher nicotine level. The proposal reduced the burden of proof after 12 years to a "preponderance of evidence." Normally, the FDA must show it has not acted "arbitrarily or capriciously" in making a new rule.

The AMERICAN LUNG ASSOCIATION attacked the advertising provisions of the agreement arguing the provisions still allowed images in ads that could portray the romance of smoking.

Trial lawyers, who attacked the elimination of punitive damages and class actions, argued the agreement did not address the question as to whether the tort system had been violated by granting partial immunity to the tobacco companies.

Other critics argued that with their ability to act in concert, the tobacco companies could raise prices far in excess of the amount needed to cover their annual payments under the settlement.

Other contested parts of the proposal included the fact that penalties were pegged to packs of cigarettes sold. As the companies raised prices to pay for the settlement, sales would decline but so would industry payments. Some critics felt the 62¢-a-pack price increase was not enough to cut teen smoking.

Other critics charged that the proposal terminated class-action lawsuits filed by labor management medical insurance trust funds without compensation and allowed them recovery only by filing individual lawsuits from the settlement fund.

Critics attacked the provisions for disclosure of industry documents for which companies claimed privilege. Under the proposal, a three-judge panel would review contested documents, a slow and expensive procedure.

Finally, the enormous fees of lawyers raised questions. The proposal left this matter to a separate agreement between the lawyers and the industry.

After President Bill Clinton and legislators examined the settlement during the summer, there was a feeling that more money should have been added to the amount cigarette makers would have to pay. The $368.5 billion agreement eventually grew into a $516 billion bill in Congress that denied the tobacco companies the legal immunity they wanted in return for settling. The $516 billion proposal was defeated in the Senate.

Tobacco companies, for their part, ran a $50 million advertising campaign to sink the proposed legislation. They depicted it as a tax-and-spend bill that would have taken money out of the pockets of smokers, caused cigarette prices to rise sharply, given the government regulatory power over tobacco, and denied the industry legal protections in smoking-related lawsuits. *See also* McCain Senate Tobacco Bill

Tobacco Settlement—November 1998

On November 14, 1998, the attorneys general of eight states and the nation's four biggest cigarette companies reached agreement on a $206 billion tobacco settlement. The biggest U.S. civil settlement in history, it was designed to resolve state claims over Medicaid costs of treating people with smoking-related illnesses. Unlike the earlier tobacco settlement of June 1997, this settlement involved no federal officials and did not need congressional approval, did not deal with regulation of the tobacco industry by the Food and Drug Administration, and did not shield tobacco companies from punitive damages and class-action liability suits.

The proposed settlement received the approval of all 46 states that either had lawsuits to recover smoking-related health care costs or were yet to sue. The settlement did not apply to the four states—Florida, Minnesota, Mississippi, and Texas—that had already settled their cases for $40 billion over 25 years.

The eight states involved in the talks leading to the settlement were California, Colorado, New York, North Carolina, North Dakota, Oklahoma, Pennsylvania, and Washington. The four tobacco involved in the settlement were Philip Morris Companies Inc.; R.J. Reynolds Tobacco Company, a subsidiary of RJR Nabisco Holdings Corporation; Brown and Williamson Tobacco Corporation, a unit of BAT Industries PLC; and Lorillard Tobacco Company Inc., a unit of Loews Corporation.

The nation's fifth largest cigarette maker, Liggett and Myers Tobacco Company, a subsidiary of the Brooke Group, although not directly involved in the negotiations, agreed to join the plan. Liggett and Myers previously signed settlement agreements with a number of states, but in agreeing to the November 1998 settlement, it was released from earlier agreements. Liggett and Myers would not have to contribute financially to the settlement unless its sales rose 25 percent above current levels.

Under the settlement plan, the tobacco companies would pay $206 billion over 25 years to 46 states and five U.S. territories. The companies agreed not to market to youths, but would not pay fines if underage smoking did not decline. The producers agreed to marketing restrictions including a ban on BILLBOARD and transit advertisements as well as the sale of clothing and merchandise with brand logos. They agreed to avoid cartoon figures in ads; to ban sponsorship of youth-oriented sporting events and concerts, although they could maintain at least one sports sponsorship a year; and to refrain from lobbying against state initiatives that make it harder for underage smokers to buy cigarettes.

Cigarette makers also agreed to pay $1.45 billion over five years to finance SMOKING CESSATION programs and advertisements to counter under-age tobacco use. The companies will pay an additional $25 million a year over a decade for a foundation that will research ways to reduce youth smoking. The proposal did not contain restrictions on fees for plaintiffs' lawyers who were hired by state attorneys general to pursue the claims, which are to be paid by the industry. The states also released the tobacco companies from all federal Medicaid claims.

As a result of the settlement plan, the FEDERAL TRADE COMMISSION (FTC) said it would drop its case against R.J. Reynolds Tobacco Company, which it had accused of harming children with its OLD JOE CAMEL advertising campaign.

On November 23, 1998, Philip Morris and R.J. Reynolds announced they would raise wholesale prices 45¢ a package, the largest price increase in history.

The feature of the settlement that has garnered the most attention is the money that will pour into state coffers. The fact that the money can be spent on anything state legislatures decide has led at least a third (16) of them to propose spending money on such things as property tax (Connecticut), car tax (Rhode Island), and debt (Louisiana) reduction; college scholarships (Michigan); water projects (North Dakota); prisoners' health care (South Dakota); school construction (Colorado); and teacher retirement funds (Oklahoma). Some states propose spending nothing or less than two percent of the tobacco settlement dollars they receive on tobacco prevention efforts.

The settlement requires that 80 percent of the 46 states involved, accounting for at least 80 percent of the money, receive final approval of the settlement from their state courts if any money is to be distributed in 1999. Disputes have arisen in California and New York over the ways the monies should be spent. California and New York each account for almost 13 percent of the money so the lawsuits in the two states could hold up distribution of the money. If the cases are not resolved by June 20, 2000, the money will be released. *See also* FEDERAL TRADE COMMISSION AND JOE CAMEL ADVERTISING; LEBOW, BENNETT; TOBACCO SETTLEMENT—JUNE 1997

Tobacco Trust. *See* AMERICAN TOBACCO COMPANY

Tobago

The name "tobacco" may have derived from the island of Tobago, discovered by CHRISTOPHER COLUMBUS during his third voyage in 1498 and named, according to one story, after the PIPE that the natives there were reported to have been using. Another account indicates that tobacco was named after this island because it resembled in shape a Carib pipe.

Traditional Native American Tobacco (TNAT) Seed Bank and Education Program

Housed at the University of New Mexico (UNM) in Albuquerque, the Traditional Native American Tobacco (TNAT) Seed Bank and Education Program collects, preserves, grows, and distributes the seeds of the many traditional Native American types of tobacco. It was founded in 1996 by UNM professor Joseph Winter, who is of Wampanoag descendancy; Lawrence Shorty, a Dine/Mississippi Choctaw; and a UNM School of Public Health student. TNAT provides traditional tobacco leaves for offerings at ceremonies and pow-wows, rituals, and healing sessions; for prayers; for invocations at meetings, conferences, and classes; for the elderly, prisoners, and other needy native people as well as for other events requiring the use of tobacco.

TNAT maintains a traditional tobacco seed bank and provides traditional tobacco seeds at no cost only to native people requesting them, as long as they agree to use the resulting tobacco carefully, in prayers, ceremonies, and other traditional contexts. If there is a request, TNAT tries to match it with the seeds of the tobacco type grown or collected by that individual's tribe, or from a closely related tribe.

TNAT also educates native people about the health dangers associated with tobacco abuse. It provides anti-smoking educational material relevant to Native American children, teenagers, and adults. It designs and presents education programs at schools, community centers, and other locations. It puts on SMOKING CESSATION programs and provides information at pow-wows and other occasions. TNAT presents tobacco plant exhibits that tell about the natural and cultural history of tobacco, its traditional uses, and the beliefs associated with them. *See also* NATIVE AMERICANS; PIPE SMOKING AND NATIVE AMERICANS

Trall, Russell T.

In the mid-nineteenth century, Dr. Russell T. Trall warned the struggle to quit using tobacco would be hard. He described how the process of freeing oneself from tobacco addiction would feel.

> Ghosts and goblins, spooks and apparitions, haunt his brain; and snakes and serpents of all shapes, sizes, colors, forms, and lengths dance attendance around the room, each in dumb-show chanting the praises

of Tobacco . . . . All through the long night do these fiends of a disordered nervous system play their fantastic tricks to his torment; and as the morning dawns, the wretched victim of a miserable habit feels utterly prostrated; and although he may still be determined to persevere in his abstinence and suffer through, he finds it almost impossible to think of anything but Tobacco; while every perverted, enraged, and rabid instinct is crying out, "A quid! a quid! my kingdom for a quid!" (Brooks, 1952)

Dr. Trall reported that the U.S. had the highest per capita use of tobacco in the world, that children as young as age three to six were smoking. "And more and worse than all this: Some of the ladies of this refined and fashion-forming metropolis are aping the silly ways of some pseudo-accomplished foreigners, in smoking Tobacco through a weaker and more feminine article, which has been most delicately denominated cigarette" (Brooks, 1952). *See also* ANTI-TOBACCO MOVEMENTS, UNITED STATES

References: Jerome E. Brooks, *The Mighty Leaf: Tobacco Through the Centuries*, Boston: Little, Brown and Company, 1952, pp. 220–21.

Trask, George (1798–1875)

One of the leading anti-tobacco agitators in the United States in the mid-nineteenth century, Reverend George Trask was one of a number of physicians and ministers who viewed tobacco as a deadly poison. He expressed his views in a volume published in Boston in 1852. Addressed to youth, the volum was entitled *Thoughts and Stories for American Lads: or Uncle Toby's Anti-Tobacco Advice for his Nephew Billy Bruce*. From 1859 until 1864, Trask edited and largely wrote an anti-tobacco periodical entitled *Anti-Tobacco Journal*. Published in Fitchburg, Massachusetts, it appeared quarterly. *See also* ANTI-TOBACCO MOVEMENTS, UNITED STATES; TRALL, RUSSELL T.

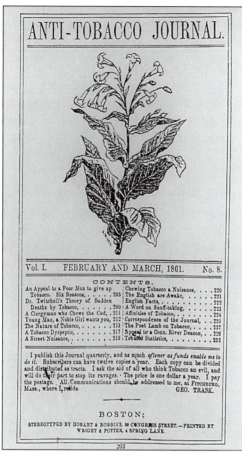

Cover of an 1861 edition of the *Anti-Tobacco Journal* edited by George Trask.

Turkey

Eastern monarchs were impressed by the opinion of their medical advisers that tobacco was an anti-aphrodisiac that would induce sterility. Around 1580, Sultan Murad II is said to have cultivated tobacco in his garden purely for its medicinal purposes, and to have sent its dried leaves to the king of Poland as a precious novelty.

Tobacco smoking spread around 1605 from Europe to Turkey, where it quickly became popular even though many attacked its use as contrary to the teachings of the Koran, which places religious taboos on a number of foodstuffs and practices including gambling, the use of narcotics, and the consumption of alcoholic beverages. One argument emphasized that the Koran forbade the use of coal, and tobacco when smoked be-

came coal. Two other concerns also influenced tobacco opponents: the fear of fires being ignited by careless smokers and the development of tobacco houses as centers of political and social unrest.

The spread of smoking divided the country into two camps. Poets praised smoking as one of the four elements (coffee, tobacco, opium, and wine) of the world of pleasure. The priests, however, were shocked and outraged by tobacco use because it was contrary to the Koran.

During the first half of the seventeenth century, Turkish rulers prohibited tobacco use. Sultan Ahmed (1603–1617) punished smokers by having a pipe stem thrust through their noses and then parading them on donkeys. MURAD IV, known to history as Murad the Cruel (1623–1640), severely punished smokers by beheading, hanging, and quartering them. Despite Murad's persecution and the mounting numbers of people he executed, including foreigners, smoking persisted. After Murad died, the prohibitory laws remained in force, but many who dreaded the penalties turned to SNUFF. The next ruler, Mohammed IV, a smoker, relaxed prohibitions and repealed strict laws. As a result, smoking increased enormously, both from

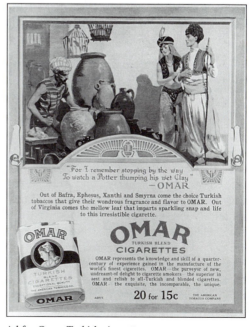

Ad for Omar Turkish cigarettes.

dry and water pipes. The cultivation of tobacco began in the Ottoman Empire and trade took on considerable importance. *See also* BUCKLEY, CHRISTOPHER; PIPE, WATER; TURKISH TOBACCO

Turkish Tobacco

During the CRIMEAN WAR of 1854–1856, French, Turkish, and Russian soldiers smoked Turkish tobacco cigarettes—the only kind available to both sides. The Turkish leaf is mild and fragrant with small leaves. It was so appealing that a veteran of the war, ROBERT GLOAG, experimented with Latakia, a smoke-cured variety of Turkish tobacco, in cigarettes made in the first full-fledged cigarette factory that he opened in 1856.

Turkish leaf was imported into NEW YORK CITY shops, which were operated by Greek and Turkish immigrants. New York, with its large foreign-born population, took to Turkish cigarettes. The vogue for Turkish cigarettes accounted for a fourth of cigarette sales between 1898 and 1903. By the turn of the century, a blended Turkish cigarette was such a popular item that cigarette packages were decorated with minarets, pyramids, and palm trees. As late as 1912, tailor-made cigarettes featured Turkish tobacco and were sold mainly in New York City and other urban markets.

The allure of Turkish tobacco was ever-present in cigarette brands introduced before WORLD WAR I that revolutionized world tobacco consumption. Although these brands evolved from domestic smoking tobaccos, CHESTERFIELD CIGARETTES were labeled "a balanced blend of the finest aromatic Turkish tobacco and the choicest of several American varieties." LUCKY STRIKE CIGARETTES was labeled "A blend of Burley and Turkish tobacco" and CAMEL CIGARETTES were a "Turkish and Domestic Blend." The emphasis on Turkish indicated the initial importance of Turkish tobacco in the cigarette market.

During the First World War, Turkish tobacco, which had played an important role in other wars, was cut off from its Western customers. This cooled the rage for Turkish cigarettes among American smokers, who switched to domestic blends. The small Turkish leaf, aromatic and light-colored, remained, however, an important "seasoning" ingredient or the "pepper and salt" of cigarettes.

Today, "Turkish" tobacco comes not only from Turkey but also from Greece, Bulgaria, and other Mediterranean countries and islands. *See also* TURKEY

Tuttle, Bill (1929–1998)

Former Major League baseball player, Bill Tuttle died of complications resulting from oral cancer. He played center field for the Detroit Tigers, Kansas City Athletics, and Minnesota Twins from 1952 to 1963. When he was 26 years old, Tuttle began using spit tobacco. Unaware of the dangers associated with its use, he chewed tobacco for the next 38 years until the fall of 1993 when squamous cell carcinoma, an oral cancer associated almost exclusively with spit tobacco users, developed inside Bill's mouth. After five bouts of surgery, the loss of his teeth, 70 radiation treatments that destroyed his taste buds, and two years of chemotherapy, Tuttle's cancer went into a brief remission.

Despite his pain, Tuttle worked with ORAL HEALTH AMERICA'S NATIONAL SPIT TOBACCO EDUCATION PROGRAM (NSTEP) to get the word out to the public, especially young people and the baseball community, that using spit tobacco was dangerous. Because of his work, Oral Health America and the Robert Wood Johnson Foundation established the Bill Tuttle Award. The award will be given each year to individuals or groups who distinguish themselves in the ongoing fight to educate Americans about the dangers of tobacco use. On May 19, 1998, Bill and Gloria Tuttle were presented with the inaugural Bill Tuttle Award at a ceremony in his honor during the Detroit Tigers/Minnesota Twins baseball game. Along with the award, Governor Arne Carlson officially pronounced May 19, 1998, as "Bill Tuttle Day" in the state of Minnesota.

Twain, Mark (1835–1910)

Samuel Clemens, better known by his pen name Mark Twain (the name he adopted when he was a reporter for the *Virginia City* [Nevada] *Territorial Enterprise*), smoked constantly, especially when writing, consuming up to 15 cigars during five hours of writing or 300 cigars a month. He said: "I smoke in moderation. Only one cigar at a time" (Conrad, 1996). Twain, who smoked cheap, smelly cigars, had a cigar named for him. The box label shows his face between two of his famous characters: Tom Sawyer and Huckleberry Finn. Twain, who began smoking at eight years of age, died of heart failure at 74. He wrote of smoking as follows:

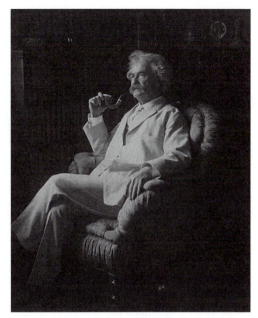

Mark Twain seated and smoking a pipe. *Library of Congress.*

> As concerns tobacco, there are many superstitions. And the chiefest of these is this—that there is a *standard* governing the matter, whereas there is nothing of the kind. Each man's own preference is the only standard for him, the only one which he can accept, the only one which can command him. A congress of all the tobacco-lovers in the world could not elect a standard which would be binding upon you or me, or would even much influence us.
>
> The next superstition is that a man had a standard of his own. He hasn't. He thinks he has, but he hasn't. He thinks he can tell what he regards as a good cigar from what he regards as a bad one—but he can't. He goes by the brand, yet imagines he goes by the flavor. One may palm off the worst counterfeit upon him; if it bears his brand he will smoke it contentedly and never suspect...
>
> No one can tell me what is a good cigar—for me. I am the only judge. People who claim to know say that I smoke the worst cigars in the world. They bring their own cigars when they come to my house. They betray an unmanly terror when I offer them a cigar; they tell lies and hurry away to meet engagements which they have not made when they are threatened with the hospitalities of my box. . . .
>
> Am I certain of my own standard? Perfectly; yes, absolutely—unless somebody fools me by putting my brand on some other kind of cigar; for no doubt I am like the rest, and know my cigar by the brand instead of by the flavor. However, my standard is a pretty wide one and covers a good deal of territory. To me, almost any cigar is good that nobody else will smoke, and to me almost all cigars are bad that other people consider good. Nearly any cigar will do me, except a Havana. (Nickels, 1994)

References: Barnaby Conrad III, *The Cigar*, San Francisco: Chronicle Books, 1996, p. 53.

Sara Nickels, *Drinking, Smoking, and Screwing: Great Writers on Good Times*, San Francisco: Chronicle Books, 1994, pp. 165–68.

U

Union City, New Jersey

Union City, New Jersey, is one of three important CIGAR manufacturing markets in the United States. Unlike MIAMI, FLORIDA, much of the Cuban population came to Union City in the 1920s and 1930s at the request of American cigar manufacturers. Labor prices had risen in CUBA because of unions, so major corporations like the AMERICAN TOBACCO COMPANY moved their operations to Union City and imported cured tobacco from Cuba. When labor prices in the United States escalated, the major manufacturers moved their operations back to the Caribbean, but the Cuban community stayed in New Jersey and made cigars for its own consumption as well as for outsiders. *See also* KEY WEST, FLORIDA

United States Tobacco (UST) Company

Founded in 1911, the United States Tobacco (UST) Company is a subsidiary of UST Inc. Headquartered in Greenwich, Connecticut, UST manufactures and markets moist smokeless tobacco products (SNUFF and CHEWING TOBACCO), PIPE tobacco, CIGARS, CIGARETTES, as well as accessories. In the 1990s, the company had about 80 percent of the U.S. smokeless tobacco market share.

Its top snuff brands include Skoal and Copenhagen. In 1983, UST launched Skoal Bandits—a milder, lower-nicotine-released "introductory" product—and in 1984 introduced Skoal Long Cut flavored tobaccos. In 1993, cherry and spearmint flavorings were added to Skoal Long Cut.

UST Inc. also has other businesses including wines and pipe tobacco products. *See also* MARSEE, SEAN; *MARSEE V. UNITED STATES TOBACCO COMPANY*

Uptown Cigarettes

In 1990, R.J. REYNOLDS TOBACCO COMPANY tried to introduce a new brand of cigarettes, Uptown, to the African-American community in Philadelphia. Through the efforts of African-American leaders like Reverend Jesse Brown and Charyn Sutton, the Uptown Coalition emerged and succeeded in banishing Uptown from stores in Philadelphia. This was the first time a community succeeded in getting a tobacco company to take a cigarette out of production.

Urban VIII (1568–1644)

In January 1642, Pope Urban VIII issued a Papal Bull that prohibited in churches "the use of the herb commonly called tobacco" because it had

> gained so strong a hold on persons of both sexes, yea, even priests and clerics, that—we blush to state—during the actual celebration of Holy Mass, they do not shrink from taking tobacco through the mouth or nostrils, thus soiling the altar linen and in-

fecting the churches with its noxious fumes, sacrilegiously and to the great scandal of the pious . . . it therefore behooves us, in order to purge our churches of this shameless abuse, to prohibit and interdict all persons of either sex, clergy or laity, collectively and individually, from using tobacco or snuff in any form whatever in the churches of the said dioceses . . . and all persons thus offending shall be punished by immediate excommunication, ipso facto, without further ado, in accordance with the terms of the present interdict. (Corti, 1931)

See also ITALY

References: Egon Caesar Corti, *History of Smoking*, London: G.G. Harry & Co. Ltd, 1931, p. 129.

U.S. Army

In 1986, the army began to deal with the fact that smoking rates in the military were much higher than in civilian life. While 52 percent of the military smoked, only 36.7 percent of American men in civilian life smoked. The army chief of staff and the secretary of the Army issued a joint proclamation aimed at reducing the level of cigarette use in the U.S. Army.

Tobacco usage impairs such critical skills as night vision, hand-eye coordination and resistance to cold weather injuries. Moreover, it increases susceptibility to disease. It has become a substantial threat to the well-being of our Army, and we must take immediate steps to eliminate its usage.

The army plan included more frequent health checks for soldiers who smoked and SMOKING CESSATION and education programs. The army now limits the places where soldiers can smoke ("Army Declares War on Smoking," 1986).

References: "Army Declares War on Smoking," *Smoking and Health Reporter*, vol. 4, no. 1 (Fall 1986), p. 5.

Utah

In 1921, the state of Utah, in accord with the official Mormon attitude, forbade the sale of cigarettes. The regulations for the public use of tobacco were so severe that one member of the state legislature threatened to introduce a law prohibiting the public sale of corned beef and cabbage because their fumes were as obnoxious to some people as tobacco smoke to others. The statute banned the advertising of cigarette and tobacco products on BILLBOARDS, street car signs, street cars, placards, and other places of display. It permitted the advertising of CIGARETTES and other tobacco products in newspapers, magazines, and periodicals.

After Utah banned cigarette billboards, its statute was challenged and upheld by the Utah Supreme Court. In *State v. Packer* (1931), the Supreme Court of Utah stated the following:

We see no reason why the state which may prohibit or limit the sale of his article, may not also limit or restrict the solicitation of the sale, especially where, as here, it has prohibited the sale to minors. Such solicitation by advertisement is for the purpose of increasing the demand for and use of tobacco. These advertisements do not appeal alone to the class of persons who may lawfully purchase and use cigarettes and tobacco; they are general in their nature, and appeal to all classes and ages of our population. *It is inconsistent to say the Legislature may lawfully prohibit the sale of tobacco to minors of both sexes, but is without power to place any restriction on the solicitation of such persons by advertisements.* Laws have been enacted in almost every state in the union prohibiting the sale of tobacco or some of its manufactured forms to minors, but, notwithstanding the enactment of these laws and the attempt to enforce them, the tobacco habit has made great inroads into the youth of the country. The reason would seem quite plain. Manufacturers and dealers have been left free to appeal to the boys and girls as well as adults with most alluring and attractive cigarette and tobacco advertisements. It is almost useless to pass laws prohibiting the sale of tobacco to minors, and at the same time make no attempt to restrict the solicitation of these same minors.

The U.S. Supreme Court in *Packer Corp. v. Utah* (1932) also upheld the constitutionality of the Utah cigarette billboard ban. Mr. Justice Louis Brandeis delivered the opinion of the Court.

> Advertisements of this sort are constantly before the eyes of the observers on the streets and in street cars to be seen without the exercise of choice or volition on their part. Other forms of advertising are ordinarily seen as a matter of choice on the part of the observer. The young people as well as the adults have the message of the billboard thrust upon them by all the arts and devices that skill can produce. In the case of newspapers and magazines, there must be some seeking by the one who is to see and read the advertisement.
>
> Most states have banned the sale of tobacco products to minors. Since the sale of tobacco can be regulated, solicitation of sales can similarly be regulated.

See also BALTIMORE BILLBOARD ORDINANCE; CINCINNATI, OHIO

Utah Clean Air Act

On April 4, 1995, tribal elders throughout Utah gathered in the Utah Capitol rotunda for the ceremonial smoking of the pipe and to celebrate the traditional use of tobacco. The ceremony also celebrated Governor Mike Leavitt's signing of HB149, a bill that exempts American Indian religious leaders from the state law prohibiting smoking in public buildings. Because there was no exemption for religious ceremonies, even in churches or at annual gatherings of American Indians at traditional powwows, the law directly infringed on American Indians' right to freedom of religion.

In sponsoring the legislation to exempt American Indian religious leaders from the smoking ban, Representative Eli H. Anderson (Republican-Tremonton), maintained the infringement of religious freedom was never the intent of the legislature. After initial opposition from the Rules Committee, the bill passed overwhelmingly. Under the provisions of HB149, those American Indians who have been designated by their tribes as religious leaders or pipe carriers are allowed to conduct pipe ceremonies in a public building at the invitation of the owner of the public place.

On April 4, 1995, the state granted permission to Pete Littlejohn, a Shoshone pipe carrier from Ft. Hall, Idaho, to smoke the pipe inside the Captiol building. Clifford Duncan, former councilman of the Ute Tribe, explained that it is not the spirit of tobacco alone that is meaningful to American Indians, but the many dreams and prayers reaching back through generations of ancestors. He said the "Great Spirit" touches the smoke rising from a traditional ceremony. *See also* NATIVE AMERICANS; PIPE SMOKING AND NATIVE AMERICANS

V

Vending Machines

Because it's so easy for children and teens to get cigarettes from vending machines, dozens of municipalities across the country have adopted ordinances banning them. Younger smokers say it's usually no problem to buy cigarettes from vending machines, even if states ban sales to anyone under 18. A 1992 study said children can buy cigarettes from vending machine placed in "adults only" areas 77 percent of the time. A 14-year-old girl proved the point right under the government's nose. In March 1996, she illegally purchased a pack of cigarettes from a vending machine located in a U.S. House of Representatives office building. The Virginia girl was lobbying in support of the 1995 FOOD AND DRUG ADMINISTRATION's proposed restrictions on tobacco advertising to children. When she purchased the cigarettes, she wore a T-shirt that said "I am 14 years old." No one stopped her.

In April 1996, a 17-year-old also proved the same point to President Bill Clinton. After the president landed at Newark International Airport, Raymond Tavarez, a junior at Perth Amboy High School, handed him a pack of Newports he bought from a vending machine at an employee cafeteria inside a smoke-free Port Authority building.

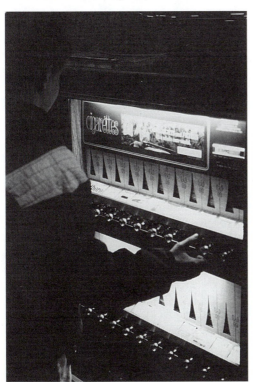

A cigarette vending machine. *Courtesy of Laurence Pringle.*

Viceroy Cigarettes

Viceroy cigarettes, introduced in 1936 by BROWN AND WILLIAMSON TOBACCO CORPORATION, used cylinders of folded paper for filters rather than hollow tubes with cotton. The brand achieved only nominal success until 1952 when the filter trend began. In 1954, Viceroy changed to a tip made of cellulose acetate, a material that quickly became the "normal" filter. *See also* FILTERED CIGARETTES

Virginia Colony. *See* JAMESTOWN, VIRGINIA COLONY

Virginia Slims Cigarettes

In 1968, PHILIP MORRIS USA introduced Virginia Slims, a new "slimmer than usual" (100 mm) cigarette for women. Its slogan, "You've Come a Long Way, Baby!" appealed to many women who were moving into more assertive, independent roles. The slogan and copy contrasted women's historical lack of rights with the modern situation in which women were no longer restricted by dated social mores. Television and magazine ads contrasted the old social order with the new by belittling dated restrictions on women.

After cigarette advertising was banned from the broadcast media effective January 2, 1971, the volume of advertising in women's magazines increased dramatically. In 1974, Philip Morris spent $8.3 million in advertising in magazines, newspapers, and Sunday supplements, making the campaign the biggest in print advertising. The themes in the ads showed liberation, independence, sophistication, and self-confidence. Many ads contrasted what women looked like hundreds of years ago next to images of thin, glamorous, free-spirited women of the 1960s.

Virginia Slims started sponsoring women's professional tennis in 1970. Free cigarettes were given away at stadium entrances, and contract players were not permitted to take any public position opposing cigarette sponsorship. Despite the broadcast ban on cigarette advertising, television coverage of the tournaments brought Virginia Slims into homes across the United States. In 1990, when Secretary of Health and Human Services Louis Sullivan, M.D., called for an end to sports sponsorship by cigarette makers, women's tennis stars opposed the effort and supported Philip Morris.

During the mid-1970s, as part of Virginia Slims' promotions, 400,000 items were distributed, including "You've come a long way, baby" T-shirts (200,000), jerseys (110,000), and sweaters (70,000). By 1985, another promotion, an appointment calendar called

the "Book of Days" that notes historic dates including the 1968 launch of Virginia Slims, had one million in distribution.

In 1976, Philip Morris began advertising Virginia Slims to British women. The tobacco company used a different blend of tobacco and modified the "Baby" slogan, which had offended *Ms.* magazine in the United States. In October, a campaign launched the anglicized version of Virginia Slims with the slogan "We've come a long, long way." Mike Daube, director of ACTION ON SMOKING AND HEALTH (ASH), the anti-smoking pressure group in England, protested to the Advertising Standards Authority (ASA). Daube claimed that the "ads deliberately attempt to exploit the women's movement and are thus trying to recruit new smokers. The Virginia Slims advertisements are directed at a specific sector of the market where there is still room for expansion" (Jacobson, 1981, p. 66). The ASA was unable, at the time, to see "how the campaign could be said to seek to persuade women to start smoking." It did express "considerable reservations" about the advertisements, which it saw as being in "doubtful taste because they exploited the campaign for women's rights." The ASA found the ads objectionable but could not find sufficient reason to reject them because there was no clause in the cigarette code that prevented Philip Morris from pursuing its line.

The cigarette code required that advertisements "should not seek to encourage people, particularly the young, to start smoking, or, if they are already smokers, to increase their level of smoking or smoke to excess; and should not exploit those who are especially vulnerable" (Jacobson, 1981, p. 64). The code also said that ads were not allowed to suggest that smoking was "a sign or proof of manliness, or that smokers were more virile or tougher than nonsmokers." The code did not prohibit appeals to femininity.

Philip Morris approached the editor of *Ms London,* a magazine aimed mainly at working women between the ages of 16 and 24, who agreed to let the company use the magazine to run a contest. Readers who saw the contest in the December 6, 1976, issue answered questions about such "female revolutionaries" as Princess Anne, and completed the slogan "Virginia Slims are perfect for the modern woman because . . ." The six best entrants won prizes, which included an elegant pen and propelling pencil set. Two members of Parliament, Laurie Pavitt and Lynda Chalker, reacted immediately and questioned the ad as did the health minister, Roland Moyle, who was concerned that the ASA did not consider the *Ms London* ad in breach of the cigarette code. Moyle said: "This strengthens our view that the present [ASA] Code does not go far enough" (Jacobson, 1981, p. 66). When the ASA code was revised in 1977, ASH made sure that there was a femininity clause alongside the virility clause to protect women against further advertising. The British Code of Advertising Practice was changed to read that advertisements are not allowed to suggest "female smokers are more glamorous or independent than non-smokers" or that "smoking enhances feminine charm."

The print advertising targeted to women continued into the 1980s. In July 1985, a Virginia Slims advertising campaign featured eight American Indian "princesses" carved on a totem pole next to a chic, sexy white woman holding a cigarette. The ad declared "Virginia Slims remembers one of many societies where the women stood head and shoulders above the men." After hundreds of angry phone calls and letters from American Indian and non-American Indian individuals and organizations, the Philip Morris Company withdrew the ad.

In her letter to Philip Morris, National Congress of American Indian executive director Suzan Shown Harjo especially objected to demeaning names like "Princess Wash and Scrub" and "Little Running Water Fetcher" ascribed to the eight women. "The terms 'Little' and 'Princess' are both diminishing and inaccurate. Indian women are not referred to by Indian men as 'the little woman' . . . and we have no princesses, historically or today" (Harjo, 1985). Michael Bush, executive director of the New York-based American Indian Community House, was of-

fended by the ad because it portrayed American Indian women as "menial servants" and perpetuated "an idiotic stereotype for the assumed amusement of the public." In his letter to the president of Philip Morris, Bush wrote "Even if the ad is superfluous, it seems ludicrous to capture a stereotype which is so erroneous." He went on to write that the Virginia Slims' portrayal of Indian women as "servile" was especially inappropriate because they "are the developers, the initiators and the planners in Indian society" (Bush, 1985).

Guy Smith, Philip Morris vice president, who stated the ad would be removed from all publications within a month, said that the ad was never intended to fuel a stereotype or to offend. Instead, he said, the ad was meant to show how women have advanced. In reply to H. Blue, editor of *The Circle,* a Minneapolis-based Indian paper, a spokeswoman for the tobacco company said Philip Morris would no longer use the ad "out of deference to the individuals and organizations who complained or wrote letters." In his editorial, Blue wrote as follows:

> This story proves that where's there's a will, there's a way. Even a giant like Philip Morris Company will bow to the pressure of the public, in this case, the American Indian public. Of course the fact that the Philip Morris Company "gave in" does not by any means excuse the ad's publication in the first place. Especially since this is supposed to be the day and age where discrimination is on the downswing, and we are all equal. (Blue, 1985)

The greatest growth of tobacco advertising aimed at women followed the introduction of Virginia Slims. Numerous women's brands were released and by 1979, magazine tobacco advertising equaled those ads targeted at men. *See also* WOMEN, UNITED STATES

References: H. Blue, "Philip Morris Co. Hasn't Come a Long Way, Baby." *The Cerole* (Boston Indian Council) vol. 8, no. 3 (August 1985), p. 1.

Michael Bush, Letter to Mr. John L. Murphy, President, Philip Morris Inc., July 25, 1985.

Suzan Shown Harjo, "NCAI Protests Virginia Slims Ad Denigrating Indian Women," *NCAI News*, vol. 50, no. 6, 1985, p. 7.

Bobbie Jacobson, *The Ladykillers: Smoking Is a Feminist Issue*, London: Pluto, 1981, pp. 64, 66.

Viscusi, W. Kip (1949–)

A Harvard University economist, W. Kip Viscusi, held that the financial cost arguments advanced in a series of lawsuits filed by states against cigarette companies to recoup smoking-related Medicaid costs do not stand up under scrutiny. According to Vicusi, smokers pay the states in advance for at least some of the costs they generate through the excise taxes the states levy on cigarettes, and cigarettes actually save states money. He reasons that because of their shorter expected life spans, cigarette smokers will incur fewer medical costs and other expenses in old age, such as pensions, nursing-home expenditures, and social security payments. By dying younger, on average, about eight years before nonsmokers, smokers actually save the nation money.

Viscusi argues that in their lawsuits, state officials calculate only one component—the increased medical costs due to smoking. The officials ignore the short life expectancy of smokers and the fact there are no medical costs generated by smokers after they are dead. States, he says, also dismiss the excise taxes that smokers pay.

Viscusi has challenged the figures of public health officials that smoking costs the nation about $100 billion a year in smoking-related hospital bills, doctor fees, drugs, nursing-home bills, as well as lost working hours and income taxes from smokers who get ill and die early. Viscusi has argued that these officials have ignored the long-term, or "lifetime" approach that amount to savings, not costs, from excise taxes paid by smokers, income taxes paid by doctors, pharmacies, and health care providers involved in caring for smokers with tobacco-related diseases.

Viscusi has also argued that several groups lose when smoking regulations are put in place to limit exposure to ENVIRONMENTAL TOBACCO SMOKE (ETS) in the workplace and smoking overall. Smokers, he says, lose a substantial benefit to their welfare when they forego an activity they enjoy; if relegated to a specific smoking area, their welfare also decreases and their productivity may be affected as well because they are impeded from smoking. The tobacco industry and its shareholders lose profits because of the decrease in smoking, and he calculates that society loses because of lost tax revenue from a reduction in smoking. Finally, Viscusi says there are other expenses associated with setting aside smoking areas including setting up ventilation systems and smoking lounges. *See also* FLORIDA MEDICAID CASE; MINNESOTA MEDICAID CASE; MISSISSIPPI MEDICAID CASE; TEXAS MEDICAID CASE

Vuelta Abajo, Cuba

An area of CUBA west of HAVANA and nearest the United States, Vuelta Abajo ("down turn"), is Cuba's finest tobacco region. It is renowned for growing a fragrant, rich leaf that Connecticut, Pennsylvania, Wisconsin, Sumatra, Jamaica, and Puerto Rico cannot imitate. Vuelta Abaja is located in the district of Pinar del Rio, 100 miles west of Havana, where about 100,000 acres of tobacco are planted. The region's combination of brown soil, bright sun, and heavy humidity is suited to cigar-leaf cultivation. A handful of villages on the Vuelta Abajo have reputations for growing great tobacco; among them are San Juan y Martinez and San Luiz. *See also* CIGAR; CUBAN TOBACCO HISTORY

W

Wafer, Lionel (c. 1660–1705)

In 1681, a British surgeon named Lionel Wafer joined a party of buccaneers on a foray across the Isthmus of Panama. Accidentally disabled, he left his companions and lived with Darien Indians. He wrote an account of his adventures in *Travels* (1681) in which he described the use of tobacco on ritual occasions—in this case the practice of an individual "smoking over" other persons and objects for religious purposes:

> These Indians have tobacco among them. When it is dried and cured they strip it from the stalks, and laying two or three leaves upon another, they roll up all together sideways into a long roll, yet leaving a little hollow. Round this they roll other leaves one after another, in the same manner, but close and hard, till the roll be as big as one's wrist, and two or three feet in length. Their way of smoking when in company together is this: a boy lights one end of the roll, burning it to a coal, wetting the part next to it to keep it from wasting too fast. The other end he puts into his mouth, and blows the smoak [sic] of the roll into the face of every one of the company or council, though there be two or three hundred of them. Then they, sitting in their usual posture, make, with their hands held hollow together, a kind of funnel round their mouths and noses. Into this they receive the smoak [sic] as it blows upon them, snuffing it up greedily and strongly, as long as ever they are able to hold their breath; and seeming

to bless themselves, as it were, with the refreshment it gives them. (Dunhill, 1969)

References: Alfred Dunhill, *The Pipe Book*, New York: Macmillan Company, 1924, 1969, p. 32–33.

War

Every major war has been associated with an increase in tobacco sales and consumption because it is believed tobacco can calm the frightened, quiet the wounded, and energize the weary and bored. Military commanders have long regarded tobacco as an essential product for soldiers.

In the late nineteenth century, during the Boer War, cigars and plug sold well. The CRIMEAN WAR of the 1850s helped popularize cigarette smoking in Great Britain and France, the troops having picked up the habit from their Turkish allies and Russian enemies.

At the end of the Civil War, Union soldiers stationed near Durham, North Carolina, acquired a taste for BRIGHT TOBACCO LEAF. A local, JOHN RUFFIN GREEN, who manufactured a high-quality smoking tobacco consumed by soldiers of both the Union and the Confederacy, profited after the war. Soldiers throughout the nation sent letters to Durham Station all desirous of getting more of his smoking tobacco made from Bright leaf.

Many American soldiers smoked their first cigarettes while stationed in territories acquired during the Spanish-American War of

1898. Initially, army and navy officers viewed the new habit with deep suspicion and tried to discourage it on the grounds that it impaired health. The U.S. Military Academy at West Point banned the sale and possession of cigarettes in 1903 and 1911. By the time U.S. soldiers entered World War I, cigarettes no longer were officially censured in military life. *See also* WORLD WAR I; WORLD WAR II

Warner, Kenneth E. (1956–)

A noted tobacco policy expert, Kenneth E. Warner, a professor at the University of Michigan's School of Public Health, has studied NICOTINE REPLACEMENT PRODUCTS. In an article, "The Emerging Market for Long-term Nicotine Maintenance," published in an October 1997 issue of the *Journal of the American Medical Association (JAMA),* he wrote that more people will be using NICOTINE products such as gums and patches, not to stop smoking, but as ongoing substitutes for nicotine.

Washington, George (1732–1799)

After the French and Indian War ended in Virginia, George Washington returned to Mount Vernon in 1759 determined to become a successful tobacco planter. Like other respectable gentlemen in Virginia, Washington's reputation depended in part on the quality of the tobacco he grew. Characteristic of other tobacco planters, Washington ran into debt. No matter how hard his slaves worked the soils of Mount Vernon, his land could not grow tobacco leaves that compared favorably with the plants of other Tidewater plantations. In April 1761, he wrote to Robert Cary, an English merchant, complaining: "I am at a loss to conceive the Reason why Mr. Wormeleys, and indeed some other Gentlemen's Tobaccos should sell at 12d last year and mine . . . only fetch 11½. Certain I am no Person in Virginia takes more pains to make their Tobo. Fine than I do and tis hard then I should not be well rewarded for it" (Breen, 1985).

In 1762, Washington judging himself by the conventions of Virginia culture that price provided a measure of a planter's skills as a producer, confessed that growing tobacco was "an Art beyond my skill, to succeed in making good Tobo. as I have used my utmost endeavors for that purpose this two or 3 years past; and am once again urged to express my surprise at finding that I do not partake of the best prices that are going" (Breen, 1985).

Descending into debt like other Tidewater planters, in September 1765, he wrote Cary that the price he got for his tobacco was "worse than many of my Acquaintances upon this River, Potomack" (Breen, 1985). Reluctantly, in 1767, Washington stopped growing tobacco and turned to wheat, a plant that required little labor from the planter.

References: T.H. Breen, *Tobacco Culture: The Mentality of the Great Tidewater Planters on the Eve of Revolution*, Princeton: Princeton University Press, 1985, p. 81.

Waxman Hearings

In March 1994, Congressman Henry Waxman (1939–), a Democrat from California and an anti-tobacco campaigner, chaired landmark hearings before the Subcommittee on Health and the Environment of the House Energy and Commerce Committee. Titled "Regulation of Tobacco Products," the hearings were memorable, not only for the televised image of seven tobacco industry executives swearing that NICOTINE was not addictive, but also for the flood of documents and informants that emerged.

The nationally televised hearings on tobacco industry practices examined the possibility of providing the FOOD AND DRUG ADMINISTRATION (FDA) with broad regulatory authority over tobacco products under the federal FOOD, DRUG AND COSMETIC ACT, including a proposal to classify nicotine in tobacco as a drug. The committee reviewed the implications for tobacco regulation of current research on the alleged highly addictive nature of nicotine and examined allegations that the tobacco industry manipulated nicotine levels in cigarettes to ensure that their products remain addictive. Representative Waxman was prompted to hold the hearings after ABC's *Day One* telecast on February 28, 1994, reported that cigarette companies controlled the content of nicotine in cigarettes and Dr. DAVID KESSLER said the FDA had received "mounting evidence" that tobacco companies controlled nicotine levels in cigarettes.

The hearings began on March 25, 1994. Witnesses included Representative Richard J. Durbin, Democrat from Illinois; Representative James E. Clyburn, Democrat from South Carolina; and Representative H. Martin Lancaster, Democrat from North Carolina. They presented differing views on the proposal to subject tobacco products to FDA regulation. FDA commissioner Kessler raised the possibility that nicotine addiction rather than consumer choice influences decisions of smokers to continue smoking. He also made allegations that the tobacco industry maintained nicotine levels in cigarettes at addictive levels. Scott D. Ballin, from the now-defunct COALITION ON SMOKING OR HEALTH; Alexander W. Spears, vice chairman and CEO of LORILLARD COMPANY INC.; Stephen M. Raffle, M.D., a psychiatrist representing the TOBACCO INSTITUTE; JOHN SLADE, M.D., representing the American Society of Addiction Medicine; Sherwin Gardner, a consultant for PHILIP MORRIS USA; and GREGORY N. CONNOLLY, M.D., director of the Massachusetts Tobacco Control Program, representing the American Public Health Association, presented differing views on the proposal to allow the FDA to regulate tobacco. Tobacco representatives refuted the allegations that the tobacco industry manipulates nicotine in cigarettes.

On April 14, 1994, seven CEOs testified before Waxman's Health and Environmental Subcommittee and were asked to state their opinions for the record. "Yes or no, do you believe nicotine is addictive?"

William I. Campbell, president and CEO of Philip Morris USA, answered: "I believe nicotine is not addictive."

James W. Johnston, chairman and CEO of R.J. REYNOLDS TOBACCO COMPANY, answered: "Mr. Congressman, cigarettes and

nicotine clearly do not meet the classic definition of addiction. There is no intoxication."

Joseph Taddeo, president of U.S. Tobacco, answered: "I don't believe that nicotine or our products are addictive."

ANDREW TISCH, chairman and CEO of the Lorillard Company; Edward A. Horrigan, Jr., chairman and CEO of the Liggett Group; Donald S. Johnston, president of the AMERICAN TOBACCO COMPANY; and THOMAS E. SANDEFUR, JR., chairman and CEO of BROWN AND WILLIAMSON TOBACCO CORPORATION, each answered: "I believe that nicotine is not addictive" (Hilts, 1996).

On April 28, 1994, VICTOR DeNOBLE, former associate senior scientist at the Philip Morris Research Center, accompanied by Paul Mele, former research scientist at the Philip Morris Research Center, testified about the research findings of behavioral and psychological effects of nicotine in rats that demonstrated the reinforcing properties of nicotine in cigarette smoke. The rats experienced a decrease of susceptibility to the effects of the nicotine resulting in their need to increase the drug dosage to achieve the effects experienced previously. The scientists testified that the Philip Morris response was not to allow publication of their findings and to discontinue the research.

On May 17, 1994, JOSEPH A CALIFANO, JR., president of the Center on Addiction and Substance Abuse, Columbia University, testified about the health care problems associated with cigarette smoking and made recommendations for policy actions.

On May 26, 1994, James F. Glenn, M.D., chairman of the COUNCIL FOR TOBACCO RESEARCH (CTR), testified and refuted allegations that CTR provided misinformation to the public about tobacco use and disease. He clarified CTR's purpose and procedures and responded to allegations regarding CTR's role in cigarette promotion.

On June 21, 1994, FDA commissioner Kessler testified about the findings of an FDA investigation of alleged tobacco industry manipulation of cigarette nicotine levels, including Brown and Williamson's development of a genetically altered high-nicotine yielding tobacco plant.

On June 23, 1994, Thomas E. Sandefur, Jr., chairman and CEO of Brown and Williamson, acknowledged there were differing scientific opinions regarding the addictive nature of nicotine in cigarettes. He clarified the reason for his company developing a genetically altered tobacco plant with increased levels of nicotine.

On November 29, 1994, Michael P. Eriksen, director of the Office on Smoking and Health; JACK E. HENNINGFIELD, chief of the Clinical Pharmacological Branch, National Institute on Drug Abuse; and Gregory N. Connolly, representing the now-defunct Coalition on Smoking or Health, testified about trends in SMOKELESS TOBACCO use, findings of NIDA research on nicotine levels in smokeless tobacco, and claims regarding the UNITED STATES TOBACCO COMPANY's use of marketing ploys and graduated nicotine levels to promote initial use of SNUFF and progression to increasingly potent brands.

On July 24, 1995, Congressman Waxman read into the *Congressional Record* excerpts of dozens of previously secret TOBACCO DOCUMENTS from the nation's largest tobacco company, Philip Morris. Waxman felt the documents made a compelling case for regulation of tobacco to protect children. The subcommittee's study was cut short because of the presidential election, but Congressman Waxman continued his own investigation of Philip Morris. He said:

> One of the most significant revelations in the documents is that Philip Morris conducted pharmacological research specifically targeted at children and college students.
>
> One of the longest-running studies in the documents addresses the "hyperkinetic child as a prospective smoker." In this study, Philip Morris collaborated with the Chesterfield County school system in Richmond, Virginia to determine whether hyperkinetic and borderline hyperkinetic children will become cigarette smokers in their teenage years. The researchers explained:

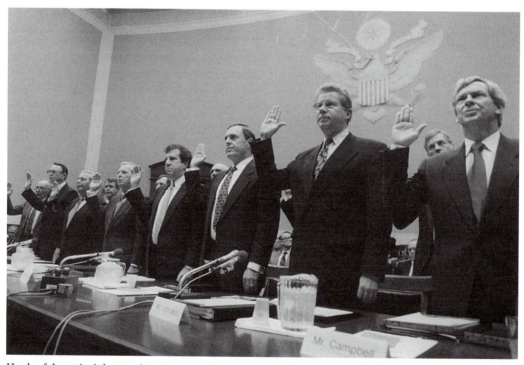

Heads of the nation's largest cigarette companies are sworn in before a hearing of a House Energy Subcommittee in April 1994. *AP Photo/John Duricka.*

"It has been found that amphetamines, which are strong stimulants, have the anomalous effect of quieting these children down. Many children are therefore regularly administered amphetamines throughout grade school years . . . . We wonder whether such children may not eventually become cigarette smokers in their teenage years as they discover the advantage of self-stimulation via nicotine. We have already collaborated with a local school system in identifying some such children in the third grade."

This research began in 1974. It continued until 1978, when it had to be terminated prematurely because of objections from the school system and physicians.

Many of the studies conducted by Philip Morris investigated the pharmacological effects of cigarettes on college students. These studies provided scientific data about the youngest segment of the cigarette market lawfully available to Philip Morris. Moreover, because there is no bright line that separates college students from underage smokers, the studies also provided Philip Morris with considerable insight into the underage market.

In one series of experiments with college students—code-named "Shock I, II, III, IV, and V"—Philip Morris administered electric shocks to the students to determine if student smoking rates increased under stressful conditions. This study began in 1969. It ultimately had to be terminated in 1972 because "fear of shock is scaring away some of our valuable students."

In another study, Philip Morris gave college students low-nicotine cigarettes in an attempt to force the students "to modify their puff volumes, inhalation volumes, and/or smoke retention times in order to obtain their usual nicotine dose."

Philip Morris maintains publicly that it does not target children in advertising, cigarette sales, or other ways. The documents undermine this claim—at least as it applies to scientific research. They show that Philip Morris has targeted children and college students, the youngest segment of the market, for specific research projects. (Congrssional Record, 1995).

References: *Congressional Record-House*, July 24, 1995, p. H7472.

Philip J. Hilts, *Smoke Screen: The Truth Behind the Tobacco Industry Cover-Up*, Reading, MA: Addison-Wesley Publishing Co., Inc., 1996, pp. 122–23.

Werner, Carl Avery (1873–1945)

In 1922, Carl Avery Werner, a tobacco trade journalist who wrote books and articles about tobacco, wrote a "creed" for smokers, urging them to respect the rights of nonsmokers. The creed read as follows:

Notwithstanding that those who derive happiness, comfort and good fellowship through the use of tobacco comprise 90 percent of the male adult population of the United States, I fully realize that the majority, counting women and children, are nonsmokers and that among this majority there are some to whom the fumes of tobacco are not agreeable. I take pleasure, therefore, in observing the following rules of courtesy and consideration:

1. I shall not smoke or carry a lighted cigar or cigarette in any place or at any time where or when, either by placard or common understanding, smoking is prohibited.

2. I shall not smoke in any place or at any time where or when the fumes of tobacco are obviously annoying to others, even though such abstinence is not compulsory.

3. I shall not smoke in any passenger elevator, public or private.

4. I shall not smoke in a dense crowd of people, indoors or out, if I discover that my smoke is annoying some one near me who, owing to the circumstances, is unable to move away.

5. I shall not smoke in any home or any room wherein I am a guest without first making sure that smoking therein is agreeable to my host and others present.

6. I shall not smoke in the presence of any lady until I have been assured that she has no objections to my doing so.

7. I shall not approve of the use of tobacco by growing boys and girls.

8. I shall exercise caution in discarding the ends of cigars and cigarettes in order

to preclude the possibility of fire.

9. I shall, in my enjoyment of the smoking privilege, be always considerate of those whose inclinations happen to differ from my own and always be guided by the finer instincts of true chivalry and American manhood.

10. I shall faithfully adhere to the forgoing self-imposed rules myself, and shall urge others to do the same, that the days of tobacco may be long and its friends legion in the land of our fathers.

White Buffalo Calf Woman

White Buffalo Calf Woman was the holy woman who brought the Lakota people the Buffalo Calf Pipe, their most sacred possession. She gave instructions on its meaning and care. The PIPESTONE bowl represented the earth, the wood stem represented all the earth's growing things, a buffalo calf carved on the bowl represented all four-legged creatures, and the pipe's 12 feathers from the spotted eagle represented all winged creatures. She instructed that those who prayed with the pipe would be joined to all others in the universe. *See also* CATLIN, GEORGE; NATIVE AMERICANS; PIPE SMOKING AND NATIVE AMERICANS

White Burley Tobacco

In 1864, George Webb, a tobacco grower in Brown County, Ohio, planted some tobacco seeds he purchased in Kentucky. As the seedlings grew, he noticed the leaves were a strange creamy color instead of green. He figured the seeds were bad and destroyed the plants. Owing to a shortage of crops the next year, Webb planted the remainder of the "bad" seeds. The crop he harvested and shipped for sale was well received by buyers. It produced a milder smoke than the standard burley tobaccos of the area.

Ever since it was discovered, the popularity of white burley grew steadily. The white burley mutation became the only type of leaf grown as BURLEY TOBACCO. By 1875, it was a popular FILLER in plug tobacco. It became the base of American smoking mixtures and a principal ingredient of CIGARETTES.

Wigand, Jeffrey S. (1943–)

Jeffrey S. Wigand was a former vice president (1989–1993) for research and development at BROWN AND WILLIAMSON TOBACCO CORPORATION, headquartered in Louisville, Kentucky. He became the highest-ranking defector in the history of the tobacco industry. Wigand was the son of a mechanical engineer who earned a doctorate in biochemistry and endocrinology. With a budget of more than $20 million, a staff of 243, and a salary of $300,000 a year, Wigand worked on two projects: a new low-tar cigarette and fire-safe cigarettes—or cigarettes that burn at lower temperatures to reduce the risk of fires.

Frustrated by his job, the company's reluctance to pursue a low-tar cigarette, and its use of coumarin as an additive in pipe tobacco, Wigand had confrontations with Brown and Williamson management. He especially clashed with the chief executive officer THOMAS E. SANDEFUR, who fired him on March 24, 1993. In exchange for signing a lifelong agreement of confidentiality, of which he would be in violation if he discussed anything he knew about the corporation, Wigand was given a severance package and medical benefits. He needed the benefits for a daughter who required expensive medical treatments. Nevertheless, Wigand agreed to help CBS research a story about fire-safe cigarettes. By the spring of 1994, he also began sharing information with DAVID KESSLER, commissioner of the FOOD AND DRUG ADMINISTRATION, and others.

In January 1995, Wigand, who became a high school science teacher in Louisville, was pressured by CBS producer of *60 MINUTES* Lowell Bergman to be interviewed for a segment. Wigand agreed, but only with the assurance of CBS protection if he were sued for breaking his agreement with Brown and Williamson. The interview was taped, but CBS made a last-minute controversial decision in October 1995 to cancel the segment featuring an interview with Mr. Wigand, who discussed potentially damaging information about the tobacco industry. CBS was fearful of legal retaliation because of Wigand's severance contract.

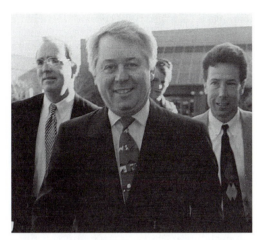

Former Brown and Williamson Tobacco Company employee Jeffrey Wigand arrives to give a deposition in Pascagoula, Mississippi, in November 1995. *AP/Wide World Photos.*

After someone at CBS leaked a transcript of the Wigand interview to the *New York Daily News,* parts of which were printed, Brown and Williamson denied the charges and sued Wigand in Jefferson County Circuit Court in Louisville, Kentucky (where the company has its headquarters). It accused Wigand of theft, fraud, and breach of contract in violating two confidentiality agreements that he made with the company. The tobacco company was also granted a temporary restraining order that prohibited Mr. Wigand from disclosing further information about Brown and Williamson. Wigand's lawyer said the researcher was discharged "on a pretext" by Brown and Williamson in 1993. The company cut off Wigand's severance package and health benefits. It also began to publicize Wigand's private life, accusing him of shoplifting (the charges had been dropped), not paying child support (the charges had been settled with his first wife), and spousal abuse (the charges had been withdrawn).

Wigand hired RICHARD F. SCRUGGS, who took him on as a pro bono client. Wigand also testified in December 1995 before a federal grand jury. RONALD MOTLEY, a South Carolina trial attorney working for MICHAEL C. MOORE (the Mississippi attorney general), deposed Wigand on November 29, 1995, as part of trial preparation in the state of Mississippi's lawsuit seeking to force tobacco companies to pay for the cost of smoking-related illnesses. In his deposition, Wigand accused Sandefur, now retired from Brown and Williamson, of lying under oath when he testified to Congress that NICOTINE was not addictive.

The details of Wigand's accusations against Brown and Williamson in a court-sealed deposition became public in January 1996 when Alix Freedman of the *Wall Street Journal* received a copy of the transcript of testimony Wigand gave in the Mississippi deposition. Freedman turned in an article, citing key sections of the transcript in which Wigand offered specifics about his beliefs that Brown and Williamson engaged in a variety of abuses, including perjury, destruction of evidence, quashing research into safer cigarettes, reckless use of possibly harmful additives, and violations of export controls. He said Sandefur repeatedly said, in private conversations, that nicotine was addictive. Wigand also spoke about Y1 TOBACCO, the high-nicotine, cross-bred tobacco plant publicized earlier by David Kessler at Henry Waxman's subcommittee hearings.

After the sealed testimony Mr. Wigand gave to the state of Mississippi was leaked to the media in January 1996, Brown and Williamson released a 500-page report entitled "The Misconduct of Jeffrey S. Wigand Available in the Public Record," which was said to be filled with a "pile of unsubstantiated slurs" (Hilts, 1996). The media, led by the *Wall Street Journal,* discovered many of the assertions in the report were petty and some of them not true. One Brown and Williamson executive quoted in the *Wall Street Journal* said: "From the moment Brown and Williamson got personal with him, they turned him into a martyr."

Towards the end of the talks between tobacco executives and state attorneys leading up to the tobacco settlement of June 1997, the issue of general protection for Wigand from a Brown and Williamson lawsuit became a big issue. The lawsuit was dropped in exchange for Wigand keeping to his confidentiality agreement for nine months. *See also* TOBACCO SETTLEMENT—JUNE 1997; WAXMAN HEARINGS

References: Philip J. Hilts, *Smoke Screen: The Truth Behind the Tobacco Industry Cover-Up*, Reading, MA: Addison-Wesley Publishing Co., Inc., 1996, pp. 122–23.

Wiley, Harvey W. (1844–1930)

Harvey W. Wiley, chief chemist for the Department of Agriculture and later the first director of the FOOD AND DRUG ADMINISTRATION, directed studies in 1892 that tested whether cigarettes from retail outlets contained narcotics. After testing 13 popular brands, Wiley reported that he found no trace of opium or its derivatives in any of them. *See also* FOOD AND DRUG ACT OF 1906

Wiley, Mildred (1935–1991)

In December 1995, a federal hearing examiner in Cleveland, Ohio, awarded death benefits to Philip E. Wiley whose wife, Mildred Wiley, died from lung cancer. It is believed to be the first award of death benefits in the nation for a workplace injury connected to SECONDHAND SMOKE. The government had awarded claims for other ailments linked to secondhand smoke.

A Veterans Administration Hospital nurse in Marion, Ohio, Mildred Wiley died a month after developing lung cancer. Her husband contended that his wife, who worked in the hospital's psychiatric ward for 18 years, was exposed to heavy secondhand smoke. On a third claim's try, Wiley's lawyers produced testimony from DAVID M. BURNS, M.D., a University of San Diego medical professor who evaluated and ruled out all possible alternative causes of the nurse's cancer, including exposure to radon and asbestos.

Mr. Wiley was awarded $1,000 in death and funeral benefits and was entitled to payments of about $21,500, half his wife's annual salary, each year for the rest of his life. Experts in workers' compensation law said the decision would have limited value as a precedent because it was issued under federal workers' compensation law. Anti-smoking advocates, however, believe the ruling was a breakthrough because employers could face claims if they did not ban smoking in the workplace. *See also* ENVIRONMENTAL TOBACCO SMOKE (ETS)

Willard, Frances (1839–1898)

Frances Willard, national director of the WOMEN'S CHRISTIAN TEMPERANCE UNION (WCTU), detested smoking, and believed that her brother's death at 43 was caused by his smoking habit. Although she abhorred tobacco in all its forms, she knew it was impossible to prohibit its use altogether, so she concentrated on battling cigarettes. At her instigation, the WCTU periodically called for the prohibition of CIGARETTE manufacturing, sales, and imports. In her last annual address to the WCTU in 1897, however, she urged the abolition of the entire tobacco industry.

Williams, Jesse (1930–1997)

In the biggest liability verdict ever against the tobacco industry, a judge ordered PHILIP MORRIS COMPANIES INC. to pay $81 million to the family of Jesse Williams who died of lung cancer after smoking MARLBORO CIGARETTES for four decades. The jury, finding Philip Morris liable for negligence and deceit, awarded $1.6 million in conpensatory damages and $79.5 million in punitive damages (later reduced to $32 million). In testimony, Williams, a former janitor with the Portland, Oregon, school system, was described as a three-pack-a day Marlboro smoker who believed the manufacturer wouldn't sell a harmful product and who was heavily addicted to NICOTINE. He died five months after being diagnosed with small-cell carcinoma of the lungs.

In closing arguments, attorneys for the Williams family cited internal Philip Morris documents to bolster their claim that the company long knew about the cancer-causing potential of cigarettes and hid the information from its customers. The documents came from a repository of internal industry documents set up by the settlement of the MINNESOTA MEDICAID CASE.

Philip Morris planned to appeal the verdict on the grounds that Multnomah County Circuit Judge Anna Brown erred in allowing the jury to see evidence that the company contends was inadmissable.

Williams, Merrell (1932–)

A paralegal at the largest law firm in Louisville, Kentucky, Merrell Williams stole BROWN AND WILLIAMSON TOBACCO CORPORATION documents because he believed that the papers revealed a cover-up of the harmful effects of smoking. After Williams turned over the papers to prominent litigation attorneys, the papers were widely disseminated in the public domain. The information contained in the papers prompted decisions by President Bill Clinton and the FOOD AND DRUG ADMINISTRATION to propose regulations regarding NICOTINE as an addictive drug and CIGARETTES and SMOKELESS TOBACCO products as drug delivery devices. Some of the documents were used in the GRADY CARTER lawsuit against Brown and Williamson.

At the end of 1987, Louisiana-born Merrell Williams, in the middle of a second divorce, took pre-law courses at the University of Louisville. He took a paralegal job, starting at $9 an hour, with the law firm of Wyatt, Tarrant, and Combs, the largest law firm in Kentucky. One of Wyatt, Tarrant's most important accounts was Brown and Williamson Tobacco Corporation, maker of Kool, Carlton, and Misty cigarettes. The corporation was the nation's third largest tobacco company and one of the state's largest companies, employing more than 600 in Louisville alone.

Williams worked, along with paralegals from two other law firms, on a project that involved sorting Brown and Williamson archive documents on product promotion and smoking and health going back to the 1950s. There were also memos and letters from other tobacco companies, and many of the documents concerned contacts with Brown and Williamson's London-based parent, BAT INDUSTRIES PLC. The documents were put into categories—those dealing with disease in the "D" category, with those covering addiction in the "DA" pile and those concerning cancer placed under "DD." Documents discuss-

ing ads targeted to minors were coded "ABEG." Williams, who had signed a confidentiality agreement, was warned that the Brown and Williamson memos were secret and must not be shared with anyone outside Wyatt, Tarrant.

While sorting the documents, Williams read them. He learned that the tobacco companies had done research about the effects of nicotine and cancer-causing agents in tobacco smoke, but had not made the research public. He felt he had uncovered a widespread cover-up of the harmful effects of smoking that included the participation of company lawyers. Williams began photocopying and stealing the documents, and for two years carried them out of the building, sometimes hidden in his shirt or old exercise back brace, and on his last day of work in a banker's box. In all, he stole more than 4,000 pages. In February 1992, Williams was told the project at Wyatt, Tarrant was being cut back and his job had ended.

In March 1993, Williams, a Kool smoker since he was 19 years old, underwent major heart surgery. He felt his heart attack was a sign from God that he should use the stolen documents to punish cigarette makers. He turned his bypass surgery into a personal injury lawsuit against Brown and Williamson. He claimed his heart condition had been caused by the stress of reviewing the documents as well as a lifetime of smoking Brown and Williamson cigarettes. His lawyer, Fox DeMoisey, talked him out of filing the suit, saying his case was based on stolen documents that almost certainly would not be admissible as evidence. Williams and his attorney decided to offer the return of the documents to Wyatt, Tarrant in exchange for $2.5 million. The Wyatt firm filed a civil suit in the Circuit Court for Jefferson County, Kentucky, accusing Williams of breaching his confidentiality agreement. Williams sent the stolen documents to a friend in Florida for safekeeping.

It took Williams several months before he could interest someone in the stolen documents. He eventually met with DON BARRETT and RICHARD F. SCRUGGS, both Mississippi attorneys. Scruggs not only got Williams a job in the state, he personally transported the stolen documents in his Lear jet from Florida to a safe place in Mississippi. Soon after, Williams signed over the documents to MICHAEL C. MOORE, attorney general of Mississippi.

On January 7, 1994, Judge Thomas Wine issued an order prohibiting Williams from discussing or disseminating any of the information contained in the documents, modified three months later by the judge so Williams could speak with his attorney about the case. By then, Congress, numerous news media, and STANTON GLANTZ in California had copies of the documents. On May 7, 1994, the *New York Times* published the first report based on thousands of pages of internal company documents stolen by Williams from Wyatt, Tarrant. The University of California at San Francisco made the documents available to the public by putting them on the World Wide Web and on a CD-ROM. Within a year, half-a-million people had visited the Web page. Brown and Williamson subsequently failed in its attempts to suppress the documents. *See also* BROWN AND WILLIAMSON TOBACCO CORPORATION–MERRELL WILLIAMS DOCUMENTS

Wilner, Norwood "Woody" (1948–)

Norwood "Woody" Wilner is a Jacksonville, Florida, trial attorney who in 1996 represented GRADY CARTER and defeated BROWN AND WILLIAMSON TOBACCO CORPORATION in court. The tobacco company was ordered to pay Carter $750,000 in damages; this was the second time a tobacco company was ordered to pay a smoker. The verdict was overturned on appeal.

Wilner was born in Miami, Florida, and graduated from Yale with a degree in physics. He then graduated from the University of Florida law school, and became a partner in a small eight-lawyer firm. Wilner defended asbestos companies for nearly 20 years, but became interested in tobacco companies when he and his experts in pulmonary disease and pathology began to suspect that alleged asbestos injuries were really more closely linked to smoking. He needed clients, so in 1995 he ran advertisements in newspapers across Florida that read: "Do you have a cigarette or other product-related illness or injury?" He built an inventory of more than 200 individual cases, involving different tobacco companies; Grady Carter's was one of them.

Although Brown and Williamson attorneys fought to keep their documents sealed, arguing they were illegally obtained, Wilner won the court's approval to use documents stolen from Brown and Williamson's files by MERRELL WILLIAMS. This was the first time the Williams documents were used as evidence. Wilner produced 21 documents that showed tobacco companies' top executives were aware that cigarettes were addictive and harmful and chose to bury the research.

At the trial, Wilner preempted the tobacco company's assumption of risk defense by admitting that the smoker shared responsibility. After that admission, Wilner focused on the company's liability. Under Florida state law, the manufacturer, not the consumer, is required to possess expert knowledge of its products and to warn consumers of the hazards. Wilner blamed the company for failing to warn Carter of the hazards of smoking before warning labels went on cigarette packs in 1966. The lawyer asked for $1.5 million in compensatory damages and no punitive damages.

The tobacco company's counsel claimed there was no scientific evidence that smoking causes cancer; said that the company did not know the dangers in the 1950s when Carter started to smoke; and provided no explanation of the Merrell Williams documents that showed the company did know prior to 1966 that NICOTINE was addictive and that tobacco smoke contained carcinogens.

On August 9, 1996, six jurors found the tobacco company negligent in selling Grady Carter an "unreasonably dangerous and defective product" and they awarded Carter and his wife $750,000 in damages. In June 1998, however, a Florida appeals court struck down the jury verdict.

In 1997, Wilner represented JEAN CONNOR, who had contracted lung cancer. After her death, Connor's wrongful death civil suit was continued by her three adult children and her sister. During a trial in Jacksonville, Florida, in May 1997, the jury found R.J. Reynolds not responsible for the lung cancer death of Connor.

In 1997, Wilner represented JOANN KARBIWNYK who also had lung cancer, but was in remission. The jury again ruled in favor of R.J. REYNOLDS TOBACCO COMPANY, a second defeat in a row for Wilner.

In 1998, Wilner represented the family of ROLAND MADDOX, who died of lung cancer in May 1997. A state court jury ordered Brown and Williamson to pay both compensatory and punitive damages, the first time a jury intended to punish a tobacco company in a traditional lawsuit.

Like the Grady Carter trial, Wilner showed the *Maddox* jury industry documents pulled off the Internet that indicated the tobacco companies suppressed research on the dangers of smoking. Wilner, as head of the 40-member Tobacco Trial Lawyers Association, tries to help other lawyers prepare cases against tobacco companies. The network of lawyers shares information, exchanges documents, and streamlines tactics in lawsuits against cigarette makers. *See also* BROWN AND WILLIAMSON TOBACCO CORPORATION—MERRELL WILLIAMS DOCUMENTS; CIPOLLONE, ROSE; HOROWITZ, MILTON

Winston-Salem, North Carolina

One of the largest cities built by the tobacco industry, Winston-Salem, North Carolina, is home to R. J. REYNOLDS TOBACCO COMPANY. The company was founded in 1875 in Winston by RICHARD JOSHUA REYNOLDS. In 1918, when Reynolds died, the company employed 10,000 people in 121 buildings in Winston-Salem. Today Reynolds Tobacco has about 9,000 employees who work in two modern facilities, one in Winston-Salem, the other near it.

Women, United States

During antebellum days, women smoked pipes or chewed just as the men did. Mrs. Andrew Jackson and Mrs. Zachary Taylor smoked pipes while they lived in the White House. But by the middle of the nineteenth century, women's pipes became outdated as a romanticized image of women as dainty flowers became fashionable.

In the middle of the nineteenth century, when European women barely smoked in private, Latin American women lit up after dinner in public. An English traveler in the 1850s noted: "Every gentleman carries in his pocket a silver case, with a long string of cotton, steel, and flint, and one of the offices of gallantry is to strike a light; by doing it well, he may kindle a flame in a lady's heart" (Sobel, 1978).

The popularity of cigarettes and their identification with women was evidenced in Prosper Mérimée's novel, which was the basis for George Bizet's opera CARMEN. The heroine of the opera worked in a cigarette factory in SEVILLE, SPAIN, around 1820.

By the early 1850s, upper-class women in large eastern cities like New York smoked Turkish and Russian brands of cigarettes, but they usually did so in the privacy of their homes.

Before WORLD WAR I, females of dubious reputation smoked, not respectable women. During the early 1920s, it would have been shocking to show women in cigarette ads. At this time, it was only acceptable for women to smoke at home. If they did it in public, they were perceived as disreputable or worse. Once people got used to seeing more women smoking in public, however, ad agencies took advantage of women's new attitudes. By the second half of the 1920s, women in cigarette ads became more acceptable.

Tobacco advertisers especially recognized women's new independence as a boon to their business, so they devised ways to lure women into smoking their brands. In a 1926 CHESTERFIELD CIGARETTES ad, a woman asked her date who is smoking to "Blow some my way." Although a storm of protest greeted the ad, other tobacco companies followed suit. In

1927, MARLBORO CIGARETTES ads showed a woman's hand in silhouette holding a lit cigarette. Marlboro even had a red "fashion" tip designed to blend in with the smoker's lipstick. In 1927, CAMEL CIGARETTES put women into their ads, but didn't show them actually smoking until 1933.

Even more ads were aimed at women in the 1930s. Ads began to appear in middle-class women's magazines such as *McCalls, Ladies Home Journal,* and *Better Homes and Gardens.* Images showed wealthy-looking American women, opera stars, and athletic-looking women promoting cigarette brands. During the 1930s, Camels pictured all kinds of women in ads: college "girls," housewives, business "girls," and secretaries. Amelia Earhart, the famous airplane pilot promoted LUCKY STRIKE CIGARETTES, as did famous actress Carole Lombard who said she almost quit smoking but "her singing coach advised a light cigarette" (Stop Teenage Addition to Tobacco, n.d.). Another Lucky ad showed a prominent-looking woman in evening clothes. Although she was not smoking, she said, "I prefer Luckies and so do my daughters."

During WORLD WAR II, the government suggested it was the patriotic duty of women to leave home. About 350,000 women went into the Women's Army Corps and women's branch of the navy. Thousands of women joined assembly lines to replace the men who were overseas fighting in the war and took jobs in heavy industry working as welders, riveters, and crane operators, jobs once held by men. Tobacco companies, recognizing that women in industry were potential customers, bombarded women with advertising in *Better Homes and Gardens* and other women's magazines. Ads showing women as role models hard at work in the national effort were designed to suggest they could smoke, do a man's job, and still be totally feminine. Camel ran a series of ads picturing and naming women who worked in war industries. In one ad, a female war worker explained that she had a new war job so her cigarette had to be extra mild. Mora Schell, a war worker, said she smoked "the fighting man's favorite—Camels" and Dorothy

Canavor, a war plant worker, said "like the men in the service, *my* cigarette is Camel." Ads showed Inez Dale Myers, a naval ship-yard worker, Beatrice Cole, a draftswoman for navy ship designers, and Anne Basa, an inspector of navy binoculars all praising Camels.

Chesterfields went after feminine war workers in their "Workers in the War Effort" campaign. One window display showed a smiling female war worker with a cigarette hanging from her lips; she was dressed in blue dungarees and her helmet was tilted backwards. An open pack of Chesterfields partially appeared in her dungarees, and a banner crossing her body proclaimed "For My Taste It's Chesterfield." By the second half of the 1940s, tobacco companies portrayed women as wives and sweethearts waiting for returning husbands and boyfriends while they smoked.

For decades, the cigarette companies did everything they could to attract women to their brands. They hired female celebrities, opera stars, athletes, and young sophisticated models to appear in ads to try to entice women to buy cigarettes. In 1968, PHILIP MORRIS USA introduced VIRGINIA SLIMS, a cigarette strictly for women. Tobacco companies like Philip Morris knew the time was right for them to target women. In the early 1970s, a survey noted that in a two-year period, the number of college students who felt that women were oppressed had doubled. The Virginia Slims slogan, "You've come a long way, Baby," appealed to women who wanted to be independent. One of the obvious ways to assert independence was to smoke. Since the 1920s, women had thought of cigarettes as torches of freedom.

Virginia Slims prompted an explosion of feminine cigarettes. Soon Eve, Capri, Misty, and other brands were competing with Virginia Slims. Brand names associated cigarettes with thinness. SuperSlims, Newport Stripes, and Misty 120's (120 pounds was considered by some to be the ideal weight for women) were manufactured long and thin. Tobacco companies gave packages and filter bands attractive designs. They even manufactured cigarettes with different-colored papers so they matched smokers' outfits. Feminine cigarettes became fashion statements.

The greatest growth of tobacco advertising aimed at women followed the introduction of Virginia Slims. During the 1970s and 1980s, cigarette advertising flooded women's magazines, newspapers, and Sunday supplements. By 1979, cigarettes were the most advertised product in some women's magazines, with as many as 20 ads in a single issue, and equaled the ads targeted to men.

In addition to advertising, coupon offers for discounts or free packs appeared in magazines and newspapers. The MORE cigarette brand was promoted by sponsorship of fashion shows in 18 shopping centers throughout the United States. Tobacco companies offered women's clothing and calendars in exchange for money and proof of cigarette purchase. Philip Morris sponsored professional women's tennis.

After cigarette companies aimed ads and promotions at women, the numbers of women smoking grew at a faster rate; the ads also influenced girls. Fewer than 8 percent of teenage girls smoked before Virginia Slims was introduced in 1968. Six years later, that figure was almost 15 percent. In 1979, surveys showed more girls smoked than boys.

The tobacco industry has been seen as a financial benefactor of the women's movement. In response to a survey published by the DEPARTMENT OF HEALTH AND HUMAN SERVICES in 1987, 13 women's organizations reported accepting donations from tobacco interests exceeding $318,000. The National Women's Political Caucus, recipient of significant tobacco money, honored Philip Morris vice president George Knox at its 1989 Good Guys Award Dinner.

The tobacco industry has admitted that it targeted women. The headline "Women Top Cig Target" appeared in a 1981 issue of *Advertising Age*. The chief operating officer of R.J. REYNOLDS TOBACCO COMPANY described the women's market as "probably the largest opportunity for the company" (Ernster, 1985). The article quoted other people who viewed the stressed-out working woman as the ideal candidate for cigarettes.

Although CIGAR smoking is predominantly a male behavior, in the 1990s, women began to smoke cigars. Cigar smoking by women has been one of the themes of cigar advertising and promotional efforts. Celebrity women and their cigars have frequently been featured on the covers and insides of cigar magazines like *Cigar Aficionado*. Newspapers, popular news magazines, and television programs have highlighted cigar smoking by women as a new trend. These activities have increased the visibility of cigar use by women.

The prevalence of smoking by women in the 1990s serves as testimony to the success of targeted tobacco advertising. Women younger than 25 years now smoke more than men.

References: Virginia L. Ernster, "Mixed Messages for Women: A Social History of Cigarette Smoking and Advertising," *New York State Journal of Medicine*, July 1985, p. 337.

Robert Sobel, *They Satisfy: The Cigarette in American Life*, Garden City: Doubleday, 1978, p. 9.

Stop Teenage Addiction to Tobacco, "Overview," to Slide Tape about cigarette Advertisements, n.d. p. 7.

Women and Girls against Tobacco (WAGAT)

Women and Girls against Tobacco (WAGAT), headquartered in Berkeley, California, was created to counteract tobacco messages that target women and girls. WAGAT's "Fact Sheet on Women and Smoking" reports that women's magazines that rely heavily on tobacco ads carry virtually no articles about the health hazards of smoking. WAGAT also points out that the tobacco industry gives generous donations to the general funds, programs, annual meetings, and research projects of women's political and leadership organizations like League of Women Voters and the American Association of University Women. Studies show groups with tobacco money rarely speak out about the dangers of women smoking, and sometimes they defend the rights of tobacco companies.

For a long time, PHILIP MORRIS COMPANIES INC. supported women's tennis through the VIRGINIA SLIMS Tennis Tournament. After the sponsorship ended, the Women's Tennis Association started a new tour called the Legends Tour, also sponsored by Philip Morris. According to WAGAT, many of the women who made their fame and fortunes from women's tennis have been reluctant to take a public stand against tobacco companies or issues.

WAGAT aims to help women's and girls' organizations get rid of tobacco industry funding and eliminate tobacco advertising in leading magazines with young readers. In 1993, the National Foundation for Women Business Owners rejected a donation from Philip Morris. A letter returning Philip Morris's check said: "[A] resolution of our Board . . . prevents the Foundation from accepting contributions from tobacco companies." *See also* WOMEN, UNITED STATES

References: "Thumbs Up/Thumbs Down." *ANR Update*, vol. 12, no. 1 (Spring 1993), p. 5.

Women's Christian Temperance Union (WCTU)

In 1874, the Women's Christian Temperance Union (WCTU) was founded; it was the largest women's organization in the United States in the late nineteenth and early twentieth centuries. Women, in general, were horrified when they saw young children hauling home pails of beer for their families, and the WCTU made it a priority to wage war on saloons and drinking (and still battles substance abuse today).

Women became equally upset when they saw children smoking, so they added tobacco to their agenda. The WCTU believed that "Smoking leads to drinking and drinking leads to the devil." The organization created a Department for the Overthrow of the Tobacco Habit in 1883, but replaced it with a Department of Narcotics in 1885. Although the department was concerned about other drugs, it devoted most of its resources to the anti-cigarette battle. The WCTU periodically called for the prohibition of cigarette manufacturing, sales, and imports. Before 1898, it approved six resolutions calling for the prohibition of CIGARETTES.

For the most part, the WCTU did not battle other forms of tobacco. At its Victory Convention in November 1919 in St. Louis (celebrating the passage by Congress of the Nineteenth Amendment giving women the right to vote), the group voted to fight against tobacco, but preferred using a general education program as its weapon. The women refused to vote for a resolution supporting legislation that banned smoking. *See also* WILLARD, FRANCES

World Boomerang Throwing Cup

In May 1988, the U.S. boomerang team won the World Boomerang Throwing Cup competition in Barooga, New South Wales, Australia. The event marked the first time an American health organization called DOCTORS OUGHT TO CARE (DOC), AMERICANS FOR NON-SMOKERS' RIGHTS, and individual donations sponsored a national sports team. Initially, the team considered but then rejected the offer of PHILIP MORRIS COMPANIES INC. for a $15,000 sponsorship. The team would have been required to wear Philip Morris magazine uniforms and pose for photos with a Philip Morris logo.

World Health Organization (WHO)

The World Health Organization (WHO) is an intergovernmental organization and specialized agency of the United Nations, headquartered in Geneva, Switzerland, with six regional offices. It is the directing and coordinating authority on international health work. In reaction to the argument that tobacco is responsible for millions of deaths a year, it created in January 1990 a global program on "tobacco or health."

One of the program's goals is to develop effective comprehensive national tobacco control programs in WHO member states, and to enforce policies adopted collectively by these member states at the World Health Assembly. The program also wishes to further collectively devise strategies, principles, and programs to make the policies effective. The activities of the Tobacco or Health program take place in member states, supported by WHO regional offices and headquarters.

The program addresses not only the medical, epidemiological, and statistical information but also the legal, sociological, and economic aspects of tobacco or health issues, such as pricing and advertising. Topics such as women and tobacco; children and smoking; the role of health services against tobacco; and the position of the media, sports, and the arts, have received special attention.

To promote the concept of tobacco-free societies and to establish the non-use of tobacco as normal social behavior, the Tobacco or Health program has developed promotional, public information, and educational activities in the following areas:

- Collaboration with governments, specialized non-governmental organizations, and organizations of the United Nations system to promote tobacco-free lifestyles to create a positive social norm and to obtain commitment to action.
- Preparation and dissemination of information and educational material to convince governments, the population at large, and relevant target groups— such as the health and teaching professions, politicians, decision makers, and youth—of the extent and seriousness of the tobacco problem and of the need to act. This effort includes furthering knowledge about SMOKING CESSATION.
- Coordination of the annual WORLD NO-TOBACCO DAY on May 31 and of other major public and media events; production of material for and communication with the media; publication of the international quarterly tobacco or health newsletter, *Tobacco Alert*, which will be used to make WHO policies and activities in the tobacco control field better known worldwide.

WHO has tried to move the tobacco and health agenda towards the problem of developing countries to help them prevent the catastrophic health, social, and economic consequences of tobacco consumption. WHO has been asked to support countries that depend on tobacco to sustain their often feeble economies and their health development. To resolve the socio-economic and health dilemmas surrounding tobacco production and consumption in these countries, WHO has mobilized United Nations agencies such as the Food and Agriculture Organization (FAO), General Agreement on Tariffs and Trade (GATT), and International Labor Organization (ILO).

Since 1967, WHO has published the proceedings of World Conferences on Smoking and Health as well as the reports of the World Health Organization.

For many years, WHO has taken a firm stand on smoking and health, and produced three major reports with strong recommendations to member governments for smoking controls. It took years before the reports focused on women and smoking. In the first, in 1971, two eminent anti-smoking campaigners expressed no thoughts about women. The second, in 1975, was compiled by a committee of nine men, and dealt with smoking mothers and harm to children. At the first World Conference on Smoking in 1967, the specific problems of female smokers was not raised at all. The third World Conference was held in 1976, and there was a sub-section entitled "women and cigarettes." In June 1979, at the fourth gathering of international anti-smoking experts, 10 of the 60 major speakers were women. *See also* GLOBAL TOBACCO USE; INTERNATIONAL UNION AGAINST CANCER (UICC)

World No-Tobacco Day

On May 31, 1988, the WORLD HEALTH ORGANIZATION (WHO) sponsored the first World No-Tobacco Day with the objective of encouraging people worldwide who smoke or chew tobacco to quit for at least 24 hours. Today, World No-Tobacco Day is an international event held on May 31 of each year to discourage tobacco users from consuming tobacco. Besides encouraging all persons who use tobacco to quit for at least 24 hours, the event organizers want governments, communities, groups, and individuals to become aware of the tobacco problem and do something about it. The day is a growing global observance, and diverse celebrations take place around the world on an individual, municipal, provincial, or national basis.

WHO sees World No-Tobacco Day as an opportunity to ask people not only to stop smoking for one day but also to initiate research on specific themes, publish information, and initiate action. In the past, themes for World No-Tobacco Day have been:

- 1989— Women and Tobacco
- 1990—Childhood and Young People and Tobacco
- 1991— Public Places and Transport
- 1992—Tobacco-Free Workplaces
- 1993—Role of Health Services
- 1994—The Media against Tobacco
- 1995—The Economics of Tobacco Control
- 1996—Sports and the Arts without Tobacco
- 1997—The United Nations and Specialized Agencies against Tobacco
- 1998—Growing Up without Tobacco.

See also GREAT AMERICAN SMOKEOUT; NATIONAL CENTER FOR TOBACCO-FREE KIDS

World War I

Once the U.S. entered World War I in 1917, efforts began to provide cigarettes to soldiers. General John J. Pershing, commanding the American Expeditionary Force, made his requirements clear: "You ask me what we need to win the war. I answer tobacco as much as bullets" (Heimann, 1960). Past military experience had indicated the value of tobacco to morale.

The use of cigarettes by servicemen was sanctioned by official edict; Congress included cigarettes in the rations issued to soldiers overseas. When deciding which cigarettes to provide to soldiers, the government awarded contracts to cigarette manufacturers based on their pre-war sales at home. Since CAMEL CIGARETTES were the best-selling cigarette at the time, most soldiers smoked that brand. The ration consisted of a choice of four manufactured cigarettes daily or enough smoking tobacco to roll 10 cigarettes, or four-tenths of an ounce of CHEWING TOBACCO. CIGARS and PIPES were not offered as rations because they were difficult to transport.

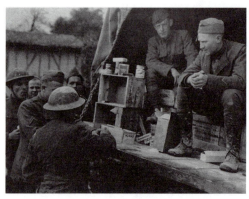

American soldiers during World War I smoking in the back of a truck. *Library of Congress.*

Congress subsidized the sale of cigarettes at military post exchange stores at home and abroad. The War Industries Board encouraged production by designating cigarette manufacturing as an essential industry, giving it access to raw materials, fuel, and transportation networks, and protecting it from any labor disputes.

The U.S. government became the single greatest tobacco buyer in the world. It shipped an average of 425 million cigarettes a month to FRANCE alone, along with a greater quantity of loose tobacco for hand-rolled cigarettes. During the last nine months of the war, the entire production of BULL DURHAM SMOKING TOBACCO was consigned to the Subsistence Division of the War Department. Altogether the government sent about 5.5 billion manufactured cigarettes overseas, along with enough tobacco to roll another 11 billion. It also bought 200 million cigars. Of nearly $80 million in federal spending on tobacco products between April 7, 1917, and May 1, 1919, more than 80 percent was used to buy cigarettes and cigarette tobacco.

The public supported cigarettes for soldiers as well. The campaign to provide "smokes for soldiers" began shortly after the first American troops reached France. It was precipitated by newspaper stories with headlines such as "Our Army in France Is Short of Tobacco." Newspapers, business groups, women's clubs, and many other civic organizations, including some that had been involved in the anti-smoking movement before the war, established funds to augment government supplies. The Red Cross gave away more than one billion cigarettes, which it purchased directly from manufacturers. Even the YMCA and Salvation Army, at one time hostile to cigarettes, shipped free packs to soldiers. Collection boxes for tobacco funds were placed in department stores, hotels, theaters, and restaurants.

During World War I, cigarette sales increased while cigar, plug, and pipe sales declined. American newspapers pictured English, French, German, and Russian soldiers smoking cigarettes. News photos showed the kaiser lighting up as well as French and Belgian politicians handing out packs of cigarettes to men on the front lines.

After a news story reported that some Belgians appealed to their minister of war "Give us worse food if you like, but let us have tobacco," Americans started the Belgian Soldiers' Tobacco Fund. It raised money for cigarettes that were distributed free to soldiers in that army. In other countries, civilian groups organized cigarette funds that sent tons of cigarettes to allied soldiers. Governments even waived tax and import restrictions so soldiers could have as many cigarettes as they wished.

The distribution of free smokes to servicemen ended after the armistice. Soldiers then had to pay for their cigarettes, and they did.

Despite the concerns of anti-cigarette crusaders who objected on moral, legal, and health grounds, cigarettes were viewed as narcotics that soothed the nerves and deadened the loneliness of men in the trenches. As one Lynn, Massachusetts, *Evening Post* reporter put it: "Whatever may be the effect under normal conditions of living, they [cigarettes] help soldiers at the front endure the strain. All anti-cigarette crusades must rec-ognize this fact and be governed accordingly" (Heimann, 1960). During the war, when outdoor smoking became more acceptable, more women appeared in public as well with cigarettes in their hands. *See also* CONFEDERATE GOVERNMENT

References: Robert K. Heimann, *Tobacco and Americans*, New York: McGraw-Hill Book Company, Inc., 1960, p. 227.

World War II

Tobacco companies encouraged World War II GIs to take up the smoking habit. One way they did this was to provide a constant flow of free cigarettes. "Smokes" were added to army K-rations (balanced rations for troops in the field and named after Dr. Ancel Keys, leader of the team that created them). Breakfast consisted of enriched biscuits, compressed graham crackers, veal luncheon meat, a fruit bar, soluble coffee, sugar, chewing gum, and four cigarettes. Lunch was much the same. Supper included biscuits, cheese, fruit-juice powder, a chocolate bar, sugar, chewing gum, and four more cigarettes. (It was not until 1975 that cigarettes were discontinued in K-rations of soldiers and sailors.)

Tobacco companies not only sent free cartons of cigarettes to soldiers overseas, they encouraged the public to send them as a show of love and support. Radio broadcasters and newspapers around the country encouraged people to support "Smokes for Yanks," so did churches, labor unions, and the Red Cross.

Several tobacco manufacturers stepped up operations so they could increase shipments of cigarettes to military forces in war zones. Cigarette production increased by almost 50 percent from 1941 to 1945. During those years, about 20 percent of the cigarettes produced in the United States were shipped to soldiers overseas, creating a shortage in the United States that forced customers to line up and wait their turn to buy cigarettes at stores. About the time World War II started, a survey showed 48 percent of men and 36 percent of women were smoking.

The distribution of free cigarettes during the war contributed to the massive growth of the smoking habit, but so did advertising campaigns. According to a survey, Americans listened to radios an average of four and a half hours a day during the war. Tobacco advertisers injected their messages directly into radio programs. In the fall of 1942, millions of Americans heard a radio broadcaster announce "Lucky Strike Green—(pause for a trumpet blast and a drum roll)—Has Gone to War!" CAMEL CIGARETTES ran a "Thanks to Yanks" radio campaign. Contestants who answered game show questions correctly could send 2,000 Camels to the serviceman of their choice. If game contestants could not answer a question correctly, 2,000 cigarettes went into the "Thanks to Yanks" duffle bag. By January 1943, 29,250 packs of Camels had been shipped to servicemen free of charge.

Tobacco companies created ad campaigns that linked smoking, war, and patriotism. At first, cigarette manufacturers showed men in service uniforms using cigarettes. Then Camel ads showed men in action—in torpedo rooms in submarines, breaking through barbed wire, and lugging anti-tank guns. CHESTERFIELD CIGARETTES had a "Workers in the War Effort" campaign. PALL MALL CIGARETTES used military themes and Raleigh offered cheap prices on gift cigarettes sent to soldiers overseas. Twenty-five dollars purchased a case of 10,000 cigarettes. BROWN AND WILLIAMSON TOBACCO CORPORATION offered to donate another case of Raleigh with each order of 10 cases or more.

Many young soldiers and women who began to smoke in the service during both World Wars kept up the habit in civilian life. *See also* LUCKY STRIKE CIGARETTES; RADIO AND CIGARETTE ADVERTISING; U.S. ARMY; WORLD WAR I

Worldwide Tobacco Use. *See* GLOBAL TOBACCO USE

Wynder, Ernst L. (1922–1999)

Dr. Ernst L. Wynder maintained his belief that there was a link between smoking and lung cancer, and his persistence led to a landmark research study with EVARTS A. GRAHAM. Dr. Wynder, the son of a German-born physician who fled Nazi persecution and settled his family in New Jersey, graduated from New York University (NYU) in 1943 and then served in the U.S. Army intelligence section. As a medical student at Washington University in St. Louis, Missouri, Wynder displayed great intelligence. During a summer internship at NYU after two years of medical school, he attended an autopsy of a lung cancer victim. After he learned from the widow that her husband had smoked two packs of cigarettes a day, he began to suspect that the relationship between smoking and lung cancer had been underestimated because of the absence of that information in the autopsy report.

Wynder approached the head of Bellevue Hospital's chest service and got permission to conduct in-depth interviews with people stricken with lung cancer. His questionnaire not only aimed to find out about the patient's smoking history, but also other possible related factors such as occupational exposures and the cause of parents' deaths.

After Wynder returned to medical school, he approached and received permission from famed thoracic surgeon Dr. Evarts A. Graham, head of the chest service at Barnes Hospital (closely affiliated with Washington University Medical School), to continue data gathering with Graham's patients. During his last two years of medical school, Wynder also collected data from separate sites whenever possible. He was given access to state hospital patients in California by Dr. Lester Breslow. It was reported by one of Breslow's assistants that his "questioning was crude and the record-keeping inconsistent" (Kluger, 1996). Nevertheless, Breslow ordered his department to undertake an investigation into the smoking-cancer link and the findings were almost identical to Wynder's and Graham's.

In 1950, Dr. Wynder and Dr. Graham (who placed his name as second author) published an influential scientific study in the *Journal of the American Medical Association (JAMA)* titled "Tobacco Smoking as a Possible Etiological Factor in Bronchiogenic Carcinoma: A Study of 684 Proved Cases." The study showed that smokers had a greater risk of lung cancer than did nonsmokers. This article is now regarded as a classic in epidemiology due to the size and geographic spread of its sample. The data were collected from personal interviews, not hospital records or other secondhand sources, and the doctors broke down their subjects into five clear categories of smoking—ranging from none to chain smoking. Among its chief findings were that 96.5 percent of the lung cancer patients interviewed were moderately heavy to chain smokers, that almost all those with lung cancer had smoked for 20 or more years, and that 98.7 percent of the cigarette smokers inhaled. There were no nonsmokers among the lung cancer patients. Only 14 percent of the non-cancer hospital patients covered in the study were nonsmokers.

In 1953, the doctors published another article in *Cancer Research* ("Experimental Production of Carcinoma with Cigarette Tar") showing that mice who had cigarette TAR painted on their backs were more likely to develop malignant tumors than control mice that were not painted with tobacco tar. (The mouse skin painting model became the cigarette industry's standard for assessing the carcinogenicity of cigarette smoke condensate.) The results were widely published in newspapers and magazines.

In 1957, Wynder testified before Congress that cigarette filters did not remove toxins to any greater degree than they removed harmless smoke components. He also criticized some cigarette manufacturers for blending tobaccos in their filter cigarette brands so that they produced smoke with higher levels of tar than came from the non-filtered brands of the same manufacturer. Dr. Wynder wrote or contributed to more than 700 papers and received many honors in the United States and in Europe. *See also* DOLL, RICHARD AND HILL, A. BRADFORD; FILTERED CIGARETTES; LARTIGUE, FRANK

References: Richard Kluger, *Ashes to Ashes*, New York: Alfred A. Knopf, 1996, p. 136.

X Cigarettes

In February 1995, X brand cigarettes were introduced to the Boston marketplace (and in at least 19 other states). The black box, with a large white X surrounded by a red square and the word "Menthol" spelled out in green letters (a color combination rarely used in American culture), outraged tobacco control advocates in Boston's African-American community. They felt the X was reminiscent of the X used in Spike Lee's movie on Malcolm X. Along with other concerned citizens throughout the nation, they demanded that production and distribution of X cigarettes be stopped. Within a month, X cigarettes were removed from store shelves. The distributor denied the cigarettes had anything to do with Malcolm X or that the brand targeted African-Americans.

Xanthi Tobacco

One of the ORIENTAL TOBACCOS deemed by some to be the finest of the Turkish blends used in PIPE tobacco, Xanthi is grown around the city of Xanthi, in eastern Greece. The tiny tissue thin leaves add flaver to English-Scottish pipe tobacco mixtures.

Y

Ybor City, Florida

A section of Tampa, Florida, Ybor City owes its origins to Vicente Martinez Ybor, who immigrated to CUBA in 1832 when he was 14 years old. In 1853, he started his own CIGAR factory in HAVANA, but labor problems, the high tariff on Cuban cigars, and the start of the Cuban Revolution in 1868 forced Ybor to move his plant and workers to KEY WEST, FLORIDA.

Labor problems, the lack of a fresh water supply, and no transportation system for distributing the cigars led Ybor to move his operation to Tampa. Two men helped in this decision. Gavino Gutierrez went from Spain to the United States in 1868. Although he settled in NEW YORK CITY, he traveled often to Cuba, Key West, and Tampa in search of exotic fruits. During a visit to Key West in 1884, he convinced Ybor and Ignacio Haya, a cigar owner from New York who was visiting Ybor, to travel to Tampa to investigate its potential for cigar manufacturing. Besides fresh water and a warm, humid climate, Tampa had a rail line that connected it to major transcontinental railroads. In addition, it had an improved shipping port that would make it easier to import tobacco from Cuba as well as to distribute the finished products. In 1885, both Ybor and Haya decided to build cigar factories in the area. Ybor constructed a three-story factory two miles northeast of Tampa in 1886. The area, known as Ybor City, became part of Tampa in 1887.

Ybor City, which grew to become the center of worldwide cigar production, became home to diverse groups of people for whom English was a second language. Cubans made up the largest group, followed by Spaniards, who came in large numbers after 1890. These two groups dominated the cigar industry and set the cultural tone for the community. Most cigar workers in Ybor City lived in houses that were built and owned by factory owners.

The men and women of Ybor City who made hand-rolled cigars earned good wages for the times. They were paid by the number of cigars they turned out each day rather than by the hour. Workers called "strippers" would select and strip from the tobacco plant the leaves that were carried to the cigar makers. Those workers had two tools, a blade (a thin, wedge-shaped steel knife) and a wood board.

After the cigar was rolled and sealed with a dab of gum tragacanth, the sap of a tree grown in Iran, the cigar was ready for storage for up to three years. Workers, called pickers, sorted the finished cigars according to size, color, and shade to ensure all cigars in a box would look roughly the same. Packers than placed a paper ring on each cigar and put them in boxes that were ready to be shipped.

While the cigar rollers worked, a reader sat on a platform above the workers and read aloud from several daily newspapers, Spanish poets, and the works of Miguel de

Cervantes Saavedra—the author of plays and novels, including *Don Quixote*. The readers, well-paid and talented, used different voices to indicate different characters in the poems and novels they read. Cigar makers were permitted to smoke while they worked.

After work hours, most cigar workers took advantage of Ybor City's Spanish, Italian, or German mutual aid societies. These social and cultural organizations were founded by different ethnic groups to help members hold on to their cultural traditions as well as adapt to a new land. These societies provided more than entertainment. For a small fee collected weekly from members, they contracted with doctors and hospitals to provide care for their members, with patients paying no extra charge. The societies also ran pharmacies and burial services for members.

Ybor City became a manufacturing center of quality cigars, eventually out-producing Havana. Both Ybor and Haya offered plant sites to lure other cigar factory owners away from Cuba and Key West. By 1900, Tampa's Ybor City had become known as the "Cigar Capital of the World." Through the 1920s and 1930s, the city grew, but several factors caused Ybor's decline. The growing popularity of CIGARETTES, the Great Depression, and improved machinery for rolling cigars produced a product that rivaled the workmanship of the hand-rolled variety. Large factories either mechanized or went out of business. As machines replaced people, many of Ybor City's residents moved elsewhere in Tampa to find work.

In the 1960s, Ybor City was split apart by an urban renewal project. Seventy acres of the old city were leveled to make way for an interstate highway. But a number of civic organizations banded together and preserved what was left of the city's historic building and ethnic heritage. Today, Ybor City is a National Historic Landmark District.

Y-1 Tobacco

The BROWN AND WILLIAMSON TOBACCO CORPORATION embarked on a project in the 1980s as part of a strategy to develop a low-TAR cigarette that would have high levels of NICOTINE.

It hired DNA Plant Technology Corporation (DNAP) of Oakland, California, which created a genetically engineered tobacco plant, code-named Y-1. It had nicotine levels twice as high as that in regular tobacco leaf and low tar.

In 1993, Brown and Williamson used the Brazilian grown Y-1 in five brands of American cigarettes: Viceroy King Size, Viceroy Lights King Size, Richland King Size, Richmond Lights King Size, and Raleigh Lights King Size.

In 1994, FOOD AND DRUG ADMINISTRATION (FDA) investigators learned from an anonymous phone tip that Brown and Williamson had created Y-1. Through an investigation of patent documents and shipping records, the FDA found U.S. Customs Service invoices showing that Y-1 tobacco was shipped to Brown and Williamson in 1992. The tobacco company, which stopped using Y-1 in 1994 because of FDA concerns, said that the higher-potency tobacco was one of a variety of tobaccos blended into the unique recipes of each brand. It said that products using Y-1 had the same or lower nicotine content as regular CIGARETTES.

In January 1997, the Justice Department brought the first criminal action in its investigation of the tobacco industry, accusing DNAP of conspiring with Brown and Williamson to produce Y-1 tobacco. In the court papers, the government charged that the aim of the conspiracy was to provide Brown and Williamson with a reliable source of high-nicotine tobacco that it would use to manipulate cigarettes' nicotine strength. The court also charged that DNAP and Brown and Williamson secretly devised a scheme to improve high-nicotine tobacco in BRAZIL and other countries because federal regulations ban commercial growing of high-nicotine tobacco in the United States. The government also charged DNAP with hiding information about shipping the genetically altered seeds, breaking a law that prohibited the export of any tobacco seeds without a permit. In September 1998, DNAP was fined $100,000 by U.S. District Court Judge Norma Holloway Johnson for illegally exporting the seeds. *See also* VICEROY CIGARETTES

Z

Zyban

Zyban is a smoking-cessation prescription product that was released in July 1997. It eases withdrawal symptoms by acting on the same brain receptors affected by NICOTINE. What makes Zyban different from other prescription and nonprescription products is that it contains no nicotine. Containing the same chemical as the antidepressant Wellbutrin, Zyban aims to reduce the cravings, anxieties, and depression associated with nicotine withdrawal. One of its advantages is that smokers can safely smoke during the one or two weeks it takes the drug to become effective. Smoking can be dangerous while using a nicotine patch, gum, or nasal spray. *See also* NICOTINE REPLACEMENT PRODUCTS; SMOKING CESSATION

APPENDIX 1

Contributed Essays

Women, Tobacco, and Health
Michele H. Bloch, M.D., Ph.D.

Smoking and Women's Health

In the twentieth century, tobacco use has become the single largest cause of preventable, premature death among women. Of the more than 440,000 deaths attributed annually to tobacco in the United States, about one-third occur in women. Women who smoke die of lung and other cancers, ischemic heart disease, respiratory diseases, and other causes. Lung cancer among women, which increased by more than 550 percent between 1950 and 1991, surpassed breast cancer as the leading cancer killer of women in 1986. In addition, women incur additional risks from smoking, including a greater risk of cervical cancer, osteoporosis, early menopause, and infertility.

Half of all women (and men) who smoke can expect to die from tobacco-related illness. Of those who die, half will die in old age (70 years or older), losing 5 to 10 years of normal life expectancy, while half will die in middle age (35–69 years of age), losing 20 to 25 years of normal life expectancy.

Many women of reproductive age smoke. Smoking during pregnancy jeopardizes the life and health of the developing child. Tobacco use—the most significant preventable cause of poor pregnancy outcome—is a cause of low birth weight, decreased mean birth weight, placental abnormalities, premature delivery, spontaneous abortion, and perinatal death. Tobacco use is also an important cause of Sudden Infant Death Syndrome (SIDS), the number one cause of death in infants under one year of age.

Lastly, women who do not themselves smoke can be injured by exposure to environmental tobacco smoke (ETS). ETS is estimated to cause approximately 40,000 deaths annually in nonsmokers from lung cancer and heart disease. In addition, ETS exposure exacerbates asthma and other lung diseases and may cause pregnancy complications in nonsmoking pregnant women.

Demographics

Despite the enormous negative health effects of smoking, about one in four American women smoke. However, smoking is far more common among women with lower levels of education, and those living in poverty. In 1994, approximately 10 percent of women with 16 or more years of schooling (college graduates) smoked; in contrast, 32 percent of women without a high school diploma smoked. The prevalence of smoking among white and black women is similar while that of Hispanic and Asian/Pacific Islander women is significantly lower.

The 1990s saw a significant increase in smoking by girls (and boys). In 1997, 35 percent of high school girls were current cigarette smokers; 16 percent were already frequent smokers. In re-

*Michele H. Bloch is a health policy consultant and physician who focuses on tobacco-related health issues of women and girls.

cent years, an increase in smoking has also been noted among college students, both men and women. This is of great concern because college graduates have been a group with lower smoking rates.

Smoking—More Than Nicotine Addiction

Cigarettes and other tobacco products are addictive because they contain nicotine. Tobacco products meet the criteria for addiction developed by the American Psychiatric Association. The U.S. surgeon general has concluded that: "The pharmacological and behavioral processes that determine tobacco addiction are similar to those that determine addiction to drugs such as heroin and cocaine."

Nonetheless, smoking is far more than physiological addiction to nicotine. Smoking, and its associated rituals, are ingrained in the daily life of women. Cigarette use in certain circumstances has become automatic, an over-learned behavior. While not consciously thinking of smoking a cigarette, the behavior occurs reliably and predictably under certain circumstances, such as while driving, or talking on the phone.

Smoking may also be viewed as a response to women's social, cultural, and economic disadvantage, relative to men. Many women use smoking to deal with stress and negative emotions, such as anger, anxiety, sadness, or loneliness. Women commonly "invest" their cigarettes with meaning. In a real way, the cigarette has become a trusted friend, a source of solace, stability, companionship, and reliability. While such "investment" is probably most common among women in difficult life circumstances, it is also present to a degree in other women smokers.

Tobacco Industry Efforts to Promote Smoking among Women

In the early 1900s, few women smoked cigarettes because of social conventions and legal restrictions. However, tobacco companies recognized the potential value of the female market. George Washington Hill, president of the American Tobacco Company, said of the female market, "It will be like opening a new gold mine right in our front yard." By the late 1920s, tobacco companies' fears of backlash for advertising to women had diminished, and women became "fair" game for sophisticated marketing schemes. In a piece

published in a special issue of the *Journal of the American Medical Women's Association* (January/April 1996), Dr. Allan Brandt described the role cigarette marketers played in promoting women's smoking as follows:

Cigarette advertisers and public relations experts recognized the significance of women's changing roles and the rising culture of consumption, and worked to create specific meaning for the cigarette to make it appeal to women. The cigarette was a flexible symbol, with a remarkably elastic set of meanings; for women it represented rebellious independence, glamour, seduction, and sexual allure, and served as a symbol for both feminists and flappers. The industry, with the help of advertisers and public relations experts, effectively engineered consent for women as smokers.

Marketing themes, which have changed little over the years, include weight control, independence/autonomy, glamour, beauty, relaxation, and rebellion. They are supplemented by promotional events and sponsorship of community events and organizations. More than 70 years of marketing targeted to women have helped create an epidemic of smoking and smoking-caused disease among them.

Reversing the Trend

Solving the problem of women and smoking will require concerted action in many areas, including smoking cessation, public education, school-based health education, litigation, and public policy solutions. Effective smoking cessation should become the standard of care in medical practice, and health professionals should become more knowledgeable about women smokers' specific needs. Increased public knowledge of the extraordinary health hazards of tobacco, and the role the tobacco industry plays in promoting tobacco use will help "demoralize" tobacco use. Comprehensive, intensive, K–12 school-based health education, can help protect youth from smoking. Litigation promises to help hold the tobacco industry accountable for decades of lies and deceit. Lastly, public policy measures have enormous power to decrease tobacco use. Some specific policy measures are especially important to women. These include restrictions on indoor smoking and restrictions or bans on tobacco marketing efforts.

Unions: Labor's Role in Tobacco Control

Regina Carlson

Unions, like other sectors of society, increasingly support smoke-free policies. Decision makers creating smoke-free policies need to be cognizant of unions because a significant percentage of employees (approximately 16 percent of all wage and salary workers in the United States) are union members and about half of private-sector, non-agricultural jobs are in worksites where a majority of either the production employees or the non-production employees are unionized. The National Education Association (NEA), for instance, represents more than 2.2 million school employees in 70 percent of the nation's school districts (*New Solutions, a Journal of Environmental and Occupational Health Policy*, Summer 1996, published by the Oil, Chemical, and Atomic Workers International Union, AFL-CIO. That volume contained the proceedings of a conference, "Smokefree or Free to Smoke? Labor's Role in Tobacco Control," Washington, D.C., September 1995. It is an excellent resource).

Unions are not uniform in their response to smoke-free policies. The Bakery, Confectionary and Tobacco Workers Union has opposed smoke-free policies, believing that more smoke-free policies mean fewer jobs for its members, and has asked other unions to join it in solidarity on this issue. Yet other unions support smoke-free policies, both to support the health of their members and to further the professional goals of their members.

Musicians in California fought legislation that postponed until 1998 the original 1997 implementation date for state legislation banning smoking in bars. This was an issue of workplace health for singers and musicians who play in bars and clubs. Flight attendants were one of the first groups of employees to work for nonsmoking policies in their workplaces. Unions that advocate smoke-free policies to protect the health of their members, also ask other unions to join *them* in solidarity.

Some unions that have taken a proactive position on smoking include: Fire Fighters (the issue of presumptive laws on cancer and heart disease); nurses (encourage programs of positive health education); and teachers (responsibility to educate young people). Some of these unions have supported far-reaching positions such as not investing in tobacco company stocks, eliminating federal tobacco subsidies, increasing cigarette taxes, encouraging legislative initiatives, and opposing coercion of other nations to accept U.S.-produced tobacco (*New Solutions*, 1996)

The NEA supports smoke-free policies in its members' workplaces and in public places, in addition to many anti-tobacco measures, including controls on tobacco advertising. In California, all labor unions, including building trade unions, supported state legislation to ban smoking in all workplaces.

The first nationwide, systematic study of unions on this question, surveying almost 200 unions, national, international, and local, was conducted in 1995 by the Dana-Farber Cancer Institute. It determined that 17 percent of national unions supported a complete ban on smoking in the workplace; 26 percent supported restrictions; only 3 percent actively opposed nonsmoking policies. Among local unions, 15 percent supported a complete ban; 33 percent supported restrictions; and 8 percent actively opposed nonsmoking policies. Most national unions had eliminated or restricted smoking in their offices; 52 percent were smoke free and 25 percent allowed smoking only in designated areas. Among local unions, 31 percent were entirely smoke free and 12 percent had limited smoking to designated areas (*New Solutions*, 1996).

Just as unions differ in their response to questions about tobacco use, individual union members differ in their tobacco use. This poses a dilemma for some unions. "This is a very touchy area," one official said. "I file grievances for nonsmokers. I file grievances for smokers. Arguing both sides undermines the arguments" (Carlson, 1997).

A primary role of unions is to protect the health and safety of union members. In 1991, the National Institute for Occupational Safety and Health, responding to increasing evidence that environmental tobacco smoke (ETS) is a health hazard, recommended that workers be protected. Unions have a responsibility.

Some union leaders fear that the smoking issue might obscure other problems in the workplace, that management might use a smoking ban as an

---

* Regina Carlson is executive director of New Jersey Group Against Smoking Pollution (GASP).

excuse not to clean up other health hazards in the workplace. "Just eliminating smoke is not going to take care of indoor air quality," one union official commented (Carlson, 1997). Some union leaders also worry that employers will maintain that employee health problems result from smoking rather than workplace exposure.

This ambiguity has led some unions to adopt a position of "no position" on smokefree policies. But that surrenders union's role on the issue. With employers conscious of health care dollars spent because of tobacco, unions can be at a disadvantage. As one of the participants of the Washington, D.C. labor conference put it, ". . . when we have to put an extra 50 cents into your health and welfare contribution [to pay for smoking-related illnesses], it truly does come out of the wage negotiation" (Carlson, 1997).

The National Labor Relations Board (NLRB) has ruled that regulation of smoking by management is a "term of condition of employment" and a subject for collective bargaining (304 NLRB 957, 1991, quoted in *New Solutions*, 1996). *New Solutions* cites an evaluation of 92 published decisions in which management prevailed in upholding proposed policies on smoking twice as frequently as unions succeeded in blocking them. Relatively few unions have taken employers to court over this question, compared to the thousands of employers who have implemented smoke-free workplaces.

The primary benefit of a smoke-free environment for unions is that it protects union members from ETS. A smoke-free policy also encourages members who smoke to reduce their smoking or become nonsmokers, thereby improving their health and reducing the exposure of their families to secondhand smoke. These efforts result in lower health care costs for everyone. Another plus for unions: Studies have found that when tobacco control policies are well defined and consistently enforced, they minimize polarization between smoking and nonsmoking members.

References: Regina Carlson, *Smoke Free Air Everywhere: Why and Here for Decision Makers in Workplaces and Public Places*, Montclair: New Jersey Group Against Smoking Pollution (GASP), 1997, p. 30.

The Tobacco Products Liability Project's Top 10 Tobacco Cases
Mark Gottlieb

1. ***Green v. American Tobacco Company*** (Florida 1957): Lung cancer victim and Lucky Strike smoker sued based on breach of warranty, misrepresentation, battery, and violation of Florida and federal pure food and drug law. A Florida jury found that smoking caused plaintiff's lung cancer after hearing from 16 medical experts. But the jury also found that the defendant could not have known of that danger prior to the plaintiff's diagnosis in 1956. On appeal, the Court found that the defendant's knowledge of the product's propensity to cause cancer was a relevant factor, but, on further appeal to the Florida Supreme Court, American Tobacco's knowledge of cancer risks was, in 1963, overturned as "wholly irrelevant" to the issue of manufacturer's liability. Yet the case was remanded for a second jury trial in which, again, the defendant prevailed. The appeals process finally ended in 1969 after a U.S. Court of Appeals panel affirmed the second trial decision. This leading case in the "First Wave" of tobacco litigation came close to winning.

2. ***Marsee v. U.S. Tobacco Company*** (Oklahoma 1986): Wrongful death action seeking $37 million in damages for the death of plaintiff's son from oral cancer allegedly cause by smokeless tobacco (snuff). The *Marsee* case was the first and only product liability case involving smokeless tobacco to be tried by a jury, which found for the defendant. The case, however, led to federal warnings on smokeless tobacco products and a ban on television and radio advertising. *See also* MARSEE, SEAN

3. ***Horton v. American Tobacco Company*** (Mississippi 1986*)*: Nathan Horton smoked

*Mark Gottlieb is a staff attorney at the Tobacco Control Resource Center.

Note: Legal developments are unfolding very rapidly in 1999 and several cases may supplant some of these listed here. Cases are listed chronologically and not necessarily by order of importance. Dates indicate year of trial or settlement.

Pall Malls for 30 years before succumbing to lung cancer. His case was tried twice. The first effort was declared a mistrial and the second resulted in a plaintiff's verdict, although no damages were ever awarded (unheard of in a wrongful death verdict for the plaintiff). Rumors about jury tampering started to spread when reports surfaced that the American Tobacco Company representatives had come to Holmes County, where the trial was held, to hand out money. These rumors about the defendant's behavior inspired John Grisham's best seller *The Runaway Jury. See also* HORTON, NATHAN

4. ***Cipollone v. Liggett Group*** (New Jersey 1988): A leading second wave case, it went on for more than nine years. The case had everything: perhaps 100 published opinions, a huge cache of documents that is still being used, a jury verdict for the plaintiff that was reversed on appeal, a favorable Supreme Court preemption opinion, and more. In the end, the original plaintiffs had died and the firm representing them felt pressure to stop spending money to bring the case to trial for a second time. *Cipollone* was voluntarily dismissed in 1992. *See also* CIPOLLONE, ROSE

5. ***Helling v. McKinney*** (Nevada 1993): Although not against a tobacco defendant, this case saw a convicted felon persuade the U.S. Supreme Court that forced exposure to secondhand smoke could violate the Eighth Amendment protection from cruel and unusual punishment. McKinney was forced to reside within a cell (6 by 8 feet) with an inmate who smoked five packs of cigarettes a day. McKinney did not complain of serious health risks at the time of the exposure but feared future health problems as a result of the exposure. The case has led to the establishment of smoke-free policies at many prison facilities.

6. ***Horowitz v. Lorillard Tobacco Company*** (California 1995): First successful case involving Kent's early asbestos-based "micronite" filter. Milton Horowitz smoked Kents with the asbestos-laden filter and developed a fatal, asbestos-specific lung cancer. Plaintiff received, and was paid, both compensatory and punitive damages. These payments were the first ever paid to a successful tobacco plaintiff by a defendant as a result of a jury verdict. Payment was made by wire transfer during a national holiday, allegedly to avoid Wall Street's attention and a physical check that could create negative publicity for Lorillard. *See also* FILTERED CIGARETTES; HOROWITZ, MILTON

7. ***Castano v. American Tobacco Company et al.*** (Louisiana 1996): National class action for addicted smokers, though decertified by appellate court, led to many state class actions. Sixty law firms from around the country combined resources to fight the industry and in the late 1990s began pursuing more than two dozen state-based class actions. All these cases are based on the common injury of addiction to nicotine from cigarette smoking. *See also* CASTANO, PETER

8. ***Carter v. Brown and Williamson Tobacco Corporation*** (Florida 1996): First third wave cigarette case where plaintiff was awarded damages. Tobacco stocks plummeted, inspiring efforts towards "global settlement" by tobacco executives. Jury verdict overturned when appeals court ruled that plaintiff filed his case two days late. That decision has been appealed. *See also* CARTER, GRADY

9. ***Broin v. Philip Morris et al.*** (Florida 1997): Class-action suit filed in 1991 by flight attendants who were exposed to secondhand tobacco smoke. The first class action against tobacco companies, this case was once considered the longest of long shots. However, after years of wrangling over whether the case could proceed as a class action, a trial commenced in 1997 only to end when the defendants agreed to a $350 million settlement, including attorney fees. The funds are to be used for tobacco and health research.

10. ***State of Minnesota et al. v. Philip Morris Inc. et al.*** (Minnesota 1998): Of the more than 40 states to sue the tobacco industry, Minnesota's case was the most important. After Mississippi, Minnesota became the second state to sue the tobacco industry for recovery of Medicaid expenses related to treating indigent smokers suffering from tobacco-related disease. The state was joined by Blue Cross, Blue Shield of Minnesota as co-plaintiff. Over 30 million pages of tobacco industry documents were

discovered by the state, and are now housed in a public depository in Minnesota. The 1998 trial, which took five months, resulted in a $6.1 billion settlement for the state as well as powerful public health concessions. *See also* MINNESOTA MEDICAID CASE; GOTTLIEB, MARK; KELDER, GRAHAM; SWEDA, EDWARD L.; TOBACCO LITIGATION: FIRST, SECOND, AND THIRD WAVES

SmokeLess States Coalitions and Tobacco Control
Thomas P. Houston, M.D.

The idea for the SmokeLess States National Tobacco Prevention and Control Program grew out of California's successes in tobacco control in the 1980s. The idea was to take the lessons learned in the post–Proposition 99 period in California and apply them in many other states.

SmokeLess States was the brainchild of the Robert Wood Johnson Foundation (RWJF), the nation's largest philanthropy organization devoted exclusively to health and health care. The Princeton, New Jersey-based foundation asked the nation's largest physician group—the American Medical Association (AMA)—to administer the program from its headquarters in Chicago, Illinois, where the SmokeLess States National Program Office (NPO) is based.

The RWJF established the SmokeLess States program in 1993 with a $13-million grant that funded statewide coalitions in 19 states and a youth-specific project in Tucson, Arizona. Two years later, a $20-million grant brought 13 new grantees on board and established a $3-million Special Opportunities Grant Program. And in 1998, the SmokeLess States program received another $6 million to continue grants in eight states that originally were funded for four years each.

SmokeLess States today include Alaska, Arizona, California, Colorado, Connecticut, Delaware, Florida, Georgia, Hawaii, Illinois, Iowa, Kansas, Kentucky, Maryland, Minnesota, Nebraska, New Jersey, New York, North Carolina, Ohio, Oklahoma, Oregon, Utah, Vermont, Virginia, Washington, West Virginia, Wisconsin, and the District of Columbia. With 30 grantees, SmokeLess States is the largest non-governmentally funded national effort in tobacco control and prevention.

The goals of the program are three-fold: (1) to promote public awareness of the dangers of tobacco use; (2) to educate the public regarding policy options related to tobacco; and (3) to en-

hance local prevention and treatment programs. The work is carried out through statewide coalitions made up of major voluntary health organizations, such as the American Cancer Society, American Heart Association, and American Lung Association; tobacco control organizations; state medical, dental, and hospital associations; state government agencies; educational and civic groups; and businesses.

The coalition structure that is at the heart of SmokeLess States grants has been crucial to the program's effectiveness. This is because each coalition member organization brings to the table different strengths and resources that, when taken together, make many victories possible. And even when some of the efforts fall short of their mark, the lessons learned become valuable resources for others. War stories often are shared at Smokeless States meetings through case study presentations and round-table discussions so that pitfalls experienced by one grantee may be avoided by others.

SmokeLess States grantees have enjoyed numerous successes since the program's founding in 1993. Powerful media educational campaigns, both earned and paid, have helped change community norms and improve the lives of millions of Americans. In Alaska, for example, the Alaska Tobacco Control Alliance spent two years educating the public, legislators, and the media about tobacco use in the state. The alliance used news conferences, billboards, paid ads, and surveys to keep the issue before Alaska voters. The alliance built on this educational media campaign by promoting policy changes, including increasing the state's tobacco excise tax in an effort to bring down use rates, especially among youth. Individual member organizations that were free to lobby worked on this portion of the campaign, which in 1997 ended with the passage of a record 71¢-per-pack cigarette excise tax. The increase was the largest ever passed in the United States and brought the excise tax to $1 per pack.

* Thomas P. Houston, M.D., is director of the SmokeLess States National Program Office and director of Science and Public Health Advocacy and Programs, American Medical Association.

Promoting policy initiatives that help reduce tobacco use is high on the agenda of many SmokeLess States coalitions. In all cases, these policy efforts are funded with matching money that coalition member organizations contribute as a condition to receiving the SmokeLess States grant. SmokeLess States funds never are used for lobbying activities.

Since the first of the grants were awarded in 1994, 12 states have increased their tobacco excise taxes, led by Alaska's record 71¢-per-pack increase in 1997. That same year, the Hawaii State Legislature also voted to increase the state's cigarette excise tax to $1 per pack over two years. Other states passing tobacco excise taxes include Arizona, which increased taxes from 40¢ to 58¢ per pack; California, which increased taxes from 50¢ to 87¢ per pack; Illinois' twin 14¢ increases in 1995 and 1997 to the current 58¢ per pack; New Jersey's 40¢ increase to 80¢; Oregon's 30¢ increase to 68¢; Rhode Island's 10¢ increase to 71¢; Utah's 25¢ increase to 51¢; Vermont's 24¢ increase to 44¢; Washington's 48¢ increase to 82¢; and Wisconsin's 15¢ increase to 59¢ per pack.

Hundreds of counties, municipalities, and towns across SmokeLess States have achieved additional policy victories—including passing strong youth access laws and clean indoor air ordinances. In Minnesota, for example, a powerful collaboration among health care groups—including the State Medical Society, HMOs, and Blue Cross/Blue Shield of Minnesota—was instrumental in winning passage of a strong youth access law. In New Jersey, member organizations of the New Jersey Breathes Coalition have helped shape local ordinances on youth access, vending machines, and billboard bans. And in Maryland, the Smoke Free Maryland Coalition has helped advance statewide workplace smoking regulations that are among the most protective of workers and the public in the United States.

Many of these accomplishments would not have been possible if the SmokeLess States coalitions did not strive to be inclusive and representative of the different groups that make up their state's population. Groups that traditionally are singled out as targets by the tobacco industry—such as Native Americans, African Americans, Hispanics, Asian Americans, and Pacific Islanders—actively participate in many SmokeLess States coalitions.

The SmokeLess States program recognizes that the society's understanding and support of tobacco prevention and control issues does not happen overnight; that it takes years to build a strong foundation for future successes. The program, therefore, puts great emphasis, when deciding which coalitions to fund, on identifying states that have the best potential for bringing about long-term reduction of tobacco use, particularly among children and teens.

Grants are awarded to coalitions that have a clear vision of what needs to be done and have a roadmap of how to get there. The most successful coalitions in the program have been those whose memberships mirror their states' populations, including minority and other ethnic groups, and who pull together to advance a united agenda rather than promoting those of their individual organizations.

Yet great coalitions require great leaders, and that's one of the key skills the National Program Office staff works to develop and nurture in each SmokeLess State. Because once the Smokeless States grant ends, the coalition will survive and thrive only if it has strong leaders who have vision and are resourceful enough to find new ways to keep the coalition going.

Safe Cigarettes

John Slade, M.D.

Since the early 1950s, cigarette manufacturers have marketed brands that have the appearance of being less poisonous. First there were filtered brands, and then "low tar" or "light" brands. In neither instance were the manufacturers required to actually show that their new products were less dangerous; no governmental agency regulated tobacco products. Filtered brands came in at a time when smoking was on the decline out of concern about cancer caused by cigarettes. Smoking rates rose as ads for filtered brands poured out of television sets and the pages of leading magazines.

---

*Dr. John Slade is a practicing internist specializing in addiction medicine at St. Peter's Medical Center in New Brunswick, New Jersey.

Similarly, "light" brands, from the mid-1960s on, provided reassurance to smokers who otherwise might have quit. This has been explicitly acknowledged in once-secret industry documents.

Because consumers smoke cigarettes of different machine-measured delivery so that the nicotine dose they receive is similar to actual cigarettes, the supposed advantage of "light" cigarettes is illusory. However, the marketing campaigns for these products kept customers in the market who would otherwise have stopped.

Several major tobacco companies have tried to develop what would appear to have the potential to be genuinely less poisonous cigarettes and related devices. Special filters, special tobaccos, radical designs, (Ariel, Premier, Eclipse) have been employed in both prototypes and in products tested in the marketplace.

Whether any of these products are actually less poisonous in use (unlike filtered and "light" cigarettes) is only half of the public health issue. The other part of the equation is whether the sale of products like this would expand the market for nicotine delivery devices and so actually place more people at risk of illness and death. This is an especially important concern since none of these novel products is risk-free.

Up to now, there has been no accountability on the part of manufacturers for the effects of smoking on their customers. The cigarette makers have not had to prove or even stand behind their claims of safety and reduced risk to anyone. The government of Canada now has the authority to regulate tobacco products. Health Canada can force manufacturers who want to bring supposedly less poisonous products to market to prove that they are better. Moreover, if a product does not live up to expectations, or if it turns out to be more of a problem than a help for public health, the government can force the maker to change it or to stop selling it. These measures of accountability have long been matters of routine for many consumer products. Cigarettes and other tobacco products have escaped regulation, however, to the detriment of public health.

Any claim that a tobacco product is safer must be backed up by governmental oversight. This is already the law in Canada and should be so in the United States and elsewhere as well. Until the manufacturers are accountable for what their products do, the term "safe cigarette" has no practical meaning. *See also* ARIEL, PREMIER, ECLIPSE

Warning Labels: Legal Protection for the Tobacco Industry
Elizabeth M. Whelan

Government warning labels, currently on cigarette packages, while presumably well intended, have done nothing to discourage smoking, but have provided extraordinary legal protection for the tobacco industry. During the mid-1960s, when the hazards of smoking finally became undeniable to policy makers, nearly 30 years after the scientific community had reached consensus on the issue, public health activists and the tobacco industry both lobbied Congress for warning labels.

Health advocates thought they were "doing good." The industry acted to ensure survival. First, because as more states proposed different warning labels, the potential for chaos in interstate commerce was a looming nightmare. Better to have a single standard label they reasoned. There was a second reason as well. By agreeing to the labels the industry figured it was buying immu-

nity from the lawsuits that would be brought by the families of people who become ill and die from smoking cigarettes. In other words, as a direct result of the 1965 congressionally mandated "health" label (which was extended to include advertisements in 1969), the industry was given a unique and privileged legal status. As a result, the cigarette industry has never paid a cent in liability damages.

The threat of litigation is a clear and powerful incentive for an industry to keep its products safe, or to be very, very specific about the dangers associated with their use. Given their congressionally bestowed litigation shield, however, cigarette manufacturers have no incentive to be honest about the consequences of smoking. For example, despite 60,000 medical citations to the contrary, industry spokespeople continue to maintain that there is no evidence that smoking adversely af-

*Elizabeth M. Whelan, Sc.D., is president and founder of the American Council on Science and Health in New York City.

fects health. In November 1993, during sworn pretrial testimony in a Miami lawsuit, Michael Rosenbaum, vice president of the holding company that owns Liggett Group Inc., manufacturer of Chesterfield, L and M, and other cigarette brands, when asked if cigarettes cause cancer responded, "I'm not a medical doctor. I don't have a clue."

Tobacco companies spend $4 billion annually to promote cigarettes as healthy, invigorating, and part of the good life, a clear distortion of the grim medical realities. Only an industry that perceives itself as immune from lawsuits would have the gall to offer "free" designer clothing (Virginia Slims attire, fashions any young woman would die for) in return for proof of purchase of 975 packs of cigarettes in a six-month period, a consumption rate in excess of five packs a day.

Advocates for tobacco control frequently contend that the solution to our nation's pandemic of cigarette related diseases—now accounting for one in four deaths annually—is more government intervention, a ban on advertising, a hike in the excise tax, and restrictions on smoking in public places. But the real solution lies in the opposite direction, because if government had not meddled in the first place, cigarette companies would conduct business on the same legal turf as every other industry. They would have been sued by smokers made ill by their deadly products and by the loved ones of people who had died from their use. The industry would have paid, and paid big.

If Congress had not legislated the label and the legal immunity it spawned, cigarettes might still be available, but the industry would be totally forthright about risks and might even require written, informed consent from smokers as a means of protecting itself against further liability. If free-market forces and an unfettered judicial system had prevailed, the cigarette might now be an anachronism, simply because it would be too expensive to buy and too unprofitable to produce.

APPENDIX 2

Surgeon General's Reports 1964–1998

In 1964, the Public Health Service established a small unit called the NATIONAL CLEARINGHOUSE FOR SMOKING AND HEALTH. Through the years, the clearinghouse and its successor organization, the OFFICE ON SMOKING AND HEALTH, have been responsible for reporting on the health consequences of smoking. Listed below are the titles of the reports published from 1964 to 1998 as well as brief summaries of their conclusions.

- **1964:** *Smoking and Health: Report of the Advisory Committee to the Surgeon General of the Public Health Service* was the first official report of the federal government on smoking and health. It concluded that "Cigarette smoking is a health hazard of sufficient importance in the United States to warrant appropriate remedial action."

- **1967:** *The Health Consequences of Smoking: A Public Health Service Review* confirmed and strengthened the conclusions of the 1964 report. It stated that "The case for cigarette smoking as the principal cause of lung cancer is overwhelming." While the 1964 report described the relationship between smoking and coronary heart disease as an "association," the 1967 report found that evidence "strongly suggests that cigarette smoking can cause death from coronary heart disease." The report also concluded that "Cigarette smoking is the most important of the causes of chronic non-neoplastic bronchiopulmonary diseases in the United States."

- **1968:** *The Health Consequences of Smoking: 1968 Supplement to the 1967 Public Health Service Review* updated information presented in the 1967 report. It estimated that the smoking-related reduction of life expectancy among young men was eight years for "heavy smokers" (over two packs per day) and four years for "light" smokers (less than a half pack per day).

- **1969:** *The Health Consequences of Smoking: 1969 Supplement to the 1967 Public Health Service Review* also supplemented the 1967 report. It confirmed the association between maternal smoking and infant low birth weight. It identified evidence of increased incidence of prematurity, spontaneous abortion, stillbirth, and neonatal death.

- **1971:** *The Health Consequences of Smoking: A Report of the Surgeon General* reviewed the entire field of smoking and health, emphasizing the most recent literature. It discussed new data, including associations between smoking and peripheral vascular disease, atherosclerosis of the aorta and coronary arteries, increased incidence and severity of respiratory infections, and increased mortality from cerebrovascular disease and nonsyphilitic aortic aneurysm. It concluded that smoking is associated with cancers of the oral cavity and esophagus. It found that "Maternal smoking during pregnancy exerts a retarding influence on fetal growth."

- **1972:** *The Health Consequences of Smoking: A Report of the Surgeon General* examined evidence on immunological effects of tobacco and tobacco smoke, harmful constituents of tobacco smoke, and "public exposure to air pollution from tobacco smoke." The report stated tobacco may impair protective mechanisms of the immune system; nonsmokers' exposure to tobacco smoke may exacerbate allergic symptons; and carbon monoxide in smoke-filled rooms may harm the health of persons with chronic lung or heart disease. The report found that tobacco smoke contains hundreds of compounds, several of which have been shown to act as carcinogens, tumor initiators, and tumor promoters. Finally, carbon monoxide, nicotine, and tar are identified as smoke constituents most likely to produce the health hazards of smoking.

- **1973:** *The Health Consequences of Smoking, 1973*, presented evidence on the health effects of smoking pipes, cigars, and "little cigars." It found that the mortality rates of pipe and cigar smokers was higher than those of nonsmokers but lower than those of cigarette smokers. It found that cigarette smoking impairs exercise performance in healthy young men. The report presented additional evidence on smoking as a risk factor in peripheral vascular disease and problems of pregnancy.

- **1974:** *The Health Consequences of Smoking, 1974*,the 10th anniversary report, reviewed and strengthened evidence on the major hazards of smoking. It reviewed evidence on the association between smoking and atherosclerotic brain infarction and on the synergistic effect of smoking and asbestos exposure in causing lung cancer.

- **1975:** *The Health Consequences of Smoking, 1975*, updated information on the health effects of involuntary (passive) smoking. It noted evidence linking parental smoking to bronchitis and pneumonia in children during the first year of life.

- **1976:** *The Health Consequences of Smoking: Selected Chapters from 1971 to 1975.*

- **1978:** *The Health Consequences of Smoking, 1977–1978*, was a combined two-year report focusing on smoking-related health problems unique to women. It cited studies showing that use of oral contraceptives potentiates harmful effects of smoking on the cardiovascular system.

- **1979:** *Smoking and Health: A Report of the Surgeon General*, the 15th anniversary report, presented the most comprehensive review of the health effects of smoking ever published. It was the first surgeon general's report to carefully examine the behavioral, pharmacological, and social factors influencing smoking. It also was the first report to consider the role of adult and youth education in promoting nonsmoking as well as the first report to review the health consequences of smokeless tobacco. One new section identified smoking as "one of the primary causes of drug interactions in humans."

- **1980:** *The Health Consequences of Smoking for Women: A Report of the Surgeon General*, devoted to the health consequences of smoking for women, reviewed evidence that strengthened previous findings and permitted new ones. It noted projections that lung cancer would surpass breast cancer as the leading cause of cancer mortality in women. It identified the trend towards increased smoking by adolescent females.

- **1981:** *The Health Consequences of Smoking–The Changing Cigarette: A Report of the Surgeon General* examined the health consequences of "the changing cigarette," i.e., lower tar and nicotine cigarettes. It concluded that lower-yield cigarettes reduced the risk of lung cancer but found no conclusive evidence that they reduced the risk of cardiovascular disease, chronic obstructive pulmonary disease, and fetal damage. The report noted the possible risks from additives and their products of combustion. It discussed compensatory smoking behaviors that might reduce potential risk reductions of lower-yield cigarettes. It emphasized that there is no safe cigarette and that any risk reduction associated with lower-yield cigarettes would be small compared with the benefits of quitting smoking.

- **1982:** *The Health Consequences of Smoking–Cancer: A Report of the Surgeon General* reviewed and extended an understanding of the health consequences of smoking as a cause or contributing factor of numerous cancers. The report included the first surgeon general's report consideration of emerging epidemiological evidence of increased lung cancer risk in nonsmoking wives of smoking husbands. It did not find evidence at that time sufficient to conclude that the relationship was causal, but labeled it *"a possible serious public health problem."* The report discussed the potential for low-cost smoking cessation interventions.

- **1983:** *The Health Consequences of Smoking—Cardiovascular Disease: A Report of the Surgeon General* examined the health consequences of smoking for cardiovascular disease. It concluded that cigarette smoking was one of three major independent causes of coronary heart disease (CHD) and, given its prevalence, *"should be considered the most important of the known modifiable risk factors for CHD."* It discussed relationships between smoking and other forms of cardiovascular disease.

- **1984:** *The Health Consequences of Smoking—Chronic Obstructive Lung Disease: A Report of the Surgeon General* reviewed evidence on smoking and chronic obstructive lung disease (COLD). It concluded that smoking was the major cause of COLD, accounting for 80 to 90 percent of COLD deaths in the United States. It noted that COLD morbidity has greater social impact than COLD mortality because of extended disability periods of COLD victims.

- **1985:** *The Health Consequences of Smoking—Cancer and Chronic Lung Disease in the Workplace: A Report of the Surgeon General* examined the relationship between smoking and hazardous substances in the workplace. It found that for the majority of smokers, smoking is a greater cause of death and disability than their workplace environment. The report characterized the risk of lung cancer from asbestos exposure as multiplicative with smoking exposure. It observed the special importance of

smoking prevention among blue-collar workers because of their greater exposure to workplace hazards and their higher prevalence of smoking.

- **1986:** *The Health Consequences of Involuntary Smoking: A Report of the Surgeon General* concluded that "Involuntary smoking is a cause of disease, including lung cancer, in healthy nonsmokers." It also found that, compared with children of nonsmokers, children of smokers have higher incidence of respiratory infections and symptoms and reduced rates of increase in lung function. It presented a detailed examination of growth in restrictions on smoking in public places and workplaces. It concluded that simple separation of smokers and nonsmokers within the same airspace reduces but does not eliminate exposure to environmental tobacco smoke.

- **1988:** *The Health Consequences of Smoking—Nicotine Addiction: A Report of the Surgeon General* established nicotine as a highly addictive substance, comparable in its physiological and psychological properties to other addictive substances of abuse.

- **1989:** *Reducing the Health Consequences of Smoking—25 Years of Progress: A Report of the Surgeon General* examined the fundamental developments over the past 25 years in smoking prevalence and in mortality caused by smoking. It highlighted important gains in preventing smoking and smoking-related diseases, reviewed changes in programs and policies designed to reduce smoking, and emphasized sources of continuing concern and remaining challenges.

- **1990:** *The Health Benefits of Smoking Cessation: A Report of the Surgeon General* concluded that smoking cessation has major and immediate health benefits for men and women of all ages. Benefits apply to persons with and without smoking-related disease. It noted that former smokers live longer than continuing smokers. For example, persons who quit smoking before age 50 have one-half the risk of dying in the next 15 years compared with continuing smokers. The report explained that smoking cessation decreases the risk of lung cancer, other cancers, heart attack, stroke, and chronic lung disease. Women who stop smoking before pregnancy or during the first three or four months of pregnancy reduce their risk of having a low–birth weight baby to that of women who never smoked. Finally, the report concluded that the health benefits of smoking cessation far exceed any risks from the average 5-pound weight gain or any adverse psychological effects that may follow quitting.

- **1992:** *Smoking in the Americas: A Report of the Surgeon General*, developed in collaboration with the Pan American Health Organization, examined epidemiological, economic, historical, and legal aspects of tobacco use in the Americas. The report concluded that the prevalence of smoking in Latin America and the Caribbean varies but is 50 percent or more among young people in some urban areas. It noted that substantial numbers of women have begun smoking in recent years. The report explained that in Latin America and the Caribbean, the tobacco industry restricts smoking-control efforts and that economic arguments for support of tobacco production are offset by the long-term economic effects of smoking-related diseases. Finally, the report concluded that a commitment to surveillance of tobacco-related factors (prevalence of smoking; morbidity and mortality; knowledge, attitudes, and practices; tobacco consumption and production; and taxation and legislation) is crucial to the development of a systematic program for prevention and control of tobacco use.

- **1994:** *Preventing Tobacco Use Among Young People: A Report of the Surgeon General* focused on the adolescent ages of 10 through 18 when most users start smoking, chewing, or dipping and become addicted to tobacco. It examined the health effects of early smoking and smokeless tobacco use, the reasons that young men and women begin using tobacco, the extent to which they use it, and efforts to prevent tobacco use by young people.

- **1998:** *Tobacco Use Among U.S. Racial/ Ethnic Minority Groups—African Americans, American Indians and Alaska Natives,*

Asian Americans and Pacific Islanders, and Hispanics: A Report of the Surgeon General concluded that cigarette smoking is a major cause of disease and death in each of the four population groups studied, with African Americans bearing the greatest health burden. It reported that tobacco use varies within and among racial/ethnic groups. Among adults, American Indians and Alaska Natives have the highest prevalence of tobacco use, and African American and Southeast Asian men also have a high prevalence of smoking. Asian American and Hispanic women have the lowest prevalence. Among adolescents, cigarette smoking prevalence increased in the 1990s among African Americans and Hispanics after several years of substantial decline among adolescents of all four racial/ethnic groups. The report concluded that tobacco use is the result of multiple factors, including socioeconomic status, cultural characteristics, acculturation, stress, biological elements, targeted advertising, price of tobacco products, and varying capabilities of communities to mount effective tobacco control initiatives.

Following are conclusions for each of the U.S. racial/ethnic groups profiled in the 1998 report:

African Americans. In the 1970s and 1980s, death rates from respiratory cancers (mainly lung cancer) increased among African-American men and women. 1990 to 1995, these rates declined substantially among African-American men and leveled off in African-American women.

Middle-aged and older African Americans are far more likely than their counterparts in the other major racial/ethnic groups to die from coronary heart disease, stroke, or lung cancer.

Smoking declined dramatically among African-American youths during the 1970s and 1980s, but has increased substantially during the 1990s.

Declines in smoking have been greater among African American men with at least a high school education than among those with less education.

American Indians and Alaska Natives. Nearly 40 percent of American Indian and Alaska Native adults smoke cigarettes, compared with 25 percent of adults in the overall U.S. population. They are more likely than any other racial/ethnic minority group to smoke tobacco or use smokeless tobacco.

Since 1983, little progress has been made in reducing tobacco use among American Indian and Alaska Native adults. The prevalence of smoking among American Indian and Alaska Native women of reproductive age has remained strikingly high since 1978.

American Indians and Alaska Natives were the only one of the four major U.S. racial/ethnic groups to experience an increase in respiratory cancer death rates from 1990 to 1995.

Asian Americans and Pacific Islanders. Estimates of the smoking prevalence among Southeast Asian American men range from 34 percent to 43 percent—much higher than among other Asian American and Pacific Islander groups. Smoking rates are much higher among Asian American and Pacific Islander men than among women, regardless of country of origin.

Asian American and Pacific Islander women have the lowest rates of death from coronary heart disease among men or women in the four major U.S. racial/ethnic minority groups.

Factors associated with smoking among Asian Americans and Pacific Islanders include having recently moved to the United States, living in poverty, having limited English proficiency, and knowing little about the health effects of tobacco use.

Hispanics. After increasing in the 1970s and 1980s, death rates from respiratory cancers decreased slightly among Hispanic men and women from 1990 to 1995.

In general, smoking rates among Mexican American adults increase as they learn and adopt the values, beliefs, and norms of American culture.

Declines in the prevalence of smoking have been greater among Hispanic men with at least a high school education than among those with less education.

Factors that are associated with smoking among Hispanics include drinking alcohol, working and living with other smokers, having poor health, and being depressed.

Bibliography

U.S. Department of Health and Human Services. *The Health Consequences of Smoking for Women: A Report of the Surgeon General*. Washington, DC: DHHS, PHS, Office on Smoking and Health, 1980.

——. *The Health Consequences of Smoking—The Changing Cigarette: A Report of the Surgeon General*. Washington, DC: DHHS, PHS, Office on Smoking and Health, 1981.

——. *The Health Consequences of Smoking—Cancer: A Report of the Surgeon General*. Washington, DC: DHHS, PHS, Office on Smoking and Health, 1982.

——. *The Health Consequences of Smoking—Cardiovascular Disease: A Report of the Surgeon General*. Washington, DC: DHHS, PHS, Office on Smoking and Health, 1983.

——. *The Health Consequences of Smoking—Chronic Obstructive Lung Disease: A Report of the Surgeon General*. Washington, DC: DHHS, PHS, Office on Smoking and Health, 1984.

——. *The Health Consequences of Smoking—Cancer and Chronic Lung Disease in the Workplace: A Report of the Surgeon General*. Washington, DC: DHHS, PHS, Office on Smoking and Health, 1985.

——. *The Health Consequences of Involuntary Smoking: A Report of the Surgeon General*. Atlanta: DHHS, PHS, CDC, Office on Smoking and Health, 1986.

——. *The Health Consequences of Smoking—Nicotine Addiction: A Report of the Surgeon General*. Atlanta: DHHS, PHS, CDC, Office on Smoking and Health, 1988.

——. *Reducing the Health Consequences of Smoking—25 Years of Progress: A Report of the Surgeon General*. Atlanta: DHHS, PHS, CDC, Office on Smoking and Health, 1989.

———. *The Health Benefits of Smoking Cessation: A Report of the Surgeon General*. Atlanta: DHHS, PHS, CDC, Office on Smoking and Health, 1990.

———. *Smoking in the Americas: A Report of the Surgeon General*. Atlanta: DHHS, PHS, CDC, Office on Smoking and Health, 1992.

———. *Preventing Tobacco Use Among Young People: A Report of the Surgeon General*. Atlanta: DHHS, PHS, CDC, Office on Smoking and Health, 1994.

———. *Tobacco Use Among U.S. Racial/Ethnic Minority Groups—African Americans, American Indians and Alaska Natives, Asian Americans and Pacific Islanders, and Hispanics: A Report of the Surgeon General*. Atlanta: DHHS, PHS, CDC, Office on Smoking and Health, 1998.

U.S. Department of Health, Education, and Welfare. *The Health Consequences of Smoking: A Report of the Surgeon General*. Washington, DC: DHEW, PHS, Health Services and Mental Health Administration, 1971.

———. *The Health Consequences of Smoking: A Report of the Surgeon General*. Washington, DC: DHEW, PHS, Health Services and Mental Health Administration, 1972.

———. *The Health Consequences of Smoking*. Washington, DC: DHEW, PHS, Health Services and Mental Health Administration, 1973.

———. *The Health Consequences of Smoking*. Washington, DC: DHEW, PHS, CDC, 1974.

———. *The Health Consequences of Smoking, 1975*. Washington, DC: DHEW, PHS, CDC, 1975.

———. *The Health Consequences of Smoking*. Washington, DC: DHEW, PHS, CDC, 1976.

———. *The Health Consequences of Smoking, 1977-1978*. Washington, DC: DHEW, PHS, Office on Smoking and Health, 1978.

———. *Smoking and Health: A Report of the Surgeon General*. Washington, DC: DHEW, PHS, Office on Smoking and Health, 1979.

U.S. Public Health Service. *Smoking and Health: Report of the Advisory Committee to the Surgeon General of the Public Health Service*. Washington, DC: DHEW, PHS, CDC, 1964.

———. *The Health Consequences of Smoking: A Public Health Service Review*. Washington, DC: DHEW, PHS, 1967.

———. *The Health Consequences of Smoking: 1968 Supplement to the 1967 Public Health Service Review*. Washington, DC: DHEW, PHS, 1968.

———. *The Health Consequences of Smoking: 1969 Supplement to the 1967 Public Health Service Review*. Washington, DC: DHEW, PHS, 1969.

APPENDIX 3

Secondhand Smoke Timeline

1971

The Interstate Commerce Commission (ICC) issued orders restricting smoking on interstate buses.

United Airlines became the first carrier to institute separate smoking and nonsmoking sections.

1972

The first report of the surgeon general identified involuntary smoking as a health risk.

The Civil Aeronautics Board (CAB) ruled all airlines must create smoking/ nonsmoking sections for all commercial carriers.

1973

Arizona became the first state to pass a law prohibiting smoking in select public places (elevators, theaters, libraries, museums, art galleries, and buses).

1974

British study by Harlap and Davies showed infants and children of smoking parents were at risk for pneumonia and bronchitis.

1975

Legislators from both parties in Minnesota passed a Clean Indoor Air Act, a law that became a model for other states.

1976

The ICC banned smoking in dining cars on trains and banned the use of cars containing both smoking and nonsmoking sections.

In *Shimp v. New Jersey Bell,* the New Jersey Superior Court ruled that an ITT office worker allergic to tobacco smoke had the right to work in a smoke-free office.

The National Park Service banned smoking in federally owned caves saying smoking and radioactivity were unhealthy.

1977

The CAB banned pipe and cigar smoking on planes and banned all smoking when aircraft ventilation is not fully operational.

1978

Health, Education, and Welfare Secretary Joseph Califano issued a no-smoking policy in all HEW buildings except in designated areas.

1981

The first epidemiological study by Takeshi Hirayama found that nonsmoking wives of smoking husbands had increased lung cancer risk.

The Tobacco Institute took out full-page ads in major national publications denouncing Hirayama's findings as scientifically unfounded.

1982

Surgeon General C. EVERETT KOOP released his first report that reviewed evidence on environmental tobacco smoke (ETS) and lung cancer. The report concluded that involuntary smoking (secondhand smoke) may pose a carcinogenic risk to the nonsmoker.

1986

The National Academy of Sciences reported that secondhand smoke was linked to an approximately 30 percent increased risk for lung cancer in nonsmokers and respiratory problems in infants and young children.

The surgeon general's report, *The Health Consequences of Involuntary Smoking*, concluded that ETS is a cause of disease, including lung cancer in healthy nonsmokers; the children of smoking parents have an increased frequency of respiratory infections; and the simple separation of smokers and nonsmokers in the same air space may reduce but does not eliminate ETS exposure for nonsmokers.

Americans for Nonsmoking Rights, a national organization that initiated a grassroots campaign for the airline smoking ban was founded. It evolved from Californians for Nonsmoking Rights, founded in 1976.

1988

Congress banned smoking on domestic flights of two hours or less. Northwest Airlines voluntarily banned smoking on all flights in North America.

1990

Smoking was banned on interstate buses and on domestic flights of six hours or less, effectively eliminating smoking on over 99 percent of all domestic flights.

1993

The Environmental Protection Agency (EPA) issued its final report titled *Respiratory Health Effects of Passive Smoking: Lung Cancer and Other Disorders*. The agency classified ETS as a Group A carcinogen.

Representatives of the tobacco industry filed suit against the EPA challenging the findings of its ETS risk assesment.

The White House and U.S. Postal Service went smoke free.

The U.S. House of Representatives banned smoking in its public areas except for designated, separately ventilated areas.

1994

The U.S. Congress banned smoking in most of the nation's schools, except in designated areas closed to children.

Amtrak banned smoking on short- and medium-distance trips.

1997

President Bill Clinton ordered a ban on smoking in all federal workplaces.

1998

California banned smoking in bars, taverns, and gaming clubs.

APPENDIX 4

Tobacco Taxation in Countries of the European Union

Listed below are prices and tax incidence on a pack of 20 cigarettes of the most popular price category in the European Union countries in U.S. dollars as of January 1, 1998.

Austria	2.40 (74%)
Belgium	2.86 (74%)
Denmark	4.41 (82%)
France	3.23 (75%)
Finland	4.11 (76%)
Germany	2.94 (69%)
Greece	2.13 (73%)
Ireland	4.39 (78%)
Italy	2.11 (75%)
Luxembourg	2.00 (69%)
Netherlands	2.28 (76%)
Portugal	1.76 (82%)
Spain	1.26 (73%)
Sweden	5.81 (76%)
United Kingdom	5.37 (76%)

APPENDIX 5

Workplace and Smoking: Selected Landmark Cases

1. Unemployment Insurance

a. *Hochman, N.Y.S. Department of Labor, F.A. Russo Incorp.* (1976). The New York State Unemployment Appeal Board affirmed the decision of the referee who had found that a sensitive nonsmoker should not be disqualified for unemployment compensation for leaving his or her job as a result of experiencing extreme discomfort caused by a fellow employee's cigar smoking.

b. *Meyer v. C.P. Clare and Company et al.* (1978). The Industrial Commission of Idaho found that an employee had good cause for leaving her employment, and that she was therefore eligible for unemployment benefits. She left her job because exposure to cigar smoke in her work area caused her to have headaches and nausea, and her only choices were to quit or to continue to work under those conditions.

c. *Rottenberg v. Industrial Commission* (1979). A Colorado court denied unemployment compensation where a nonsmoking employee had presented no evidence that his working conditions were unsatisfactory or hazardous.

d. *Alexander v. Unemployment Insurance Board Appeals* (1980). A California court held that a smoke-sensitive employee was eligible to receive unemployment compensation while seeking other employment. She testified that there were medical offices in which smoking was prohibited and that she was willing to accept, and was looking for work, in such an office rather than in one in which smoking was permitted.

e. *Ruckstuhl v. Commonwealth Unemployment Compensation Board of Review* (1981). A Pennsylvania court held that an employee who left her job because of exposure to tobacco smoke had left "without cause" and consequently was not entitled to unemployment compensation. The only evidence produced by the employee was a doctor's certificate dated a month after she left her job stating that she had a tobacco and nicotine allergy and was unable to work in a smoky environment.

f. *Ennis* and *Stroehmann Brothers* (1983). The Pennsylvania Unemployment Compensation Board of Review granted benefits to an employee with a tobacco smoke allergy who voluntarily terminated her employment because exposure to smoke at work had an adverse effect on her health.

g. *McCrocklin v. Employment Development Department et al.* (1984). A California Court of Appeals held that an employee left work for "good cause" and was entitled to unemployment benefits when he feared harm to his health as a result of exposure to tobacco smoke in an unventilated room.

h. *Billman v. Sumrall* (1985). A Louisiana court denied unemployment compensation on the ground that the employee did not have "good cause" to leave. The employee had an allergy before she took the job, and did not inform the employer of her allergy. There was no tobacco smoke in the area where she worked, and her condition did not deteriorate during the course of her employment.

i. *Lapham v. Commonwealth Unemployment Compensation Board* (1987). A Pennsylvania court held that an employee with chronic bronchitis resigned from her job for "good cause" when the employer had failed to provide "reasonable accommodation." The employer had relocated her 10 to 15 feet from a heavy smoker and 20 feet from another smoker.

2. Workers' Compensation

a. *Brooks v. Trans World Airlines et al.* (1977). A California workers' compensation judge held that a flight attendant sustained an industrial injury consisting of an allergic reaction to the air in the aircraft in which she worked, including smoke, and awarded her $3,657.50 disability indemnity plus medical costs and attorney's fees.

b. *Schober v. Mountain Bell Telephone* (1981). An employee in New Mexico was found to be entitled to workers' compensation because he collapsed at work as a result of an allergic reaction to tobacco smoke.

c. *Batchelor v. Fresno County* (1982). A smoke-sensitive county employee in Fresno, California, settled a workers' compensation suit for $17,500. Surrounded by smokers on the job, she had suffered from headaches, stuffiness, chronic nosebleeds, and general "flu-like" symptoms.

d. *In the Matter of the Compensation of Marlene W. Ritchie* (1985). The Oregon Workers' Compensation Board ordered an employer corporation to accept an employee's claim that on-the-job exposure to tobacco smoke had caused the employee to develop rhinosinusitis and bronchitis. The board found that these were occupational diseases and made the corporation pay for benefits.

e. *In the Matter of the Compensation of Mary A. Downey* (1985). The Oregon Workers' Compensation Board remanded an employee's claim to the employer corporation for processing and closure, and ordered payment to the employee's attorney. The employee proved that her sensitivity to cigarette smoke, and her underlying rhinosinusitis condition, had worsened as a result of her exposure to tobacco smoke in the workplace.

f. *Mack v. County of Rockland* (1988). A New York Court of Appeals held that an employee was not entitled to workers' compensation for eye irritation (as a result of being exposed, for two years, to cigarette smoke in a badly ventilated room) on the ground that such exposure constituted "environmental conditions" and not an occupational disease.

g. *J and R Electric* (1988). A New York Workers' Compensation Board held that a general manager of a retail store was entitled to compensation where a smoke-filled environment caused her to collapse from an asthmatic condition. Her collapse was held to be an accident arising out of and "in the course of" employment.

h. *Johannesen v. New York City Department of Housing Preservation and Development* (1989). An employee who developed bronchial asthma as a result of exposure to tobacco smoke in a crowded office was held to have suffered an "accidental injury as a result of the repeated trauma of exposure to cigarette smoke," and received compensation.

i. *ATE Fixture Fab v. Wagner* (1990). A Florida Court of Appeals denied a nonsmoking employee's claim for disability benefits for alleged acceleration or aggravation of his obstructive lung disease by tobacco smoke in the workplace on the ground that he had not produced enough evidence of the causal connection between his illness and his exposure to tobacco smoke.

j. *Kufahl v. Wisconsin Bell Inc.* (1990). The Wisconsin Labor and Industrial Review Commission awarded a nonsmoking employee $23,400 because her workplace exposure to tobacco smoke caused illness, with consequential absence from work that resulted in her being fired.

k. *Ubhi v. State Compensation Insurance Fund, Cat 'N' Fiddle Restaurant* (1990). A California Workers' Compensation Appeals Board granted the claim of a nonsmoking waiter who suffered a heart attack as a result of working for five years in a smoke-filled bar. A settlement of $410,000 was awarded to him together with an $85,000 reimbursement for medical bills.

l. *Bena v. Massachusetts Turnpike Authority* (1991). An employee, a former smoker who had smoked one pack of cigarettes a day for 29 years before quitting, was awarded workers' compensation when she developed chronic obstructive pulmonary disease as a result of exposure to tobacco smoke in the workplace. The employee was found to have sustained a personal injury arising out of and in the course of her employment.

m. *Seiwert v. the Child Center* (1992). The Workers' Compensation Board of Indiana awarded compensation for lost work time, medical expenses, and attorney's fees to an employee who was seven months pregnant, who had suffered four or five asthma attacks as a child, and who suffered an attack of asthmatic bronchitis at work triggered by environmental tobacco smoke. The board found that the smoking of a coworker combined with the lack of fresh air and the configuration of the offices with low ceilings caused an elevated level of smoke beyond that to which the general public is exposed.

n. *Riddle, Sharon K. v. Ampex Corp.* (1992). The Colorado Court of Appeals denied the workers' compensation claim of a smoker who alleged that she had been disabled by stress because her employer had introduced a workplace smoking ban.

o. *Schiller v. Los Angeles Unified School District* (1992). A teacher who developed chronic obstructive lung disease was awarded $29,999 in workers' compensation against her employer, the Los Angeles Unified School District, in proceedings that were settled by compromise agreement. Her injury was caused by her exposure, over a five-year period, to tobacco smoke that traveled up a stairwell from a first-floor smoking area into her second-floor classroom. Despite her complaints to the school principal, the problem was ignored, although the school eliminated indoor smoking after Ms. Schiller filed her claim.

3. Negligence

a. *McCarthy v. Department of Social Health Services* (1988). An employee who developed chronic obstructive lung disease because of exposure to tobacco smoke in the workplace was entitled to bring common law action for negligence when the workers' compensation board found that her injury was not compensable under a Washington act.

b. *Scholem v. Department of Health* (1992). A New South Wales, Australia, court found negligence on the part of an employer, the New South Wales Department of Health, for its failure to provide a smoke-free workplace for an employee psychologist who developed acute asthma attacks and emphysema as a result of exposure to smoking in the workplace. A jury awarded the employee the Australian equivalent of $64,500.

4. Federal Rehabilitation Act Cases (Disability and Handicap)

a. *Flaniken v. Office of Personnel Management* (1980). The U.S. Merit Systems Protection Board found that a smoke-sensitive federal government employee was entitled to a disability retirement annuity when she contracted chronic laryngitis caused by cigarette smoke and environmental pollution.

b. *Pletten v. Department of the Army* (1981). The U.S. Merit Systems Protection Board found that a smoke-sensitive civilian army employee was a "handicapped person" for the purpose of the Federal Rehabilitation Act and that he was accordingly entitled to reasonable accommodation of his handicap.

c. *Parodi v. Merit Systems Protection Board* (1982). The Ninth Circuit Court held that a federal government employee who suffered from exposure to tobacco smoke in the workplace was entitled to disability benefits unless the government could show that an appropriate substitute position was available. In an out-of-court settlement, the employee received a disability pension of $500 per month plus a $50,000 lump sum payment.

d. *Vickers v. The Veterans Administration* (1982). A court held that a federal government employee whose hypersensitivity to tobacco smoke limited his capacity to work in any environment that was not completely smoke-free was a "handicapped person" under the Federal Rehabilitation Act, but that the Veterans Administration had already made a reasonable accommodation.

e. *Weir v. Office of Personnel Management* (1986). The Dallas, Texas, Merit System Protection Board held that an employee who suffered severe asthma attacks when exposed to tobacco smoke while working as a secretary with the Federal Aviation Administration (FAA) was entitled to receive disability retirement when her employer was unable to provide her with a smoke-free environment, which, her doctors reported, her condition required.

f. *White v. United States Postal Service* (1987). The Equal Employment Opportunity Commission held that the employer had not furnished reasonable accommodation to an employee who suffered from rhinitis sinusitis and tracheitis merely by offering to provide him with a face mask and to move his desk. The commission ordered the employer to establish a no-smoking policy in the area where the employee worked.

5. OSHA

Federal Employees for Nonsmokers' Rights et al v. United States et al. (1978). Nonsmoking employees who complained of injury because of exposure to tobacco smoke in federal buildings were held by the court not to be entitled, under the Occupational Safety and Health Act, to bring actions against the federal agencies involved.

6. Common Law

a. *Shimp v. New Jersey Bell Telephone Company* (1976). A telephone company employee who was allergic to tobacco smoke was held by the court to have a common-law right to a safe working environment that would be enforced by the prohibition of smoking in work areas.

b. *Gordon v. Raven Systems and Research Inc.* (1983). The District of Columbia Court of Appeals held that, in the absence of legislation limiting workplace smoking, an employer in the District of Columbia was under no common-law duty to provide a smoke-free workplace when a smoke-sensitive employee requesting smoke-free accommodation presented no scientific evidence of the deleterious effects of tobacco smoke on nonsmokers in general.

c. *Smith v. Western Electric Company* (1983). A complaint filed by a smoke-sensitive employee against his employer—alleging irreparable physical injuries because of exposure to smoke in the workplace—was held by a Missouri court to state a claim for breach of the employer's common-law duty to provide a safe workplace. The trial court later refused to find that tobacco smoke at the employee's workplace had been harmful to his health.

d. *Bernard v. Cameron and Colby Co. Inc.* (1986). A Massachusetts court ruled that an allergic employee's right to a smoke-free area would not be implied in an employment contract, and that the employee had waited too long to establish an employer's duty to provide a safe and healthful working environment.

7. Discrimination against Non-smokers

a. *Tari Way v. Area Agency on Aging* (1977). An investigator of the Madison, Wisconsin, Equal Employment Opportunities Commission found that there was probable cause to believe that a smoke-sensitive employee had been discriminated against as a handicapped person, in violation of the Madison Equal Opportunities Ordinance. She had been discharged from employment following her continuous requests that her coworkers should refrain from smoking in her work area, and her report of the situation to the City Attorney's Office.

b. *GASP v. Mecklenburg County* (1979). The Court of Appeals of North Carolina dismissed a complaint that smoke-sensitive nonsmokers were handicapped persons who were denied access to public buildings by the pressure of tobacco smoke on the ground that anti-discrimination statutes did not apply to smoking.

c. *Department of Fair Employment and Housing v. Fresno County* (1984). Under terms of a settlement agreement, a smoke-sensitive county employee was awarded $27,396.59 back pay plus interest, and compensatory damages of $10,000 plus interest when the employer had violated the California Fair Employment and Housing Act by failing to accommodate the employee's smoke sensitivity.

d. *County of Fresno v. Fair Employment and Housing Commission of the State of California; Brooks and Capo, Real Parties in Interest* (1991). The California Court of Appeals found that Fresno County had failed to accommodate reasonably the physical handicaps (severe respiratory problems) of two employees, and discriminated against them by placing them in inadequately ventilated rooms filled with cigarette smoke.

e. *Ryan v. Springfield Housing Authority* (1992). The Massachusetts Commission against Discrimination ruled that a nonsmoking employee who alleged that she had been unjustly discharged because of her inability to tolerate tobacco smoke was not discriminated against as a handicapped person. Although she had testified that she left work with a headache and nausea and that her physician had written a statement saying that she should not be exposed to tobacco smoke, she had provided no evidence that exposure to smoke in the office had "substantially limited any of her major life activities."

8. Constitutional Rights

a. *Anderson v. Anoka County Welfare Board et al.* (1981). The U.S. District Court, District of Minnesota, Fourth Division, awarded a smoke-sensitive Welfare Board employee $4,282 compensatory damages and $200 exemplary damages against the acting director of the Anoka County Social Service Department. The employer had dismissed the employee, without affording her an opportunity to be heard, in retaliation for her attempts to enforce the MINNESOTA CLEAN INDOOR AIR ACT in her workplace. Such a dismissal violated the employee's exercise of both her First Amendment (free speech) and Fourteenth Amendment (due process) rights.

b. *Kensell v. State of Oklahoma* (1983). The U.S. Court of Appeals for the Tenth Circuit denied the claim of a smoke-sensitive nonsmoking employee who alleged that his employer, the Oklahoma Department of Human Services, had violated his First, Fifth, Ninth, and Fourteenth Amendment rights by refusing to ban smoking in the workplace.

9. Assault and Battery

a. *McCracken v. Sloane* (1979). Although a doctor had testified that a Postal Service employee in North Carolina had severe respiratory problems when exposed to tobacco smoke, a court held that there had been no competent evidence presented that the employee had suffered an assault or battery by exposure to tobacco smoke in the workplace. The employee's supervisor had smoked a cigar at a meeting to discuss the problem of smoking in the workplace, and the employee had become ill and had to miss work and seek medical care.

10. Infliction of Emotional Distress

a. *Carroll v. Tennessee Valley Authority* (1988). A U.S. District Court refused to dismiss a smoke-sensitive nonsmoker's claim (which was settled later) for intentional infliction of emotional distress when her employer failed to provide her with a smoke-free workplace and her supervisor orally harassed her.

11. Labor/Management Relations

a. *American Federation of Government Employees, Council of District Office Locals, Local 147 and Department of Health, Education and Welfare, Social Security Administration, San Francisco Region, Palm Springs Office* (1979). The management of the Palm Springs Office of the Social Security Administration was found by the arbitrator to have properly and reasonably applied the Health, Education and Welfare Policy on Smoking by declaring a nonsmoking work area but allowing reasonable smoking breaks outside the office. Negotiated arrangements would, however, have to be made to shelter smokers in inclement weather.

b. *Social Security Administration and American Federation of Government Employees, AFL-CIO, Local No. 1923* (1980). The arbitrator, in applying the Health, Education and Welfare Policy on Smoking, found that the entire quadrant of the floor on which a smoke-sensitive employee worked was a common "work area," and therefore that smoking had to be prohibited entirely in that quadrant where there were no floor-to-ceiling partitions. That area was approximately 100 feet long and 70 feet wide, or 7,000 square feet. (The award was subsequently sustained by the Federal Labor Relations Authority in 1981.)

c. *Social Security Administration Headquarters Bureaus and Office* and *Local 1923 American Federation of Government Employees, AFL-CIO* (1982). An arbitrator ruled that the agency had violated its policy on smoking and that smoking must be prohibited in the work area of the entire floor where the grievant, a smoke-sensitive employee, worked in an "open-space" office.

d. *Commonwealth of Pennsylvania v. Commonwealth of Pennsylvania Labor Relations Board; Council 13, American Federation of State, County, and Municipal Employees* (1983). The Commonwealth Court of Pennsylvania held that the Commonwealth of Pennsylvania, an employer of unionized workers, should have complied with the bargaining procedures prescribed by the Collective Bargaining Agreement for matters concerning wages, hours, and other terms and conditions of employment. The court believed the commonwealth should have considered the agreement before imposing a ban on tobacco smoking by employees at their workstations thereby unilaterally discontinuing a more permissive practice previously applicable.

e. *San Mateo County Firefighters Local 2400 v. City of San Mateo* (1983). An action brought by a firemen's union in San Mateo, California, against the employer for recision of a rule to bar new firefighters from smoking on or off duty was settled by the collective bargaining process. The terms were that no one would be hired as a firefighter who had smoked in the one year preceding his or her employment application.

f. *Shattuck v. County of Orange* (1983). The arbitrator found that the employer, County of Orange, California, had required the grievant, a smoke-sensitive employee, to work in a smoke-contaminated atmosphere under conditions dangerous to her health and safety. Under the provision of a memorandum of understanding between the County of Orange and the American Federation of State, County, and Municipal Employees, Council 36, Local 2076, AFL-CIO, the employee was therefore entitled to work in an immediate work area that was free of tobacco smoke.

g. *Social Security Administration, Baltimore, Maryland v. American Federation of Government Employees, AFL-CIO, Local 1923* (1984). Jack Clare, an arbitrator, in applying a policy on smoking directed the agency to declare the entire floor in which the desk of a tobacco sensitive employee was located—his working environment—consisting of a space approximately 75 by 150 feet, to be a no smoking area. The employee had testified that being subjected to tobacco smoke bothered him physically and mentally, that cigarette smoke, sometimes caused him to be nauseated, and that he was concerned for injury to his health caused by being subjected to tobacco smoke and the contaminants contained in it.

h. *In re Honeywell Inc.* and *International Association of Machinists and Aerospace Workers, Lodge 570* (1989). An arbitrator in Louisiana ruled that an employer might impose a unilateral rule prohibiting all smoking in its facilities where the rule was reasonable and necessary to protect nonsmokers from secondhand smoke.

i. *Department of Health and Human Services, Indian Health Service, Oklahoma City v. Federal Labor Relations Authority* (1989). The U.S. Court of Appeals for the District of Columbia held that the Indian Health Service ban of smoking in its hospitals was a subject for negotiation under the collective bargaining agreement, unless it could be shown that the union's proposals would be detrimental to the health of Native Americans.

j. *Department of Health and Human Services Family Support Administration et al. v. Federal Labor Relations Authority and National Treasury Employees Union* (1990). The U.S. Court of Appeals for the District of Columbia upheld a decision of the Federal Labor Relations Authority, which had rejected the assertion of the Department of Health and Human Services (DHHS) that there was a compelling need for an agency-wide ban on smoking within DHHS facilities. The court ordered DHHS to bargain with local chapters of the National Treasury Employees Union regarding the agency's smoking regulations.

12. Enforcement of, and Complaints Related to, Workplace Smoking Limitation Laws and Policies

a. *Rossie v. Wisconsin Department of Revenue* (1985). The Circuit Court of Dane County, Wisconsin, held that the state employer could sue for an injunction, the method prescribed by statute to enforce a workplace smoking limitation law that was being violated by a pipe smoker. But the court could not enforce the statute by internal disciplinary procedures.

b. *Riddle v. Ampex Corporation* (1992). A Colorado Court of Appeals found that workers' compensation was not available to an employee, with a 24-year smoking habit, who claimed that a workplace smoking ban caused her to develop a stress-related disability.

c. *Quinn, Gent et al. v. Unemployment Compensation Board of Review* (1992). The Commonwealth Court of Pennsylvania ruled that a paralegal employee who smoked was not entitled to unemployment compensation when she left work because her employer had introduced a total ban on workplace smoking. There was no evidence that the employee suffered any pressure to terminate her employment, and she was the only employee to leave in response to the smoking ban.

APPENDIX 6

Ten Selected Tobacco Advertising Agencies

The following ad agencies create advertising campaigns for cigarettes:

- **Bates USA, New York City:** This agency creates ads for Brown and Williamson's Lucky Strike cigarettes.

- **Leo Burnett, Chicago, Illinois:** This agency created Philip Morris's Marlboro Man and handles more tobacco brands in more countries than any other company. It creates ads for six Marlboro brands; Basic, Benson and Hedges, Merit, and Virginia Slims (all Philip Morris); Players Navy Cut brand (Philip Morris); and Bucks and Alpine.

- **Compton Partners, New York City:** This unit of the London, England, Cordiant, parent company of Saatchi and Saatchi Advertising and Bates Worldwide ad agencies, creates ads for Lorillard's Newport cigarettes.

- **Euro RSCG Tatham, Chicago, Illinois:** A unit of France's Havas Advertising, this agency creates ads for Misty and Capri, as well as for GPC, a private-label brand—all Brown and Williamson Tobacco Corporation brands.

- **Grey Advertising, New York City:** This agency creates ads for Brown and Williamson's Carlton and Kool brands.

- **Gyro Advertising, Philadelphia, Pennsylvania:** This ad agency creates ads for Red Kamel cigarettes for R.J. Reynolds, a brand that was discontinued in 1936 but revived in the 1990s.

- **Long Haymes Carr, Winston-Salem, North Carolina:** This agency creates ads for Winston cigarettes.

- **Mezzina/Brown, New York City:** This ad agency creates ads for R.J. Reynold's Camel cigarettes.

- **Trone Advertising, Greensboro, North Carolina:** This agency creates ads for R.J. Reynold's Salem, More, and Now brands.

- **Young and Rubicam, New York City:** This agency creates ads for Philip Morris's Parliament and Dave brands of cigarettes.

CHRONOLOGY

1492	Christopher Columbus and his crew reported seeing people who "drank smoke."
1560–1561	Jean Nicot, France's ambassador to Portugal, learned that court physicians prized tobacco for its curative powers. In 1561, Nicot presented some tobacco plants to the French queen, Catherine de Medici. Nicot's name was later used to name nicotine, an element in tobacco.
1604	King James I of England issued *A Counterblaste to Tobacco*, calling smoking "a custom loathesome to the eye, hateful to the nose, harmful to the brain, dangerous to the lungs."
1614	In June, John Rolfe of the Virginia Colony shipped his first cargo of Virginia tobacco to London where it became an immediate success. The popularity of the tobacco crop made the colony, near financial collapse, economically viable.
1769	Pierre Lorillard established a plant in New York City for processing tobacco, which became the first tobacco company in the colonies.
1794	The U.S. Congress passed its first tobacco tax; it applied only to snuff.
1839	Tobacco manufacturers in North Carolina used charcoal for the first time in the process of flue curing tobacco leaves, turning them into a "bright leaf" and making tobacco milder in taste when smoked.
1850s	Philip Morris opened a shop in England to sell Turkish cigarettes.
1870s–1910	Cigarette manufacturers inserted series of colorful picture cards with various subjects, especially baseball, into cigarette packs. Used to stiffen packs, the cards were also a marketing device to attract buyers who wanted to collect all the images in a series.
	Hand rolling of cigarettes was being done by skilled female "rollers" in Virginia factories.
1875	Richard Joshua Reynolds founded R.J. Reynolds Tobacco Company in Winston, North Carolina, to make chewing tobacco.

1881	James Albert Bonsack, a Virginian, patented a cigarette-rolling machine that produced more than 70,000 cigarettes in a 10-hour day.
1884	On April 30, called the "birthday" of the modern cigarette, the Bonsack machine successfully operated for a full day turning out 120,000 cigarettes—the equivalent of 40 hand rollers rolling five cigarettes a minute for 10 hours.
1890	James Buchanan Duke formed the American Tobacco Company, a monolithic tobacco enterprise that gobbled up competitors.
	Anti-cigarette leagues were organized in the American heartland.
1892	Portable matches were invented that permitted smokers to light up whenever and wherever they wished.
1893	State legislatures began to pass anti-cigarette laws. Some states totally outlawed the sale, manufacture, possession, advertising, or use of cigarettes; others outlawed sales to minors.
1902	British tobacco companies united to fight James Buchanan Duke by forming the Imperial Tobacco Group.
1906	Brown and Williamson Tobacco Corporation was formed by a group of farmers in Winston-Salem, North Carolina. It made plug, snuff, and pipe tobacco.
	The Food and Drug Act of 1906, the first federal food and drug law, made no express reference to tobacco products. The definition of a drug included medicines and preparations listed in the *U.S. Pharmacoepia* or National Formulary.
1911	The U.S. Supreme Court ruled the American Tobacco Company violated the 1890 Sherman Anti-Trust Act and ordered James Buchanan Duke to break up his company.
1912	Liggett and Myers introduced Chesterfield cigarettes.
1913	On October 13, R.J. Reynolds Tobacco Company introduced Camels, the first "modern" blended cigarette, and launched the first national cigarette-advertising campaign in the nation.
1914	The Federal Trade Commission Act was passed to "prevent persons, partnerships, or corporations . . . from using unfair or deceptive acts or practices in commerce."
1917–1918	During World War I, soldiers smoked cigarettes that were part of their daily rations.
1921	Iowa was the first state to levy a tax on cigarettes.
	Cigarettes became the main form of tobacco consumed, over pipes, snuff, chewing tobacco, and cigars.
1927	State anti-cigarette laws were all repealed.
	British-American Tobacco bought Brown and Williamson Tobacco Corporation.

1928   George Washington Hill and Albert Lasker, an advertising executive, launched one of the most profitable ad campaigns in advertising history: "Reach for a Lucky Instead of a Sweet." Sales of Lucky Strike cigarettes zoomed up by 47 percent two months after radio listeners first heard commercials on the air.

1933   On May 12, President Franklin Delano Roosevelt signed the Agricultural Adjustment Act. It was the first law aimed at providing immediate relief to growers of "basic" crops such as wheat and tobacco, and preventing crop prices from collapsing.

            Brown and Williamson introduced Kool menthol cigarettes.

1938   The Wheeler-Lea Act gave the Federal Trade Commission (FTC) power to regulate "unfair or deceptive acts or practices in commerce." Since 1938, the FTC has acted 51 times against tobacco companies.

            The Food, Drug, and Cosmetic Act of 1938 defined "drugs" as "articles intended for use in the diagnosis, cure, mitigation, treatment, or prevention of disease in man or other animals" and "articles (other than food) intended to affect the structure or any function of the body of man or other animals."

            On February 16, the Agricultural Adjustment Act gave relief to tobacco farmers by controlling the number of acres planted and setting quotas on crops to be marketed. Marketing quotas have been in effect ever since.

            Biological statistician Raymond Pearl made a pioneering study that concluded heavy smokers did not live as long as light smokers and that nonsmokers outlived both.

1940s   Almost 20 percent of the cigarettes produced in the United States were shipped to soldiers overseas, as well as added to army K-rations; a domestic shortage resulted.

1947   Lucky Strikes began sponsoring televised college football games.

1948   Camels sponsored the televised "Camel News Caravan."

1950   American scientists Ernst L. Wyndner and Evarts A. Graham published a report that 96.5 percent of lung-cancer patients were moderate-to-heavy smokers.

1952   Reacting to lung cancer publicity, Lorillard introduced its new "micronite" filter-tip Kent cigarettes in full-page advertisements. Filters were supposed to protect smokers from nicotine and tar. Competing brands soon developed their own filter versions.

            A study by Alton Ochsner, a renowned thoracic surgeon, and Michael DeBakey, renowned heart surgeon, concluded that the increase in smoking was largely responsible for the increase of pulmonary carcinoma.

1953   A landmark study by Ernst L. Wynder showed that painting cigarette tar on the backs of mice created malignant tumors.

1954   The tobacco industry established the Tobacco Industry Research Council (later renamed the Council for Tobacco Research). On January 4, it issued a "Frank Statement" to the public, a nationwide two-page advertisement that stated cigarette makers did not believe their products were injurious to a person's health.

1954 (*cont.*)
Philip Morris hired attorney David Hardy to defend the company in litigation, beginning the company's association with Shook, Hardy and Bacon. Philip Morris won the first case handled by Hardy.

1955
In January, the Marlboro Man appeared for the first time in ads. Leo Burnett, advertising genius, changed the Marlboro image from "Mild as May" to the "Marlboro Man." At the time, Marlboro cigarettes only had 1 percent of the U.S. market.

1957
Philip Morris began diversifying by acquiring Milprint Inc., a packaging products firm. The same year, R.J. Reynolds established a diversification committee.

1958
Major cigarette manufacturers formed the Tobacco Institute to counter the adverse effects of health studies as well as to emphasize the inconclusiveness of the research on smoking and disease, the contribution of tobacco products to the national economy, and the individual rights of smokers.

Philip Morris Incorporated made its first grant to support the arts. The tobacco company now operates the leading corporate arts support program in the world.

1962
Every one of the 20 baseball teams in the Major League had either tobacco or alcoholic-beverage sponsorship, or both.

1964
On January 11, U.S. Surgeon General Luther Terry issued the first report on smoking and health. The landmark report linked smoking to cancer and increased mortality and identified it as a contributing factor in several diseases.

Philip Morris decided to concentrate on the cowboy as the only Marlboro Man. The image now is the most widely recognized advertising image in the world.

1966
The Cigarette Labeling and Advertising Act of 1965 took effect January 1, requiring a nine-word health warning on cigarette packages: "Caution: Cigarette smoking may be hazardous to your health." The act required no labels on advertisements for three years.

1967
The Federal Communications Commission ruled that the Fairness Doctrine applied to cigarette advertising. Stations broadcasting cigarette commercials had to donate air time to anti-smoking messages.

1968
Philip Morris introduced Virginia Slims, a cigarette strictly for women. Soon after, other cigarettes for women appeared on the market.

1969
The Public Health Cigarette Smoking Act of 1969 required the following package label "warning": The Surgeon General Has Determined that Cigarette Smoking is Dangerous to Your Health." The act prohibited cigarette advertising on television and radio after January 1, 1971.

1970s
Tobacco industry marketed its products to countries in Africa, Asia, and Latin America.

1970s *(cont.)*	Tobacco sponsorship of sporting events put tobacco ads back on television.
1970	The Controlled Substances Act of 1970 excluded tobacco from the definition of a "controlled substance."
1971	The Public Health Cigarette Smoking Act went into effect banning cigarette ads from television and radio on midnight January 1, 1971. Print ads zoomed up after the ban.
	The Fairness Doctrine anti-smoking messages ended when cigarette advertising ended on television and radio.
	Surgeon General Jesse Steinfeld called for a national Bill of Rights for the Nonsmoker, touching off the environmental tobacco smoke (ETS) movement. During the 1970s, nonsmoking sections began to appear on buses, airplanes, trains, and in other public places.
1972	Cigarette advertising health warnings in print ads began.
	The Consumer Product Safety Act of 1972 did not include tobacco or tobacco products.
1973	Arizona became the first state to pass a comprehensive law protecting nonsmokers by prohibiting smoking in select public places.
	The Little Cigar Act banned little cigar advertisements from television and radio.
1975	The military stopped providing cigarettes in K-rations and C-rations given to soldiers and sailors.
1976	The Toxic Substances Control Act of 1976 did not include tobacco or any tobacco products.
1977	Berkeley, California, enacted the first modern ordinance limiting smoking in restaurants and other public places.
	The American Cancer Society sponsored its first national Great American Smokeout.
1978	Utah enacted the first state law banning tobacco ads on any billboard, street car sign, or bus.
1979	Minneapolis and St. Paul, Minnesota, became the first cities to ban free distribution of cigarette samples in the streets.
	Cigarettes were the most advertised product in some women's magazines, with as many as 20 ads in a single issue.
1980s	Studies by the American Council on Science and Health showed that magazines with tobacco ads rarely carried articles about health dangers of smoking.
1980	The surgeon general's report was devoted to the health consequences of smoking for women.
1982	Surgeon General C. Everett Koop's report on smoking and cancer made headlines everywhere: "Cigarettes Blamed for 30 Percent of All Cancer Deaths." (Bangor, Maine *News*, February 23, 1982)

1984	On January 13, the FDA approved Nicorette® Gum, a nicotine gum, as a smoking-cessation product. Once available only by prescription, its sale is now restricted to those over 18 years of age.
	On October 12, President Ronald Reagan signed the Comprehensive Smoking Education Act of 1984 instituting four rotating health warning labels on cigarette packages and advertisements.
1985	Aspen, Colorado, became the first city to ban smoking in restaurants.
	Philip Morris bought General Foods; R.J. Reynolds purchased Nabisco Brands Inc.
1986	Surgeon General C. Everett Koop crusaded against smokeless tobacco and passive smoking.
	The Comprehensive Smokeless Tobacco Health Education Act of 1986 instituted three rotating health warnings on smokeless tobacco packages and advertisements. The act prohibited smokeless tobacco advertising on television and radio.
1987	A workplace smoking ban went into effect at the Department of Health and Human Services, the first smoke-free federal agency.
	Public Law 100-202 banned smoking on domestic airline flights scheduled for two hours or less.
1988	R.J. Reynolds Tobacco Company launched its "Old Joe" ad campaign featuring a "smooth character" cartoon camel.
	Surgeon General C. Everett Koop declared nicotine a highly addictive substance
	The 15th Winter Olympic games in Calgary, Canada, were the first to have a smoke- free program.
	The Canadian government passed the Tobacco Products Control Act that banned tobacco advertising in Canada. It was struck down by the Canadian Supreme Court in 1995.
	On February 1, a Newark, New Jersey, federal district court ruled, for the first time in history, that cigarette manufacturers were liable for the death of a smoker, Rose Cipollone. She died of lung cancer in 1984. Liggett and Myers was ordered to pay Cipollone $400,000 in compensatory damages.
	On April 23, Northwest Airlines became the first nonsmoking airline. It banned smoking on all of its domestic flights in North America regardless of length.
	The first World No-Tobacco Day, an internationally coordinated event, was held to discourage tobacco users from consuming tobacco. Now a growing global observance, diverse celebrations take place every May 31.
1989	Public Law 101-164 banned smoking on domestic airline flights scheduled for six hours or less (except the cockpit) and on intercity buses.
	The Minnesota Timberwolves basketball team opened the first major smoke-free stadium in the nation.

1989 (*cont.*)   The Tobacco Institute launched an anti-smoking youth campaign, "It's the Law."

Don Barrett, a Mississippi attorney representing Nathan Horton, won the case against the American Tobacco Company but his client was not awarded money.

1991   Researchers found that Camel cigarette's cartoon camel was as familiar to six-year-olds as Mickey Mouse.

1992   The Synar Amendment required states to enact and enforce laws prohibiting the sale of cigarettes to children under 18 years.

The Supreme Court handed down a landmark decision in *Cipollone v. Liggett Group Inc.,* ruling that the federal Cigarette Labeling and Advertising Act of 1965 does not shield tobacco manufacturers from liability.

Cigar Aficionado was launched celebrating the pleasures of cigar smoking. One of the most successful magazine start-ups of the 1990s, it has also been credited with launching the cigar craze of the late 1990s.

1993   The Environmental Protection Agency released its report linking environmental tobacco smoke (ETS) with cancer and other diseases among nonsmokers. It classified ETS as a "Group A" (known human) carcinogen.

1994   In her surgeon general's report (the first devoted solely to young people), Joycelyn Elders reported that most smokers become addicted by age 18, and emphasized the importance of preventing smoking among children and teenagers.

Baltimore, Maryland, became the first city to ban tobacco ads on billboards in most neighborhoods.

The Pro-Children Act of 1994 required all federally funded children's services to become smoke-free.

The Department of Defense (DOD) banned smoking in DOD workplaces.

On February 28, ABC's news magazine *Day One* reported that cigarette companies controlled the content of nicotine in cigarettes to keep smokers hooked.

On March 29, a national class-action suit, know as the *Castano* lawsuit, filed on behalf of nicotine-addicted smokers, evolved into the largest class action in U.S. judicial history. The case was dismissed in May 1996.

On April 14, in a widely televised broadcast, seven executives of the largest American tobacco companies testified under oath before a House subcommittee that they did not believe cigarettes and nicotine are addictive.

On May 5, the nation's second class action lawsuit brought by smokers, *Engle v. R.J. Reynolds Tobacco Company et al.,* was filed. The trial started October 14, 1998.

On May 7, the *New York Times* published its first report on internal tobacco company documents stolen by Merrell Williams, a former employee of a law firm doing work for Brown and Williamson Tobacco Corporation.

1994 (*cont.*)　　On May 23, Mississippi became the first state to file a lawsuit suing tobacco companies for reimbursement of the costs of treating smoking-related illnesses incurred by Medicaid and other public health care programs in the state.

In June, Geoffrey Bible was named Philip Morris's president and chief executive, replacing Michael Miles.

1995　　Delta Airlines banned smoking aboard its international flights, the first and only U.S. airline to provide a completely smoke-free environment worldwide.

The Department of Justice reached an agreement with the Philip Morris Companies Inc. to remove from sports arenas and stadiums tobacco advertisements seen regularly on telecasts of football, basketball, baseball, or hockey games.

The *New York Times* disclosed that it obtained some 2,000 pages of documents showing that Philip Morris studied nicotine and found it affected the body, brain, and behavior of smokers.

Philip Morris announced a comprehensive program to curb under-age smoking. Called "Action against Access," Philip Morris said the program reflected the company's concern about the tobacco industry's negative image caused by young people who smoke.

In January 1995, Dr. Jeffrey Wigand, a former top scientist at Brown and Williamson Tobacco Corporation who had become a whistle blower, providing tobacco industry secrets to CBS's *60 Minutes* and later that year to Mississippi lawyers.

On July 1, at 12:01 A.M. Pacific Standard Time, the University of California Library posted documents on the Internet stolen by Merrell Williams from the law firm doing work for Brown and Williamson Tobacco Corporation.

In August, President Bill Clinton announced his support for the Food and Drug Administration's proposal to regulate tobacco sales and marketing aimed at youth under 18. Clinton was the first president in history to make smoking prevention among youth a national priority.

In August, the nation's five largest tobacco companies filed a lawsuit in Federal District Court in Greensboro, North Carolina, to block the Food and Drug Administration's (FDA) rule-making procedure. Six trade groups, including the National Advertisers and the American Association of Advertising Agencies, filed separate lawsuits in North Carolina challenging the FDA's regulations.

In October, Steven Goldstone was named chief executive of RJR Nabisco Holdings Corporation, after having served as president and general counsel.

In December, the nation's largest retailer and wholesaler associations announced the "We Card" program to provide training and educational materials to retailers to prevent the sale of tobacco products to under-age customers.

1995 (*cont.*) In December, a federal hearing examiner awarded death benefits to Philip E. Wiley, whose wife died from lung cancer. This was believed to be the first award of death benefits in the nation for a workplace injury connected to secondhand smoke.

1996 The *Washington Post* disclosed a 1973 R.J. Reynolds Tobacco Company marketing memo from Claude E. Teague, then RJR assistant director of research and development. The memo proposed marketing cigarettes to underage smokers, suggesting that teenage rebellion might make the risks of smoking more attractive to that market.

In January, the *Wall Street Journal* published excerpts of a sealed deposition from Jeffrey Wigand (former Brown and Williamson Tobacco Corporation employee) that was leaked to the paper. Wigand claimed that former Brown and Williamson CEO Thomas Sandefur repeatedly acknowledged that nicotine was addictive, comments that directly contradicted Sandefur's testimony before Congress on April 14, 1994.

In March, the Liggett Group became the first tobacco company to settle unilaterally, out of court, a lawsuit with *Castano* class-action lawyers and five states suing tobacco companies for the Medicaid costs of treating smoking-related diseases.

In April, Nicorette® gum became available for nonprescription sale as a smoking-cessation aid.

In May, a federal appellate court in New Orleans, Louisiana, disqualified the *Castano* suit as a national class action on the grounds that it involved too many different state laws and too many plaintiffs. The ruling overturned a 1995 decision that would have allowed almost any smoker in the country to sue the tobacco industry on the grounds that tobacco companies manipulated nicotine levels to addict smokers.

In July, the Food and Drug Administration approved the Nicotrol transdermal patch for nonprescription sale. The patch became available over the counter starting July 18.

In August, a Florida circuit court awarded $750,000 to 66-year-old Grady Carter, who sued the maker of Lucky Strikes after he lost part of a lung to cancer in 1991. This was the second time the tobacco industry was ordered to pay damages in a liability case.

On August 23, President Clinton announced the nation's first comprehensive program to prevent children and teens from smoking cigarettes or smokeless tobacco. The provisions of the Food and Drug Administration rule are aimed at reducing youth access to tobacco products and the appeal of tobacco advertising to young people.

1997 On February 28, the FDA ban on tobacco sales to minors went into effect requiring retailers to card all cigarette and smokeless tobacco customers under 27 years of age.

On March 20, the Liggett Group signed a new, broader settlement with 22 states. As part of the settlement, the Liggett Group, the smallest of the major U.S. cigarette companies, acknowledged that smoking causes cancer and other diseases, that nicotine is addictive, and that it and other major tobacco companies deliberately targeted their products to teens. The settlement provided evidence implicating other tobacco companies.

1997 (*cont.*)   On April 25, Federal District judge William L. Osteen, Sr., upheld the Food and Drug Administration's (FDA) power to regulate nicotine in tobacco as a drug, but he said the FDA lacked authority to control advertising and promotions. The FDA and the tobacco industry appealed the ruling.

On May 28, the FTC filed an unfair advertising complaint against the R.J. Reynolds Tobacco Company alleging that its Joe Camel advertising campaign illegally promoted cigarettes to minors. This was the first time the FTC accused the tobacco industry of aiming its products at youngsters.

On June 20, the tobacco companies and state attorneys general announced the landmark $368.5 billion settlement agreement in Washington, D.C., the largest proposed payout in U.S. history. The settlement later collapsed.

On July 3, Mississippi settled its lawsuit against the tobacco industry for $3.4 billion.

On August 25, Florida settled its lawsuit against the tobacco industry for $11.3 billion.

In October, four major tobacco companies settled *Broin v. Philip Morris Companies Inc.*, the first major class-action lawsuit over the effects of secondary smoke by flight attendants.

1998   In January, Texas settled its lawsuit against the tobacco industry for at least $14 billion.

On March 30, Senator John McCain (R-AZ) offered a comprehensive tobacco bill that would toughen the June 1997 settlement reached with state attorneys general and public health groups. The bill was killed in the Senate in June.

On May 8, Minnesota settled its lawsuit against the tobacco industry for $6.5 billion. As a result of the suit, the Council for Tobacco Research was disbanded.

On November 14, the attorneys general of eight states and the nation's four biggest cigarette companies reached agreement on a $206 billion tobacco settlement, the biggest U.S. civil settlement in history. Unlike the earlier June 1997 tobacco settlement, this one did not need congressional approval. The proposed settlement received the approval of all 46 states that either had lawsuits or were yet to sue.

1999   On April 23, all cigarette billboards were removed and replaced with anti-smoking ads, a result of the November 1998 settlement.

On July 7, the first class action lawsuit to go to trial, *Engle v. R.J. Reynolds Tobacco Comany et al.,* was decided. A Florida jury ruled against the tobacco company.

BIBLIOGRAPHY
AND WEB SITES

Books and Articles

Allen, Steve, and Adler, Bill, Jr. *The Passionate Nonsmokers' Bill of Rights*. New York: William Morrow and Co., 1989.

American Medical Women's Association. Special Issue: Smoking and Women's Health. *Journal of the American Medical Women's Association,* vol. 51, nos. 1 and 2 (January/April 1996).

American Tobacco Company. *"Sold American!" The First Fifty Years*. The American Tobacco Company, 1954.

Austin, Gregory A. *Perspectives on the History of Psychoactive Substance Abuse.* NIDA Research Issues, no. 24. Washington, DC: U.S. Government Printing Office, 1978.

Badger, Anthony J. *Prosperity Road: The New Deal, Tobacco and North Carolina*. Chapel Hill: University of North Carolina Press, 1980.

Barth, Ilene. *The Smoking Life*. Columbus, MS: Genesis Press, 1997.

Bernays, Edward. *Biography of an Idea: Memoirs of Public Relations Counsel Edward L. Bernays*. New York: Simon and Schuster, 1965.

Blum, Alan, ed. *The Cigarette Underworld*. Secaucus, NJ: Lyle Stuart, 1985. (Previously published as a special edition of the *New York State Journal of Medicine,* December 1983.)

Brecher, Edward M., and the editors of *Consumer Reports. Licit and Illicit Drugs*. Boston: Little, Brown, and Co., 1972.

Breen, T.H. *Tobacco Culture: The Mentality of the Great Tidewater Planters on the Eve of Revolution*. Princeton: Princeton University Press, 1985.

British Medical Association. *Smoking Out the Barons: The Campaign Against the Tobacco Industry: A Report of the British Medical Association Public Affairs Division*. New York: Wiley, 1986.

Brooks, Jerome. *Green Leaf and Gold Tobacco in North Carolina*. Chapel Hill: North Carolina Archives, 1975.

———. *The Mighty Leaf: Tobacco Through the Centuries*. Boston: Little, Brown, and Co., 1952.

Buckley, Christopher. *Thank You for Smoking*. New York: Random House, 1994. (Novel.)

Califano, Joseph A., Jr., *Governing America. An Insider's Report from the White House and the Cabinet*. New York: Simon and Schuster, 1981.

Campbell, Tracy. *The Politics of Despair: Power and Resistance in the Tobacco Wars*. Lexington: University of Kentucky Press, 1993.

Candre, Hipólito. *Cool Tobacco, Sweet Coca: Teachings of an Indian Sage from the Columbian Amazon*. London: Themis Books, 1996.

Casey, Karen. *If Only I Could Quit: Recovering from Nicotine Addiction*. Center City, MN: Hazelden, 1996.

Chapman, Simon. *Great Expectorations: Advertising and the Tobacco Industry.* London: Comedia, 1986.

Corina, Maurice. *Trust in Tobacco: The Anglo-American Struggle for Power.* New York: St. Martin's Press, 1975.

Corti, Egon Caesar. *A History of Smoking.* London: George A. Harrap and Co. Ltd., 1931.

Cunningham, Rob. *Smoke and Mirrors: The Canadian Tobacco Wars.* Ottawa: IDRC Books, 1996.

Degh, Linda. *People in the Tobacco Belt: Four Lives.* North Stratford, NH: Ayer, 1980.

Dillow, Gordon L. *The Hundred-Year War against the Cigarette.* New York: American Heritage Publishing Co., 1981.

Duke, Maurice, and Jordan, Daniel P. *Tobacco Merchant: The Story of Universal Leaf Tobacco Company.* Lexington: University Press of Kentucky, 1995.

Dunhill, Alfred H. *The Gentle Art of Smoking.* London: Max Reinhardt, 1954.

———. *The Pipe Book.* London: Arthur Barker Ltd., 1969.

Durden, Robert F. *The Duke of Durham 1865–1929.* Durham, NC: Duke University Press, 1975.

Ehwa, Carl, Jr. *The Book of Pipes and Tobacco.* New York: Random House, 1974.

Evans, Nicola, et al. "Influence of Tobacco Marketing and Exposure to Smokers on Adolescent Susceptibility to Smoking." *Journal of the American Cancer Institute,* October 18, 1995.

Eysenck, Hans J. *Smoking, Health, and Personality.* New York: Basic Books, 1965.

Ferrence, Roberta G. *Deadly Fashion: The Rise and Fall of Cigarette Smoking in North America.* New York: Garland, 1989.

Fisher, Ronald A. *Smoking: The Cancer Controversy.* London: Oliver and Boyd, 1959.

Fitzgerald, Jim. *The Joys of Smoking Cigarettes.* New York: Holt, Rinehart and Winston, 1983.

Flannagan, Roy C. *The Story of Lucky Strike.* Richmond, VA: Richmond News Leader, 1938.

Ford, Barry J. *Smokescreen: A Guide to the Personal Risks and Global Effects of the Cigarette Habit.* North Perth, Australia: Halcyon Press, 1994.

Fox, Maxwell. *The Lorillard Story.* New York: P. Lorillard Company, 1947.

Glantz, Stanton A. *Tobacco, Biology and Politics.* Waco, TX: WRS Group, 1994.

Glantz, Stanton A.; Slade, John; Bero, Lisa A.; Hanauer, Peter; and Barnes, Deborah E. *The Cigarette Papers.* Berkeley: University of California Press, 1996.

Gompers, Samuel. *Seventy Years of Life and Labor: An Autobiography.* New York: E.P. Dutton and Company, 1957.

Goodman, Jordan. *Tobacco in History: The Cultures of Dependence.* New York: Routledge, 1995.

Greaves, Loraine. *Smoke Screen: Women's Smoking and Social Control.* Alpine, TX: LPC Inbook; Scarlet Press, United Kingdom, 1996.

Grossman, Michael, and Price, Philip. *Tobacco Smoking and the Law in Canada.* Charlottesville, VA: Lexis Law Library, 1992.

Harvard Institute for the Study of Smoking Behavior and Policy. *The Cigarette Excise Tax.* Cambridge, MA: Harvard University Press, 1987.

Heimann, Robert K. *Tobacco and Americans.* New York: McGraw-Hill Book Company Inc., 1960.

Henningfield, Jack E., *Nicotine: An Old-Fashioned Addiction.* New York: Chelsea House, 1992.

Hilts, Philip. *Smokescreen: The Truth Behind the Tobacco Industry Cover-Up.* Reading, MA: Addison-Wesley Press, 1996.

Houston, Thomas P., ed. *Tobacco Use: An American Crisis.* Chicago: American Medical Association, 1993.

Infante, Guillermo Cabrera. *Holy Smoke.* London: Faber and Faber, 1985.

Institute of Medicine. *Growing Up Tobacco Free.* Washington, DC: National Academy Press, 1984.

Jacobson, Bobbie. *The Ladykillers: Why Smoking Is a Feminist Issue.* London: Pluto Press, 1981; New York: Continuum Publishing Co., 1982.

———. *Beating the Ladykillers: Women and Smoking.* London: Gollancz, 1988.

Jacobson, Peter D., and Wasserman, Jeffrey. *Tobacco Control Laws: Implementation and Enforcement.* Santa Monica, CA: Rand Corporation, 1997.

Jahn, Raymond. *Tobacco Dictionary.* New York: Philosophical Library, 1954.

Johnson, Paul. *The Economics of the Tobacco Industry.* New York: Praeger, 1984.

Journal of the American Medical Association, vol. 253, May 24/31, 1985. Special Issue devoted to smoking and health.

Kasper, Rhona. *A Woman's Guide to Cigar Smoking: Everything You Need to Know to Be the Ultimate Cigar Aficionada.* New York: St. Martin's Press, 1988.

Kaufman, Stuart Bruce. *Samuel Gompers and the Origins of the American Federation of Labor, 1848–1896.* Westport, CT: Greenwood Press, 1973.

Keyishian, Elizabeth. *Everything You Need to Know about Smoking.* New York: Rosen Group, 1995.

Kirchner, Wendy. *Dying to Smoke: One Family's Struggle with America's Deadliest Drug.* Melbourne, FL: Starr Publishing, 1997.

Klein, Richard. *Cigarettes Are Sublime.* Durham, NC: Duke University Press, 1993.

Kluger, Richard. *Ashes to Ashes: America's Hundred-Year War, the Public Health, and the Unabashed Triumph of Philip Morris.* New York: Alfred A. Knopf, 1996.

Koop, C. Everett. *Koop: The Memoirs of America's Family Doctor .* New York: Random House, 1991.

Koven, Edward L. *Smoking: The Story Behind the Haze.* Commack, NY: Nova Science Publishers, 1996.

Krantzler, Nora, and Miner, Kathleen Rae. *Tobacco: Health Facts.* Santa Cruz, CA: ETR Associates, 1995.

Krogh, David. *Smoking, The Artificial Passion.* New York: W.H. Freeman and Co., 1991.

Kulikoff, Allan. *Tobacco and Slaves: The Development of Southern Cultures in the Chesapeake, 1680–1800.* Durham: University of North Carolina Press, 1988.

Lee, P.N. *Environmental Tobacco Smoke and Mortality: A Detailed Review of Epidemiological Evidence Relating Environmental Tobacco Smoke to the Risk of Cancer.* Farmington, CT: S. Karger, 1992.

Lewine, Harris. *Good-bye to All That.* New York: McGraw-Hill Book Company, 1970.

Lloyd, Barbara B., et al. *Smoking in Adolescence: Images and Identities.* New York: Routledge, 1998.

Mandel, Bernard. *Samuel Gompers: A Biography.* Antioch, OH: The Antioch Press, 1963.

Marrero, Eumelio Espino. *Cuban Cigar Tobacco: Why Cuban Cigars Are the World's Best.* Neptune, NJ: TFH Publications, 1997.

McFarland, J. Wayne, and Folkenberg, Elman J. *How to Stop Smoking in Five Days.* Englewood Cliffs, NJ: Prentice-Hall Inc., 1962.

McGrath, Sally V., and McGuire, Patricia J., eds. *The Money Crop: Tobacco Culture in Calvert County, Maryland.* Crownsville, MD: Division of History and Culture Programs, 1992.

McKeen, W.E. *Blue Mold of Tobacco.* St. Paul, MN: American Phytopathology Society, 1989.

McLaurin, Tim. *Cured by Fire.* New York: G.P. Putnam's Sons, 1995.

Middleton, Arthur Pierce. *Tobacco Coast: A Maritime History of the Chesapeake Bay in the Colonial Era.* Baltimore: Johns Hopkins, 1984.

Miles, Robert H. *Coffin Nails and Corporate Strategies.* Englewood Cliffs, NJ: Prentice-Hall Inc., 1982.

Mollenkamp, Carrick; Levy, Adam; Menn, Joseph; and Rothfeder, Jeffrey. *The People vs. Big Tobacco: How the States Took on the Cigarette Giants.* Princeton, NJ: Bloomberg Press, 1998.

Moore, James. *Very Special Agents: The Inside Story of America's Most Controversial Law Enforcement Agency—The Bureau of Alcohol, Tobacco and Firearms.* Norristown, PA: PB, 1997.

Mullen, Chris. *Cigarette Pack Act.* London: Gallery Press, 1979.

Neuberger, Maurine B. *Smoke Screen: Tobacco and the Public Welfare.* Englewood Cliffs, NJ: Prentice-Hall Inc., 1963.

New York State Journal of Medicine vol. 83, 12, December 1983. Special issue devoted to "The World Cigarette Pandemic—Part 1.

New York State Journal of Medicine vol. 85, 7, July 1985. Special issue devoted to "The World Cigarette Pandemic—Part II."

Nuttall, Floyd H. *Memoirs in a Country Churchyard: A Tobaccoman's Plea—Clean Up Tobacco Row!* Lawrenceville, VA: Brunswick Publishers, 1996.

Orleans, C. Tracy, and Slade, John, eds. *Nicotine Addiction: Principles and Management.* New York, Oxford University Press, 1993.

Ortiz, Fernando. *Cuban Counterpoint: Tobacco and Sugar.* Durham, NC: Duke University, 1995.

Pan American Health Organization. *Tobacco or Health: Status in the Americas.* Scientific Publication No. 536. Washington, DC: Pan American Health Organization, 1992.

Paper, Jordan. *Offering Smoke: The Sacred Pipe and Native American Religion.* Moscow: University of Idaho Press, 1988.

Pomerleau, Ovide F., and Pomerleau, Cynthias S., eds. *Nicotine Replacement: A Critical Evaluation.* Binghamton, NY: Haworth Publishers, 1992.

Pringle, Peter. *Cornered: Big Tobacco at the Bar of Justice.* New York: Henry Holt and Company Inc., 1998.

Raw, Martin; White, Patti; and McNeill, Ann. *Clearing the Air: A Guide for Action on Tobacco.* London: World Health Organization, 1990.

Read, Melvyn D. *The Politics of Tobacco: Policy Networks and the Cigarette Industry.* Brookfield, VT: Ashgate Publishing Co., 1996.

Reynolds, Patrick, and Shachtman, Tom . *The Gilded Leaf: Triumph, Tragedy and Tobacco.* New York: Little, Brown, 1989.

Robert, Joseph C., *The Story of Tobacco in America.* Chapel Hill: University of North Carolina Press, 1949, 1967.

Robicsek, Francis. *The Smoking Gods: Tobacco in Mayan Art, History, and Religion.* Norman: University of Oklahoma Press, 1978.

Rogozinski, Jan. *Smokeless Tobacco in the Western World: 1550–1950.* Santa Cruz, CA: Devin, 1990.

Roleff, Tamar L., and Williams, Mary, eds. *Tobacco and Smoking: Opposing Viewpoints.* San Diego: Greenhaven, 1998.

Schmitz, Cecilia M., and Gray, Richard A. *Smoking: The Health Consequences of Tobacco Use: An Annotated Bibliography with Analytical Introduction.* Ann Arbor, MI: Pierian, 1995.

Selig, Louis. *Tobacco, Peace Pipes, and Indians.* Palmer Lake, CO: Filter Press, 1971.

Simonich, William L. *Government Antismoking Policies.* New York: Peter Lang Publishers, 1991.

Smith, Jane Webb. *Smoke Signals: Cigarettes, Advertising and the American Way of Life.* Richmond, VA: Valentine Museum, 1990. (An exhibition catalogue from the Valentine Museum.)

Sobel, Robert. *They Satisfy: The Cigarette in American Life.* New York: Anchor Press/Doubleday, 1978.

Storrino, Louis. *Chewing Tobacco Tin Tags, 1870–1930.* Atglen, PA: Schiffer, 1997.

Sullum, Jacob. *For Your Own Good: The Anti-Smoking Crusade and the Tyranny of Public Health.* New York: Free Press, 1998.

Tate, C. Cassandra. The *American Anti-Cigarette Movement,1880–1930.* (Ph.D. Dissertation at the University of Washington) Ann Arbor, MI: UMI Dissertation Services, 1995.

Tate, C. Cassandra. "In the 1800s, Antismoking Was a Burning Issue." *Smithsonian,* July 1989, pp. 107–17.

Taylor, C. Barr, and Killen, Joel D., *The Facts About Smoking.* Yonkers, NY: Consumer Reports Books, 1991.

Taylor, Peter. *The Smoke Ring: Tobacco, Money, and Multinational Politics.* New York: Pantheon Books, 1984.

Tennant, Robert E. *The American Cigarette Industry: A Study in Economic Analysis and Public Policy.* New Haven, CT: Yale University Press, 1950.

Tilley, Nannie Mae. *The Bright Tobacco Industry: 1860–1929.* Chapel Hill: University of North Carolia Press, 1948.

———. *The R.J. Reynolds Tobacco Company.* Chapel Hill: University of North Carolina Press, 1948.

Tobias, Andrew. *Kids Say Don't Smoke.* New York: Workman Press, 1991.

Troyer, Ronald J., and Markle, Gerald E., *Cigarettes: The Battle Over Smoking.* New Brunswick, NJ: Rutgers University Press, 1983.

Van Willigen, John, and Eastwood, Susan C. *Tobacco Culture: Farming Kentucky's Burley Belt.* Lexington: University of Kentucky Press, 1998

Viscusi, W. Kip. *Smoking: Making the Risky Decision.* New York: Oxford University Press, 1991.

Vizzard, William J. *In the Cross Fire: A Political History of the Bureau of Alcohol, Tobacco and Firearms.* Boulder, CO: Lynne Rienner, 1997.

Voges, Ernst, ed. *Tobacco Encyclopedia.* Mainz, Germany: Mainzer Verlagsanstalt, 1984.

Wagner, Susan. *Cigarette Country: Tobacco in American History and Politics.* New York: Praeger, 1971.

Wald, Nicholas, and Froggatt, Sir Peter. *Nicotine, Smoking, and the Low Tar Programme.* New York: Oxford University Press, 1989.

Walker, Ellen. *Smoker: Self-Portrait of a Nicotine Addict.* San Francisco: Harper and Row, 1990.

Warner, Kenneth E. *Selling Smoke: Cigarette Advertising and Public Health.* Washington, DC: American Public Health Association, 1986.

Warren, Robert Penn. *Night Rider.* Nashville, TN: J.S. Sanders, 1992.

Wekesser, Carol, ed. *Smoking (Current Controversies).* San Diego: Greenhaven, 1997.

Werner, Carl A. *Tobaccoland.* New York: The Tobacco Leaf Publishing Co., 1922.

Wetherall, Charles F. *Quit for Teens/Read This Book and Stop Smoking.* Kansas City, MO: Andrews and McMeel, 1995.

Whelan, Elizabeth M. *A Smoking Gun: How the Tobacco Industry Gets Away with Murder.* Philadelphia: George F. Stickley Co., 1984.

———. *Cigarettes: What the Warning Label Doesn't Tell You.* Amherst, NY: Prometheus Books, 1997.

White, Larry. *Merchants of Death: The American Tobacco Industry.* New York: Beech Tree Books/ William Morrow and Co. Inc., 1988.

Whiteside, Thomas. *Selling Death:Cigarette Advertising and Public Health.* New York: Liveright, 1971.

Wilbert, Johannes. *Tobacco and Shamanism in South America.* New Haven, CT: Yale University Press, 1987.

Zalis, Marian. *Dictionary of Tobacco Terminology.* New York: Philip Morris Inc., 1980.

Web Sites

Action on Smoking and Health: <http://www.ash.org>

Advocacy Institute: <http://www.advocacy.org/>

American Cancer Society: <http://www.cancer.org/>

American Council on Science and Health: <http://www.acsh.org/>

American Health Foundation: <http://www.ahf.org/>

American Heart Association: <http://www.amhrt.org/>

American Lung Association: <http://www.lung.usa.org/>

American Medical Association: <http://www.ama-assn.org/>

American Medical Women's Association: <http://www.amwa-doc.org/>

Americans for Nonsmokers Rights: <http://www.no-smoke.org/>

Bureau of Alcohol, Tobacco, and Firearms: <http://www.atf.treas.gov/>

Centers for Disease Control and Prevention: <http://www.cdc.gov/tobacco>

Department of Health and Human Services: <http://www.hhs.gov/>

Environmental Protection Agency: <http://www.epa.gov/>

Federal Trade Commission: <http://www.ftc.gov/index.html>

Food and Drug Administration: <http://www.fda.gov/>

FORCES (Fight Ordinances and Restrictions to Control and Eliminate Smoking: <http://www.forces.com>

Globallink: <http://www.globalink.org/>

INFACT: <http://www.infact.org/>

National Cancer Institute: <http://www.nci.nih.gov/>
National Center for Tobacco-Free Kids: <http://www.tobaccofreekids.org/>
National Smokers Alliance: <http://www.speakup.org/>
Office on Smoking and Health: <http://www.cdc.gov/nccdphp/osh/>
Public Health Service: <http://www.phs.os.dhhs.gov/>
QUITNET: <http://www.quitnet.org/>
Smokefree Educational Services, Inc.: <http://www.smokefree.org/>
Stop Teenage Addiction to Tobacco: <http://www.stat.org/>
Tobacco Bulletin Board System: <http://www.tobacco.org>
Tobacco Control Resource Center: <http://www.tobacco.neu.edu/>
Tobacco Settlement: State Updates <http://www.tcsg.org/tobacco/settlement/updates.htm>
U.S. Department of Agriculture: <http://www.usda.gov/>
World Health Organization: <http://www.who.int/>

INDEX

by Virgil Diodato